AF737200

Bioprocess Technologies for Environmental Sustainability

This book provides a comprehensive overview of current trends and advancements in bioprocess technologies for sustainable development. It discusses the objectives of environmental sustainability, including the methods used to carry out various biological processes, pertinent aspects of biochemical engineering, and how these are applied to solve environmental issues. The focus is on waste valorization using advanced chemical and bioprocess technologies. It also highlights the technological perspectives of biorefineries in achieving zero-waste management.

- Emphasizes bioprocessing related to waste and carbon dioxide
- Presents state-of-the-art chemical and biochemical technologies for producing value-added products from biowaste
- Reviews potential valorization techniques for resource recovery from various biological feedstocks
- Outlines integrated techniques for producing high-value bioproducts from diverse waste resources
- Discusses bioprocess aspects for a clean and green environment

This book is intended for researchers and graduate students in bioprocessing, sustainability, and environmental biotechnology.

Bioprocess Technologies for Environmental Sustainability

Trends and Developments

Edited by
Jerold Manuel and Ramani Kandasamy

CRC Press
Taylor & Francis Group
Boca Raton London New York

CRC Press is an imprint of the
Taylor & Francis Group, an **informa** business

Designed cover image: © Jerold Manuel and Ramani Kandasamy

First edition published 2027
by CRC Press
2385 NW Executive Center Drive, Suite 320, Boca Raton FL 33431

and by CRC Press
4 Park Square, Milton Park, Abingdon, Oxon, OX14 4RN

CRC Press is an imprint of Taylor & Francis Group, LLC

© 2027 selection and editorial matter, Jerold Manuel and Ramani Kandasamy; individual chapters, the contributors

Reasonable efforts have been made to publish reliable data and information, but the author and publisher cannot assume responsibility for the validity of all materials or the consequences of their use. The authors and publishers have attempted to trace the copyright holders of all material reproduced in this publication and apologize to copyright holders if permission to publish in this form has not been obtained. If any copyright material has not been acknowledged please write and let us know so we may rectify in any future reprint.

The Open Access version of this book, available at www.taylorfrancis.com, has been made available under a Creative Commons Attribution-Non Commercial-No Derivatives (CC-BY-NC-ND) 4.0 International license.

Any third party material in this book is not included in the OA Creative Commons license, unless indicated otherwise in a credit line to the material. Please direct any permissions enquiries to the original rightsholder.

The electronic version of this book was funded to publish Open Access through Taylor & Francis' Pledge to Open, a collaborative funding open access books initiative. The full list of pledging institutions can be found on the Taylor & Francis Pledge to Open webpage.

For Product Safety Concerns and Information please contact our EU representative GPSR@taylorandfrancis.com. Taylor & Francis Verlag GmbH, Kaufingerstraße 24, 80331 München, Germany.

Trademark notice: Product or corporate names may be trademarks or registered trademarks and are used only for identification and explanation without intent to infringe.

ISBN: 9781032796840 (hbk)
ISBN: 9781032815800 (pbk)
ISBN: 9781003500483 (ebk)

DOI: 10.1201/9781003500483

Typeset in Times
by codeMantra

Contents

Editors' biography vii
List of contributors ix
Preface xiii

Chapter 1 Treatment of industrial wastewater with bacteria, fungi, microalgae, and cyanobacteria 1

Diaz-Parra Karen Lizette and Martínez-Roldán Alfredo de Jesús

Chapter 2 Bioremediation of emerging pollutants, options, and challenges 25

Morales-Romero Juan Manuel, Rodríguez-Oloño Brenda Michell, Reynoso-Cuevas Liliana, and Martínez-Roldán Alfredo de Jesús

Chapter 3 Fungal biorefinery and bioprocessing: advanced strategies for waste valorization 54

Damián Reyes-Jáquez, Itza Nallely Cordero-Soto, Sergio Valle-Cervantes, María Dolores Josefina Rodríguez-Rosales, and María Gorety Contreras-Hernández

Chapter 4 Novel materials for bioelectrodes 72

Abinash Kumararaj, Geetha Arunachalam, Rekha Pachaiappan, Divyadharshini Satheesh, Rathika Rajendran, Kovendhan Manavalan, and Tri Khoa Nguyen

Chapter 5 Napier grass grown in arid and saline water conditions for biochar production and its applications 92

Ramachandran Subramanian, Souvik Kumar Paul, and Prakash Kumar B G

Chapter 6 Natural biopolymer-derived porous materials as super adsorbents for wastewater treatment 101

Akhtar Alam, Atikur Hassan, and Neeladri Das

Chapter 7 Separation processes in valorization of biomass for circular bioeconomy 127

Anju Tomy, Sree Priya S, and Rakesh K Yasarla

Chapter 8 Polyhydroxyalkanoates production from effluents – cheap renewable resources 146

Poorna Chandrika Sabapathy, Koushika Saravanan and Preethi Kathirvel

Chapter 9 Production of biofuels from biomolecules obtained from microbial consortium: a review 160

Sindhu S and Krishna Prasad R

Chapter 10 Plastics and microplastics: the state-of-the-art in advanced treatment technologies 201

Sheikh Mohammed, Karmuhil Mathimozhiyazh Vetriselvan, Sekaran Ganesan, and Ramani Kandasamy

Chapter 11 Biodegradation mechanisms and its applications in wastewater treatment 214

Sarojini Devi Nagesh, Renuka Devi Ravi, Rekha Pachaiappan, Padmavathi Rajangam, Geetha Arunachalam, and Kovendhan Manavalan

Chapter 12 Biopolymers types, characterization, and application: an overview 237

Padmavathi Rajangam, Sarojinidevi Nagesh, and Rekha Pachaiappan

Chapter 13 Unravelling the multifaceted applications of biofilms for environmental sustainability 272

Tarun Suryarajan, Naveen Nair, Shivangi Dutta, Swathi Krishnan Venkatesan, Maseed Uddin, Sekaran Ganesan, and Ramani Kandasamy

Chapter 14 Nanocomposites for clean water 287

Radha K. V. and Selvi V. S.

Chapter 15 An overview of cathode development for microbial fuel cell 309

Neeraj V. S., Muthukumar K., and Samsudeen Naina Mohamed

Index 319

Editors' biography

Jerold Manuel is an academician and researcher in the field of Biochemical Engineering. Currently, he is serving as an Assistant Professor in the Department of Biotechnology at NIT Warangal. His research interest includes biorefineries, waste valorization, and biomaterials. He has embarked his research potential for the clean and green environment. He is the recipient of "IEI Young Engineers Award" by the Institution of Engineers (India) for the year 2020–2021 in Environmental Engineering discipline. He has received various sponsored projects worth 80 lakhs from several funding agencies. He has been awarded with Dr. D.G.S. Dhinakaran fellowship for his postgraduate education and MoE Fellowship by the Government of India for his doctoral studies. In addition, he has been honoured with gold medals for his higher academic credentials by Karunya University during his higher studies. In addition to his research, he is involved in teaching for B.Tech. and M.Tech. students. He has handled various subjects related to Biotechnology and Biochemical Engineering. He has published 32 research and review papers at international and national peer-reviewed journals. In addition, Jerold has authored six book chapters in reputed book publishers. He has guided many B.Tech. and M.Tech. students for their dissertation work. He is currently guiding three doctoral students. To his credit, he has edited three books which are published in CRC Press, Taylor and Francis Group, and Springer Nature. He is a reviewer for various peer-reviewed journals at international and national levels. He is a life member of Biotech Research Society of India (BRSI), International Society for Technical Education (ISTE), India, Indian Institute of Chemical Engineers (IIChE), and IEI Institution of Engineers (India).

Ramani Kandasamy is a Professor in the Department of Biotechnology, Faculty of Engineering and Technology, SRM Institute of Science and Technology (SRMIST), Kattankulathur, Chennai, India, and holds 20 years of extensive academic, research, and industrial collaborative experience. She received her Ph.D. in Microbiology-Environmental Technology from the Council of Scientific and Industrial Research-Central Leather Research Institute (CSIR-CLRI), Chennai, where she specialized in Microbiology-driven environmental solutions. Her research is centred on developing sustainable, eco-efficient biotechnological strategies for industrial solid and liquid waste management including the bioremediation of emerging pollutants from petrochemical industries, refineries, leather processing, and municipal waste sectors. She has significantly contributed to advancing microbial fermentation technologies for the conversion of industrial wastes into high-value-added biomolecules such as biosurfactants, industrial enzymes, and biocatalysts. Her research work also spans strain improvement technologies, biosurfactant-assisted hydrocarbon remediation, production of magnetic nanoparticles through green synthesis and surface-functionalized carrier materials for enhanced pollutant removal. Her research extends to the remediation of hydrocarbon-contaminated soils and process development for the treatment of toxic landfill leachates enabling resource recovery within circular bioeconomy frameworks. She has successfully executed multiple government- and industry-funded research projects and has authored numerous articles in international high-impact journals, conference proceedings, and edited volumes. Her strong commitment to translational research has led to active collaborations with industrial partners for pilot-scale demonstration of eco-efficient solutions. She serves as research mentor to postgraduate and doctoral researchers facilitating multidisciplinary innovations aligned with sustainable development priorities. She continues to contribute immensely to the real-field through her research outreach, scientific evaluations, and technology transfer activities aimed at achieving scalable environmental remediation technologies. She has published 65 research papers in the peer-reviewed international journals and authored eight book chapters with reputed publishers. She is the recipient of Tamil Nadu Women Scientist Award from the Department of Higher Education, Government of Tamil Nadu. She is a member of Association of Microbiologists in India (AMI) and International Water Association (IWA).

Contributors

Akhtar Alam,
Department of Chemistry, IIT Patna, India.

Geetha Arunachalam,
Department of Physics and Nanotechnology, SRM Institute of Science and Technology, Kattankulathur, Chengalpattu, Tamil Nadu, India.

Prakash Kumar B.G.,
Department of Chemical Engineering, BITS Pilani, Dubai Campus, Dubai International Academic City, Dubai, United Arab Emirates.

Rodríguez-Oloño Brenda Michell,
National Technological Institute of Mexico/ IT Durango, Durango, México.

María Gorety Contreras-Hernández,
National Technological Institute of Mexico, Technological Institute of Durango, Department of Chemical and Biochemical Engineering, Durango, Mexico.

Itza Nallely Cordero-Soto,
National Technological Institute of Mexico/ Durango Technological Institute, CONAHCyT National Laboratory for Evaluation of Biotic Products (LaNAEPBi), Department of Chemical-Biochemical Engineering, Durango, Durango, Mexico.

Neeladri Das,
Associate Professor, Department of Chemistry, IIT Patna, India.

Karen Lizette Diaz-Parra,
National Technological Institute of Mexico/IT Durango, Nueva Vizcaya, Durango, México.

Shivangi Dutta,
Industrial and Environmental Sustainability Laboratory, Department of Biotechnology, School of Bioengineering, SRM Institute of Science and Technology, Kattankulathur, Tamil Nadu, India.

Sekaran Ganesan,
Department of Biotechnology, School of Bioengineering, SRM Institute of Science and Technology, Kattankulathur, Tamil Nadu, India, and SRM Institute of Science and Technology, Ramapuram Campus, Chennai, Tamil Nadu, India.

Atikur Hassan,
Department of Chemistry, IIT Patna, India.

Morales-Romero Juan Manuel,
Center of Investigation in Advanced Materials, Ejido Arroyo Seco, Durango, México.

Muthukumar K.
Department of Chemical Engineering, National Institute of Technology Tiruchirappalli, India.

Ramani Kandasamy,
Industrial and Environmental Sustainability Laboratory, Department of Biotechnology, School of Bioengineering, SRM Institute of Science and Technology, Kattankulathur, Tamil Nadu, India.

Preethi Kathirvel,
Department of Microbial Biotechnology, Bharathiar University, Coimbatore, Tamil Nadu, India.

Swathi Krishnan Venkatesan,
Industrial and Environmental Sustainability Laboratory, Department of Biotechnology, School of Bioengineering, SRM Institute of Science and Technology, Kattankulathur, Tamil Nadu, India.

Abinash Kumararaj,
Department of Physics and Nanotechnology, SRM Institute of Science and Technology, Kattankulathur, Chengalpattu, Tamil Nadu, India.

Radha K. V.,
Bioproducts Laboratory, Department of Chemical Engineering, AC. Tech., Anna University, Chennai, Tamil Nadu, India.

Reynoso-Cuevas Liliana,
SECIHTI-TecNM, National Technological Institute of Mexico/IT Durango, Chemical and Biochemical Engineering, Durango, México.

Kovendhan Manavalan,
Department of Physics and Nanotechnology, SRM Institute of Science and Technology, Kattankulathur, Chengalpattu, Tamil Nadu, India.

Alfredo de Jesús Martínez-Roldán,
SECIHTI-TecNM, National Technological Institute of Mexico/IT Durango, Chemical and Biochemical Engineering, México.

Sheikh Mohammed,
Industrial and Environmental Sustainability Laboratory, Department of Biotechnology, School of Bioengineering, SRM Institute of Science and Technology, Kattankulathur, Tamil Nadu, India.

Sarojinidevi Nagesh,
Department of Physical Sciences, SIMATS Engineering, Thandalam, Chennai, Tamil Nadu, India.

Samsudeen Naina Mohamed,
Department of Chemical Engineering, National Institute of Technology Tiruchirappalli, India.

Naveen Nair,
Industrial and Environmental Sustainability Laboratory, Department of Biotechnology, School of Bioengineering, SRM Institute of Science and Technology, Kattankulathur, Tamil Nadu, India.

Tri Khoa Nguyen,
NTT Hi-Tech Institute, Nguyen Tat Thanh University, Ho Chi Minh City, Vietnam.

Rekha Pachaiappan,
Departamento de Ingeniería Mecanica, Facultad de Ingeniería Mecanica, Universidad de Tarapaca, Arica, Chile; Energy Center, FCFM, University of Chile, Santiago, Chile.

Souvik Kumar Paul,
Department of Chemical Engineering, BITS Pilani, Dubai Campus, Dubai International Academic City, Dubai, United Arab Emirates.

Padmavathi Rajangam,
Department of Chemistry, Vel Tech Multi Tech Dr. Rangarajan Dr. Sakunthala Engineering College, Avadi, Chennai, Tamil Nadu, India.

Rathika Rajendran,
Department of Physics, St. Theresa's Arts & Science College for Women, Tharangambadi, Mayiladuthurai, Tamil Nadu, India.

Renuka Devi Ravi,
Department of Physical Sciences, SIMATS Engineering, Thandalam, Chennai, Tamil Nadu, India.

Damián Reyes-Jáquez,
National Technological Institute of Mexico, Technological Institute of Durango, Department of Chemical and Biochemical Engineering, Durango, Mexico.

Krishna Prasad R.,
Department of Chemical Engineering and Materials Science, Center of Excellence in Advanced Materials and Green Technologies, Amrita School of Engineering, Coimbatore, Amrita Vishwa Vidyapeetham, Coimbatore, Tamil Nadu, India.

María Dolores Josefina Rodríguez-Rosales
National Technological Institute of Mexico, Technological Institute of Durango, Department of Chemical and Biochemical Engineering, Durango, Mexico.

Poorna Chandrika Sabapathy,
Department of Microbial Biotechnology, Bharathiar University, Coimbatore, Tamil Nadu, India.

Koushika Saravanan,
Department of Microbial Biotechnology, Bharathiar University, Coimbatore, Tamil Nadu, India.

Divyadharshini Satheesh,
Department of Physics and Nanotechnology, SRM Institute of Science and Technology, Kattankulathur, Chengalpattu, Tamil Nadu, India.

Sindhu S.,
Department of Chemical Engineering and Materials Science, Center of Excellence in Advanced Materials and Green Technologies, Amrita School of Engineering, Coimbatore, Amrita Vishwa Vidyapeetham, Coimbatore, Tamil Nadu, India.

Sree Priya S.,
Microbial Processes and Technology Division, CSIR – National Institute for Interdisciplinary Science and Technology, Thiruvananthapuram, Kerala, India.

Ramachandran Subramanian,
Department of Biotechnology, BITS Pilani, Dubai Campus, Dubai International Academic City, Dubai, United Arab Emirates.

Tarun Suryarajan,
Industrial and Environmental Sustainability Laboratory, Department of Biotechnology, School of Bioengineering, SRM Institute of Science and Technology, Kattankulathur, Tamil Nadu, India.

Anju Tomy,
Microbial Processes and Technology Division, CSIR – National Institute for Interdisciplinary Science and Technology, Thiruvananthapuram, Kerala, India.

Maseed Uddin,
Industrial and Environmental Sustainability Laboratory, Department of Biotechnology, School of Bioengineering, SRM Institute of Science and Technology, Kattankulathur, Tamil Nadu, India.

Sergio Valle-Cervantes,
National Technological Institute of Mexico, Technological Institute of Durango, Department of Chemical and Biochemical Engineering, Durango, Mexico.

Karmuhil Mathimozhiayazh Vetriselvan,
Industrial and Environmental Sustainability Laboratory, Department of Biotechnology, School of Bioengineering, SRM Institute of Science and Technology, Kattankulathur, Tamil Nadu, India.

Neeraj V. S.,
Department of Chemical Engineering, National Institute of Technology Tiruchirappalli, Tamil Nadu, India.

Selvi V. S.,
Bioproducts Laboratory, Department of Chemical Engineering, AC. Tech., Anna University, Chennai, Tamil Nadu, India.

Rakesh K. Yasarla,
Microbial Processes and Technology Division, CSIR – National Institute for Interdisciplinary Science and Technology, Thiruvananthapuram, Kerala, India.

Preface

The unprecedented escalation of industrialization, rapid population growth, and intensified resource consumption has significantly debilitated global ecosystems. Most importantly, the aquatic zones are increasingly contaminated with complex industrial effluents, persistent organic pollutants, and emerging contaminants such as microplastics and hydrocarbons. Simultaneously, the pressing drive toward renewable energy and circular bioeconomy necessitates new and novel technological interventions that are efficient, sustainable, and economically viable and high-value-added resource recoverable. Conventional chemical and physical treatment methods often struggle to meet these requirements due to high operational costs, excessive energy demands, and secondary pollution generation.

In this context, bioprocess technologies have emerged as transformative tools capable of mitigating environmental pollution while recovering valuable resources. By leveraging the capabilities of microorganisms, natural biomaterials, nanotechnology, and engineered bioreactors, these strategies offer hybrid, integrated, and eco-friendly technological solutions aligned with the United Nations Sustainable Development Goals (SDGs).

This edited volume, *Bioprocess Technologies for Environmental Sustainability: Trends and Developments* compile cutting-edge research and comprehensive reviews from leading experts globally. The 15 chapters collectively address modern methods and breakthroughs in wastewater treatment, industrial waste valorization, biopolymer and biofuel production, nanomaterials engineering, and the remediation of plastics and microplastics. Each chapter contributes innovative perspectives and technological advancements that could structurally devise the future of sustainable industrial practices and practical applicability.

CHAPTER OVERVIEW

Chapter 1 provides an in-depth assessment of wastewater characteristics from major industrial sectors and explores biological treatment strategies utilizing bacteria, fungi, microalgae, and cyanobacteria.

Chapter 2 presents state-of-the-art physicochemical and biotechnological processes for the removal of emerging pollutants along with the challenges associated with their implementation.

Chapter 3 discusses fungal biorefineries and bioprocessing innovations emphasizing the waste valorization and scalable bioreactor design for a circular economy.

Chapter 4 introduces novel materials and advanced fabrication routes for high-performance bioelectrodes used in microbial fuel cells and energy storage systems.

Chapter 5 presents biochar production from Napier grass grown under saline and arid conditions and its potential applications in the environmental remediation.

Chapter 6 describes natural biopolymer-derived porous adsorbents, their adsorption mechanisms, and their role in wastewater purification.

Chapter 7 highlights the industrially relevant separation processes that are essential for biomass valorization and sustainable bioprocess integration.

Chapter 8 focuses on the polyhydroxyalkanoate (PHA) production from low-cost wastewater substrates alongside addressing economic feasibility and industrial prospects.

Chapter 9 reviews biofuel generation from microbial consortia encompassing biodiesel, bioethanol, biobutanol, biogas, and biohydrogen technologies.

Chapter 10 emphasis advanced treatment strategies for plastics and microplastics, including catalytic oxidation, photocatalysis, and biodegradation.

Chapter 11 describes biodegradation kinetics, pathways, and environmental applications in degrading persistent pollutants, petrochemical wastewaters, and plastics.

Chapter 12 provides an extensive overview of biopolymers including classification, characterization, sources, sustainability considerations, and emerging applications.

Chapter 13 explores the structural complexity and multifunctional applications of microbial biofilms in wastewater treatment, soil remediation, and bioenergy systems.

Chapter 14 details nanocomposite synthesis and their deployment in advanced wastewater treatment reactors such as membrane and fluidized-bed systems.

Chapter 15 reviews recent innovations in cathode materials for microbial fuel cells, addressing material performance, design optimization, and future research directions.

By integrating foundational principles with emerging trends and technological advancements emphasized in this book chapters, this volume is expected to serve as a practical guide and inspiration for undertaking short-term and economically feasible research projects that foster innovation in environmental biotechnology. In addition, this book incorporates real-world case studies, scalable experimental approaches, and emerging technological solutions, aiming to build confidence among early career researchers, students, industrial scientists, and academic professionals onto value-added products recovery upon devising innovative waste remediation technologies. More importantly, the content presented herein is anticipated to catalyse stronger industry-academia partnerships, encouraging the translation of laboratory findings into field applications and pilot-scale demonstrations. Ultimately, this volume aspires to contribute meaningfully to sustainable environmental remediation, clean energy generation, and the advancement of circular bioeconomy initiatives of eco-efficient bioprocess technologies.

Place: Warangal, Telangana State, India
Kattankulathur, Tamil Nadu, India

Editors

Prof. Dr. M Jerold
Prof. Dr. Ramani Kandasamy
Bioprocess Technologies for Environmental Sustainability 2025

1 Treatment of industrial wastewater with bacteria, fungi, microalgae, and cyanobacteria

Diaz-Parra Karen Lizette and
Martínez-Roldán Alfredo de Jesús

1.1 INTRODUCTION

Water is a scarce resource and necessary for human and animal consumption, other daily activities, agriculture, and several productive processes. The World Health Organization (WHO) estimates that approximately 2 billion people worldwide live in countries with limited availability of water, which is projected to worsen because of climate change in the next few years (WHO, 2023). The use of water causes the loss of its original quality (i.e., it becomes wastewater) and necessitates its treatment. The actual situation with respect to wastewater generation and treatment is not clear because there are regions of the world where reports of wastewater generation and treatment do not exist. This makes it difficult to know the actual status and does not allow the generation of projections and future scenario development. Worldwide, there are 14 countries with situational reports regarding wastewater issues, and with this information, the United Nations estimates that only 30% of industrial wastewater receives some type of treatment; this percentage is higher in European countries, reaching values close to 100% in some nations (UNESCO, 2021). The global tendency is to improve not only the efficiency of treatment processes but also employment efficiency and the elimination of leaks (WHO, 2023); nevertheless, there are many challenges that are specific to every country and region. Technology for the treatment of industrial effluents cannot be easily developed because the composition of the wastewater is specific for every sector or even for each company, and in many cases, the guidelines that are applicable for one process do not work for another.

Wastewater includes municipal runoff, agricultural runoff, stormwater, industrial effluents, and other types (Kunhikrishnan et al., 2012). At the global level, the industrial sector uses approximately 20% of the tap water available worldwide. The industrial sector impacts the environment through not only the generation of wastewaters but also the emission of greenhouse gases (GHGs) and soil pollution, which reduce biodiversity and impact human health and quality of life. Industrial effluents are produced at a global scale continuously but with very diverse compositions and pollutant concentrations, resulting in very distinct physicochemical properties, such as color, odor, temperature, suspended solids (SS), foam, conductivity, pH, dissolved oxygen, nitrogen and phosphorus concentrations, heavy metals or even organic compounds (Table 1.1) (Koncagül et al., 2024; Martínez-Frías, 2011; Thomas & Thomas, 2022).

Effluents that contain organic matter, such as chemical oxygen demand (COD) or biochemical oxygen demand (BOD) with a high biodegradability ratio, normally cause eutrophication, diversity losses, or GHG emissions. Effluents containing other types of pollutants, such as heavy metals, colorants, chlorinated compounds, and hydrocarbons, are normally associated with problems such

DOI: 10.1201/9781003500483-1

This chapter has been made available under a (CC-BY-NC-ND) 4.0 license

TABLE 1.1
Composition and impacts caused by diverse types of industrial wastewater

Industrial sector	Pollutants in the effluent	Impacts on the environment	References
Food • **Dairy products** • **Beverages** • **Meat processing**	Oils Sugars Inorganic compounds Fats Detergents BOD (mainly) and COD	Deterioration of ecosystems Eutrophication GHG emission	Milenković (2021)
Mining and metallurgy • **Mining** • **Batteries production** • **Steel**	Alkalis Cyanide Mercury Lead and other heavy metals COD	Bioaccumulation through the trophic chain GHG emission	Nemerow (2006)
Paper and pulp	Chlorinated compounds TSS BOD	Eutrophication Pollution of bodies of water with BOD Emission of nitrogenized and sulfated compounds to the atmosphere	Nemerow (2006)
Petroleum • **Refinery** • **Gas**	Hydrocarbons Heavy metals Inorganic compounds BOD and COD (mainly)	Affectation in aquatic ecosystems Emission of GHG	Muralikrishna and Manickam (2017)
Chemical • **Plastics** • **Pesticides** • **Pharmaceutics**	Acids Alkalis Heavy metals Solvents BOD and COD	Pollution of waterbodies GHG emissions Chronic toxicity	Muralikrishna and Manickam (2017)
Textile • **Fabrics** • **Garments**	Acids Alkalis Colorants Turbidity BOD and COD	Diminution of dissolved oxygen in bodies of water caused by reduced transparency of the water Chronic toxicity GHG emissions	Nemerow (2006)

as magnification and chronic toxicity even at low concentrations; at very high concentrations, industrial effluents cause imbalances in the environment and death of ecosystems (Table 1.1).

The alimentary and textile industries are in the first and second places in the rankings in terms of use or resources required, and both cause greater impacts on the environment because of the enormous amount of water needed per unit produced. The negative impacts of the alimentary and textile industries include not only water consumption and wastewater generation but also GHG emissions; according to the United Nations Environment Program (UNEP), the textile industry alone accounts for 8% of the global carbon emissions and nearly 20% of wastewater generation (Bailey et al., 2022).

1.2 CHARACTERISTICS OF THE WASTEWATER PRODUCED IN SOME INDUSTRIAL SECTORS

1.2.1 Food industry

The food industry uses high amounts of resources such as soil, water, and energy because many processes are intensive. Specifically, the use of water by this industrial sector is important because the water is involved in not only the raw material production phase but also the production and processing phases. The major problem is that the food industry produces high amounts of wastewaters, and

TABLE 1.2
Wastewater produced by final products commercialized from some common products in the food industry

Produced unit		Wastewater produced	References
Tuna fish	1 kg	13 L	Uttamangkabovorn et al. (2005)
Cheese	1 kg	9 L	Padin-Gonzalez and Diaz-Fernandez (2009)
Mezcal	1 L	11–15 L	Bermeo-Garay et al. (2017)
Fruit juice	1 L	10 L	Rashid et al. (2023)

because these effluents have high concentrations of BOD, nitrogen, and phosphorus, their potential to contaminate superficial bodies of water is very high (Carpenter, 2008; UNEP, 2013).

In the food industry, some of the processes with high potential for contamination include the use of canned tuna fish, processed seafood, cheese and dairy products, alcoholic drinks such as beer, liquors, ancestral fermented beverages such as tequila and mezcal, fruit juices, and gassed beverages. The pollution potential of these industries is due to not only their physicochemical properties (low pH, high DQO, nitrogen, and phosphorus concentrations) but also the high amount of wastewater produced per unit of final product (Table 1.2). The volume of wastewater produced by the food industry has reached millions of cubic meters per year, and its treatment has high costs for productive processes (Bermeo-Garay et al., 2017; Hermosilla et al., 2014; Padin-Gonzalez & Diaz-Fernandez, 2009; Sridang et al., 2008; Vieira-Costa et al., 2021).

1.2.2 Textile industry

The textile industry contributes an important fraction of the gross domestic product, mainly in Asiatic countries. Regardless of the economic impact, the amount of contaminated effluents caused by this industry is very high. In addition, the wastewater generated contains important amounts of COD, TSS, heavy metals, intense and deep colors, and high pH values; moreover, the textile industry generates high GHG emissions (Christian et al., 2023; Imran et al., 2023).

The raw materials of the textile sector include different fibers, some of which are natural (renewable and biodegradable), but others are synthetic and are produced mainly as derived petroleum (nonrenewable and difficult to biodegrade). Some of natural fibers include cotton, bamboo, soy, linen, wool, and leather, and some oil-derived fibers include polyester, nylon, and rayon; cotton and polyester fibers are in the greatest demand worldwide (Holkar et al., 2016).

For the production of cloth, the fibers pass through a drying process that mainly impacts the environment by the emission of GHG due to the energy used in the phases of spinning, weaving, cutting, and other processes. The generation of wastewater mainly occurs in the wet process, in which the consumption of water can be close to 200 L of water per kg of cloth. The wastewater produced can contain very diverse types of pollutants, some of which are listed in Table 1.3. The amount of wastewater is high, as is its toxicity because of the presence of toxic or even carcinogenic compounds (Holkar et al., 2016; Shenoy et al., 2022).

Compared with natural pigments such as curcuma, carmine, and chlorophyll, azo dyes are very common in the textile industry and are used in the dyeing process; these dyes are preferred because of their high degree of fixation and resistance to UV radiation. Because of the advantages of synthetic colorants over natural pigments, synthetic colorants cover more than 50% of the demand and include more than 3000 different molecules, according to Zafar et al. (2022). The principal disadvantage of synthetic dyes is their tendency to accumulate in ecosystems because complex molecules make biotransformation or mineralization difficult. The low mineralization efficiency

TABLE 1.3
Risk derived from compounds used in different phases of the wet process into the textile sector

Step in the wet process	Chemical compound used	Consequences
Gluing	Starch Enzymes (mainly amylases) Polyvinyl alcohol (PVA) NaOH	Effluents with persistent compounds Holkar et al. (2016); Reddy et al. (2014).
Bleaching	Acetic anhydride H_2O_2 Per-acetic acid NaClO	Effluents with elevated pH, high amounts of BOD, and risk of the generation of chlorinated organic compounds Gürsoy and Dayioğlu (2000); Holkar et al. (2016).
Mercerization	NaOH	Alkaline effluent with risk to cause environmental imbalance Holkar et al. (2016); Sharma and Sharma (2014).
Dyeing – Printmaking	Azo dyes as • Congo red • Direct Brown 78 • Direct Blue 1 • Basic Red 18 Surfactants	Effluents with high COD and deep colors that can cause interferences in the entrance of light to the aquatic environments Alzain et al. (2023); Ramamurthy et al. (2024).
Finishing phase	Solvents Softeners	Recalcitrant wastewaters with toxic compounds, many of which are classified as emerging pollutants with the risk of biomagnification in the aquatic ecosystems Badmus et al. (2021).

stimulates the biomagnification of these molecules through the feed chain, causing teratogenic and carcinogenic risks for humans and animals.

1.2.3 Petroleum Extraction and Refining Industry

Petroleum-related industries are among the main industries that were originally used for illumination and heating, after being used for transportation; today, petroleum is used to obtain thousands of molecules and products, including plastics, detergents, cloths, chemical materials, and raw materials. This industrial sector generates high amounts of effluents (solids, liquids, and gases) with elevated concentrations of BDO, CO_2, and sulfur; therefore, it is considered one of the most contaminant-producing industries today (Clews, 2016; Rani et al., 2019).

The number of petroliferous fields worldwide is close to 70,000, according to recent estimations. In all of them, water is used for extraction (water injection), hydraulic fracking, machine cooling, refining, steam generation for distillation and cracking, and elimination of impurities (Johnston et al., 2019). Another risk derived from the petroleum industry is accidents (i.e., leaks and spills); authors such as Zhang et al. (2019) estimate that thousands of petroleum-related accidents every day worldwide affect aquatic and terrestrial ecosystems. In some cases, the impact is so strong that natural regeneration processes require many years to restore the ecosystem.

1.2.4 Chemical Industrial Sector

The chemical industry is the most important industry worldwide. This sector is closely related to the exploitation of nonrenewable sources, and petroleum is the principal raw material for obtaining plastics and chemical products such as fibers, colorants, pesticides, cosmetics, and drugs. Because of this, the chemical industry is imperative for the proper function of many other industries. The most important disadvantage of the chemical sector is derived from the long lives of some of the molecules produced, their high toxicity, their resistance to degradation, and their negative impact on the environment (Petruccioli et al., 2019; Santos et al., 2019).

1.2.5 Pharmaceutic industry

The production of drugs and pharmaceutical products has an important role in the prevention, diagnosis, and treatment of chronic diseases such as diabetes, arterial hypertension, cancer, and cardiovascular issues. Additionally, the production of drugs and pharmaceutical products contributes to eliminating ailments such as pain, headache, fever, and fatigue and can even heal infections caused by pathogenic bacteria, fungi, or viruses (Boxall, 2004).

The sizing of the environmental effects of these types of products is very recent; thus, the presence of pharmaceutical products has not been detected. Nevertheless, the concentrations of some of these products as well as health care/cosmetics products have recently started to reach alarming concentrations. Both drugs and health care products have been named as emerging contaminants, and their concentrations are becoming high in some bodies of water or wastewater treatment plants. Analgesics, antibiotics, and hormones can be found in superficial bodies of water and reach concentrations ranging from 340 to 1200 ng/L for analgesics, from 30 to 1900 ng/L for antibiotics and 4.3 ng/L for contraceptives, many of which are difficult to degrade and have the potential to cause physiological modifications to aquatic fauna (Boxall, 2004; Geissen et al., 2015).

1.2.6 Health care products and cosmetics

The beauty and personal care industry includes diverse compounds, some of which are obtained from natural sources and others produced by chemical synthesis from petroleum derivatives (Table 2.3). The variability of these compounds causes problems because the classic process used to treat wastewater works to eliminate only some of these compounds and because many of these compounds have antibiotic or antifungal activities, which affects the population dynamics in bodies of water. Health care products include components from soaps, body gels, deodorants, toothpastes, makeups, eye shadows, lipsticks, nail polishes, creams, solar filters, hair dyes, shampoos, conditioners, mascaras, perfumes, and colognes, many of which include azo dyes, fragrances, surfactants, essential oils, antioxidants, emulsifiers, excipients, solvents, antifungals, thickening gums, astringents, and other components. Table 1.4 lists some products included in different health care/cosmetics products. The daily use of health care/cosmetic products results in effluents with high DQO, variable pH, and very diverse composition. Many of these compounds remain intact throughout the treatment process and tend to accumulate in natural bodies of water (Cubas et al., 2022; Khalid & Abdollahi, 2021; Pereira-Lima et al., 2022).

1.2.7 Metallurgical sector

The mining and metal processing industries have caused environmental effects, and an important fraction is related to the emission of particulate material, CO_2, CH_4, NOx, and SOx to the atmosphere, as well as wastewater generation. Estimations indicate that this sector consumes 5% to 10% of the water used by the industrial sector worldwide. In 2013, Kunz et al. reported that close to 70% of the total operations in the mining sector were carried out by only six companies. The activities of these companies include the extraction and processing of iron, copper, lead, arsenic, precious metals such as gold, silver, and platinum, and metals involved in energetic processes such as nickel, cobalt, and zinc. The contribution of this sector to the gross domestic product is very important, and for developing countries, it is even fundamental.

TABLE 1.4
Chemical compounds normally found in health care/cosmetic products

Compound	Type of products				
	Personal hygiene	Cosmetics	Fragrances	Skincare	Haircare
1,4 Dichlorobenzene	Soaps Toothpaste Deodorants				
Carboxylic acids	Soaps Deodorants	Cleaners		Body creams Solar protector	
Amines	Soaps Deodorants	Face cleaners Makeup		Body creams Solar protector	Shampoo
Bisphenol A (BPA)	Soaps	Nail polishes	Colognes	Body creams Solar protector	Shampoo Conditioner
Ketones	Soaps Deodorants	Nail polishes Face cleaners	Colognes Perfumes		
Cicloxiloxanes (Silicone oil)	Deodorants	Nail polishes	Perfumes Colognes	Hydrating creams Solar protector	Shampoo Conditioner
Glycol esters			Colognes	Solar protector	
Phenols	Soaps		Perfumes Colognes	Solar protector	Hair dyes
Phthalate	Soaps	Nail polishes	Perfumes	Hydrating creams	Shampoo
Parabens		Blush Mascara Makeup		Solar filter	

Water is used for extraction, processing, melting, refining, cooling, and cleaning of equipment. The level of pollution generated in some of these phases results in effluents with high toxicity and recalcitrance (Conejo et al., 2020; Kunz et al., 2013). The toxicity of the effluents from mining is caused mainly by the presence of heavy metals (such as Ni, Cu, Co, Cd, Pb, or As), and the compounds used as emulsifiers or antifoam products are very resistant to biodegradation and have the potential to accumulate in aquatic ecosystems or even in the soil. Therefore, spills involving this type of wastewater are restricted, and treatment is mandatory to reduce the risk of affecting plants, animals, or even human communities (Wood et al., 1978).

1.2.8 Paper and Pulp Industry

This sector is ranked 6th regarding the consumption of natural resources, but the use of productive soils for tree cultivation, water consumption in the productive process, energy cost, and the amount of chemical compounds are very important. In 2022, a production of 400 million tons worldwide was reported, and an estimated growth rate close to 90 million tons per year was noted, with China being the major producer (Bajpai, 2016; Moussavi et al., 2022; Yang et al., 2023).

Considering the volume of water used by this sector, the estimation is that it represents 4% to 10% of the water used by the industrial sector. The most water-consuming stages include pulping, bleaching, and paper laminating. The wastewaters produced by this sector typically contain BOD and COD (mainly BOD), heavy metals, metalloids, and organic compounds derived from the wood, such as lignin and dioxins. In the pulping and delignifying phases, chlorinated compounds are sometimes used, a fraction is discarded in the wastewater, and these compounds make the treatment of the effluents even more difficult. Lignin causes very serious problems, mainly because it is difficult to degrade, whereas chlorinated compounds are very toxic, as are dioxins (Kunhikrishnan et al., 2012; Salamanca-Torres et al., 2009).

Currently, the treatment of industrial wastewater by microorganisms (e.g., bacteria, algae, and fungi) is considered a sustainable and environmentally friendly alternative for transforming or mineralizing organic compounds, which makes their use in wastewater treatment possible. Recently, the proposal to focus on wastewater treatment processes to obtain high-value products has gained importance in biotechnology. The processes developed into a circular economy concept include the generation of products such as biogas, biofuels, biomass, and high-value molecules, in addition to the environmental benefit of reducing GHG emissions and treating wastewater (Amjith & Bavanish, 2022; Borowitzka, 2013; Diaz-Parra et al., 2024; Rani et al., 2019).

1.3 BIOTECHNOLOGICAL PROCESSES FOR THE TREATMENT OF INDUSTRIAL WASTEWATER

The central criteria in the development of biotechnological processes for the treatment of wastewater are the selection of the microorganism to be used (i.e., bacteria, fungi, cyanobacteria, microalgae, or a mixture of them), the operational conditions (pH, temperature, light, humidity, atmospheric pressure, etc.) and even the bioreactor configuration (closed or open system) and operation strategy (batch, continuous, fed-batch, or cyclic batch) (Martínez-Roldán, 2024; Masojídek & Torzillo, 2008; Rani et al., 2019). In wastewater, the phases used to eliminate organic matter normally include aerobic or anaerobic processes, whereas the polishing steps (tertiary treatment) include microalgae, fungi, or mixed cultures. Tertiary microorganisms are employed for the elimination of specific pollutants, such as nitrogen, phosphorus, heavy metals, and coliforms (Diaz-Parra et al., 2024).

1.3.1 Bacteria

Bacteria are prokaryotic microorganisms that are useful in the treatment of wastewater because of their efficient consumption of macronutrients (mainly organic matter such as BOD). The reduction of BOD can be carried out through different metabolic pathways, such as aerobic respiration, fermentation, or anaerobic routes. The application of bacterial technologies normally includes the use of different bioreactor configurations depending on the objective of the process. The most popular bacteria used for the treatment of industrial effluents are *Escherichia coli, Bacillus thuringiensis, Bacillus mycoides, Bacillus subtilis, Bacillus* sp., *Lactobacillus, Clostridium, Chromobacterium vaccinii, Enterobacter asburiae,* and *Klebsiella pneumoniae* (Rani et al., 2019; Silva-Bedoya et al., 2016).

Bacteria can be used in processes such as upflow anaerobic sludge blanket (UASB), anaerobic filter (AF), anaerobic fluidized bed (AFB), moving bed biofilm reactor (MBBR), membrane bioreactor (MBR), multistage fluidized bed bioreactor (M-FBBR), aerobic lagoons, biologic filters, sequential arrangements of anoxic–aerobic (AnASBR), or a combination of these processes in sequential series. The use of bacteria in aerobic or anaerobic systems is normally very efficient for the elimination of organic matter, reaching efficiencies close to 50% within a large interval of hydraulic retention time (Chatzipaschali & Stamatis, 2012; Chowdhury et al., 2010; Jena et al., 2020).

1.3.2 Bioremediation of food industry effluents

The use of bacteria, whether aerobic, anaerobic, or facultative, for the treatment of effluents from the fishing and dairy sectors, is very common because these effluents normally contain large amounts of organic matter. Higher efficiencies of removing COD and BOD by bacteria normally occur in anaerobic or aerobic systems, which are typically employed as single phases or sequentially, depending on the characteristics of the wastewater.

TABLE 1.5
Bacteria used to treat wastewater from the food industry

Industrial sector	Inoculum	Effluent	BR (h HRT)	Removal efficiency (%)		References
Fishing	*Anaerobic bacteria*	Fishing effluent	UASB 7.2 h	COD	80–95	Chowdhury et al. (2010)
Fishing	*Anaerobic bacteria*	Fishing effluent	AF 36 days	COD	78–84	Chowdhury et al. (2010)
Dairy	*Anaerobic bacteria*	Whey	AF 4 days	COD	97	Chatzipaschali and Stamatis (2012)
Dairy	*Facultative bacteria*	Whey	AnASBR	COD $\mathbf{PO_4^{-3}}$	80 90	Jena et al. (2020)

TABLE 1.6
Bacteria used to treat wastewater from the textile industry

Bacteria	Effluent	Bioreactor type	Reduction (%)		References
Pseudomonas luteola	Textile	Anaerobic reactor 96 h	RBB RP2B Red G	93 92 37	Hu (1994)
Klebsiella pneumoniae	Textile	Anaerobic reactor	DB-284	95	Mustafa et al. (2021)
Bacillus subtilis	Textile	M-FBBR	Congo red	92	Shalini and Pydi-Setty (2019)
Escherichia coli	Textile	Aerobic reactor	Red 22	N.R	Chang and Kuo (2000)

The removal efficiencies for COD and BOD of bacteria-based processes can reach values of 80–95% (Table 1.5). In the case of anaerobic processes, obtaining methane is possible, and the methane obtained can be commercialized or used in the process, significantly reducing the cost (Chowdhury et al., 2010; Jena et al., 2020).

1.3.3 Bioremediation of Textile Effluents

The use of conventional processes for the treatment of effluents from the textile industry is not the best option because the dyes employed are very recalcitrant and difficult for bacteria to degrade. The elimination of the color of this kind of effluent is normally due to the breaking of double or triple bonds in the colored portion of the molecule (called the chromophore). This rupture is normally caused by enzymatic activity in the membrane of the cell, but in many cases, the compound produced after this rupture has a higher toxicity level than the original molecule does; thus, this process should be performed carefully (Table 1.6) (Cortazar-Martínez et al., 2012). Bacteria such as *Escherichia coli* and different species of *Pseudomonas* genera, such as *P. putida, P. mendocina, P. cepacia,* and *P. luteola,* are very efficient in the discoloration process and, at times, are also able to degrade azo dyes such as reactive red G (Red G), reactive blue black (RBB), reactive red RP2B (RP2B), reactive blue 19 (DB-284), acid red 22 (Red 22), and Congo red. This process is carried out at pH values ranging from seven to nine at temperatures of 20 to 45°C; increasing the temperature normally causes an increase in the efficiency of the discoloration (Chang & Kuo, 2000; Hu, 1994).

1.3.4 Bioremediation of hydrocarbons

The environmental impact of the extraction, refining, and transportation of hydrocarbons produced from petroleum is very high and sometimes includes not only the effects on soils and bodies of water but also the generation of wastewaters. Physicochemical processes are typically used because of the high toxicity caused by this kind of effluent, but these processes are expensive, and in some cases, bioremediation is preferred. Recently, almost 25 species of marine bacteria capable of living while employing hydrocarbons as the sole carbon source have been described (Table 1.7); these bacteria have shown the ability to degrade saturated hydrocarbons, aromatic molecules, phenols, ketones, esters, quinolones, and amides.

Compared with monocultures, the process of bioremediation of petroleum-derived compounds is most efficient because of the use of biostimulation and bioaugmentation processes or by cocultures or mixed inocula (Table 1.8). This is because the bacteria show better responses and an increased metabolic rate when the culture includes different species, according to Das and Chandran (2011), Perdigão et al. (2021), and Wu et al. (2023).

TABLE 1.7
Bacteria employed for the treatment of effluents from the petroleum industry

Bacteria	Effluent	(d HRT)	Reduction (%)		References
Marine bacteria	Oil spill	Batch 15 d	TPH		Perdigão et al. (2021)
Bacillus subtilis	Crude	Batch 30 d	Alkanes 42 Aromatics 21		Li et al. (2021)
Bacillus subtilis	Crude	Batch 7 d	TPH 32		Wu et al. (2023)
Pseudomonas aeruginosa	Crude	Batch 7 d	TPH 54		Wu et al. (2023)
Coculture of Bacillus subtilis and Pseudomonas aeruginosa	Crude	Batch 7 d	TPH	63	Wu et al. (2023)

TABLE 1.8
Bacteria used in the elimination of emerging contaminants

Bacteria	Effluent	HRT	Removal (%)		References
Aerobic bacteria	Pharmaceutical effluent	MBR 140 d	Naproxen DQO PO_4^{3-} $N\text{-}NO_3$	92 95 60 89	Mokhtariazar et al. (2024)
Aerobic bacteria	Pharmaceutical effluent	FBMBR 140 d	Naproxen DQO PO_4^{3-} $N\text{-}NO_3$	94 96 60 89	Mokhtariazar et al. (2024)
Aerobic bacteria	Pharmaceutical effluent	ASSBR 24 h (145 d)	Ibuprofen Ketoprofen DQO $N\text{-}NO_3$	63–90 13–92 88–89 35–92	Abu-Hasan et al. (2016)
Aerobic bacteria	Synthetic pharmaceutical effluent	CBR 18 h (40 d)	ATC DQO	98 95	Khoshvaght et al. (2021)

1.3.5 Bioremediation of emerging contaminants

Emerging contaminants are a group of recently defined compounds derived from daily life; these molecules are persistent, and conventional wastewater treatment plants do not eliminate them, so they start to accumulate in the environment. Emerging contaminants include antibiotics, anti-inflammatories, disinfectants, fragrances, and hormones. Bacteria-based elimination processes for the elimination of emerging contaminants from pharmaceutical, domestic, or municipal effluents have yielded good results. Additionally, the use of bacteria is less expensive than physicochemical methods, such as adsorption and absorption processes. Bacteria such as *Bacillus pseudomycoides, Rhodococcus ruber,* and *Vibrio mediterranei* are used to eliminate emerging pollutants in different bioreactor configurations (Abu-Hasan et al., 2016; Mokhtariazar et al., 2024; Rivera-Utrilla et al., 2013).

1.3.6 Bioremediation of industrial effluents containing heavy metals

Heavy metal elimination from wastewater is not easy because heavy metals are non-degradable and persistent in the environment. The processes used to eliminate heavy metals usually include only removal from water or a change in the oxidation number because some metals have different toxicity levels depending on the oxidation state. The biotechnological processes for the treatment of wastewater containing heavy metals normally take advantage of the ability of biomass to absorb ions even at very low concentrations. Microorganisms also have metabolic mechanisms to reduce the toxicity of heavy metals, which bind them to functional groups or send them to specific organelles. The efficiency of detoxification processes can be improved by manipulating operational conditions such as the carbon source, pH, temperature, and heavy metal concentration (e.g., Cu, Cr, Pb, Ni, Co, and Hg). Many bacterial genera stand out, such as *Pseudomonas, Bacillus, Vibrio, Klebsiella,* and *Enterobacter,* for processes of sorption, adsorption, and bioaccumulation, with removal efficiencies ranging from 60 to almost 100% (Table 1.9) (Igiri et al., 2018; Pham et al., 2022).

1.3.7 Bioprocessing of wastewater with microalgae and cyanobacteria

The microalgae group includes both prokaryotic and eukaryotic microorganisms, all of which have the ability to carry out photosynthesis, absorb light, and transform it into chemical energy (Diaz-Parra et al., 2024). Photosynthetic microorganisms can grow using different metabolic pathways and can be autotrophic, mixotrophic, or heterotrophic depending on the carbon source consumed. The metabolic flexibility of microalgae makes it possible to employ them in different wastewater

TABLE 1.9
Heavy metal biosorption and bioaccumulation in bacterial-based biotechnological processes

Bacteria	Effluent	HRT (h)	Efficiency (%)		References
Vibrio fluvialis	Industrial effluent	Batch 48	Hg	60	Saranya et al. (2017)
Vibrio parahaemolyticus	N.R	Batch 50	Hg	90	Jafari et al. (2015)
Pseudomonas alcaliphila	Synthetic	Batch 48	Cu	99	El-Naggar et al. (2020)
Bacillus megaterium	Synthetic	Batch 48	Cu	70	Roşca et al. (2023)

bioremediation processes. The microalgae are proposed as options for the removal/degradation of heavy metals, colorants, antibiotics, and other contaminants. Some of the most employed microalgae are *Chlorella vulgaris, Chlorella* sp., *Desmodesmus* sp., *Stigeoclonium nanum, Pleurococcus* sp., *Spirulina platensis, Calotrix,* and *Synechocytis aquatilis*, which reach efficiencies greater than 50% in the elimination of nitrogenized or phosphorus compounds; COD; heavy metals; pesticides; and colorants. Bioremediation processes based on microalgae can be carried out in a very diverse group of bioreactors with open or closed configurations called photobioreactors (PBRs) because of the necessity of adding light as another nutrient to cultures. There are tubular, stirred tanks, column cylinders, flat panels, and special configurations designed to satisfy the specific necessities of every strain (Egbo et al., 2018; Martínez-Roldán & Cañizares-Villanueva, 2015; Martínez-Roldán et al., 2024; Masojídek & Torzillo, 2008; Vela-García et al., 2019).

1.3.8 Phycoremediation of wastewater from the food industry

The use of microalgae and cyanobacteria as alternatives to the biological treatment of wastewater produced in the food industry is considered a sustainable alternative because of their high tolerance to the concentration of inorganic and organic compounds in this kind of effluent. Additionally, microalgae can eliminate turbidity, color, acidity, and other undesirable conditions. Some of the effluents treated with microalgal cultures include beverages, molasses/vinasses, and whey. The action of these microorganisms causes reductions in nitrogen compounds ($N\text{-}NH_3$ and $N\text{-}NO_3$), phosphorus salts ($P\text{-}PO_4$), COD, fats, and carbohydrates, reaching efficiencies greater than 50% (Table 1.10). The operation is typically batch, and the duration of the process can be 7 or 15 days; however, semicontinuous operation allows the processes to be maintained for 37 days. Changes in the PBR configuration, duration of the process, strain used, and addition of specific nutrients can stimulate the culture to improve the process, increasing the removal efficiency. Recently, the exploitation of the biomass produced (e.g., proteins, carbohydrates, carotenoids, and pigments) during the treatment process was proposed with the objective of promoting a circular economy and improving the financial balance of the wastewater process (Rojo-Gómez, 2022; Ruiz-Reza et al., 2024).

TABLE 1.10
Microalgae and cyanobacteria used to treat food industry effluents

Microalga	Effluent	PBR (HRT d)	Removal (%)		References
Chlorella vulgaris	Molasses	Cylindrical 15 d	DQO	30	Olarte-Gómez and Valencia-Giraldo (2016)
			TP	75	
			TN	84	
Stigeoclonium nanum	Mezcal vinasse	Column 11 d	DQO	56	Ruiz-Reza et al. (2024)
			TP	88	
			$N\text{-}NO_3$	97	
Stigeoclonium nanum	Mezcal vinasse	Flat-panel 37 d	DQO	6	Diaz-Parra et al. (2024)
			$P\text{-}PO_4$	87	
			$N\text{-}NO_3$	59	
Stigeoclonium nanum	Whey	Flat-panel 7 d	DQO	99	Rojo-Gómez (2022)
			$P\text{-}PO_4$	60	
			$N\text{-}NO_3$	98	
Calotrix	Whey	Flat-panel 7 d	DQO	93	Rojo-Gómez (2022)
			$P\text{-}PO_4$	67	
			$N\text{-}NO_3$	97	

1.3.8.1 Phycoremediation of dyes

Contamination by dyes in bodies of water has a very important impact because it affects the dynamics of light absorption and employment by photosynthetic microorganisms (Hernández-Zamora et al., 2014). The effluents of the textile industry are normally alkaline, and microalgae prefer to grow under these conditions rather than at acidic pH. If microalgae are exposed to effluents containing colorants used in the textile industry, they can adsorb/absorb or even degrade the colorants, and if other contaminants such as COD or nitrogen are present in the effluent, these contaminants can also be eliminated. Typically, the use of microalgae to treat textile effluents can reach efficiencies ranging from 60% to 90% in the elimination of nitrogen and phosphorus compounds as well as CDO and color. Effluents containing alanine blue, Congo red, indigo blue, malachite green, and methylene blue can be discolored by employing microalgal cultures with efficiencies ranging from approximately 60–90% (Table 1.11). The process of discoloration can involve the transformation of a molecule (i.e., the loss of its color), the use of the compound in physiological processes (i.e., as an energy source or precursor), or only its elimination by adsorption/absorption processes (Allende-Valera et al., 2021; M. Hernández-Zamora et al., 2015; Martínez-Roldán et al., 2024; Premaratne et al., 2021).

1.3.8.2 Phycoremediation of hydrocarbons

The ability of microalgae and cyanobacteria to adsorb/absorb organic molecules is due to the presence of an extracellular polymeric matrix (mainly polysaccharides). Additionally, some genera are able to produce enzymes that are useful for the degradation of molecules derived from petroleum; in some cases, these molecules are employed as carbon sources (Dell' Anno et al., 2021). Microalgae, such as *Chlamydomonas, Chlorella, Dunaliella, Scenedesmus,* and *Spirulina,* are able to reduce the concentration of polycyclic aromatic hydrocarbons (PAHs) (Table 1.12), and according to Hamouda et al. (2023), this process can be combined with the production of biofuels. The phycoremediation of petroleum-related pollution or for the treatment of wastewater from oil refining systems is very efficient; in some cases, the removal of very toxic molecules, such as anthracene, phenanthrene, fluoranthene, naphthalene, and pyrene, with efficiencies ranging from 35% to 80%, is highly efficient, and the reported values depend on the strains and operational conditions used (Stepanova, Gladkov, Osipova et al., 2022).

TABLE 1.11
Microalgae and cyanobacteria employed in the treatment of textile wastewater

Microalga	Contaminant	PBR/HRT (d)	Removal (%)		References
Chlorella vulgaris	Congo red	Column 4 d		58–83	Hernández-Zamora et al. (2015)
Chlorella vulgaris	Alanine blue	Column 11 d		~60	Carbajo-Arteaga et al. (2018)
Chlorella pyrenoidosa	Congo red DQO	Continuous operation 10 d	Congo red DQO	100 87	Premaratne et al. (2021)
Scenedesmus quadricauda	Indigo blue	Column 4 d		100	Premaratne et al. (2021)
Oscillatoria sp.	N-NO_3 N-NO_2 P-PO_4 SO_4^{2-}	21 d			Mathimani et al. (2024)
Phormidium sp.	N-NO_3 N-NO_2 P-PO_4 SO_4^{2-}	21 d			Mathimani et al. (2024)

TABLE 1.12
Microalgae and cyanobacteria used to treat effluents from the petroleum refining industry

Microalga	Effluent	Operational mode	Removal (%)		References
Chlorella vulgaris	Crude oil	Batch 5 d	TOC	~80	Kuttiyathil et al. (2021)
Nitzschia sp.	Synthetic	Batch 196 h	PHE	~55	Hong et al. (2008)
Skeletonema costatum	Synthetic	Batch 195 h	PHE FLA	~48 ~8	Hong et al. (2008)
Anabaena sp.	Synthetic	Batch 60 d	n-C18 PHE DBT	29 51 30	Ibraheem (2010)
Nostoc sp.	Synthetic	Batch 60 d	n-C18 PHE DBT	10 43 44	Ibraheem (2010)
Synechocystis aquatilis	Synthetic	Batch 60 d	n-C18 PHE DBT	78 46 21	Ibraheem (2010)

TOC Total organic carbon
PHE Phenanthrene
FLA Fluoranthene
n-C18 n-octadecane
DBT Dibenzothiophene

1.3.8.3 Phycoremediation of heavy metals

Microalgae are able to remove not only nitrogen, phosphorus, and carbon from wastewaters but also ions such as Fe, Cu, Zn, and Mn; the absorption of ions is necessary for the optimal function of metabolic processes because they are cofactors of different enzymes. Metallic ions are scarce in nature, which has led to the development of efficient strategies to obtain microalgae from the environment. Additionally, highlighting the importance of the negative functional groups of the cell walls of microalgae is important because these groups also permit the adhesion of metals. Both these characteristics, the strategies used to obtain them from the environment and the chemical interactions with the functional groups, allow microalgae very high efficiencies in the removal of heavy metals from liquid effluents.

The efficiencies of removing metals and metalloids remain regardless of whether live or dead biomass is employed (Liu et al., 2021; Martínez-Roldán et al., 2024). Table 1.13 shows examples of metal and metalloid removal by microalgae and cyanobacteria. The reported efficiencies range from 30% to 80%, highlighting the importance of operational conditions such as temperature, pH, the presence of other ions, and the strain used; if live biomass is used, the optimal growth conditions must also be considered (Abinandan et al., 2019; Martínez-Roldán et al., 2024).

1.3.9 Fungi and yeast technologies

Fungi are a very diverse group of eukaryotic microorganisms with a filamentous or unicellular configuration and heterotrophic metabolism. These microorganisms normally have many adaptations that allow them to degrade many different molecules through the use of extracellular enzymes in biotechnological processes known as mycoremediation. Fungi are used for the elimination of compounds such as pharmaceutical products, pesticides, colorants, complex organic compounds, or even the accumulation of heavy metals. Research on mycoremediation includes studies using strains of *Penicillium Candida, Geotrichum, Trichoderma, Trichosporon, Rhodotorula, Aspergillus,* and some white rot fungi that present laccases, manganese peroxidases, or cellulase activities that are useful for degrading pollutants in industrial wastewaters (Buratti et al., 2022; Dinakarkumar et al., 2024).

TABLE 1.13
Phycoremediation of heavy metals

Microalgae	Effluent	Operation condition	Removal (%)		References
Spirulina sp.	Synthetic	Column 14 d	Cd	73	Soeprobowati and Hariyati (2012)
Chlorella sp.	Synthetic	Column 14 d	Pb Cd Cu	90 62 93	Soeprobowati and Hariyati (2012)
Porphyridium sp.	Synthetic	Column 14 d	Cd Cu	70 96	Soeprobowati and Hariyati (2012)
Pseudochlorococcum typicum	Synthetic	24 h	Hg^{+2} Pb^{+2}	98 61	Shanab et al. (2012)
Pleurococcus sp.	Mining	Airlift 20 d	Hg N-NO_3 P-PO_4	86 ~90 ~90	Vela-García et al. (2019)
Chlorella sp.	Mining	Airlift 20 d	Hg N-NO_3 P-PO_4	83 ~85 ~85	Vela-García et al. (2019)
Scenedesmus sp.	Mining	Airlift 20 d	Hg N-NO_3 P-PO_4	64 ~83 ~80	Vela-García et al. (2019)

1.3.9.1 Mycoremediation of effluents from the food industry

The effluents of the food industry include high amounts of organic matter, such as sugars, proteins, and lipids, which make them ideal growth media for fungi and yeast. Their use in the wastewater treatment of dairy and distillated beverage effluents is common. The application of fungi in wastewater treatment normally occurs in aerobic submerged cultures, regardless of whether the system is open or closed; the operation strategy can be continuous, semicontinuous, or batch. The fungi normally grow, forming pellets that are very easy to separate from the treated effluent. Table 1.14 shows the different fungal strains used to treat wastewater from different sectors of the food industry. The removal efficiency sometimes exceeds 80% regardless of whether the compounds are COD, sugars, or most complex compounds, such as proteins, vitamins, or others (Bansfield et al., 2024; González-Benito et al., 1997; Veiter et al., 2018).

1.3.9.2 Mycoremediation of textile effluents

Fungi and yeast have a high diversity of organisms, many of which are unspecific and produce secondary metabolites such as organic acids that favor the degradation of recalcitrant molecules; this allows the use of fungi and yeast for the treatment of effluents from the textile industry containing colorants. The success of bioprocesses based on fungi for the degradation/removal of synthetic colorants such as azo, silicone, phthalocyanine, and heterocyclic compounds is due to the excretion of oxidative enzymes such as oxidases, catalases, manganese peroxidases, and peroxidases. However, as for the biotechnological processes, the efficiency varies depending on the strain, culture conditions, operational conditions, and presence of other molecules. (Allende-Valera et al., 2021; Singh et al., 2013). Table 1.15 shows cases of different strains used in the degradation of synthetic colorants, and in the majority of cases, the best efficiencies are reached at concentrations lower than 600 ppm (Faraco et al., 2009; Salem et al., 2019). Fungi normally show high efficiencies in the removal/degradation of colorants; nevertheless, ensuring the absence of toxicity in the treated effluent is important. This is because some colorant degradation can produce residues with greater toxicity than the original molecules (Chen et al., 2019; Sosa-Martínez et al., 2020).

TABLE 1.14
Remediation of effluents from the food industry

Fungi	Effluent	Operational condition	Removal (%)		References
Trametes sp.	Molasses	Batch 7 d	COD Discoloration	61 73	González et al. (2000)
Tremetes versicolor	Molasses	Batch	COD Discoloration $N\text{-}NH_4^+$	77 82 36	González-Benito et al. (1997)
Aspergillus niger	Molasses	ABR 4 d	COD Discoloration	72 69	Peña Miranda et al. (1996)
Geotrichum candidum	Whey	Batch, 1 L	COD TOC PT	16–26 6–11 22	Bansfield et al. (2024)
Penicillium corylophilum	Whey	Batch, 1 L	COD TOC PT	16–26 6–11 ~41	Bansfield et al. (2024)

TABLE 1.15
Mycoremediation of effluents from the textile industry

Fungi	Effluent	Operational condition	Removal (%)		References
Aspergillus niger	Textile	Batch 7 d	RY RD	98 92	Salem et al. (2019)
Aspergillus flavus	Textile	Batch 6 d	Red[S2-B] Blue [FN-R] Orange [FN-R] Black[-G]	~65 ~98 ~98 ~52	Karim et al. (2020)
Pleurotus flabellatus	Synthetic	Batch 6 h	DB14	90	Singh et al. (2013)
Phanerochaete chrysosporium	Textile	Batch 2 d	AR299 DY_3	90 100	Faraco et al. (2009)
Pleurotus ostreatus	Textile	Batch 10 d	RBI5 DB1	90 80	Faraco et al. (2009)
Penicillium simplicissimum	Triphenylmethane dyes		Crystal Violet, Methyl Violet, Malachite Green, Cotton Blue	>95%	Chen et al. (2019)

RY Reactive yellow
RD Reactive red
DB14 Direct blue 14
S2-B Benzema red
FN-R Novacron brilliant blue
FN-R Novacron orange
Black-G Novacron super black
AR299 Acid red 299
DY_3 Disperse yellow 3
RBI5 Reactive black 5
DB1 Disperse blue 1

1.3.9.3 Mycoremediation of petroleum-derived effluents

Fungi are a group of heterotrophic microorganisms that grow if the organic matter content is high, regardless of whether the ecosystem is aquatic or soil. This allows their application for the removal of hydrocarbons from both soil and wastewater containing crude oil. Fungi-based technology is used because its operational cost is low, and it normally has high efficiency for the removal of many petroleum-derived products, such as diesel, paraffin, and phenanthrene (Table 1.16). Fungi can use

TABLE 1.16
Mycoremediation of petroleum industry wastewater

Fungi	Effluent	Operational condition	Removal (%)		References
Pycnoporus sanguineus	Synthetic	Batch 14 d	ANT	67	Imam et al. (2021)
Ganoderma lucidum	Crude oil	Batch 30 d	PHE PY	99.6 99.5	Agrawal et al. (2018)
Aspergillus niger	Wastewater from petroleum reservoir	21 d	PAHs	73	Obire et al. (2020)
Aspergillus sydowii	Wastewater from petroleum reservoir	21 d	PAHs	73	Obire et al. (2020)
Fusarium lichenicola	Wastewater from petroleum reservoir	21 d	PAHs	65	Obire et al. (2020)
Mix culture	Wastewater from petroleum reservoir	21 d	PAHs NAP	85 100	Obire et al. (2020)

PHE Phenanthrene NAP Naphthalene
PY Pyrene PAHs Polycyclic aromatic hydrocarbons
ANT Anthracene

these compounds as the sole carbon source or as a cometabolite and use a very digestible carbon source, such as carbohydrates (Rani et al., 2024). The process of hydrocarbon degradation normally includes the production of extracellular laccases and peroxidases, which facilitate elimination by fungi.

The most common fungi used in the degradation of hydrocarbons are *Aspergillus, Talaromyces,* and *Gramphium,* regardless of whether the process is *in situ* or *ex situ,* and the strategies used can include bioaugmentation, mixing of fungi or cocultures with bacteria, reaching efficiencies higher than 80% in the removal of polycyclic aromatic hydrocarbons or total hydrocarbons. For the removal of pure compounds such as naphthalene and chrysene from wastewater from the petroleum industry, the efficiency can reach 100% in the treatment of mixed cultures (Benguenab & Chibani, 2021; Das & Chandran, 2011; Imam et al., 2021; Obire et al., 2020).

1.3.9.4 Mycoremediation of heavy metals

As occurs for other types of effluents, the presence of extracellular enzymes involved in the excretion of organic acids favors the elimination of heavy metals from wastewaters. This is because they normally act as chelators, favor elimination, or reduce toxicity because they precipitate or are less readily available for microorganisms. These advantages make fungi the most employed microbial group for the removal of metallic elements such as As, Cr, Pb, Cd, Zn, and Cu present in effluents from the crude oil extraction, mining, or metallurgic industries. According to Anahid et al. (2011) and Bayramoğlu et al. (2003), the most common fungi used for the sorption of heavy metals such as Cr or Ni are *Aspergillus niger, Trametes versicolor, Penicillium simplicissimum,* and *Rhizopus arrhizus* (Table 1.17). *A. niger* and *P. simplicissimum* produce high amounts of organic acids, which makes them useful for biolixiviation processes developed for the recovery of metals from tailings or wastewaters with high concentrations of metals. The high efficiency shown by fungi remains regardless of pH or temperature; this is because the cell wall of fungi has functional groups that ensure removal (Dong et al., 2023).

TABLE 1.17
Bioremediation of effluents from the metallurgic and mining industries

Fungi	Effluent	Operational condition	Metal	Removal (%)	References
Rhizopus arrhizus	Metallurgic effluent	60–90 min	Cu Ni	~97% ~75%	Subudhi and Kar (1996)
Aspergillus niger DDN	Mining effluent	15 h 200 rpm	Cr^{+6} 2.8 g	0,0574 mg/g	Ume et al. (2022)
Aspergillus flavus	Water contaminated by mining activities	10 d 160 rpm	Mg/L Cr 3.1 Cd 24.5 Zn 75.6 Mg 124	% MBR 25 43 30 23	Anupong et al. (2022)
Penicillium simplicissimum immobilized in zeolite	Gold mining effluent	180 min 150 rpm	Cr^{+3}	525 mmol/kg	Bakatula et al. (2011)

1.3.10 Mixed cultures

In the majority of cases, the use of monospecific cultures normally results in low removal/degradation efficiencies compared with those of mixed cultures. There are many possible combinations to employ: prokaryote–eukaryote (bacteria–microalga or bacteria–fungi) or eukaryote–eukaryote (fungi–microalgae), which typically improve biotechnological processes for wastewater treatment (Mahlangu et al., 2024; Masojídek & Torzillo, 2008). This is because there is a synergistic relationship and an interchange of macro- and micronutrients that favor the simultaneous growth of both organisms. An example is the symbiosis of fungi and microalgae when the fungi form pellets. This microalgal biomass is immobilized; the mycelium barrier reduces the exposure of the microalgae to the pollutant and favors their growth and the removal of the biomass after treatment. This approach is useful in the treatment of industrial effluents containing emerging contaminants, aromatic hydrocarbons, and heavy metals. According to Wang et al. (2023), a coculture of *Aspergillus fumigatus* and *Synechocystis* sp. can eliminate Cd^{+2} and C^{+6} with efficiencies close to 98%, and the high efficiency is attributed to the formation of crystals of insoluble salts on the surface of the pellets formed by the fungi and algae.

In the case of processes based on the interaction of microalgae and bacteria, these systems have the potential to be used to treat wastewater for the elimination of heavy metals, nitrogen, phosphorus compounds, and COD/BOD (Ovis-Sánchez et al., 2023; Romero-Frasca et al., 2024). This symbiosis occurs because bacterial metabolism results in the production of CO_2, which can be fixed by microalgae, converted into biomolecules, and produce oxygen, some of which can be used by bacteria for growth. Nevertheless, the diffusion processes involved in the entrance of nutrients to the pellets and the population dynamics of the components of the mixed culture are not clear (Romero-Frasca et al., 2024).

Chlorella vulgaris and *Pseudomonas putida* are commonly used in treatment processes because they are very useful for the removal of nitrogen, phosphorus, and organic matter, with values higher than 60%. The process shows better performance if the bacteria and the microalgae are coimmobilized because their close interaction stimulates the metabolism of both and increases the efficiency of the process (Mujtaba et al., 2017; Zhao et al., 2023).

1.4 CONCLUSIONS

The microbial groups have the potential to help us reduce the impact of productive processes, whether by eliminating the impact of the processes on the environment, prior to the discharge of the effluents, or when an impact is caused by the spill of wastewater into a body of water. Importantly, every group of microorganisms has characteristics that increase their applicability to specific bioremediation processes. Whereas bacteria are very efficient at reducing the pollutant charge of effluents rich in organic matter, microalgae are very efficient at removing nitrogen, phosphorus, and fungi to transform/degrade very recalcitrant molecules as synthetic colorants or emerging contaminants. This makes decision-making easier if the effluent has a specific composition or is a production process wastewater; however, in the case of real wastewater (or municipal wastewater), the composition is not constant or even unknown. In the case of this kind of effluent, the use of mixed cultures to stimulate the microorganisms present in the wastewater is always beneficial because these cultures normally have tolerance to pollutants, which could improve the process in a very straightforward manner. Therefore, the selection of the microbial group to be used must be careful and multifactorial to ensure a bioremediation process with low operational costs and high removal efficiency.

ACKNOWLEDGMENTS

To TecNM/IT Durango for the financial support provided, and to SECIHTI for the scholarship of Diaz-Parra (CVU 1266356) to achieve the master's degree.

REFERENCES

Abinandan, S., Subashchandrabose, S. R., Venkateswarlu, K., Perera, I. A., & Megharaj, M. (2019). Acid-tolerant microalgae can withstand higher concentrations of invasive cadmium and produce sustainable biomass and biodiesel at pH 3.5. *Bioresource Technology, 281*, 469–473. https://doi.org/10.1016/j.biortech.2019.03.001

Abu-Hasan, H., Sheikh-Abdullah, S. R., Al-Attabi, A. W. N., Nash-Hassoon, D. A., Anuar, N., Rahman, N. A., & Titah, H. S. (2016). Removal of ibuprofen, ketoprofen, COD and nitrogen compounds from pharmaceutical wastewater using aerobic suspension-sequencing batch reactor (ASSBR). *Separation and Purification Technology, 157*, 215–221. https://doi.org/10.1016/j.seppur.2015.11.017

Agrawal, N., Verma, P., & Shahi, S. K. (2018). Degradation of polycyclic aromatic hydrocarbons (phenanthrene and pyrene) by the ligninolytic fungi *Ganoderma lucidum* isolated from the hardwood stump. *Bioresources and Bioprocessing, 5*, 11. https://doi.org/10.1186/s40643-018-0197-5

Allende-Valera, G., Pancho-Márquez, A. M., Sánchez-Cerón, B., López-Candelaria, G., Vásquez-Jiménez, O., Rodríguez, R., Almanza-Orea, F. E., Mendoza-Hernández, J. C., & Pérez-Osorio, G. (2021). Sistemas de biorremediación de colorantes textiles: una perspectiva. *Revista Latinoamericana el Ambiente y las Ciencias, 12*(31), 38–61.

Alzain, H., Kalimugogo, V., & Hussein, K. (2023). A review of environmental impact of azo dyes. *International Journal of Research and Review, 10*(6), 64–689. https://doi.org/10.52403/ijrr.20230682

Amjith, L. R., & Bavanish, B. (2022). A review on biomass and wind as renewable energy for sustainable environment. *Chemosphere, 293*, 133579. https://doi.org/10.1016/j.chemosphere.2022.133579

Anahid, S., Yaghmaei, S., & Ghobadinejad, Z. (2011). Heavy metal tolerance of fungi. *Scientia Iranica, 18*(3 C), 502–508. https://doi.org/10.1016/j.scient.2011.05.015

Anupong, W., Jutamas, K., On-uma, R., Alshiekheid, M., Sabour, A., Krishnan, R., Lan Chi, N. T., Pugazhendhi, A., & Brindhadevi, K. (2022). Bioremediation competence of *Aspergillus flavus* DDN on pond water contaminated by mining activities. *Chemosphere, 304*, 135250. https://doi.org/10.1016/j.chemosphere.2022.135250

Badmus, S. O., Amusa, H. K., Oyehan, T. A., & Saleh, T. A. (2021). Environmental risks and toxicity of surfactants: Overview of analysis, assessment, and remediation techniques. *Environmental Science and Pollution Research, 28*(44), 62085–62104. https://doi.org/10.1007/s11356-021-16483-w

Bailey, K., Basu, A., & Sharma, S. (2022). The environmental impacts of fast fashion on water quality: A systematic review. *Water (Switzerland), 14*, 11. https://doi.org/10.3390/w14071073

Bajpai, P. (2016). Global pulp and paper production and consumption. In P. Bajpai (Ed.), *Pulp and paper industry* (9–14). Elsevier Ltd. https://doi.org/10.1016/b978-0-12-803411-8.00002-0

Bakatula, E. N., Cukrowska, E. M., Straker, C. J., Weiersbye, I. M., & Tutu, H. (2011). Biosorption of metals from gold mine wastewaters by *Penicillium simplicissimum* immobilized on zeolite: Kinetic, equilibrium and thermodynamic studies. In T. R. Rüde, A. Freund, & C. Wolkersdorfer (Eds.), *11th International mine water association congress: Mine water–managing the challenges* (271–276). International Mine Water Association.

Bansfield, D., Spilling, K., Mikola, A., & Piiparinen, J. (2024). An investigation into the ability of three fungi and one yeast to grow and capture nutrients in cheese whey. *Bioresource Technology Reports, 26*, 101854. https://doi.org/10.1016/j.biteb.2024.101854

Bayramoğlu, G., Bektaş, S., & Arica, M. Y. (2003). Biosorption of heavy metal ions on immobilized white-rot fungus *Trametes versicolor*. *Journal of Hazardous Materials, 101*(3), 285–300. https://doi.org/10.1016/S0304-3894(03)00178-X

Benguenab, A., & Chibani, A. (2021). Biodegradation of petroleum hydrocarbons by filamentous fungi (*Aspergillus ustus and Purpureocillium lilacinum*) isolated from used engine oil contaminated soil. *Acta Ecologica Sinica, 41*(5), 416–423. https://doi.org/10.1016/J.CHNAES.2020.10.008

Bermeo-Garay, M., Bonilla-Albarca, L., Yagual-Romero, A., & Alvarez-Macias, D. (2017). *Tratamientos de vinaza aplicando procesos fisico-químicos y electrocoagulación*. Grupo Compas.

Borowitzka, M. A. (2013). High-value products from microalgae-their development and commercialisation. *Journal of Applied Phycology, 25*(3), 743–756. https://doi.org/10.1007/s10811-013-9983-9

Boxall, A. B. A. (2004). The environmental side effects of medication. *EMBO Reports*, *5*(12), 1110–1116. https://doi.org/10.1038/sj.embor.7400307

Buratti, S., Girometta, C. E., Baiguera, R. M., Barucco, B., Bernardi, M., De Girolamo, G., Malgaretti, M., Oliva, D., Picco, A. M., & Savino, E. (2022). Fungal diversity in two wastewater treatment plants in north Italy. *Microorganisms, 10*(6), 1096. https://doi.org/10.3390/microorganisms10061096

Carbajo-Arteaga, L., Ponce-Zavaleta, M., Moreno-Eustaquio, W., & Mendoza-Bobadilla, J. (2018). Removal of aniline blue dye using live microalgae *Chlorella vulgaris*. *Journal of Energy & Environmental Sciences, 2*(1), 6. https://doi.org/10.32829/eesj.v2i1.51

Carpenter, S. R. (2008). Phosphorus control is critical to mitigating eutrophication. *Proceedings of the National Academy of Sciences of the United States of America, 105*, 11039–11040. https://doi.org/10.1073/pnas.0806112105

Chang, J. S., & Kuo, T. S. (2000). Kinetics of bacterial decolorization of azo dye with *Escherichia coli* NO3. *Bioresource Technology, 75*(2), 107–111. https://doi.org/10.1016/S0960-8524(00)00049-3

Chatzipaschali, A. A., & Stamatis, A. G. (2012). Biotechnological utilization with a focus on anaerobic treatment of cheese whey: Current status and prospects. *Energies, 5*(9), 3492–3525. https://doi.org/10.3390/en5093492

Chen, C., Guo, W., & Ngo, H. H. (2019). Pesticides in stormwater runoff—A mini review. *Frontiers of Environmental Science and Engineering*, *13*(5). https://doi.org/10.1007/s11783-019-1150-3

Chowdhury, P., Viraraghavan, T., & Srinivasan, A. (2010). Biological treatment processes for fish processing wastewater - A review. *Bioresource Technology, 101*(2), 439–449. https://doi.org/10.1016/j.biortech.2009.08.065

Christian, D., Gaekwad, A., Dani, H., Shabiimam, M. A., & Kandya, A. (2023). Recent techniques of textile industrial wastewater treatment: A review. *Materials Today: Proceedings, 77*, 277–285. https://doi.org/10.1016/j.matpr.2022.11.301

Clews, R. J. (2016). Fundamentals of the petroleum industry. In R. J. Clews (Ed.), *Project finance for the International Petroleum Industry* (83–99). Academic Press. https://doi.org/10.1016/b978-0-12-800158-5.00005-0

Conejo, A. N., Birat, J. P., & Dutta, A. (2020). A review of the current environmental challenges of the steel industry and its value chain. *Journal of Environmental Management, 259*, 109782. https://doi.org/10.1016/j.jenvman.2019.109782

Cortazar-Martínez, A., González-Ramírez, C. A., Coronel-Olivares, C., Escalante-Lozada, J. A., Castro-Rosas, J., & Villagómez-Ibarra, J. R. (2012). Biotechnology applied to the degradation of textile industry dyes. *Universidad y Ciencia, 28*(2), 187–199. https://www.scielo.org.mx/scielo.php?pid=S0186-29792012000200009&script=sci_arttext&tlng=pt%0Awww.universidadyciencia.ujat.mx

Cubas, A. L. V., Bianchet, R. T., Reis, I. M. A. S. dos, & Gouveia, I. C. (2022). Plastics and microplastic in the cosmetic industry: Aggregating sustainable actions aimed at alignment and interaction with UN Sustainable Development Goals. *Polymers, 14*(21), 4576. https://doi.org/10.3390/polym14214576

Das, N., & Chandran, P. (2011). Microbial degradation of petroleum hydrocarbon contaminants: An overview. *Biotechnology Research International*, *2011*(1), 1–13. https://doi.org/10.4061/2011/941810

Dell' Anno, F., Rastelli, E., Sansone, C., Dell' Anno, A., Brunet, C., & Ianora, A. (2021). Bacteria, fungi and microalgae for the bioremediation of marine sediments contaminated by petroleum hydrocarbons in the omics era. *Microorganisms, 9*(8), 1695. https://doi.org/10.3390/microorganisms9081695

Diaz-Parra, K. L., Contreras-Hernández, M. G., Ayala-García, V. M., Hernández-Melchor, D. J., & Martínez-Roldán, A. J. (2024). Microalgae and cyanobacteria in the biological treatment of effluents. *Revista de Gestão Social e Ambiental, 18*(10), 1–13. https://doi.org/10.24857/rgsa.v18n10-010

Dinakarkumar, Y., Ramakrishnan, G., Gujjula, K. R., Vasu, V., Balamurugan, P., & Murali, G. (2024). Fungal bioremediation: An overview of the mechanisms, applications and future perspectives. *Environmental Chemistry and Ecotoxicology, 6*, 293–302. https://doi.org/10.1016/j.enceco.2024.07.002

Dong, Y., Zan, J., & Lin, H. (2023). Bioleaching of heavy metals from metal tailings utilizing bacteria and fungi: Mechanisms, strengthen measures, and development prospect. *Journal of Environmental Management, 344,* 118511. https://doi.org/10.1016/j.jenvman.2023.118511

Egbo, M. K., Okoani, A. O., & Okoh, I. E. (2018). Photobioreactors for microalgae cultivation – An Overview. *International Journal of Scientific & Engineering Research, 9*(11), 65–74.

El-Naggar, N. E. A., El-khateeb, A. Y., Ghoniem, A. A., El-Hersh, M. S., & Saber, W. E. I. A. (2020). Innovative low-cost biosorption process of Cr^{6+} by *Pseudomonas alcaliphila* NEWG-2. *Scientific Reports, 10*(1), 14043. https://doi.org/10.1038/s41598-020-70473-5

Faraco, V., Pezzella, C., Giardina, P., Piscitelli, A., Vanhulle, S., & Sannia, G. (2009). Decolourization of textile dyes by the white-rot fungi *Phanerochaete chrysosporium* and *Pleurotus ostreatus*. *Journal of Chemical Technology and Biotechnology, 84*(3), 414–419. https://doi.org/10.1002/jctb.2055

Geissen, V., Mol, H., Klumpp, E., Umlauf, G., Nadal, M., Van der Ploeg, M., Van de Zee, S. E. A. T. M., & Ritsema, C. J. (2015). Emerging pollutants in the environment: A challenge for water resource management. *International Soil and Water Conservation Research, 3*(1), 57–65. https://doi.org/10.1016/j.iswcr.2015.03.002

González-Benito, G., Peña-Miranda, M., & Rodríguez de los Santos, D. (1997). Decolorization of wastewater from an alcoholic fermentation process with *Trametes versicolor. Bioresource Technology, 61*(1), 33–37. https://doi.org/10.1016/S0960-8524(97)84695-0

González, T., Terrón, M. C., Yagüe, S., Zapico, E., Galletti, G. C., & González, A. E. (2000). Pyrolysis/gas chromatography/mass spectrometry monitoring of fungal- biotreated distillery wastewater using *Trametes* sp. I-62 (CECT 20197). *Rapid Communications in Mass Spectrometry, 14*(15), 1417–1424.

Gürsoy, N. Ç., & Dayioğlu, H. (2000). Evaluating peracetic acid bleaching of cotton as an environmentally safe alternative to hypochlorite bleaching. *Textile Research Journal, 70*(6), 475–480. https://doi.org/10.1177/004051750007000602

Hamouda, R. A., Alhumairi, A. M., & Saddiq, A. A. (2023). Simultaneous bioremediation of petroleum hydrocarbons and production of biofuels by the micro-green alga, cyanobacteria, and its consortium. *Heliyon, 9*(6). https://doi.org/10.1016/j.heliyon.2023.e16656

Hermosilla, D., Merayo, N., Gascó, A., & Blanco, Á. (2014). The application of advanced oxidation technologies to the treatment of effluents from the pulp and paper industry: A review. *Environmental Science and Pollution Research, 22*, 168–191 https://doi.org/10.1007/s11356-014-3516-1

Hernández-Zamora, M., Cristiani-Urbina, E., Martínez-Jerónimo, F., Perales-Vela, H. V., Ponce-Noyola, T., Montes-Horcasitas, M. C., & Cañizares-Villanueva, R. O. (2015). Bioremoval of the azo dye Congo Red by the microalga *Chlorella vulgaris. Environmental Science and Pollution Research, 22*(14), 10811–10823. https://doi.org/10.1007/s11356-015-4277-1

Hernández-Zamora, M., Perales-Vela, H. V., Flores-Ortíz, C. M., & Cañizares-Villanueva, R. O. (2014). Physiological and biochemical responses of *Chlorella vulgaris* to Congo Red. *Ecotoxicology Environmental Safety*, *108*, 72–77. https://doi.org/10.1016/j.ecoenv.2014.05.030

Holkar, C. R., Jadhav, A. J., Pinjari, D. V., Mahamuni, N. M., & Pandit, A. B. (2016). A critical review on textile wastewater treatments: Possible approaches. *Journal of Environmental Management, 182*, 351–366. https://doi.org/10.1016/j.jenvman.2016.07.090

Hong, Y.-W., Yuan, D. X., Lin, Q. M., & Yang, T. L. (2008). Accumulation and biodegradation of phenanthrene and fluoranthene by the algae enriched from a mangrove aquatic ecosystem. *Marine Pollution Bulletin, 56*(8), 1400–1405. https://doi.org/10.1016/j.marpolbul.2008.05.003

Hu, T. L. (1994). Decolourization of reactive azo dyes by transformation with *Pseudomonas luteola. Bioresource Technology, 49*(1), 47–51. https://doi.org/10.1016/0960-8524(94)90172-4

Ibraheem, I. B. M. (2010). Biodegradability of hydrocarbons by cyanobacteria. *Journal of Phycology, 46*(4), 818–824. https://doi.org/10.1111/j.1529-8817.2010.00865.x

Igiri, B. E., Okoduwa, S. I. R., Idoko, G. O., Akabuogu, E. P., Adeyi, A. O., & Ejiogu, I. K. (2018). Toxicity and bioremediation of heavy metals contaminated ecosystem from tannery wastewater: A review. *Journal of Toxicology*, *2018*(1). https://doi.org/10.1155/2018/2568038

Imam, A., Kanaujia, P. K., Ray, A., & Suman, S. K. (2021). Removal of petroleum contaminants through bioremediation with Integrated concepts of resource recovery: A review. *Indian Journal of Microbiology, 61*(3), 250–261. https://doi.org/10.1007/s12088-021-00928-4

Imran, S., Mujtaba, M. A., Zafar, M. M., Hussain, A., Mehmood, A., Farwa, U. E., Korakianitis, T., Kalam, M. A., Fayaz, H., & Saleel, C. A. (2023). Assessing the potential of GHG emissions for the textile sector: A baseline study. *Heliyon, 9*(11). https://doi.org/10.1016/j.heliyon.2023.e22404

Jafari, S. A., Cheraghi, S., Mirbakhsh, M., Mirza, R., & Maryamabadi, A. (2015). Employing response rurface rethodology for optimization of mercury bioremediation by vibrio parahaemolyticus PG02 in coastal sediments of Bushehr, Iran. *Clean - Soil, Air, Water, 43*(1), 118–126. https://doi.org/10.1002/clen.201300616

Jena, J., Narwade, N., Das, T., Dhotre, D., Sarkar, U., & Souche, Y. (2020). Treatment of industrial effluents and assessment of their impact on the structure and function of microbial diversity in a unique Anoxic-Aerobic sequential batch reactor (AnASBR). *Journal of Environmental Management, 261*, 110241. https://doi.org/10.1016/j.jenvman.2020.110241

Johnston, J. E., Lim, E., & Roh, H. (2019). Impact of upstream oil extraction and environmental public health: A review of the evidence. *Science of the Total Environment, 657*, 187–199. https://doi.org/10.1016/j.scitotenv.2018.11.483

Karim, M. E., Dhar, K., Moniruzzaman, M., Hossain, M. U., Das, K. C., & Hossain, M. T. (2020). Decolorization of synthetic dyes by *Aspergillus flavus* Strain EF-3 isolated from textile dyeing sludge. *Bangladesh Journal of Microbiology, 37*(1), 7–13. https://doi.org/10.3329/bjm.v37i1.51203

Khalid, M., & Abdollahi, M. (2021). Environmental distribution of personal care products and their effects on human health. *Iranian Journal of Pharmaceutical Research, 20*(1), 216–253. https://doi.org/10.22037/ijpr.2021.114891.15088

Khoshvaght, H., Delnavaz, M., & Leili, M. (2021). Optimization of acetaminophen removal from high load synthetic pharmaceutical wastewater by experimental and ANOVA analysis. *Journal of Water Process Engineering, 42*, 102107. https://doi.org/10.1016/j.jwpe.2021.102107

Koncagül, E., Connor, R., & Abete, V. (2024). *Informe Mundial de las Naciones Unidas sobre el Desarrollo de los recursos hídricos 2024: agua para la prosperidad y la paz; datos, cifras y planes de acción (11).* UNESCO.

Kunhikrishnan, A., Bolan, N. S., Müller, K., Laurenson, S., Naidu, R., & Kim, W. I. (2012). The influence of wastewater irrigation on the transformation and bioavailability of heavy metal(loid)s in soil. *Advances in Agronomy, 115*, 215–297. https://doi.org/10.1016/B978-0-12-394276-0.00005-6

Kunz, N., Williams, H., Nyhan-Jones, V., & Hamilton, R. (2013). *Agua compartida, responsabilidad compartida, enfoque compartido: El agua en el Sector Minero.* International Finance Corporation.

Kuttiyathil, M. S., Mohamed, M. M., & Sulaiman, A.-Z. (2021). Using microalgae for remediation of crude petroleum oil–water emulsions. *Biotechnology Progress, 37*(2), e3098. https://doi.org/10.1002/btpr.3098

Li, H., Li, Y., Bao, M., & Li, S. (2021). Solid inoculants as a practice for bioaugmentation to enhance bioremediation of hydrocarbon contaminated areas. *Chemosphere, 263*, 128175. https://doi.org/10.1016/j.chemosphere.2020.128175

Liu, T., Wang, Y., Zeng, Y., Li, J., Yu, Q., Wang, X., Gao, D., Wang, F., & Cai, S. (2021). Effects from fe, p, ca, mg, zn and cu in steel slag on growth and metabolite accumulation of microalgae: A review. *Applied Sciences (Switzerland), 11*(14), 6589. https://doi.org/10.3390/app11146589

Mahlangu, D., Mphahlele, K., De Paola, F., & Mthombeni, N. H. (2024). Microalgae-mediated biosorption for effective heavy metals removal from wastewater: A review. *Water (Switzerland), 16*(5), 718. https://doi.org/10.3390/w16050718

Martínez-Frías, M. (2011). *Los metales en los efluentes líquidos industriales.* Thesis. Universidad de Zaragoza.

Martínez-Roldán, A. J. (2024). Introduction to environment-friendly bioprocesses by microalgae and cyanobacteria. In A. J. Martínez-Roldán (Ed.), *Biotechnological processes for green energy, and high value bioproducts by microalgae, and cyanobacteria cultures* (1–3). Springer Nature Switzerland AG. https://doi.org/10.1007/978-3-031-43969-8_1

Martínez-Roldán, A. J., Villanueva-García, R. P., Rodríguez-Rosales, M. D. J., Valle-Cervantes, S., & Perales-Vela, H. V. (2024). Wastewater treatment by microalgae and cyanobacteria. The reduction of the contaminant potential of real domestic wastewater: A case study. In A. J. Martínez-Roldan (Ed.), *Biotechnological processes for green energy, and high value bioproducts by microalgae, and cyanobacteria cultures* (31–42). Springer Nature Switzerland AG. https://doi.org/10.1007/978-3-031-43969-8

Masojídek, J., & Torzillo, G. (2008). Mass cultivation of freshwater microalgae. *Encyclopedia of Ecology*, 2226–2235. https://doi.org/10.1016/b978-0-12-409548-9.09373-8

Mathimani, T., Alshiekheid, M. A., Sabour, A., Le, T. H. T., & Xia, C. (2024). Appraising the phycoremediation potential of cyanobacterial strains *Phormidium* and *Oscillatoria* for nutrient removal from textile wastewater (TWW) and synchronized biodiesel production from TWW-tolerant biomass. *Environmental Research, 241*, 117628. https://doi.org/10.1016/j.envres.2023.117628

Milenković, L., Ra đenović, T., & Baljošević, A. (2021). The importance of wastewater treatment plants for sustainable development. *Economics of Sustainable Development, 5*(2). https://doi.org/10.5937/esd2102049m

Mokhtariazar, A., Hassani, A. H., Borghei, M., & Massoudinejad, M. (2024). A comparative study on performance of the conventional and fixed-bed membrane bioreactors for treatment of naproxen from pharmaceutical wastewater. *Scientific Reports, 14*(1), 9944. https://doi.org/10.1038/s41598-024-52872-0

Moussavi, A., Bonhivers, J. C., Filho, R. M., Mariano, A. P., & Stuart, P. R. (2022). Applications of Process Integration Methodologies in the pulp and paper industry. In J. J. Klemeš (Ed.), *Handbook of Process Integration (PI): Minimisation of energy and water use, waste and emissions* (2nd ed., pp.783–810). Elsevier Ltd. https://doi.org/10.1016/B978-0-12-823850-9.00032-3

Mujtaba, G., Rizwan, M., & Lee, K. (2017). Removal of nutrients and COD from wastewater using symbiotic co-culture of bacterium *Pseudomonas putida* and immobilized microalga *Chlorella vulgaris*. *Journal of Industrial and Engineering Chemistry, 49*, 145–151. https://doi.org/10.1016/j.jiec.2017.01.021

Muralikrishna, I. V., & Manickam, V. (2017). Industrial wastewater treatment technologies, recycling, and reuse. *Environmental management, 13*, 295–336.

Mustafa, G., Tariq Zahid, M., Ali, S., Zaghum-Abbas, S., & Rafatullah, M. (2021). Biodegradation and discoloration of disperse blue-284 textile dye by *Klebsiella pneumoniae* GM-04 bacterial isolate. *Journal of King Saud University - Science, 33*(4), 101442. https://doi.org/10.1016/j.jksus.2021.101442

Nemerow, N. L. (2006). Industrial waste treatment: contemporary practice and vision for the future. in industrial waste treatment: Contemporary practice and vision for the future. https://doi.org/10.1016/B978-0-12-372493-9.X5031-5

Obire, O., Aleruchi, O., & Wemedo, S. A. (2020). Fungi in biodegradation of polycyclic aromatic hydrocarbons in oilfield wastewater. *Acta Scientific Microbiology, 3*(4), 220–224. https://doi.org/10.31080/asmi.2020.03.0572

Olarte-Gómez, E. A., & Valencia-Giraldo, M. J. (2016). *Evaluación del uso de la microalga Chlorella vulgaris en el tratamiento de aguas residuales (Vinazas)*. (Research project) Universidad Abierta y a Distancia. Escuela de ciencias Agrarias, Pecuarias y del Medio Ambiente.

Ovis-Sánchez, J. O., Perera-Pérez, V. D., Buitrón, G., Quintela-Baluja, M., Graham, D. W., Morales-Espinosa, R., & Carrillo-Reyes, J. (2023). Exploring resistomes and microbiomes in pilot-scale microalgae-bacteria wastewater treatment systems for use in low-resource settings. *Science of The Total Environment, 882*, 163545. https://doi.org/10.1016/J.SCITOTENV.2023.163545

Padin-Gonzalez, C., & Diaz-Fernandez, M. (2009). Fermentacion alcoholica del lactosuero por *Kluyveromyces marxianus* y solventes organicos como extractantes. *Revista de la Sociedad Venezolana de Microbiologia, 29*(2), 110–116.

Peña Miranda, M., González Benito, G., San Cristobal, N., & Heras Nieto, C. (1996). Color elimination from molasses wastewater by *Aspergillus niger*. *Bioresource Technology, 57*(3), 229–235. https://doi.org/10.1016/S0960-8524(96)00048-X

Perdigão, R., Almeida, C. M. R., Magalhães, C., Ramos, S., Carolas, A. L., Ferreira, B. S., Carvalho, M. F., & Mucha, A. P. (2021). Bioremediation of petroleum hydrocarbons in seawater: Prospects of using lyophilized native hydrocarbon-degrading bacteria. *Microorganisms, 9*(11), 2285. https://doi.org/10.3390/microorganisms9112285

Pereira-Lima, J. P., Dias-Melo, E., & Aguiar, A. (2022). Characteristics and ways of treating cosmetic wastewater generated by Brazilian industries: A review. *Process Safety and Environmental Protection, 168*, 601–612. https://doi.org/10.1016/j.psep.2022.10.031

Petruccioli, M., Raviv, M., Di Silvestro, R., & Dinelli, G. (2019). Agriculture and agro-industrial wastes, by-products, and wastewaters: Origin, characteristics, and potential in bio-based compounds production. In M. Moo-Young (Ed.), *Comprehensive biotechnology* (3rd ed., pp. 477–490). Elsevier B.V. https://doi.org/10.1016/B978-0-444-64046-8.00375-X

Pham, V. H. T., Kim, J., Chang, S., & Chung, W. (2022). Bacterial biosorbents, an efficient heavy metals green clean-up strategy: Prospects, challenges, and opportunities. *Microorganisms, 10*(3), 610. https://doi.org/10.3390/microorganisms10030610

Premaratne, M., Nishshanka, G. K. S. H., Liyanaarachchi, V. C., Nimarshana, P. H. V., & Ariyadasa, T. U. (2021). Bioremediation of textile dye wastewater using microalgae: Current trends and future perspectives. *Journal of Chemical Technology and Biotechnology, 96*(12), 3249–3258. https://doi.org/10.1002/jctb.6845

Ramamurthy, K., Priya, P. S., Murugan, R., & Arockiaraj, J. (2024). Hues of risk: Investigating genotoxicity and environmental impacts of azo textile dyes. *Environmental Science and Pollution Research, 31*(23), 33190–33211. https://doi.org/10.1007/s11356-024-33444-1

Rani, N., Sangwan, P., Joshi, M., Sagar, A., & Bala, K. (2019). Microbes: A key player in industrial wastewater treatment. In M. P. Shah & S. Rodriguez-Couto (Eds.), *Microbial wastewater treatment* (1st ed., pp. 83–102). Elsevier. https://doi.org/10.1016/B978-0-12-816809-7.00005-1

Rashid, N., Abdelnabi, M. N. A., Vincent, A. S., & Mackey, H. R. (2023). Simultaneous treatment of fruit juice industry wastewater and single-cell protein synthesis using purple non-sulfur bacteria. *Biomass Conversion and Biorefinery, 13*, 16321–16332. https://doi.org/10.1007/s13399-022-03669-6

Reddy, N., Chen, L., Zhang, Y., & Yang, Y. (2014). Reducing environmental pollution of the textile industry using keratin as alternative sizing agent to poly (vinyl alcohol). *Journal of Cleaner Production, 65*, 561–567. https://doi.org/10.1016/j.jclepro.2013.09.046

Rivera-Utrilla, J., Sánchez-Polo, M., Ferro-García, M. A., Prados-Joya, G., & Ocampo-Pérez, R. (2013). Pharmaceuticals as emerging contaminants and their removal from water. A review. *Chemosphere, 93*(7), 1268–1287. https://doi.org/10.1016/j.chemosphere.2013.07.059

Rojo-Gómez, E. (2022). *Valorización de lactosuero para la obtención de biomasa de microalgas y cianobacterias.* Master thesis (Dissertation) Centro de Investigación y de Estudios Avanzados del Instituto Politécnico Nacional.

Romero-Frasca, E., Galea-Outón, S., Coronado-Apodaca, K. G., Milferstedt, K., Jimenez, J., Hamelin, J., & Buitrón, G. (2024). Bioaccessibility characterization of organic matter, nitrogen, and phosphorus from microalgae-bacteria aggregates. *Waste and Biomass Valorization, 15*(9), 5137–5150.

Roşca, M., Silva, B., Tavares, T., & Gavrilescu, M. (2023). Biosorption of hexavalent chromium by *Bacillus megaterium* and *Rhodotorula* sp. inactivated biomass. *Processes, 11*(1), 179. https://doi.org/10.3390/pr11010179

Ruiz-Reza, C. L., Rodríguez-Rosales, M. D. J., Martínez-Casillas, D. C., Hernández-Melchor, D. J., Peña-arellano, L. A., & Martínez-Roldan, A. J. (2024). Evaluation of mezcal distillery vinasse at various concentrations as a culturing medium for *Stigeoclonium nanum. Chemical Engineering Transactions, 110*, 469–474. https://doi.org/10.3303/CET24110079

Salamanca-Torres, A., Geissler, G., & Sánchez-Salas, J. L. (2009). Tratamiento de aguas provenientes de la industria papelera por medio de la combinación de un proceso fotooxidativo y un proceso microbiológico. *Revista Latinoamericana de Recursos Naturales, 5*(1), 50–57.

Salem, S. S., Mohamed, A. A., Gl-Gamal, M. S., Talat, M., & Fouda, A. (2019). Biological decolorization and degradation of azo dyes from textile wastewater effluent by *Aspergillus niger. Egyptian Journal of Chemistry, 62*(10), 1799–1813.

Santos, A., Barbosa-Póvoa, A., & Carvalho, A. (2019). Life cycle assessment in chemical industry – a review. *Current Opinion in Chemical Engineering, 26*, 139–147. https://doi.org/10.1016/j.coche.2019.09.009

Saranya, K., Sundaramanickam, A., Shekhar, S., Swaminathan, S., & Balasubramanian, T. (2017). Bioremediation of mercury by *Vibrio fluvialis* screened from industrial effluents. *BioMed Research International, 2017*(1), 6509648. https://doi.org/10.1155/2017/6509648

Shalini, & Pydi-Setty, Y. (2019). Multistage fluidized bed bioreactor for dye decolorization using immobilized polyurethane foam: A novel approach. *Biochemical Engineering Journal, 152*, 107368. https://doi.org/10.1016/j.bej.2019.107368

Shanab, S., Essa, A., & Shalaby, E. (2012). Bioremoval capacity of three heavy metals by some microalgae species (Egyptian isolates). *Plant Signaling and Behavior, 7*(3), 392–399. https://doi.org/10.4161/psb.19173

Sharma, D. K., & Sharma, S. (2014). Effects of caustic recovery on pollution and cost of production in a cotton textile industry. *Journal on Today's Ideas - Tomorrow's Technologies, 2*, 133–143.

Shenoy, A., Shukla, B. K., & Bansal, V. (2022). Sustainable design of textile industry effluent treatment plant with constructed wetland. *Materials Today: Proceedings, 51*, 537–542. https://doi.org/10.1016/j.matpr.2022.01.308

Silva-Bedoya, L. M., Sánchez-Pinzón, M. S., Cadavid-Restrepo, G. E., & Moreno-Herrera, C. X. (2016). Bacterial community analysis of an industrial wastewater treatment plant in Colombia with screening for lipid-degrading microorganisms. *Microbiological Research, 192*, 313–325. https://doi.org/10.1016/j.micres.2016.08.006

Singh, M. P., Vishwakarma, S. K., & Srivastava, A. K. (2013). Bioremediation of direct blue 14 and extracellular ligninolytic enzyme production by white rot fungi: *Pleurotus* spp. *BioMed Research International, 2013*(1). https://doi.org/10.1155/2013/180156

Soeprobowati, T. R., & Hariyati, R. (2012). The potential used of microalgae for heavy metals remediation. *Proceeding ISNPiNSA, 3*, 274–278.

Sosa-Martínez, J. D., Balagurusamy, N., Montañez, J., Peralta, R. A., Moreira, R. de F. P. M., Bracht, A., Marina Peralta, R., Morales-Oyervides, L. (2020). Synthetic dyes biodegradation by fungal ligninolytic enzymes: Process optimization, metabolites evaluation and toxicity assessment. *Journal of Hazardous Materials*, *400*, 123254. https://doi.org/10.1016/J.JHAZMAT.2020.123254

Sridang, P. C., Pottier, A., Wisniewski, C., & Grasmick, A. (2008). Performance and microbial surveying in submerged membrane bioreactor for seafood processing wastewater treatment. *Journal of Membrane Science, 317*, 43–49. https://doi.org/10.1016/j.memsci.2007.11.011

Stepanova, A. Y., Gladkov, E. A., Osipova, E. S., Gladkova, O. V., & Tereshonok, D. V. (2022). Bioremediation of soil from petroleum contamination. *Processes, 10*(6), 1224. https://doi.org/10.3390/pr10061224

Subudhi, E., & Kar, N. R. (1996). Decontamination of metals from metallurgical effluent utilizing *Rhizopus arrhizus* biomass. *International Journal of Environmental Studies, 50*(2), 111–116. https://doi.org/10.1080/00207239608711046

Thomas, O., & Thomas, M. F. (2022). Industrial wastewater. In O. Thomas & C. Burgess (Eds.), *UV-Visible spectrophotometry of waters and soils* (3rd ed., pp. 385–416). https://doi.org/10.1016/B978-0-323-90994-5.00013-7

Ume, L. O., Ekeoma, B. C., Yusuf, M., Al-Kahtani, A. A., Ubaidullah, M., & Sillanpää, M. (2022). Batch studies of hexavalent chromium biosorption from mining wastewater using *Aspergillus niger. Results in Chemistry, 4*, 100490. https://doi.org/10.1016/j.rechem.2022.100490

UNESCO. (2021). UN World Water Development Report 2021 | UN-Water. UN World Water Development Report 2021.

Uttamangkabovorn, M., Prasertsan, P., & Kittikun, A. H. (2005). Water conservation in canned tuna (pet food) plant in Thailand. *Journal of Cleaner Production, 13*, 547–555. https://doi.org/10.1016/j.jclepro.2003.12.003

Veiter, L., Rajamanickam, V., & Herwig, C. (2018). The filamentous fungal pellet—relationship between morphology and productivity. *Applied Microbiology and Biotechnology, 102*(7), 2997–3006. https://doi.org/10.1007/s00253-018-8818-7

Vela-García, N., Guamán-Burneo, M., & González-Romero, N. (2019). Efficient bioremediation from metallurgical effluents through the use of microalgae isolated from the amazonic and highlands of Ecuador. *Revista Internacional de Contaminacion Ambiental, 35*(4), 917–929. https://doi.org/10.20937/RICA.2019.35.04.11

Vieira-Costa, J. A., Cruz-González, C., & Centeno da Rosa, A. P. (2021). Insights into the technology utilized to cultivate microalgae in dairy effluents. *Biocatalysis and Agricultural Biotechnology*, *35*, 102106. https://doi.org/10.1016/j.bcab.2021.102106

Wang, J., Tian, Q., Zeng, W., Qiu, G., & Shen, L. (2023). Insights about fungus-microalgae symbiotic system in microalgae harvesting and wastewater treatment: A review. *Renewable and Sustainable Energy Reviews, 182*, 113408. https://doi.org/10.1016/j.rser.2023.113408

Wood, J. M., Fanchiang, Y. T., & Ridley, W. P. (1978). The biochemistry of toxic elements. *Quarterly Reviews of Biophysics, 11*(4), 467–479. https://doi.org/10.1017/S0033583500005643

WHO. (2023). World health statistics 2023: monitoring health for the sdgs, sustainable development goals. In *The Milbank Memorial Fund quarterly* (Vol. 27).

Wu, B., Xiu, J., Yu, L., Huang, L., Yi, L., & Ma, Y. (2023). Degradation of crude oil in a co-culture system of *Bacillus subtilis* and *Pseudomonas aeruginosa. Frontiers in Microbiology, 14*, 1132831. https://doi.org/10.3389/fmicb.2023.1132831

Yang, M., Li, J., Wang, S., Zhao, F., Zhang, C., Zhang, C., & Han, S. (2023). Status and trends of enzyme cocktails for efficient and ecological production in the pulp and paper industry. *Journal of Cleaner Production, 418*, 138196. https://doi.org/10.1016/j.jclepro.2023.138196

Zafar, S., Bukhari, D. A., & Rehman, A. (2022). Azo dyes degradation by microorganisms – An efficient and sustainable approach. *Saudi Journal of Biological Sciences, 29*(12), 103437. https://doi.org/10.1016/j.sjbs.2022.103437

Zhang, B., Matchinski, E. J., Chen, B., Ye, X., Jing, L., & Lee, K. (2019). Marine oil spills-oil pollution, sources and effects. In C. Sheppard (Ed.), *World seas: An environmental evaluation volume III: Ecological issues and environmental Impacts* (2nd ed., pp. 391–406). Elsevier Ltd. https://doi.org/10.1016/B978-0-12-805052-1.00024-3

Zhao, D., Cheah, W. Y., Lai, S. H., Ng, E. P., Khoo, K. S., Show, P. L., & Ling, T. C. (2023). Symbiosis of microalgae and bacteria consortium for heavy metal remediation in wastewater. *Journal of Environmental Chemical Engineering, 11*(3), 109943. https://doi.org/10.1016/j.jece.2023.109943

2 Bioremediation of emerging pollutants, options, and challenges

Morales-Romero Juan Manuel, Rodríguez-Oloño Brenda Michell, Reynoso-Cuevas Liliana, and Martínez-Roldán Alfredo de Jesús

2.1 INTRODUCTION

In recent years, technological development, the demand for goods, and population growth have led to the depletion of natural resources and the generation of waste containing polluting compounds with special physicochemical characteristics that make them persistent, toxic, and stable under environmental conditions. This has led to the accumulation of such compounds in different spheres of the environment. These pollutants are known as emerging pollutants (EPs) and have been the focus of recent attention to better understand their impact on the environment and on the health of the human population (Peña-Guzmán et al., 2019).

EPs are chemical substances of natural or synthetic origin, which can represent a risk because they tend to accumulate in the environment and are not monitored. In fact, these compounds are not recently created compounds; rather, studies on their effects and impacts are recent (Reynoso-Cuevas et al., 2020).

Different research groups have proposed the classification of these compounds according to their physicochemical characteristics, properties, and form of use to enable study and develop analytical methods that aid in their identification and, subsequently, their degradation or removal from the environment. Calvo-Flores et al. (2018) categorized EPs into eight groups: (1) pharmaceutical products (classified according to their function), (2) lifestyle products, (3) herbicides and pesticides, (4) personal care products, (5) illegal drugs, (6) surfactants, (7) industrial chemicals (e.g., flame retardants and solvents), and (8) others, including microplastics, metals, metalloids, toxins, radionuclides, and nanoparticles.

A major concern is the life cycle of EPs, which is associated mainly with the water cycle since many of these compounds are used on a daily basis and, as they are not regulated, are not monitored in water treatment systems, which is why they have become a global problem. Notably, conventional wastewater treatment processes are not designed to remove persistent pollutants such as EPs, so the effluents from treatment plants are a probable source of contamination of water bodies with these types of compounds (Lesser et al., 2018).

Various studies have been conducted on the presence of these compounds in the environment worldwide, and various sources have been identified, including agricultural (the use of pesticides and fertilizers), industrial activities (the spillage of chemical products), domestic (medicines and products of personal hygiene), and urban (wastewater from cities) activities.

The analysis and determination of EPs must be carried out with sensitive, selective, and highly precise methods; the currently used methods are gas chromatography (GC) or liquid chromatography (LC) in combination with mass spectrometry (MS). LC–MS offers an improvement over GC–MS, since derivation is not necessary, detection limits below 1 ng/L can be achieved, less sample preparation work is required, and the identification of multiple analytes is possible (Petrović et al., 2005).

DOI: 10.1201/9781003500483-2
This chapter has been made available under a (CC-BY-NC-ND) 4.0 license

Despite growing awareness of the risks associated with EPs, EP regulation is still under development. The European Union already has a monitoring base for more than 1036 compounds considered EPs (Vargas-Berrones et al., 2020). In the United States and Canada, several maximum permissible limits have been established. In Latin America, Brazil conducted the most research on these compounds, followed by Mexico (Peña-Guzmán et al., 2019).

Ahmad et al. (2022) proposed the use of microbial consortia for the removal of EPs, since some physicochemical processes transform the compounds into intermediates that can be more toxic than the parent compound; however, these processes require further study. On the other hand, Sandoval et al. (2024) proposed the use of advanced oxidation electrochemical methods for their removal. These processes combine electrochemical reactions with the generation of highly reactive oxidizing species, such as ozone or hydroxyl radicals, which have been shown to be effective in decomposing a wide range of organic pollutants and reducing their presence in wastewater.

Finally, addressing the occurrence of these compounds in the environment requires comprehensive strategies that include strengthening regulations, improving the monitoring infrastructure, and implementing sustainable waste management practices. Although progress has been made in research and in the implementation of some solutions, there is still a long way to go to ensure that the harmful effects of EPs do not negatively impact water, the environment, or the health of the population.

2.2 PHYSICOCHEMICAL PROCESSES

2.2.1 Adsorption

Activated carbon adsorption is a physicochemical process in which molecules of a substance (generally pollutants) adhere to the surface of an adsorbent material, such as activated carbon. This process is based on the interactions between the molecules of the adsorbed substance and the active sites of the adsorbent. Activated carbon has a porous structure, resulting in a large surface area, which is crucial for its adsorptive capacity. Its high specific surface area, which can reach up to 1500 m^2/g, allows it to capture a wide variety of pollutants, from organic compounds to gases and heavy metals (Bansal and Goyal, 2005).

The adsorption process occurs mainly by van der Waals forces and weak chemical bonds between the adsorbed molecules and the carbon surfaces. This phenomenon is reversible, which allows regeneration of the adsorbent material (Bansal and Goyal, 2005). Some adsorbents that have been studied for the removal of EPs, such as caffeine, ibuprofen, and paracetamol, are presented in Table 2.1.

Although the high adsorption capacity of activated carbon is widely recognized, activated carbon technology has several drawbacks:

- Active carbon is quite expensive; the higher the quality, the higher the cost.
- The different qualities of activated carbon are closely related to the raw material used and depend on the carbonization conditions and the type of activation (physical or chemical) used.

TABLE 2.1
Adsorption processes for the removal of emerging pollutants

Emerging pollutant	Adsorbent	Maximum adsorption	References
Caffeine	Hydrocarbon (HT-CO2) derived from biomass	45.60 mg/g	Dos Santos et al. (2024)
Diclofenac	Carbon xerogels	80.0 mg/g	Álvarez et al. (2015)
Paracetamol	Rice husk ashes	7.65 mg/g	Thakur et al. (2020)
Ibuprofen	Mil-101 (Fe) doped with Cu	497.3 mg/g	Xiong et al. (2021)
Ketoprofen	Wastewater treatment plant sludge	57 mg/g	Streit et al. (2021)

- Activated carbon is rapidly saturated and must be regenerated, which is expensive and difficult and results in the loss of adsorbent (Morin-Crini et al., 2022).

Therefore, finding new materials that can have the same performance as activated carbon without its disadvantages is an interesting goal.

In this context, other types of adsorbents, such as natural zeolites, which are hydrated aluminosilicate minerals with a porous structure that gives them valuable physicochemical properties for water treatment, have been studied (Wang et al., 2010). Zeolites have a high specific surface area due to their porosity, which allows them to adsorb different types of pollutants, including inorganic ions, organic compounds (such as dyes), and natural organic matter (such as humic acids).

These properties can be modified to improve their efficiency in water treatment (Wang et al., 2010). Modification methods include the following:

- Acid/Base Treatment: Acid treatment can remove pore-blocking impurities, convert zeolite to its H^+ form, and dealuminate the structure.
- Modification with surfactants: Cationic surfactants can be used to modify the surface of zeolites and increase their affinity for anions and organic compounds.

Cation exchange capacity (CEC), pore size, and specific surface area are the key physicochemical properties that make natural zeolites suitable for water treatment. These properties allow them to remove a wide range of contaminants, including ammonia, heavy metals, inorganic anions, and EPs. These adsorbents have been studied for the removal of EPs such as caffeine, ibuprofen, and paracetamol (Table 2.2).

2.2.2 Advanced oxidation processes

Advanced oxidation processes (AOPs) are a class of water treatment technologies that are based on the in situ generation of powerful oxidants, mainly hydroxyl radicals (OH), to degrade organic pollutants. These radicals are highly reactive transient species that can oxidize a wide range of pollutants, including those that are recalcitrant to conventional water treatment methods. AOPs are particularly effective in treating water contaminated with trace amounts of EPs such as pharmaceuticals, pesticides, and personal care products (Miklos et al., 2018). According to Bracamontes-Ruelas et al. (2022), AOPs can be classified according to the energy source (chemical, UV, or electrochemical) necessary to initiate the degradation of the pollutant (De Almeida et al., 2021).

2.2.3 Fenton reaction

The Fenton process uses hydrogen peroxide (H_2O_2) and ferrous (Fe^{2+}) salts to generate hydroxyl radicals at room temperature and atmospheric pressure in an aqueous solution with an acidic pH.

TABLE 2.2
Adsorption processes with zeolites for the elimination of emerging pollutants

Emerging pollutant	Adsorbent	Maximum adsorption	References
Caffeine	Clinoptilolite	0.181 mg/g	Ngeno et al. (2019)
Diclofenac	Zeolite modified with cationic surfactants	45 mg/g	Krajišnik et al. (2013)
Paracetamol	Natural Jordanian zeolite	26.6 mg/g	Mahran et al. (2019)
Ibuprofen	Zeolite hydrothermally modified in an acid medium, and impregnated with cetyltrimethylammonium bromide	14 mg/g	Ribeiro, et al. (2024)
Ketoprofen	Natural zeolites	35 mg/g	Smiljani et al. (2020)

TABLE 2.3
Advanced oxidation processes via the Fenton reaction for the removal of emerging pollutants

Emerging pollutant	Initial concentration	Removal	References
Caffeine	20 mg/L	4%	De Almeida et al. (2021)
Diclofenac	5 mg/L	65%	Bae et al. (2013)
Paracetamol	100 mg/L	100%	Velichkova et al. (2022)
Ibuprofen	10 mg/L	98%	Hussain et al. (2020)
Ketoprofen	1 mg/L	35%	Ulloa-Ovares et al. (2021)

Hydroxyl radicals are highly reactive and oxidize organic pollutants, including pharmaceuticals, breaking them down into less harmful substances (Kumar et al., 2019; Scaria et al., 2021). As shown in Table 2.3, this method has been used to degrade different EPs at various concentrations. Fenton reactions can be represented by the following equations:

$$Fe^{2+} + H_2O_2 \rightarrow Fe^{3+} + OH^- + \bullet OH \quad (1)$$

$$Fe^{3+} + H_2O_2 \rightarrow Fe^{2+} + HO_2\bullet + H^+ \quad (2)$$

$$Fe^{3+} + H_2O + hv \rightarrow Fe^{2+} + \bullet OH + H^+ \quad (3)$$

$$\bullet OH^- + H_2O_2 \rightarrow H_2O + HO_2\bullet \quad (4)$$

Some of the disadvantages of using the Fenton method are the need for an acidic pH, which may require a pH adjustment before and after treatment, increasing operating costs (Adityosulindro et al., 2018). The process generates iron sludge that requires further treatment. Although the Fenton method is effective in degrading many contaminants, toxic byproducts may be formed during the process, and the toxicity of these byproducts depends on the nature of the original contaminants and the operating conditions (Hussain et al., 2019).

Additionally, in heterogeneous Fenton processes, the adsorption of pollutants or degradation products on the catalyst surface can lead to deactivation, reducing the efficiency of the process and possibly requiring regeneration or replacement of the catalyst (Kumar et al., 2019). In terms of operating costs, as mentioned above, the Fenton method requires the continuous consumption of hydrogen peroxide, which can increase these costs.

2.2.4 Photo-Fenton process

The photo-Fenton process is an advanced oxidation technique used to treat wastewater and remove contaminants, including pharmaceuticals and other EPs. This technique is based on the Fenton reaction, which was first described by Henry John Horstman Fenton, but was not suggested for wastewater treatment until 1968 (Oller et al., 2021; Scaria et al., 2021).

The photo-Fenton process is based on the reaction between Fe^{2+} (as a catalyst) and H_2O_2 (as an oxidant), which generates Fe^{3+} and hydroxyl radicals (•OH). Hydroxyl radicals are highly reactive and can degrade a wide range of organic pollutants.

In this process, light accelerates the reactions, regenerating Fe^{2+} and producing more •OH. Light at a wavelength <580 nm is optimal, so this process can be powered by solar irradiation as a renewable energy source. The optimum pH of the reaction is 2.8, which prevents the precipitation of iron and ensures the maximum generation of active iron species ($FeOH^+$ and $Fe(OH)^{2+}$) (Lucas et al., 2015).

One of the main challenges of the photo-Fenton process is the need to operate at an acidic pH, which has limited its large-scale application. In recent years, photo-Fenton-type processes that operate at pH values close to neutral have been extensively investigated to overcome this disadvantage (Lucas et al., 2015).

The homogeneous photo-Fenton process, in which iron is dissolved in water, has several disadvantages, such as the need for an acidic pH and the generation of iron sludge. To overcome these disadvantages, different strategies have been studied, such as iron chelation, the substitution of iron for other metals, the immobilization of iron on solid surfaces (heterogeneous photo-Fenton), and the use of iron oxides (Wang et al., 2022).

The heterogeneous photo-Fenton process, in which iron is immobilized on a solid material, is considered a promising alternative to the homogeneous photo-Fenton process. This technique has advantages such as a wider operating pH range and the possibility of reusing the catalyst. However, the design of efficient heterogeneous catalysts remains a major challenge. Different materials have been explored as heterogeneous catalysts for the photo-Fenton process, such as iron oxides supported on graphitic or carbon materials, structural iron oxides on inert microporous materials, natural iron oxide semiconductors, magnetic particle mixtures, photo-Fenton ceramic membranes, and materials other than iron oxides (Wang et al., 2022). Table 2.4 shows how this method has been used for the removal of different EPs.

Despite its effectiveness in the degradation of pollutants, the photo-Fenton process has certain disadvantages that limit its applicability on a large scale. These disadvantages can be categorized as follows.

Operational limitations (Oller et al., 2021):

- Narrow pH range: The photo-Fenton process works best at an acidic pH of approximately 2.8. At neutral pH, iron precipitates, which dramatically decreases the efficiency of the process. This limitation requires an adjustment of the wastewater pH before treatment, which implies an additional step and the use of reagents. In addition, after treatment, the pH of the water must be neutralized for discharge or reuse.
- Sludge generation: The photo-Fenton process produces iron sludge as a byproduct, which represents a secondary contamination problem. This sludge must be managed properly, which entails additional costs.

Economic limitations (Lucas et al., 2015):

- Reagent cost: In the photo-Fenton process, hydrogen peroxide (H_2O_2) and iron salts are used as reagents. The cost of these reagents can be significant, especially for the treatment of large volumes of wastewater.

TABLE 2.4
Advanced oxidation processes using the photo-Fenton process for the removal of emerging pollutants

Emerging pollutant	Initial concentration	Removal	References
Caffeine	20 mg/L	51%	De Almeida et al. (2021)
Diclofenac	100 mg/L	100%	Gar et al. (2015)
Paracetamol	20 mg/L	85%	Roshanfekr et al. (2014)
Ibuprofen	178 mg/L	80%	Mendez-Arriaga et al. (2010)
Ketoprofen	101 mg/L	100%	Feng et al. (2014)

- Energy cost: The photo-Fenton process requires a light source, which can be sunlight or artificial light. The use of artificial light implies an additional energy cost.
- Reactor design and operating costs: Designing efficient reactors for the photo-Fenton process presents challenges and can be costly. In addition, the operation of the reactor requires precise control of the process parameters, which can increase operating costs.

Limitations on efficiency (Méndez-Arriaga et al., 2010):

- Low use of light energy: Despite being a photoassisted process, the homogeneous photo-Fenton process does not use light energy efficiently, due to the low absorption of light by the iron complexes in solution.
- Effect of the wastewater matrix: The efficiency of the photo-Fenton process can be affected by the presence of other compounds in the wastewater matrix, such as natural organic matter, carbonates, and phosphates. These compounds can act as hydroxyl radical scavengers, reducing the efficiency of the process.

2.2.5 Electro-Fenton process

The electro-Fenton (EF) process is an advanced, powerful oxidation electrochemical process for wastewater treatment. The EF process is based on the electrochemical generation of hydrogen peroxide (H_2O_2) at the cathode surface by reducing dissolved oxygen under acidic conditions. This reaction is accelerated by the cathodic reduction of ferric ions, regenerating the ferrous ions necessary for the Fenton reaction. The EF process has the ability to fully mineralize recalcitrant organic contaminants and improve the biodegradability of the solution (Nidheesh et al., 2022).

The EF process offers a number of significant advantages over other wastewater treatment methods, especially compared with the classical Fenton process, which minimizes reagent costs. The EF process generates the Fenton reagent in situ, which is composed of hydrogen peroxide (H_2O_2) and ferrous ions (Fe^{2+}). H_2O_2 is produced by reducing dissolved oxygen at the cathode, whereas Fe^{2+} is regenerated from the ferric ions (Fe^{3+}) formed in the Fenton reaction. This prevents the need to add large amounts of H_2O_2 and Fe^{2+} externally, which considerably reduces costs (Monteil et al., 2018).

Another advantage is the elimination and prevention of reactions that waste hydroxyl radicals (OH). In the EF process, the concentrations of H_2O_2 and Fe^{2+} remain low, since they are consumed as soon as they are formed. This minimizes reactions that waste •OH, such as reactions with H_2O_2 itself or with Fe^{2+} (Monteil et al., 2018).

The classic Fenton process can generate ferric hydroxide sludge, which requires additional treatment. In the EF process, the electrochemical regeneration of Fe^{2+} prevents the formation of such sludge, which simplifies the process and reduces treatment costs. Additionally, the electrochemical regeneration of Fe^{2+} in the EF process ensures a continuous supply of the catalyst for the Fenton reaction. This, together with the in situ generation of OH, enables high rates of removal of organic pollutants to be achieved (Monteil et al., 2018). In the context of the high removal rates of pollutants, Table 2.5 shows how they act in the presence of different EPs.

While the EF process is a promising technique for wastewater treatment, it has several drawbacks:

- Relatively high cost due to energy consumption, especially when complete mineralization of the treated solutions is needed. To achieve full mineralization of pollutants, the EF process may need to run for long periods of time, increasing energy consumption and consequently costs (Nidheesh et al., 2022).
- The need to operate at a low pH (approximately 3). This low pH is optimal for the Fenton reaction but may require pH adjustment before and after treatment, increasing the complexity and cost of the process (Gadi et al., 2022).

TABLE 2.5
Advanced oxidation processes from the electro-Fenton process for the removal of emerging pollutants

Emerging pollutant	Initial concentration	Removal	References
Caffeine	194 mg/L	100%	Gadi et al. (2022)
Diclofenac	5 a 50 mg/L	97.21%	Davarnejad et al. (2021)
Paracetamol	5.75 mg/L	99.5%	Ahmadzadeh et al. (2018)
Ibuprofen	400 ppm	98.29%	Davarnejad et al. (2017)
Ketoprofen	101 mg/L	100%	Feng et al. (2014)

TABLE 2.6
Flocculation coagulation processes for the removal of emerging pollutants

Emerging pollutant	Initial concentration	Removal	References
Caffeine	2–12 mg/L	85%	Ghecham et al. (2018)
Diclofenac	0.5 and 46.5 μg/L	46%	Suarez et al. (2009)
Ibuprofen	90 ng/L	71.3%	Azzouz and Ballesteros (2013)
Acetaminophen	140–232 ng/L	12%	Boleda et al. (2011)
Bisphenol A	1 μg/L	4–7%	Choi et al. (2006).

- Ferrous sludge generation. The low solubility of Fe(III) in aqueous solution can cause the precipitation of ferric sludge, which must be managed and disposed of properly (Méndez-Arriaga, et al., 2010).

These disadvantages have led to the investigation of modifications and hybrid processes to improve the efficiency and profitability of the EF process.

The selection of the most appropriate AOP depends on several factors, including water quality, the type and concentration of the contaminants, treatment requirements, operating costs, and the potential for byproduct formation. It is important to conduct treatability studies to evaluate the efficacy of different AOPs for specific applications.

2.2.6 Flocculation and coagulation

Flocculation and coagulation are processes widely used in water treatment and have been shown to be effective in eliminating EPs, especially those of higher molecular weights. In this process, coagulating agents, such as aluminum or iron salts, are added, which neutralize the electrical charges of the suspended particles, allowing them to agglomerate and settle. The list of various EP treated with flocculation and coagulation is listed in Table 2.6. According to Mahmood et al. (2022), this method has shown good results for the removal of residues from pharmaceutical products, although it generally needs to be combined with other processes, such as filtration, to maximize its effectiveness.

2.3 ELIMINATION OF EMERGING POLLUTANTS VIA BIOTECHNOLOGICAL PROCESSES

Various investigations have reported that aquatic organisms, such as fish, can be affected by the presence of these compounds. The removal of these pollutants has become a complex issue to address and manage because of their low concentration in aquatic environments, their chemical stability, and their ability to withstand conventional treatments. Therefore, biological processes are promising solutions, particularly the use of bacteria, fungi, cyanobacteria, and microalgae, which can offer a sustainable and economical alternative to traditional methods (Ayilara and Babalola, 2023).

2.3.1 Biotechnological processes using bacteria

Benson (1998) describes bacteria as single-celled organisms that have different shapes, sizes, and structures. Bacteria are characterized by morphological diversity, most commonly spheres, rods, and spirals. Spherical bacteria are usually 0.2–2 μm in size, whereas elongated bacteria are 0.2–2 μm wide and 2–10 μm long (Levin and Angert, 2015; Ryan, 2018; Zhou and Li, 2015). They can also be found in groupings of four, in chains, in clusters, and in pairs. Despite their complexity, bacteria lack internal structures and cytoskeletons and consist of up to 70% water. The basic bacterial structures are the cell wall and membrane, the cytoplasm, and genetic material (Hobot, 2015). Like other microorganisms, bacteria are scattered throughout the planet, and their presence constantly affects the ecosystem that surrounds them. The effects that these organisms have on their environment can be beneficial or harmful. One of these effects with the most positive impact on the environment is the use and biotransformation of primary compounds such as nitrogen, oxygen, and carbon, which in turn serve as sources of nutrients (Gupta et al., 2017). Over the years, the metabolic capacity of bacteria has been studied and used as an alternative to conventional treatment systems for the removal of EPs.

Bioremediation by bacteria presents an ecological alternative for the treatment of effluents and contaminated solids. These microorganisms are among the most important microbial systems for bioremediation (Vaishnav and Demain, 2009). Bacteria use various types of mechanisms for the degradation of pollutants, such as biosorption and bioaccumulation, but biotransformation and biomineralization are also noteworthy (Patil et al., 2024). The bacteria most commonly used in this process are aerobic bacteria such as *Alcaligenes*, *Pseudomonas*, *Rhodococcus*, *Sphingomonas*, and *Mycobacterium*.

Biomineralization is a process in which bacteria stimulate the formation of minerals through the precipitation of organic and inorganic compounds (Castro-Alonso et al., 2019). This mechanism facilitates the degradation and stabilization of pollutants since bacteria can metabolize them, generating byproducts such as carbon dioxide and other chemical compounds (Meng et al., 2014). Biomineralization allows the precipitation of minerals into stable compounds such as carbonates, phosphates, or sulfides, favoring their safe disposal in the environment (Hoffmann et al., 2021).

Bioadsorption is a process in which bacteria capture and retain pollutants on the cell wall through chemical interactions (Beveridge and Murray, 1976). In this process, the pollutant is not metabolized but rather adheres to the cell surface, allowing the bacteria to act as biological filters. The functional groups, including carboxyl, hydroxyl, and amine groups, in the cell walls of these microorganisms are responsible for the link between the contaminants and the bacterial cell (McLean et al., 1992; Van Der Wal et al., 1997; Vijayaraghavan and Yun, 2008). Bioabsorption, on the other hand, is an active and natural metabolic process by which contaminants accumulate and are absorbed by living bacterial cells with the help of their own intracellular proteins (Mishra and Malik, 2013). This process requires energy, which is provided through the cellular metabolic cycle and is carried out in two stages: the pollutants are first adsorbed on the surface of the cells and then transported to the cell interior, where they can be captured by proteins. This process uses the lipid bilayer of the bacteria as a transport system and peptide ligands for the storage of compounds such as heavy metals (Pham et al., 2022). Both processes are key to bioremediation, as they help reduce the mobility and toxicity of pollutants in the environment.

Bacterial enzymatic processes are a fundamental mechanism for the remediation of contaminated systems (Xu et al., 2021). Bacteria can produce a wide variety of enzymes that help catalyze the degradation of organic and inorganic compounds present in the soil, water, and sediment, allowing the transformation of toxic pollutants into less harmful or harmless products (Karigar and Rao, 2011; Scott et al., 2008). Among the pollutants that can be degraded by bacterial enzymes are hydrocarbons and heavy metals, which are converted into less toxic substances through oxidation and reduction reactions, among other biochemical processes (Husain, 2006; Verma and Kuila, 2019). Bacteria react to the presence of certain compounds and activate specific enzymatic pathways that facilitate the transformation of the contaminants with which they come into contact (Mousavi et al., 2021). Enzymes such as oxygenases and hydrolases have shown efficacy in the degradation of hydrocarbons and pesticides, respectively, which are examples of biotechnology applied to environmental bioremediation (Baffi et al., 2024; Gianfreda and Rao, 2004). Some examples of biotechnological processes based on bacteria are listed in Table 2.7.

TABLE 2.7
Bacteria-based processes for the removal of emerging pollutants

	Emerging pollutants	Bacteria	Metabolic pathway	Referencess
Insecticides, herbicides, and pesticides	Imidacloprid	*Bacillus alkalinitrilicus*	Via 6-chloronictinic acid nitrosamine.	Sharma et al. (2014)
	Fipronil	*Bacillus firmus*	Via fipronil sulfide, fipronil sulfone, and fipronil amide.	Mandal et al. (2013)
	Malathion	*Bacillus cereus PU*	Via malathion monocarboxylic and dicarboxylic acid.	Singh et al. (2012)
	Metribuzin	*Bacillus* sp. *N1*	Used as a source of nitrogen.	Zhang et al. (2014)
	Organophosphates	*Bacillus pumilus W1*	Hydrolysis of organophosphates by the enzyme encoded by opdA	Ali et al. (2012)
Polyaromatic hydrocarbons	Naphthalene	*Bacillus fusiformis*	Dioxygenase activity	Lin et al. (2010)
	Pyrene	*Bacillus subtilis DM-04*	Enzymatic pathway	Das and Mukherjee (2007)
	Phenanthrene	*Bacillus subtilis 3KP*	Dioxygenase activity	Ni'Matuzahroh et al. (2017)
Pharmaceuticals	Naproxen	*Bacillus thuringiensis B1*	Via catechol 1,2-dioxygenase	Górny et al. (2019)
	Ibuprofen	*Bacillus thuringiensis B1*	Via enzymatic, dioxygenase	Marchlewicz et al. (2017)
	Acetaminophen	*Bacillus drentensis S1*	Via 4-aminophenol to hydroquinone	Chopra and Kumar (2020)

2.3.2 Biotechnological processes using fungi

Fungi are eukaryotic organisms that lack chlorophyll and vascular filaments; they generally spread through spores that can be produced asexually or sexually, depending on the species (Hawksworth and Wiltshire, 2011). They have the ability to decompose and absorb organic matter from various sources, both living and dead (Walker and McGinnis, 2014). They are also noteworthy for their potential to recycle carbon, nitrogen, dry plant nutrients, and essential minerals (Volk, 2013). A limited number of fungal species can use pectin, cellulose, and hemicelluloses as carbon sources. The enzymes that allow fungi to degrade different types of compounds are amylases, lipases, and proteases via the use of certain types of substrates, such as starches, fats, and proteins. Some fungi are capable of degrading complex polymers such as keratin, chitin, and lignin, which are resistant to microbial processes (Vijaya Kumar, 2017). The secretion of extracellular enzymes allows these organisms to transform pollutants such as hydrocarbons, pesticides, and heavy metals into less toxic substances that are easily assimilated by the ecosystem in which they develop (Zhao et al., 2021). The enzymes produced by some fungi are often used as biotechnological tools in the bioremediation of EPs; mycoremediation can be applied to compounds from pesticides, industrial products, pharmaceuticals, and personal care products (Amobonye et al., 2023; Arun et al., 2023; Vaksmaa et al., 2023). Examples of fungi-based processes are listed in Table 2.8.

The accumulation of pharmaceutical products, such as antibiotics, analgesics, anti-inflammatory agents, and hormones, in wastewater treatment plants is due to the low efficiency of elimination in conventional systems. This allows toxic compounds to be released into the environment, leading to risks for both aquatic ecosystems, including endocrine alterations in some organisms, and human health. In addition, it facilitates the development of bacteria resistant to antibiotics. In this context, some studies have focused on seeking alternatives for the removal and decomposition of these compounds. Gould (2009) reported that basidiomycete white-rot fungi, which can decompose

TABLE 2.8
Fungi-based processes for the removal of emerging pollutants

	Emerging pollutant	Fungus	Metabolic pathway	References
Pharmaceuticals	Diclofenac	*Trametes versicolor*	Cytochrome P450 inhibitor 1-aminobenzotriazole and purified laccase	Marco-Urrea et al. (2010)
	Ibuprofen, ketoprofen, and naproxen	*Trametes versicolor*	Oxidative enzyme system	Torán et al. (2017)
	13 pharmaceutical compounds	*Trametes versicolor* *Ganoderma lucidum*	Redox cycling mechanism	Vasiliadou et al. (2019)
	Acetaminophen, bisphenol A, carbamazepine, and sulfamethoxazole	*Bjerkandera adusta*	Enzymes	Kang et al. (2021)
Pesticides	Chlorpyrifos, dicofol, and cypermethrin	*Trametes versicolor*	Laccase activity	Hu et al. (2020)
	Atrazine	*Bjerkandera adusta*	Lignin peroxidase and laccase enzyme activity	Dhiman et al. (2020)
	16 organochlorine pesticides	*Phanerochaete chrysosporium*	Hydrogen peroxidase activity	Wang et al. (2014)
	Chlorpyrifos, methyl parathion, and profenofos	*Aspergillus sydowii CBMAI 935*	Cytochrome P450, methylation reaction, enzymatic activity	Soares et al. (2021)

wood, can also decompose pharmaceutical products such as azithromycin, erythromycin, simvastatin, sulfamethoxazole, and valsartan (Kózka et al., 2023). Eibes et al. (2011) reported 100 and 80% removal of diclofenac and naproxen, respectively, through enzymatic oxidation using lignin peroxidase, which facilitated their rapid degradation by breaking bonds in the presence of water.

On the other hand, personal care products, such as sunscreen, perfumes, and some preservatives, are pollutants that persist in the environment and pose risks to human health and different ecosystems. These compounds, including triclosan and various parabens, have been shown to have toxic effects and endocrine disruption activity in aquatic organisms (Benlaassri et al., 2023; Maadani Mallak et al., 2020). In particular, bioremediation with ligninolytic fungi, such as *Trametes versicolor* and *Pleurotus ostreatus*, has been shown to be effective in degrading and reducing the toxicity of personal care products (Kang et al., 2021; Murugesan et al., 2010). Caffeine is considered an EP because it is one of the most consumed stimulant substances globally. This alkaloid is known mainly for being a component present in soft drinks, energy drinks, and foods, among other products (Glade, 2010; Graham, 2009). It is also common to find it in anti-cellulite, facial, and hair creams because of its stimulating and antioxidant properties, which can improve the appearance of the skin and hair (Carvalho Neto et al., 2021). However, the excessive use of these products has increased the presence of caffeine in the environment, and it is now considered an EP because of its ability to be potentially active in aquatic systems (Vieira et al., 2022). Hakil et al. (1998) used filamentous fungi to reduce the levels of caffeine in coffee pulp by solid-state fermentation, with dimethylxanthine used as a source of nitrogen; 67.2% caffeine removal using *Aspergillus tamarii* and 58.8% using *Penicillium commune* were achieved in 48 h.

Salicylic acid belongs to a group of molecules called salicylates, which are phenolic compounds that are naturally synthesized by plants and have an aromatic ring and a hydroxyl group (Maruri-López et al., 2019). In addition to being used as an ingredient in aspirin, which is used to reduce fever, pain, and inflammation and to treat cardiovascular symptoms such as heart attack and stroke in humans (Barry et al., 2020; Sirois et al., 2012), salicylic acid is also widely used in the cosmetic industry for its exfoliating, antiseptic, antiaging, and general skin care properties (Merinville et al., 2009; White, 2020). Although salicylic acid has been used in many agricultural processes, including seed germination, floral and root stimulation, and the response to abiotic and biotic stress, as a salicylate compound, it has a negative impact on marine ecosystems as an EP (Klessig et al., 2016; Zhao et al., 2024). *Fusarium graminearum* is an ascomycete fungus with the ability to damage cereal crops (Yang et al., 2013), including wheat, barley, rice, and oats, and causes ear and stalk rot in corn due to the segregation of mycotoxins in the body (Geng et al., 2014; Kant et al., 2017). However, a study by Rocheleau et al. (2019) revealed that this fungus has the ability to use salicylic acid as a carbon source to grow and possesses enzymes such as monooxygenase, dioxygenase, and decarboxylase for the degradation of salicylic acid in liquid media.

Endocrine-disrupting compounds are chemical compounds, both natural and synthetic, that have the ability to mimic, block, or interfere with the hormonal activity of the endocrine system (Dickerson and Gore, 2007). These compounds can alter hormonal synthesis and the normal physiological functions of the male and female reproductive organs, mainly by binding to the receptors for hormones such as estrogen, progesterone, and androgen (Gupta et al., 2010; Pan et al., 2024). As a result, they can induce reproductive abnormalities, stimulate the growth of certain types of cancer, and contribute to dysfunction of the nervous and immune systems (Hwang and Choi, 2015). These substances, which are present in the environment, are associated with a wide range of health problems in humans and wildlife (Gore et al., 2015). In aquatic environments, toxic effects have been reported in mammals, birds, reptiles, fish, and mollusks in regions such as Europe and North America (Vos et al., 2000). The changes observed vary, including permanent alterations such as mutations in sexual organs, feminization or masculinization, alterations in sexual behavior, and dysfunction of the immune and reproductive systems.

Chaetomium brasiliense, a thermophilic fungus, was shown to have a high degradation capacity for endocrine-disrupting compounds such as 17α-ethinylestradiol and 4-tert-butylphenol. Under optimal conditions at 50°C, the laccase enzyme degraded up to 60% of the 4-tert-butylphenol present in 2 h. Redox mediators such as TEMPO and syringaldehyde were also tested, and removal rates of close to 90% were achieved (Daâssi and Alharbi, 2023). On the other hand, *Pleurotus ostreatus*, an edible white-rot fungus, achieved 90% elimination of contaminants such as bisphenol A, estrone, 17β-estradiol, and triclosan in 12 days in laboratory experiments. Those experiments were validated in pilot-scale bioreactors in wastewater treatment plants, and up to 76% elimination of the endocrine compounds present in the medium was achieved, even in the presence of bacterial microflora (Křesinová et al., 2018). Likewise, *Irpex lacteus* was noteworthy in the degradation of bisphenol A, with 99.4% removal in just 3 h and 100% removal in 12 h. This process was carried out mainly by the enzymatic activities of laccase and manganese peroxidase, indicating that biodegradation was the predominant mechanism in this process (Shin et al., 2007). Finally, experiments carried out with the basidiomycete fungus *Phlebia tremellosa* have made it possible to reduce the estrogenic activity of endocrine compounds through the purification of laccase (Kim et al., 2008).

2.3.3 Biotechnological processes using cyanobacteria

Cyanobacteria are photosensitive prokaryotic organisms that can produce oxygen from CO_2 and perform oxygenic photosynthesis through photosystems I and II (Yannarell and Kent, 2009). Commonly known as blue–green algae, cyanobacteria belong to a group of gram-negative autotrophic bacteria with capacities and adaptation mechanisms that include nitrogen and carbon fixation, allowing them to grow in various environments (Stal, 2007). These microorganisms occupy terrestrial and aquatic habitats, including seas, rivers, and lakes, and can also grow in extreme environments such as hot springs, deserts, rocks, and frozen areas (Jansson and Northen, 2010). Morphologically, cyanobacteria present a wide variety of cell forms, ranging from rods, spirals, and single-cell spheres to multicellular colonies and filaments. The cells of these microorganisms lack membranous organelles but have thylakoids distributed throughout the cytoplasm, where photosynthesis takes place (Mareš et al., 2019). Thylakoids are associated with photosynthetic pigments such as chlorophyll a and phycobilins, which are responsible for the characteristic colors of cyanobacteria (Collins et al., 2012).

The metabolism of cyanobacteria enables the use of at least four mechanisms for the removal of EPs: adsorption, enzymatic biodegradation, intracellular accumulation, and chemical transformation. Adsorption is one of the simplest but most effective mechanisms by which cyanobacteria can remove EPs from the environment (Bilal et al., 2018). This process is carried out through physicochemical interactions between pollutants and components of the cyanobacterial cell surface (Dutta et al., 2022). Many species release exopolysaccharides, which are substances relevant for adsorption because their composition is rich in functional groups such as carboxyls, hydroxyls, and amines (De Philippis et al., 2011). These groups allow the formation of active sites that facilitate the binding of contaminants, particularly heavy metals, pesticides, drugs, and other compounds (Shabana et al., 2019).

The adsorption capacity varies according to the physicochemical properties of each pollutant. Heavy metals interact electrostatically with negatively charged functional groups on the cyanobacterial surface (Diaz-Uribe et al., 2021; Mota et al., 2016). Likewise, species such as *Anabaena flos-aquae* and *Aphanocapsa elachista* have been shown to have a high capacity to adsorb dyes and other organic pollutants (El-Sheekh et al., 2018; Touliabah et al., 2022). The pH of the system significantly influences the efficiency of adsorption since it affects both the ionization of functional groups and the solubility of contaminants. Additionally, cyanobacteria can adjust exopolysaccharide production in response to stressful environmental conditions, increasing their ability to capture EPs (Singh et al., 2019). Although adsorption does not destroy pollutants, it serves as an essential initial stage that concentrates and reduces their mobility, facilitating their subsequent elimination.

Intracellular bioaccumulation in cyanobacteria is a crucial mechanism that allows cyanobacteria to mitigate the toxicity of heavy metals and other persistent pollutants by capturing and storing them intracellularly (Pogrzeba and Poliwoda, 2024; Rakic et al., 2023). This process not only protects cyanobacteria from the adverse effects of these compounds but also contributes to their effective removal from the environment. Cyanobacteria can internalize contaminants and confine them to specialized organelles or protected cytoplasmic areas. For example, *Spirulina platensis* is known for its ability to accumulate metals such as arsenic, chromium, and cadmium (Al-Homaidan et al., 2015). This mechanism also includes intracellular detoxification processes, such as the chelation of metals by specific proteins or the formation of insoluble compounds that minimize cell damage (Cassier-Chauvat and Chauvat, 2014).

Another mechanism by which cyanobacteria remove pollutants is chemical transformation via photosynthesis (Cheng et al., 2023). This process uses reactive oxygen species (ROS) generated during the photolysis of water during photosynthesis to oxidize and breakdown pollutants into less toxic compounds (Latifi et al., 2009). ROS, such as hydrogen peroxide and hydroxyl radicals, are highly reactive and can attack the complex chemical bonds present in pesticides, phenols, and synthetic dyes (Parikh and Madamwar, 2005; Sachu et al., 2023; Tiwari et al., 2017). This mechanism depends on factors such as the light intensity and the photosynthetic efficiency of the cyanobacteria. In environments with high light availability, ROS are produced in greater quantities, increasing the rate of transformation of pollutants. For example, *Synechococcus elongatus* can oxidize triazine organophosphate pesticides such as atrazine and terbutryn, reducing their toxicity and environmental impact (González-Barreiro et al., 2006; Singh et al., 2011). Furthermore, this process is particularly beneficial in bioremediation applications in open systems, such as oxidation ponds, where natural conditions favor photosynthesis. However, controlling ROS production is crucial, as excessive concentrations can harm cyanobacteria and limit their effectiveness (He and Häder, 2002).

Enzymatic biodegradation is a process in which cyanobacteria transform various types of pollutants into less toxic compounds via metabolic enzymes (Tamagnini et al., 2002). These enzymes act as catalysts that break the complex chemical bonds present in pollutants, allowing their partial or complete mineralization. This process depends on the metabolism of cyanobacteria, which allows them to attack organic pollutants, such as drugs, pesticides, and endocrine disruptors (Chen et al., 2020). Among the most prominent enzymes are peroxidases, monooxygenases, hydrolases, and ligases (Sharma et al., 2024). For example, peroxidases are essential for degrading the aromatic structures present in dyes and pesticides, whereas monooxygenases catalyze oxidation reactions that modify recalcitrant compounds such as polycyclic aromatic hydrocarbons (Rios-Miguel et al., 2022).

Ferreira et al. (2023) reported that *Synechocystis sp.* can biodegrade diclofenac, ibuprofen, and paracetamol, which are commonly used nonsteroidal anti-inflammatory drugs, in aquatic environments through the enzymatic processes of hydroxylation and oxidation. Enzymatic biodegradation not only transforms pollutants but also integrates them into metabolic pathways to generate compounds useful for cyanobacteria as carbon or energy sources (Hamouda et al., 2016). This approach is notable for its specificity and sustainability, since cyanobacteria can be adapted to synthesize enzymes specific to new contaminants through natural selection or genetic engineering, thus expanding its usefulness in bioremediation. Some examples of microalgae-based processes for the elimination of EP are listed in Table 2.9.

2.3.4 Biotechnological processes from microalgae

Microalgae are unicellular organisms that can take advantage of sunlight as an energy source and CO_2 as a carbon source to carry out photosynthesis (Barsanti and Gaultieri, 2006). Over the years, microalgae have attracted interest for their practicality as biotechnological tools, from the production of food supplements to the generation of energy sources (Guldhe et al., 2016; Louw et al., 2016). Owing to the adaptability of these organisms and their potential to generate high-added-value products, such as antioxidants, polyunsaturated fatty acids, and immunostimulating polysaccharides, microalgae are environmentally friendly alternatives from an industrial perspective (Barsanti and Gualtieri, 2018; Borowitzka, 2013; Martínez-Roldán and Lozano-Gómez, 2022; Rahman, 2020). These microorganisms are part of the primary production chain in aquatic systems and help reduce

TABLE 2.9
Cyanobacteria-based processes for the removal of emerging pollutants

Emerging pollutant	Cyanobacteria	Metabolic pathway	References
Organochlorine pesticide	*Anabaena* sp.	Nitrogenase activity	Chaurasia et al. (2013)
Malachite green dye	*Synechococcus elongatus*	Enzymatic activity: Triphenylmethane reductase	Han et al. (2020)
Metronidazole, rosuvastatin, and codeine phosphate	*Synechocystis sp*	Extracellular and intracellular enzymatic mechanism	Bahman et al. (2022)
Diclofenac, ibuprofen, and paracetamol	*Anabaena* sp. and *Chroococcidiopsis thermalis*	Biosorption	Pogrzeba and Poliwoda (2024)
Aromatic compounds	*Synechocystis* sp., *Anabaena fertilissima*, and *Nostoc muscorum*	Antioxidant enzymatic activity: Biosynthesis	Patel et al. (2015)

greenhouse gas emissions, capturing CO_2 from the atmosphere and transforming it into organic compounds that are easily assimilated by ecosystems (Chapman, 2013). In wastewater treatment processes, microalgae mainly take advantage of nitrogen and phosphorus as sources of nutrients for their growth and development, releasing oxygen into the system; the generated oxygen is then used by the bacteria in the effluent responsible for the oxidation of organic matter, resulting in an algae–bacteria symbiosis (Saravanan et al., 2021). Likewise, these organisms present an opportunity to reduce the presence of EPs in the environment (Martínez-Roldán and Cañizares-Villanueva, 2020).

Among the main mechanisms of microalgae for the bioremediation of EPs are bioadsorption, bioaccumulation, and biodegradation.

The bioadsorption process occurs when pollutants are attached to the components of the cell wall of the microalgae or to the organic substances that they produce. Among secreted substances, the amino, carboxyl, hydroxyl, and phosphate functional groups are most prominent and are found mainly in lipids and polysaccharides. These functional groups allow contaminants to bind to microalgae through physical or chemical processes, such as the formation of ionic or covalent bonds, hydrogen bonds, hydrophobic interactions, or van der Waals forces (Abdelfattah et al., 2023; Ramesh et al., 2023). Some of the functions of exopolysaccharides include the protection of microalgal cells against biotic and abiotic stresses, dehydration, or toxic substances (Morais et al., 2022). The removal rates of pharmaceutical products such as diclofenac, ibuprofen, paracetamol, and carbamazepine, among others, using microalgae such as *Chlorella sorokiniana* are close to 20% according to de Wilt et al. (2016), whereas the removal rates of nitrogen and phosphorus are close to 100%. Some of the EPs treated with microalgae are summarized in Table 2.10. Some antibiotics, such as tetracycline, which is used to treat respiratory and urinary infections and diarrhea, are found in soil, water, and sediments (Amangelsin et al., 2023; Antos et al., 2024; Daghrir and Drogui, 2013). This type of compound can alter microbial communities, promoting the development of antibiotic resistance and disrupting the food chain (Fiaz et al., 2021). Similarly, some compounds, such as metals, are essential sources of nutrients for plants, animals, and microorganisms but present risks to the ecosystem in high concentrations because of their toxicity, high density, and low degree of biological degradability (Ali et al., 2019). Among the microalgal species capable of removing heavy metals are *Chlorella*, *Desmodesmus*, *Scenedesmus*, and *Spirulina*, as well as some cyanobacterial species (Cañizares-Villanueva et al., 2017).

The bioaccumulation of pollutants in microalgae is carried out through the transfer of toxic compounds into the cells of the microorganism, where they interact with different intracellular components (Gobas et al., 2016; Yang et al., 2015). This process occurs because of the ability of microalgae

TABLE 2.10
Microalgae-based processes for the removal of emerging pollutants

Pollutant	Microalgal species	% removal/chemical modification	References
Cu	*Chlorella pyrenoidosa*	> 80, > 80	Zhou et al. (2012)
Zn	*Scenedesmus obliquus*	> 80, > 80	
Cu	*Chlorella vulgaris*	< 20, < 15	Lau et al. (1999)
Nor	*Chlorella miniata*	> 20, > 20	
Cd	*Dunaliella*	> 70	Imani et al. (2011)
Hg		< 70	
Pb		< 70	
Pb	*Spirulina platensis*	< 90	Malakootian et al. (2016)
As, Cd, Co, Cr, Pb, Ni, Zn	*Chlorella minutissima*	> 90 (for all metals used)	Roy et al. (1993)
Alfuzosin Atenolol Atracurium Bisoprolol Bupropion Citalopram Clarithromycin Metoprolol	*Dictyosphaerium*	Biodegradation	Ismail et al. (2017)
Amoxicillin	*Chlorella sp.*	Photodegradation by algae, decomposition and adsorption	Shi et al. (2018)
Carbamazepine Sulfamethoxazole Tramadol	*Chaetoceros muelleri*	Biodegradation and bioaccumulation	Mojiri et al. (2020)
Flutamide	*Chlorella vulgaris*	Biosorption	Habibzadeh et al. (2018)
Bisphenol A	*Chlorella vulgaris*	Photodegradation and biodegradation by algae	Peng et al. (2006)
Climbazole	*Scenedesmus obliquus*	Hydrogenation	Pan et al. (2018)
Progesterone and norgestrel	*Scenedesmus obliquus* and *Chlorella pyrenoidosa*	Hydroxylation, reduction, oxidation, and chain breakdown	Peng et al. (2014)
Naproxen	*Cymbella* sp. and *Scenedesmus quadricauda*	Hydroxylation, decarboxylation, demethylation, tyrosine conjunction, and glucuronidation	Ding et al. (2017)
Benzalkonium chloride	*Tetraselmis suecica*	Hydroxylation and dehydration	Ding et al. (2020)
Bezafibrate	*Navicula* sp.	Hydroxylation, demethylation, and glucuronidation	Jaén-Gil et al. (2020)
Polluting	**Microalgae**	**Adsorbent type**	**References**
Caffeine	*Sargassum* sp.	Synthesized activated carbon	Francoeur et al. (2021)
Caffeine	*Stigeoclonium nanum*	Dry biomass	Morales-Romero et al. (2024)
Diclofenac	*Synechocystis* sp. and *Scenedesmus* sp.	Freeze-dried biomass	Coimbra et al. (2018)
Paracetamol	*Synechocystis* sp.	Freeze-dried biomass	Escapa et al. (2017)
Tetracycline	*Chlorella* sp.	Dry biomass without lipids	Suárez-Martínez et al. (2022)
Tetracycline	*Sargassum* sp.	Stratified carbon particles	Li et al. (2017)
Tramadol	*Scenedesmus obliquus*	Dry biomass	Ali et al. (2018)

to absorb and retain the chemicals present in their aquatic environment, such as drugs, pesticides, personal care products, and other pollutants that are difficult to remove via conventional methods such as wastewater treatment (Abdelfattah et al., 2023; Martínez-Roldán et al., 2024; Sonali and Gayathri Krishnaswamy, 2023). Once inside the cell, pollutants can adhere to proteins, lipids, or carbohydrates or even be metabolized by specific enzymes in the organism (Rajamani et al., n.d.; Sutherland and Ralph, 2019). This process depends not only on the physicochemical properties of the pollutants, such as their solubility or affinity for certain cellular receptors, but also on the physiological and genetic characteristics of each microalgal species, which determine their ability to accumulate these pollutants (Avila, Carrero, et al., 2021; Avila, Peris, et al., 2021). Similarly, external factors such as the concentration of pollutants in the system, temperature, pH, and nutrient availability can significantly influence the efficiency of this process (Alaidaroos, 2023).

The biodegradation of EPs by microalgae occurs via the enzymatic transformation of complex compounds into less toxic or simpler products (Li et al., 2023). This process is carried out through metabolic pathways and specific enzymes, such as monooxygenases and peroxidases, which participate directly in the conversion of organic pollutants (Chu et al., 2022). Microalgae, like other organisms such as fungi and bacteria, are noteworthy for their ability to biotransform recalcitrant compounds from pharmaceuticals, endocrine disruptors, and pesticides into metabolites with a higher degree of biodegradability (Chang et al., 2023; Sun et al., 2023). Unlike passive removal systems, such as biofilters, microalgae not only accumulate pollutants in their cells but also metabolize them (Ghasemi et al., 2011), which reduces the possibility of releasing pollutants into the environment. Peng et al. (2014) used *Chlorella pyrenoidosa* and *Scenedesmus obliquus* to remove progesterone and norgestrel through degradation methods such as hydroxylation and oxidation. Santaeufemia et al. (2018) used a live culture of *Phaeodactylum tricornutum* to remove ibuprofen from liquid medium.

In addition to the use of live microalgal cultures, the dry biomass of these microorganisms has been studied in recent years as an adsorption tool in the elimination of EPs. This process uses the active sites of the cell wall of microalgae, which is rich in polysaccharides, alginates, and proteins and has functional groups capable of interacting with contaminants. Recent studies have shown that the dry biomass of *Chlorella vulgaris* and *Spirulina platensis* can adsorb compounds such as bisphenol A, diclofenac, and synthetic estrogens (Ali et al., 2022; Pedrosa et al., 2022; Rahmani et al., 2024). This type of technique is attractive because of its low cost, the ease of obtaining biomass from massive cultures, and the possibility of regeneration and reuse of the adsorbent material (Kumar et al., 2021). Unlike enzymatic processes, adsorption is a passive mechanism that does not require specific cultivation conditions, which broadens its applicability in wastewater treatment systems. However, more studies are still needed to optimize the adsorption capacity of the dry microalgal biomass and address issues such as competition between multiple pollutants. This process represents an alternative to the removal of EPs in aquatic environments.

2.4 CONCLUSION

The presence of so-called EPs in aquatic ecosystems is increasingly significant, even reaching levels toxic to living organisms. The absence of treatment processes enabling their elimination or degradation is an important aspect to which attention must be paid, along with the creation of regulations related to maximum permissible limits. However, the greatest challenge is related to the fact that EPs are not found in high concentrations, under constant conditions, or in an isolated manner; rather, their presence in wastewater (especially domestic wastewater) is inconstant and intermittent, and various pollutants are present simultaneously. Therefore, the development of efficient and low-cost treatments is even more difficult, and their development is thus still a great challenge to overcome. Biotechnological processes require the action of mixed cultures that contain fungi, bacteria, microalgae, and cyanobacteria so that joint work and synergy allow efficient elimination at low cost, increasing the feasibility of these processes.

ACKNOWLEDGMENT

To TecNM/IT Durango for the financial support provided, and to SECIHTI for the scholarship of Rodríguez-Oloño to achieve the master's degree.

REFERENCES

Abdelfattah, A., Ali, S. S., Ramadan, H., El-Aswar, E. I., Eltawab, R., Ho, S.-H., Elsamahy, T., Li, S., El-Sheekh, M. M., Schagerl, M., Kornaros, M., and Sun, J. (2023). Microalgae-based wastewater treatment: Mechanisms, challenges, recent advances, and future prospects. *Environmental Science and Ecotechnology, 13*, 100205. https://doi.org/10.1016/J.ESE.2022.100205

Adityosulindro, S., Julcour-Lebigue, C., Barthe, L., Adityosulindro, S., Julcour-Lebigue, C., Barthe, L., and Fenton, H. (2018). Heterogeneous Fenton oxidation using Fe-ZSM5 catalyst for removal of ibuprofen in wastewater. *Journal of Environmental Chemical Engineering, 6*(5), 5920–5928. https://doi.org/10.1016/j.jece.2018.09.007

Ahmad, H. A., Ahmad, S., Cui, Q., Wang, Z., Wei, H., Chen, X., Ni, S., Ismail, S., Awad, H.M., and Tawfik, A. (2022). The environmental distribution and removal of emerging pollutants, highlighting the importance of using microbes as a potential degrader: A review. *Science of The Total Environment, 809*, 151926. https://doi.org/10.1016/j.scitotenv.2021.151926.

Ahmadzadeh, S., and Dolatabadi, M. (2018). Removal of acetaminophen from hospital wastewater using electro - Fenton process. *Environmental Earth Sciences, 77*, 53. https://doi.org/10.1007/s12665-017-7203-7

Alaidaroos, B. A. (2023). Advancing eco-sustainable bioremediation for hydrocarbon contaminants: Challenges and solutions. *Processes, 11*(10):3036. https://doi.org/10.3390/pr11103036

Al-Homaidan, A. A., Alabdullatif, J. A., Al-Hazzani, A. A., Al-Ghanayem, A. A., and Alabbad, A. F. 2015. Adsorptive removal of cadmium ions by *Spirulina platensis* dry biomass. *Saudi Journal of Biological Sciences 22*(6), 795–800. https://doi.org/10.1016/j.sjbs.2015.06.010

Ali, H. M., Ibrahim, O. M., Ali, A. S. M., Mohamed, M. A., Ghareeb, R. Y., Hafez, E. E., and El-Aassar, M. R. (2022). Cross-linked chitosan/gelatin beads loaded with *Chlorella vulgaris* microalgae/Zinc oxide nanoparticles for adsorbing carcinogenic Bisphenol-A pollutant from water. *ACS Omega 7*(31), 27239–27248. https://doi.org/10.1021/acsomega.2c01985

Ali, H., Khan, E., and Ilahi, I. (2019). Environmental chemistry and ecotoxicology of hazardous heavy metals: Environmental persistence, toxicity, and bioaccumulation. *Journal of Chemistry 2019*, 730305. https://doi.org/10.1155/2019/6730305

Ali, M. E. M., Abd El-Aty, A. M., Badawy, M. I., and Ali, R. K. (2018). Removal of pharmaceutical pollutants from synthetic wastewater using chemically modified biomass of green alga *Scenedesmus obliquus*. *Ecotoxicology and Environmental Safety 151*, 144–152. https://doi.org/10.1016/j.ecoenv.2018.01.012

Ali, M., Naqvi, T. A., Kanwal, M., Rasheed, F., Hameed, A., and Ahmed, S. (2012). Detection of the organophosphate degrading gene opdA in the newly isolated bacterial strain *Bacillus pumilus* W1. *Annals of Microbiology 62*(1), 233–239.

Álvarez, S., Ribeiro, R. S., Gomes, H. T., Sotelo, J. L., and García, J. (2015). Synthesis of carbon xerogels and their application in adsorption studies of caffeine and diclofenac as emerging contaminants. *Chemical Engineering Research and Design 95*(1), 229–238. https://doi.org/10.1016/j.cherd.2014.11.001

Amangelsin, Y., Semenova, Y., Dadar, M., Aljofan, M., and Bjørklund, G. (2023). The Impact of tetracycline pollution on the aquatic environment and removal strategies. *Antibiotics 12*(3), 440. https://doi.org/10.3390/antibiotics12030440

Amobonye, A., Aruwa, C. E., Aransiola, S., Omame, J., Alabi, T. D., and Lalung, J. (2023). The potential of fungi in the bioremediation of pharmaceutically active compounds: A comprehensive review. *Frontiers in Microbiology 14*, 1207792.

Antos, J., Piosik, M., Ginter-Kramarczyk, D., Zembrzuska, J., and Kruszelnicka, I. (2024). Tetracyclines contamination in European aquatic environments: A comprehensive review of occurrence, fate, and removal techniques. *Chemosphere 353*, 141519. https://doi.org/10.1016/j.chemosphere.2024.141519

Arun, K. B., Madhavan, A., Tarafdar, A., Sirohi, R., Anoopkumar, A. N., Kuriakose, L. L., Awasthi, M. K., Binod, P., Varjani, S., and Sindhu, R. (2023). Filamentous fungi for pharmaceutical compounds degradation in the environment: A sustainable approach. *Environmental Technology & Innovation 31*, 103182. https://doi.org/10.1016/J.ETI.2023.103182

Avila, R., Carrero, E., Vicent, T., and Blánquez, P. (2021). Integration of enzymatic pretreatment and sludge co-digestion in biogas production from microalgae. *International Journal of Integrated Waste Management, Science and Technology 124*, 254–263. https://doi.org/10.1016/j.wasman.2021.01.042

Avila, R., Peris, A., Eljarrat, E., Vicent, T., and Blánquez, P. (2021). Biodegradation of hydrophobic pesticides by microalgae: Transformation products and impact on algae biochemical methane potential. *Science of The Total Environment 754*, 142114. https://doi.org/10.1016/j.scitotenv.2020.142114

Ayilara, M. S., and Babalola, O. O. (2023). Bioremediation of environmental wastes: The role of microorganisms. *Frontiers in Agronomy 5*, 1183691.

Azzouz, A., and Ballesteros, E. (2013). Influence of seasonal climate differences on the pharmaceutical, hormone and personal care product removal efficiency of a drinking water treatment plant. *Chemosphere 93*(9), 2046–2054.

Bae, S., Kim, D., and Lee, W. (2013). Applied Catalysis B : Environmental degradation of diclofenac by pyrite catalyzed Fenton oxidation. *Applied Catalysis B: Environment and Energy 134–135*, 93–102. https://doi.org/10.1016/j.apcatb.2012.12.031

Baffi, M. A., de Azevedo, L. C. B., Fornazier Borges, M., and Bertini, S. B. (2024). Microbial enzymes in biodegradation of organic pollutants: Mechanisms and applications. In Amity, K., Singh J. and Basilio de Azevedo L. C. (Eds.), *Microbiome-based decontamination of environmental pollutants* (213–242). Elsevier. https://doi.org/10.1016/B978-0-443-21781-4.00010-4

Bahman, M., Jalili, H., Etesam, M., and Amrane, A. (2022). Investigation of pharmaceutical compounds (Metronidazole, Rosuvastatin and Codeine phosphate) removal by *Synechocystis* sp. PCC6803 microalga. *Journal of Water Process Engineering 47*, 102820. https://doi.org/10.1016/j.jwpe.2022.102820

Bansal, R. C., and Goyal, M. (2005). *Activated carbon adsorption*. CRC press.

Barry, A. R., Semchuk, W. M., Thompson, A., LeBras, M. H., and Koshman, S. L. (2020). Use of low-dose acetylsalicylic acid for cardiovascular disease prevention: A practical, stepwise approach for pharmacists. *Canadian Pharmacists Journal 153*(3), 153–160. https://doi.org/10.1177/1715163520909137

Barsanti, L., and Gaultieri, P. (2006). *Algae: Anatomy, biochemistry and biotechnology*. CRC Press.

Barsanti, L., and Gualtieri, P. (2018). Is exploitation of microalgae economically and energetically sustainable? *Algal Research 31*, 107–115. https://doi.org/10.1016/j.algal.2018.02.001

Benlaassri, M., Ecale, F., Crepin, A., Rodier, M. H., Venisse, N., and Cateau, E. (2023). In vitro reciprocal interactions between yeasts from human cutaneous mycobiota and parabens used in cosmetics. *FEMS Microbiology Letters 370*, 1–7. https://doi.org/10.1093/FEMSLE/FNAC124

Benson, S. A. (1998). Ultrastructure of bacteria. In Bittar, E. E. and Bittar, N. (Eds.), *Microbiology* (1–14). Elsevier. https://doi.org/10.1016/S1569-2582(97)80138-9.

Beveridge, T. J., and Murray, R. G. E. (1976). Uptake and retention of metals by cell walls of *Bacillus subtilis*. *Journal of Bacteriology 127*(3), 1502. https://doi.org/10.1128/JB.127.3.1502-1518.1976

Bilal, M., Rasheed, T., Sosa-Hernández, J. E., Raza, A., Nabeel, F., and Iqbal, H. M. N. (2018). Biosorption: An interplay between marine algae and potentially toxic elements—A review. *Marine Drugs 16*(2), 65. https://doi.org/10.3390/md16020065

Boleda, M. R., Galceran, M. T., and Ventura, F. (2011). Behavior of pharmaceuticals and drugs of abuse in a drinking water treatment plant (DWTP) using combined conventional and ultrafiltration and reverse osmosis (UF/RO) treatments. *Environmental Pollution 159*, 1584–1591. https://doi.org/10.1016/j.envpol.2011.02.051

Borowitzka, M. A. (2013). High-value products from microalgae—their development and commercialisation. *Journal of Applied Phycology 25*(3), 743–756. https://doi.org/10.1007/s10811-013-9983-9

Bracamontes-Ruelas, A. R., Ordaz-Díaz, L. A., Bailón-Salas, A. M., Ríos-Saucedo, J. C., Reyes-Vidal, Y., and Reynoso-Cuevas, L. (2022). Emerging pollutants in wastewater, advanced oxidation processes as an alternative treatment and perspectives. *Processes 10*(5), 1041.

Calvo-Flores, F. G., Isac-García, J., and Dobado, J. A. (2018). Emerging pollutants. In Calvo-Flores, F. G., Isac-García J. and Dobado J. A. (Eds.), *Emerging pollutants origin, structure and properties*. Wiley-VCH. https://doi.org/10.1201/b10505-26.

Cañizares-Villanueva, R. O., Martínez-Roldán, A. J., Perales-Vela, H. V., Vázquez-Hernández, M., and Melchy-Antonio, O. (2017). Bioremediation of copper and other heavy metals using microbial biomass. In Das S. and Dash H. R. (Eds.), *Handbook of Metal-Microbe Interactions and Bioremediation* (585–602). CRC Press.

Carvalho Neto, D. P. de, Gonot-Schoupinsky, X. P., and Gonot-Schoupinsky, F. N. (2021). Coffee as a naturally beneficial and sustainable ingredient in personal care products: A systematic scoping review of the evidence. *Frontiers in Sustainability 2*, 697092. https://doi.org/10.3389/frsus.2021.697092

Cassier-Chauvat, C., and Chauvat, F. (2014). Responses to oxidative and heavy metal stresses in cyanobacteria: Recent advances. *International Journal of Molecular Sciences 16*(1), 871–886. https://doi.org/10.3390/ijms16010871

Castro-Alonso, M. J., Montañez-Hernandez, L. E., Sanchez-Muñoz, M. A., Macias Franco, M. R., Narayanasamy, R., and Balagurusamy, N. (2019). Microbially induced calcium carbonate precipitation (MICP) and its potential in bioconcrete: Microbiological and molecular concepts. *Frontiers in Materials 6*, 458036.

Chang, X., He, Y., Song, L., Ding, J., Ren, S., Lv, M., and Chen, L. (2023). Methylparaben toxicity and its removal by microalgae *Chlorella vulgaris* and *Phaeodactylum tricornutum*. *Journal of Hazardous Materials 454*, 131528. https://doi.org/10.1016/j.jhazmat.2023.131528

Chapman, R. L. (2013). Algae: The world's most important "plants"-an introduction. *Mitigation and Adaptation Strategies for Global Change 18*(1), 5–12. https://doi.org/10.1007/s11027-010-9255-9

Chaurasia, A. K., Adhya, T. K., and Apte, S. K. (2013). Engineering bacteria for bioremediation of persistent organochlorine pesticide lindane (γ-hexachlorocyclohexane). *Bioresource Technology 149*, 439–445. https://doi.org/10.1016/j.biortech.2013.09.084

Chen, S., Zhang, W., Li, J., Yuan, M., Zhang, J., Xu, F., Xu, H., Zheng, X., and Wang, L. (2020). Ecotoxicological effects of sulfonamides and fluoroquinolones and their removal by a green alga (*Chlorella vulgaris*) and a cyanobacterium (*Chrysosporum ovalisporum*). *Environmental Pollution 263*, 114554. https://doi.org/10.1016/j.envpol.2020.114554

Cheng, J., Zhang, C., Zhang, K., Li, J., Hou, Y., Xin, J., Sun, Y., Xu, C., and Xu, W. (2023). Cyanobacteria-mediated light-driven biotransformation: The current status and perspectives. *ACS Omega 8*(45), 42062–42071. https://doi.org/10.1021/acsomega.3c05407

Choi, K. J., Kim, S. G., Kim, C. W., and Park, J. K. (2006). Removal efficiencies of endocrine disrupting chemicals by coagulation/flocculation, ozonation, powdered/granular activated carbon adsorption, and chlorination. *Korean Journal of Chemistry Engineering 23*, 399–408. https://doi.org/10.1007/BF02706741

Chopra, S., and Kumar, D. (2020). Characterization, optimization and kinetics study of acetaminophen degradation by *Bacillus drentensis* strain S1 and waste water degradation analysis. *Bioresources and Bioprocessing 7*(1), 1–18.

Chu, Y., Zhang, C., Wang, R., Chen, X., Ren, N., and Ho, S.-H. (2022). Biotransformation of sulfamethoxazole by microalgae: Removal efficiency, pathways, and mechanisms. *Water Research 221*, 118834. https://doi.org/10.1016/j.watres.2022.118834

Coimbra, R. N., Escapa, C., Vázquez, N. C., Noriega-Hevia, G., and Otero, M. (2018). Utilization of non-living microalgae biomass from two different strains for the adsorptive removal of diclofenac from water. *Water 10*(10), 1401. https://doi.org/10.3390/w10101401

Collins, A. M., Liberton, M., Jones, H. D. T., Garcia, O. F., Pakrasi, H. B., and Timlin, J. A. (2012). Photosynthetic pigment localization and thylakoid membrane morphology are altered in *Synechocystis* 6803 phycobilisome mutants. *Plant Physiology 158*(4), 1600–1609. https://doi.org/10.1104/pp.111.192849

Daâssi, D., and Alharbi, S. R. (2023). Degradation of endocrine-disrupting chemicals in wastewater by new thermophilic fungal isolates and their laccases. *3 Biotech 13*(1), 26. https://doi.org/10.1007/s13205-022-03439-1

Daghrir, R., and Drogui, P. (2013). Tetracycline antibiotics in the environment: A review. *Environmental Chemistry Letters 11*(3), 209–227. https://doi.org/10.1007/s10311-013-0404-8

Das, K., and Mukherjee, A. K. (2007). Differential utilization of pyrene as the sole source of carbon by *Bacillus subtilis* and *Pseudomonas aeruginosa* strains: Role of biosurfactants in enhancing bioavailability. *Journal of Applied Microbiology 102*(1), 195–203. https://doi.org/10.1111/J.1365-2672.2006.03070.X

Davarnejad, R., and Sabzehei, M. (2021). Sodium diclofenac removal from a pharmaceutical wastewater by electro- Fenton process sodium diclofenac removal from a pharmaceutical wastewater by electro-Fenton process. *Separation Science and Technology 54*(14), 2294–2303. https://doi.org/10.1080/01496395.2018.1540639

Davarnejad, R., Zangene, K., Fazlali, A. R., and Behfar, R. (2017). Ibuprofen removal from a pharmaceutical wastewater using electro-fenton process : An Efficient Technique. *International Journal of Engineering 30*(11), 1639–1646.

De Almeida, L. N. B., Josué, T. G., Fidelis, M. Z., Abreu, E., Bechlin, M. A., Dos Santos, O. A. A., and Lenzi, G. G. (2021). Process comparison for caffeine degradation: Fenton, photo-Fenton, UV/H_2O_2 and UV/Fe^{3+}. *Water, Air, & Soil Pollution 232*, 1–10. https://doi.org/10.1007/s11270-021-05115-1

De Philippis, R., Colica, G., and Micheletti, E. (2011). Exopolysaccharide-producing cyanobacteria in heavy metal removal from water: Molecular basis and practical applicability of the biosorption process. *Applied Microbiology and Biotechnology 92*(4), 697–708. https://doi.org/10.1007/s00253-011-3601-z

de Wilt, A., Butkovskyi, A., Tuantet, K., Leal, L. H., Fernandes, T. V., Langenhoff, A., and Zeeman, G. (2016). Micropollutant removal in an algal treatment system fed with source separated wastewater streams. *Journal of Hazardous Materials 304*, 84–92. https://doi.org/10.1016/j.jhazmat.2015.10.033

Dhiman, N., Jasrotia, T., Sharma, P., Negi, S., Chaudhary, S., Kumar, R., Mahnashi, M. H., Umar, A., and Kumar, R. (2020). Immobilization interaction between xenobiotic and *Bjerkandera adusta* for the biodegradation of atrazine. *Chemosphere 257*, 127060. https://doi.org/10.1016/j.chemosphere.2020.127060

Diaz-Uribe, C., Angulo, B., Patiño, K., Hernández, V., Vallejo, W., Gallego-Cartagena, E., Romero Bohórquez, A. R., Zarate, X., and Schott, E. (2021). Cyanobacterial biomass as a potential biosorbent for the removal of recalcitrant dyes from water. *Water 13*(22), 3176. https://doi.org/10.3390/w13223176

Dickerson, S. M., and Gore, A. C. (2007). Estrogenic environmental endocrine-disrupting chemical effects on reproductive neuroendocrine function and dysfunction across the life cycle. *Reviews in endocrine and metabolic disorders 8*(2), 143–159. https://doi.org/10.1007/s11154-007-9048-y

Ding, T., Lin, K., Yang, B., Yang, M., Li, J., Li, W., and Gan, J. (2017). Biodegradation of naproxen by freshwater algae *Cymbella* sp. and *Scenedesmus quadricauda* and the comparative toxicity. *Bioresource Technology 238*, 164–173. https://doi.org/10.1016/j.biortech.2017.04.018

Ding, T., Wang, S., Yang, B., and Li, J. (2020). Biological removal of pharmaceuticals by *Navicula* sp. and biotransformation of bezafibrate. *Chemosphere 240*, 124949. https://doi.org/10.1016/j.chemosphere.2019.124949

dos Santos, D., Moreira, W., de Araújo, T., Bernardo, M., Fonseca, I., Ostroski, I., and de Barros, M. A. (2024). Removal of emerging contaminants from water by using carbon materials derived from tingui shells. *Separations 11*(7), 215. https://doi.org/10.3390/separations11070215

Dutta, S., Ghosh, D., Lahiri, A., Chakraborty, S., and Pandit, S. (2022). Cyanoremediation. In Rodriguez-Couto, S. and Shah M. P. (Eds.), *Development in wastewater treatment research and processes* (335–354). Elsevier. https://doi.org/10.1016/B978-0-323-85839-7.00017-7

Eibes, G., Debernardi, G., Feijoo, G., Moreira, M. T., and Lema, J. M. (2011). Oxidation of pharmaceutically active compounds by a ligninolytic fungal peroxidase. *Biodegradation*, *22*(3), 539–550. https://doi.org/10.1007/S10532-010-9426-0

El-Sheekh, M., Abou-El-Souod, G., and El Asrag, H. (2018). Biodegradation of some dyes by the green alga *Chlorella vulgaris* and the cyanobacterium *Aphanocapsa elachista*. *Egyptian Journal of Botany 58*(3), 311–320.

Escapa, C., Coimbra, R., Nuevo, C., Vega, S., Paniagua, S., García, A., Calvo, L., and Otero, M. (2017). Valorization of microalgae biomass by its use for the removal of paracetamol from contaminated water. *Water 9*(5), 312. https://doi.org/10.3390/w9050312

Feng, L., Oturan, N., and Hullebusch, E. D. Van. (2014). Degradation of anti-inflammatory drug ketoprofen by electro-oxidation : Comparison of electro-Fenton and anodic oxidation processes. *Environmental Science and Pollution Research 21*, 8406–8416. https://doi.org/10.1007/s11356-014-2774-2

Ferreira, B. L., Ferreira, D. P., Borges, S. F., Ferreira, A. M., Holanda, F. H., Ucella-Filho, J. G. M., Cruz, R. A. S., Birolli, W. G., Luque, R., and Ferreira, I. M. (2023). Diclofenac, ibuprofen, and paracetamol biodegradation: Overconsumed non-steroidal anti-inflammatories drugs at COVID-19 pandemic. *Frontiers in Microbiology 14*, 1207664. https://doi.org/10.3389/fmicb.2023.1207664

Fiaz, A., Zhu, D., and Sun, J. (2021). Environmental fate of tetracycline antibiotics: Degradation pathway mechanisms, challenges, and perspectives. *Environmental Sciences Europe 33*(1), 1–17. https://doi.org/10.1186/S12302-021-00505-Y

Francoeur, M., Ferino-Pérez, A., Yacou, C., Jean-Marius, C., Emmanuel, E., Chérémond, Y., Jauregui-Haza, U., and Gaspard, S. (2021). Activated carbon synthetized from *Sargassum* (sp) for adsorption of caffeine: Understanding the adsorption mechanism using molecular modeling. *Journal of Environmental Chemical Engineering 9*(1), 104795. https://doi.org/10.1016/j.jece.2020.104795

Gadi, N., Boelee, N. C., and Dewil, R. (2022). The Electro-Fenton process for caffeine removal from water and granular activated carbon regeneration. *Sustainability 14*(21), 14313. https://doi.org/10.3390/su142114313

Gar, M., Tawfik, A., and Ookawara, S. (2015). Degradation of four pharmaceuticals by solar Photo-Fenton process: Kinetics and costs estimation. *Journal of Environmental Chemical Engineering 3*(1), 46–51. https://doi.org/10.1016/j.jece.2014.12.009

Geng, Z., Zhu, W., Su, H., Zhao, Y., Zhang, K.-Q., and Yang, J. (2014). Recent advances in genes involved in secondary metabolite synthesis, hyphal development, energy metabolism and pathogenicity in *Fusarium graminearum* (teleomorph *Gibberella zeae*). *Biotechnology Advances 32*(2), 390–402. https://doi.org/10.1016/j.biotechadv.2013.12.007

Ghasemi, Y., Rasoul-Amini, S., and Fotooh-Abadi, E. (2011). The biotransformation, biodegradation, and bioremediation of organic compounds by microalgae. *Journal of Phycology 47*(5), 969–980. https://doi.org/10.1111/j.1529-8817.2011.01051.x

Ghecham, F. Z., Guergazi, S., and Achour S. (2018). Removal of caffeine by coagulation-flocculation with aluminum sulfate and effect of metal salts. *Larhyss Journal 34*, 115–126

Gianfreda, L., and Rao, M. A. (2004). Potential of extra cellular enzymes in remediation of polluted soils: A review. *Enzyme and Microbial Technology 35*(4), 339–354. https://doi.org/10.1016/j.enzmictec.2004.05.006

Glade, M. J. (2010). Caffeine—Not just a stimulant. *Nutrition 26*(10), 932–938. https://doi.org/10.1016/j.nut.2010.08.004

Gobas, F. A., Burkhard, L. P., Doucette, W. J., Sappington, K. G., Verbruggen, E. M., Hope, B. K., Bonnell, M. A., Arnot, J. A., and Tarazona, J. V. (2016). Review of existing terrestrial bioaccumulation models and terrestrial bioaccumulation modeling needs for organic chemicals. *Integrated Environmental Assessment and Management 12*(1), 123–134. https://doi.org/10.1002/ieam.1690

González-Barreiro, O., Rioboo, C., Herrero, C., and Cid, A. (2006). Removal of triazine herbicides from freshwater systems using photosynthetic microorganisms. *Environmental Pollution 144*(1), 266–271. https://doi.org/10.1016/j.envpol.2005.12.014

Gore, A. C., Chappell, V. A., Fenton, S. E., Flaws, J. A., Nadal, A., Prins, G. S., Toppari, J., and Zoeller, R. T. (2015). EDC-2: The endocrine society's second scientific statement on endocrine-disrupting chemicals. *Endocrine Reviews 36*(6), E1–E150. https://doi.org/10.1210/er.2015-1010

Górny, D., Guzik, U., Hupert-Kocurek, K., and Wojcieszyńska, D. (2019). A new pathway for naproxen utilisation by *Bacillus thuringiensis* B1(2015b) and its decomposition in the presence of organic and inorganic contaminants. *Journal of Environmental Management 239*, 1–7. https://doi.org/10.1016/J.JENVMAN.2019.03.034

Gould, A. B. (2009). Fungi: Plant pathogenic. In Schaechter, M. (Ed.) *Encyclopedia of Microbiology, Third Edition* (457–477). Academic Press. https://doi.org/10.1016/B978-012373944-5.00347-3

Graham, D. M. (2009). Caffeine - Its identity, dietary sources, intake and biological effects. *Nutrition Reviews 36*(4), 97–102. https://doi.org/10.1111/j.1753-4887.1978.tb03717.x

Guldhe, A., Singh, B., Ansari, F. A., Sharma, Y., and Bux, F. (2016). Extraction and conversion of microalgal lipids. In Bux, F., Chisti, Y. (Eds.) *Algae Biotechnology Green Energy and Technology* (91–110). Springer. https://doi.org/10.1007/978-3-319-12334-9_6

Gupta, A., Gupta, R., and Singh, R. L. (2017). Microbes and environment. In Singh, R. (Ed.) *Principles and applications of environmental biotechnology for a sustainable future. Applied environmental science and engineering for a sustainable future* (43–84). Springer. https://doi.org/10.1007/978-981-10-1866-4_3

Gupta, R. K., Archambeault, D. R., and Yao, H. H.-C. (2010). Genetic mouse models for female reproductive toxicology studies. In McQueen, C. A. (Ed.) *Comprehensive toxicology* (561–575). Elsevier. https://doi.org/10.1016/B978-0-08-046884-6.01135-0

Habibzadeh, M., Chaibakhsh, N., and Naeemi, A. S. (2018). Optimized treatment of wastewater containing cytotoxic drugs by living and dead biomass of the freshwater microalga. *Chlorella vulgaris. Ecological Engineering 111*, 85–93. https://doi.org/10.1016/j.ecoleng.2017.12.001

Hakil, M., Denis, S., Viniegra-González, G., and Augur, C. (1998). Degradation and product analysis of caffeine and related dimethylxanthines by filamentous fungi. *Enzyme and Microbial Technology 22*(5), 355–359. https://doi.org/10.1016/S0141-0229(97)00205-6

Hamouda, R. A. E. F., Sorour, N. M., and Yeheia, D. S. (2016). Biodegradation of crude oil by *Anabaena oryzae, Chlorella kessleri* and its consortium under mixotrophic conditions. *International Biodeterioration and Biodegradation 112*, 128–134. https://doi.org/10.1016/j.ibiod.2016.05.001

Han, S., Han, W., Chen, J., Sun, Y., Dai, M., and Zhao, G. (2020). Bioremediation of malachite green by cyanobacterium *Synechococcus elongatus* PCC 7942 engineered with a triphenylmethane reductase gene. *Applied Microbiology and Biotechnology 104*(7), 3193–3204. https://doi.org/10.1007/s00253-020-10438-w

Hawksworth, D. L., and Wiltshire, P. E. J. (2011). Forensic mycology: The use of fungi in criminal investigations. *Forensic Science International 206*(1–3), 1–11. https://doi.org/10.1016/j.forsciint.2010.06.012

He, Y.-Y., and Häder, D.-P. (2002). Reactive oxygen species and UV-B: Effect on cyanobacteria. *Photochemical & Photobiological Sciences 1*(10), 729–736. https://doi.org/10.1039/b110365m

Hobot, J. A. (2015). Bacterial ultrastructure. In Tang, Y.- W., Sussman, M., Liu, D., Poxton, I. and Schwartzman, J. (Eds.) *Molecular Medical Microbiology. Second Edition* (7–32). Elsevier. https://doi.org/10.1016/B978-0-12-397169-2.00002-0

Hoffmann, T. D., Reeksting, B. J., and Gebhard, S. (2021). Bacteria-induced mineral precipitation: A mechanistic review. *Microbiology 167*(4), 001049. https://doi.org/10.1099/MIC.0.001049

Hu, K., Peris, A., Torán, J., Eljarrat, E., Sarrà, M., Blánquez, P., and Caminal, G. (2020). Exploring the degradation capability of *Trametes versicolor* on selected hydrophobic pesticides through setting sights simultaneously on culture broth and biological matrix. *Chemosphere 250*, 126293. https://doi.org/10.1016/j.chemosphere.2020.126293

Husain, Q. (2006). Potential applications of the oxidoreductive enzymes in the decolorization and detoxification of textile and other synthetic dyes from polluted water: A review. *Critical Reviews in Biotechnology 26*(4), 201–221. https://doi.org/10.1080/07388550600969936

Hussain, S., Aneggi, E., Briguglio, S., Mattiussi, M., Gelao, V., Cabras, I. L., Zorzenon, A, Trovarelli and Goi, D. (2020). Enhanced ibuprofen removal by heterogeneous-Fenton process over Cu/ZrO_2 and Fe/ZrO_2 catalysts. *Journal of Environmental Chemical Engineering 8*(1), 103586. https://doi.org/10.1016/j.jece.2019.103586

Hwang, K.-A., and Choi, K.-C. (2015). Endocrine-disrupting chemicals with estrogenicity posing the risk of cancer progression in estrogen-responsive organs. In Fishbein, J. C. and Heilman, J. M. (Eds.) *Advances in Molecular Toxicology* (1–33). Elsevier. https://doi.org/10.1016/B978-0-12-802229-0.00001-3

Imani, S., Rezaei-Zarchi, S., Hashemi, M., Borna, H., Javid, A., Zand, A. M., and Abarghouei, H. B. (2011). Hg, Cd and Pb heavy metal bioremediation by *Dunaliella* alga. *Journal of Medicinal Plants Research 5*(13), 2775–2780.

Ismail, M. M., Essam, T. M., Ragab, Y. M., El-Sayed, A. E. B., and Mourad, F. E. (2017). Remediation of a mixture of analgesics in a stirred-tank photobioreactor using microalgal-bacterial consortium coupled with attempt to valorise the harvested biomass. *Bioresource Technology 232*, 364–371. https://doi.org/10.1016/j.biortech.2017.02.062

Jaén-Gil, A., Ferrando-Climent, L., Ferrer, I., Thurman, E. M., Rodríguez-Mozaz, S., Barceló, D., and Escudero-Oñate, C. (2020). Sustainable microalgae-based technology for biotransformation of benzalkonium chloride in oil and gas produced water: A laboratory-scale study. *Science of the Total Environment 748*, 141526. https://doi.org/10.1016/j.scitotenv.2020.141526

Jansson, C., and Northen, T. (2010). Calcifying cyanobacteria—the potential of biomineralization for carbon capture and storage. *Current Opinion in Biotechnology 21*(3), 365–371. https://doi.org/10.1016/j.copbio.2010.03.017

Kang, B. R., Kim, S. Y., Kang, M., and Lee, T. K. (2021). Removal of pharmaceuticals and personal care products using native fungal enzymes extracted during the ligninolytic process. *Environmental Research 195*, 110878. https://doi.org/10.1016/J.ENVRES.2021.110878

Kant, P., Reinprecht, Y., Martin, C. J., Islam, R., and Pauls, K. P. (2017). Disease resistance. In Moo-Young, M. (Ed.) *Comprehensive Biotechnology. Third Edition* (789–805). Pergamon. https://doi.org/10.1016/B978-0-12-809633-8.09244-X

Karigar, C. S., and Rao, S. S. (2011). Role of microbial enzymes in the bioremediation of pollutants: A review. *Enzyme Research 2011*(1), 805187. https://doi.org/10.4061/2011/805187

Kim, Y., Yeo, S., Kim, M. K., and Choi, H. T. (2008). Removal of estrogenic activity from endocrine-disrupting chemicals by purified laccase of *Phlebia tremellosa*. *FEMS Microbiology Letters 284*(2), 172–175. https://doi.org/10.1111/j.1574-6968.2008.01189.x

Klessig, D. F., Tian, M., and Choi, H. W. (2016). Multiple targets of salicylic acid and its derivatives in plants and animals. *Frontiers in Immunology 7*, 206. https://doi.org/10.3389/fimmu.2016.00206

Kózka, B., Sośnicka, A., Nałęcz-Jawecki, G., Drobniewska, A., Turło, J., and Giebułtowicz, J. (2023). Various species of Basidiomycota fungi reveal different abilities to degrade pharmaceuticals and also different pathways of degradation. *Chemosphere 338*, 139481. https://doi.org/10.1016/J.CHEMOSPHERE.2023.139481

Krajišnik, D., Daković, A., Malenović, A., Milojević-Rakić, M., Dondur, V., Radulović, Ž., and Milić, J. (2013). Investigation of adsorption and release of diclofenac sodium by modified zeolites composites. *Applied Clay Science 83*, 322–326. https://doi.org/10.1016/j.clay.2013.08.011

Křesinová, Z., Linhartová, L., Filipová, A., Ezechiáš, M., Mašín, P., and Cajthaml, T. (2018). Biodegradation of endocrine disruptors in urban wastewater using *Pleurotus ostreatus* bioreactor. *New Biotechnology 43*, 53–61. https://doi.org/10.1016/j.nbt.2017.05.004

Kumar, A., Rana, A., Sharma, G., Naushad, M., Dhiman, P., Kumari, A., and Stadler, F. J. (2019). Recent advances in nano-Fenton catalytic degradation of emerging pharmaceutical contaminants. *Journal of Molecular Liquids 290*, 111177. https://doi.org/10.1016/j.molliq.2019.111177

Kumar, A., Singh, R., Kumar Upadhyay Sanjay Kumar, S., and Charaya, M. U. (2021). Biosorption: The removal of toxic dyes from industrial effluent using phytobiomass- a review. *Plant Archives 21*(1), 1320–1325. https://doi.org/10.51470/PLANTARCHIVES.2021.v21.S1.207

Latifi, A., Ruiz, M., and Zhang, C. C. (2009). Oxidative stress in cyanobacteria. *FEMS Microbiology Reviews 33*(2), 258–278. https://doi.org/10.1111/j.1574-6976.2008.00134.x

Lau, P. S., Lee, H. Y., Tsang, C. C. K., Tam, N. F. Y., and Wong, Y. S. (1999). Effect of metal interference, pH and temperature on Cu and Ni biosorption by *Chlorella vulgaris* and *Chlorella miniata*. *Environmental Technology 20*(9), 953–961. https://doi.org/10.1080/09593332008616890

Lesser, L. E., Mora, A., Moreau, C., Mahlknecht, J., Hernández-Antonio, A., Ramírez, A. I., Barrios-Piña, H. (2018). Survey of 218 organic contaminants in groundwater derived from the world's largest untreated wastewater irrigation system: Mezquital Valley, Mexico. *Chemosphere 198*, 510–521. https://doi.org/10.1016/j.chemosphere.2018.01.154.

Levin, P. A., and Angert, E. R. (2015). Small but mighty: Cell size and bacteria. *Cold Spring Harbor Perspectives in Biology 7*(7), 1–11. https://doi.org/10.1101/cshperspect.a019216

Li, G., Guo, Y., and Zhao, W. (2017). Efficient adsorption removal of tetracycline by layered carbon particles prepared from seaweed biomass. *Environmental Progress & Sustainable Energy 36*(1), 59–65. https://doi.org/10.1002/ep.12437

Li, S., Chu, Y., Ren, N., and Ho, S. H. (2023). Cytochrome P450 enzyme-based biotransformation of pharmaceuticals and personal care products (PPCPs) by microalgae in the aquatic environment. *Chemical Engineering Journal 476*, 146557. https://doi.org/10.1016/j.cej.2023.146557

Lin, C., Gan, L., and Chen, Z. L. (2010). Biodegradation of naphthalene by strain *Bacillus fusiformis* (BFN). *Journal of Hazardous Materials 182*(1–3), 771–777. https://doi.org/10.1016/J.JHAZMAT.2010.06.101

Louw, T. M., Griffiths, M. J., Jones, S. M., Harrison, S. T. (2016). Techno-economics of algal biodiesel. In Bux, F., and Chisti, Y. (Eds.) *Algae Biotechnology Green Energy and Technology* (111–141). Springer. https://doi.org/10.1007/978-3-319-12334-9_7

Lucas, M. S., and Peres, J. A. (2015). Removal of emerging contaminants by Fenton and UV-driven advanced oxidation processes. *Water, Air, & Soil Pollution 226*, 273 https://doi.org/10.1007/s11270-015-2534-z

Maadani Mallak, A., Lakzian, A., Khodaverdi, E., Haghnia, G. H., and Mahmoudi, S. (2020). Effect of *Pleurotus ostreatus* and *Trametes versicolor* on triclosan biodegradation and activity of laccase and manganese peroxidase enzymes. *Microbial Pathogenesis 149*, 104473. https://doi.org/10.1016/j.micpath.2020.104473

Mahmood, T., Momin, S., Ali, R., Naeem, A., and Khan, A. (2022). Technologies for removal of emerging contaminants from wastewater. In Ince, M. and Kaplan Ince, O. (Eds.) *Wastewater Treatment* (1–20). InTechopen.

Mahran, F. A., Mustafa, D., Rafik, K., Hani, K., and Mohannad, K. (2019). Removal of selected pharmaceuticals from aqueous solutions using natural jordanian zeolite. *Arabian Journal for Science and Engineering 44*(1), 209–215. https://doi.org/10.1007/s13369-018-3406-9

Malakootian, M., Khodashenas Limoni, Z., and Malakootian, M. (2016). The efficiency of lead biosorption from industrial wastewater by micro-alga *Spirulina platensis*. *Int J Environmental Research 10*(3), 357–366.

Mandal, K., Singh, B., Jariyal, M., and Gupta, V. K. (2013). Microbial degradation of fipronil by *Bacillus thuringiensis*. *Ecotoxicology and Environmental Safety 93*, 87–92. https://doi.org/10.1016/J.ECOENV.2013.04.001

Marchlewicz, A., Guzik, U., Smułek, W., and Wojcieszyńska, D. (2017). Exploring the degradation of ibuprofen by *Bacillus thuringiensis* B1(2015b): The new pathway and factors affecting degradation. *Molecules 22*, 1676. https://doi.org/10.3390/MOLECULES22101676

Marco-Urrea, E., Pérez-Trujillo, M., Cruz-Morató, C., Caminal, G., and Vicent, T. (2010). Degradation of the drug sodium diclofenac by *Trametes versicolor* pellets and identification of some intermediates by NMR. *Journal of Hazardous Materials 176*(1–3), 836–842. https://doi.org/10.1016/j.jhazmat.2009.11.112

Mareš, J., Strunecký, O., Bučinská, L., and Wiedermannová, J. (2019). Evolutionary patterns of thylakoid architecture in cyanobacteria. *Frontiers in Microbiology 10*, 277. https://doi.org/10.3389/fmicb.2019.00277

Martínez-Roldán, A. J., and Cañizares-Villanueva, R. O. (2020). Wastewater treatment based in microalgae. In Jacob-Lopes, E., Manzoni-Maroneze, M., Queiroz, M. I. and Queiroz-Zepka, L. (Eds.) *Handbook of microalgae-based processes and products* (165–184). Elsevier. https://doi.org/10.1016/B978-0-12-818536-0.00007-5

Martínez-Roldán, A. J., and Lozano-Gómez, B. P. (2022). Growth of *Spirulina maxima* in an optimized concentric internal tube photobioreactor. *Iranian Journal of Biotechnology 20*(3), e2985. https://doi.org/10.30498/ijb.2022.273070.2985

Martínez-Roldán, A. J., Villanueva-Garcia, R. P., Rodríguez Rosales, M. D. J., Valle Cervantes, S., and Perales Vela, H. V. (2024). Wastewater treatment by microalgae and cyanobacteria. The reduction of the contaminant potential of real domestic wastewater: A case study. In Martínez-Roldán, A. J. (Ed.) *Biotechnological Processes for Green Energy, and High Value Bioproducts by Microalgae, and Cyanobacteria Cultures* (31–41). Springer International Publishing. https://doi.org/10.1007/978-3-031-43969-8_4

Maruri-López, I., Aviles-Baltazar, N. Y., Buchala, A., and Serrano, M. (2019). Intra and extracellular journey of the phytohormone salicylic acid. *Frontiers in Plant Science 10*, 423. https://doi.org/10.3389/fpls.2019.00423

McLean, R. J. C., Beauchemin, D., and Beveridge, T. J. (1992). Influence of oxidation state on iron binding by *Bacillus licheniformis* capsule. *Applied and Environmental Microbiology 58*(1), 405–408. https://doi.org/10.1128/AEM.58.1.405-408.1992

Mendez-Arriaga, F., Esplugas, S., and Gimenez, J. (2010). Degradation of the emerging contaminant ibuprofen in water by photo-Fenton. *Water Research 44*(2), 589–595. https://doi.org/10.1016/j.watres.2009.07.009

Meng, P., Pei, H., Hu, W., Shao, Y., and Li, Z. (2014). How to increase microbial degradation in constructed wetlands: Influencing factors and improvement measures. *Bioresource Technology 157*, 316–326. https://doi.org/10.1016/J.BIORTECH.2014.01.095

Merinville, E., Laloeuf, A., Moran, G., Jalby, O., and Rawlings, A. V. (2009). Exfoliation for sensitive skin with neutralized salicylic acid? *International Journal of Cosmetic Science 31*(3), 243–244. https://doi.org/10.1111/J.1468-2494.2009.00501_2.X

Miklos, D. B., Remy, C., Jekel, M., Linden, K. G., and Hübner, U. (2018). Evaluation of advanced oxidation processes for water and wastewater treatment: A critical review. *Water Research 139*(1), 118–131. https://doi.org/10.1016/j.watres.2018.03.042

Mishra, A., and Malik, A. (2013). Recent advances in microbial metal bioaccumulation. *Critical Reviews in Environmental Science and Technology 43*(11), 1162–1222. https://doi.org/10.1080/10934529.2011.627044

Mojiri, A., Baharlooeian, M., Kazeroon, R. A., Farraji, H., and Lou, Z. (2020). Removal of pharmaceutical micropollutants with integrated biochar and marine microalgae. *Microorganisms 9*(1), 4. https://doi.org/10.3390/microorganisms9010004

Monteil, H., Péchaud, Y., Oturan, N., and Oturan, M. A. (2018). A review on efficiency and cost effectiveness of electro- and Bio-electro- Fenton processes: Application to the treatment of pharmaceutical pollutants in water *Chemical Engineering Journal 376*, 119577. https://doi.org/10.1016/j.cej.2018.07.179

Morais, M. G., Santos, T. D., Moraes, L., Vaz, B. S., Morais, E. G., and Costa, J. A. V. (2022). Exopolysaccharides from microalgae: Production in a biorefinery framework and potential applications. *Bioresource Technology Reports 18*, 101006. https://doi.org/10.1016/j.biteb.2022.101006

Morales-Romero, J. M., Martínez-Roldán, A. J., and Reynoso-Cuevas, L. (2024). Removal of emerging contaminants using microalgal biomass. *Chemical Engineering Transactions* 110, 43–48. https://doi.org/10.3303/CET24110008

Morin-Crini, N., Lichtfouse, E., Fourmentin, M., Ribeiro, A. R. L., Noutsopoulos, C., Mapelli, F., Fenyvesi, É., Vieira, M. G. A., Picos-Corrales, L. A., Moreno-Piraján, J. C., Giraldo, L., Sohajda, T., Huq, M. M., Soltan, J., Torri, G., Magureanu, M., Bradu, C., and Crini, G. (2022). Removal of emerging contaminants from wastewater using advanced treatments. A review. *Environmental Chemistry Letters 20*(2), 1333–1375. https://doi.org/10.1007/s10311-021-01379-5

Mota, R., Rossi, F., Andrenelli, L., Pereira, S. B., De Philippis, R., and Tamagnini, P. (2016). Released polysaccharides (RPS) from *Cyanothece* sp. CCY 0110 as biosorbent for heavy metals bioremediation: Interactions between metals and RPS binding sites. *Applied Microbiology and Biotechnology 100*(17), 7765–7775. https://doi.org/10.1007/s00253-016-7602-9

Mousavi, S. M., Hashemi, S. A., Iman Moezzi, S. M., Ravan, N., Gholami, A., Lai, C. W., Chiang, W.-H., Omidifar, N., Yousefi, K., and Behbudi, G. (2021). Recent advances in enzymes for the bioremediation of pollutants. *Biochemistry Research International 2021*, 599204 https://doi.org/10.1155/2021/5599204

Murugesan, K., Chang, Y. Y., Kim, Y. M., Jeon, J. R., Kim, E. J., and Chang, Y. S. (2010). Enhanced transformation of triclosan by laccase in the presence of redox mediators. *Water Research 44*(1), 298–308. https://doi.org/10.1016/J.WATRES.2009.09.058

Ngeno, E. C., Shikuku, V. O., Orata, F., Baraza, L. D., and Kimosop, S. J. (2019). Caffeine and ciprofloxacin adsorption from water onto clinoptilolite: Linear isotherms, kinetics, thermodynamic and mechanistic studies. *South African Journal of Chemistry 72*, 136–142.

Ni'Matuzahroh, Trikurniadewi, N., Pramadita, A. R. A., Pratiwi, I. A., Salamun, Fatimah, and Sumarsih, S. (2017). Biodegradation of naphthalene and phenanthren by *Bacillus subtilis* 3KP. *AIP Conference Proceedings 1854*(1), 020026. https://doi.org/10.1063/1.4985417

Nidheesh, P. V., Ganiyu, S. O., Martínez-Huitle, C. A., Mousset, E., Olvera-Vargas, H., Trellu, C., Zhou, M., Oturan, M. A., Nidheesh, P. V., Ganiyu, S. O., Martínez-Huitle, C. A., and Mousset, E. (2022). Recent advances in electro-Fenton process and its emerging applications. *Critical Reviews in Environmental Science and Technology 53*(8), 887–913. https://doi.org/10.1080/10643389.2022.2093074

Oller, I., and Malato, S. (2021). Photo-Fenton applied to the removal of pharmaceutical and other pollutants of emerging concern. *Current Opinion in Green and Sustainable Chemistry 29*, 100458. https://doi.org/10.1016/j.cogsc.2021.100458

Pan, C. G., Peng, F. J., and Ying, G. G. (2018). Removal, biotransformation and toxicity variations of climbazole by freshwater algae *Scenedesmus obliquus*. *Environmental Pollution 240*, 534–540. https://doi.org/10.1016/j.envpol.2018.05.020

Pan, J., Liu, P., Yu, X., Zhang, Z., and Liu, J. (2024). The adverse role of endocrine disrupting chemicals in the reproductive system. *Frontiers in Endocrinology 14*, 1324993. https://doi.org/10.3389/fendo.2023.1324993

Parikh, A., and Madamwar, D. (2005). Textile dye decolorization using cyanobacteria. *Biotechnology Letters 27*(5), 323–326. https://doi.org/10.1007/s10529-005-0691-7

Patel, J. G., Kumar, J. I. N., and Khan, S. R. (2015). Consequences of environmentally hazardous polycyclic aromatic hydrocarbon- anthracene treatment on cyanobacteria. *International Journal of Applied Sciences and Biotechnology 3*(3), 381–386. https://doi.org/10.3126/ijasbt.v3i3.11654

Patil, A., Chakraborty, S., Yadav, Y., Sharma, B., Singh, S., and Arya, M. (2024). Bioremediation strategies and mechanisms of bacteria for resistance against heavy metals: A review. *Bioremediation Journal,* 1–33. https://doi.org/10.1080/10889868.2024.2375204

Pedrosa, M., Ribeiro, R. S., Guerra-Rodríguez, S., Rodríguez-Chueca, J., Rodríguez, E., Silva, A. M. T., Đolic, M., and Rita Lado Ribeiro, A. (2022). *Spirulina*-based carbon bio-sorbent for the efficient removal of metoprolol, diclofenac and other micropollutants from wastewater. *Environmental Nanotechnology, Monitoring & Management 18*, 100720. https://doi.org/10.1016/j.enmm.2022.100720

Peña-Guzmán, C., Ulloa-Sánchez, S., Mora, K., Helena-Bustos, R., López-Barrera, E., Álvarez, J., and Rodríguez-Pinzón, M. (2019). Emerging pollutants in the urban water cycle in Latin America: A review of the current literature. *Journal of Environmental Management 237*, 408–423. https://doi.org/10.1016/j.jenvman.2019.02.100

Peng, F. Q., Ying, G. G., Yang, B., Liu, S., Lai, H. J., Liu, Y. S., Chen, Z. F., and Zhou, G. J. (2014). Biotransformation of progesterone and norgestrel by two freshwater microalgae (*Scenedesmus obliquus* and *Chlorella pyrenoidosa*): Transformation kinetics and products identification. *Chemosphere 95*, 581–588. https://doi.org/10.1016/J.CHEMOSPHERE.2013.10.013

Peng, Z., Wu, F., and Deng, N. (2006). Photodegradation of bisphenol A in simulated lake water containing algae, humic acid and ferric ions. *Environmental Pollution 144*(3), 840–846. https://doi.org/10.1016/j.envpol.2006.02.006

Petrović, M., Hernando, M. D., Díaz-Cruz, M. S., Barceló, D. (2005). Liquid Chromatography-Tandem mass spectrometry for the analysis of pharmaceutical residues in environmental samples: A review. *Journal of Chromatography A 1067*(1–2), 1–14. https://doi.org/10.1016/j.chroma.2004.10.110.

Pham, V. H. T., Kim, J., Chang, S., and Chung, W. (2022). Bacterial biosorbents, an efficient heavy metals green clean-up strategy: Prospects, challenges, and opportunities. *Microorganisms 10*(3), 610. https://doi.org/10.3390/MICROORGANISMS10030610

Pogrzeba, J., and Poliwoda, A. (2024). Biosorption ability of pharmaceutically active compounds by *Anabaena* sp. and *Chroococcidiopsis thermalis*. *Molecules 29*(18), 4488. https://doi.org/10.3390/molecules29184488

Rahman, K. M. (2020). Food and high value products from microalgae: Market opportunities and challenges. In Alam, M., Xu, J. L. and Wang, Z. (Eds.) *Microalgae Biotechnology for Food, Health and High Value Products* (3–27). Springer. https://doi.org/10.1007/978-981-15-0169-2_1

Rahmani, F., Sajjadi, N., Dehghani, M. H., and Zaeimdar, M. (2024). Modelling and optimization of nonylphenol biosorption by novel low-cost magnetic *Chlorella vulgaris*. *Emerging Contaminants 10*(3), 100310. https://doi.org/10.1016/j.emcon.2024.100310

Rajamani, S., Siripornadulsil, S., Falcao, V., Torres, M., Colepicolo, P., and Sayre, R. (2007). Phycoremediation of heavy metals using transgenic microalgae. In León, R., Galván, A., and Fernández, E. (Eds.) *Transgenic Microalgae as Green Cell Factories. Advances in Experimental Medicine and Biology* (99–109). Springer. https://doi.org/10.1007/978-0-387-75532-8_9

Rakic, I., Kevresan, Z., Kovac, R., Kravic, S., Svircev, Z., Djurovic, A., and Stojanovic, Z. (2023). Bioaccumulation and biosorption study of heavy metals removal by cyanobacteria *Nostoc* sp. *Chemical Industry & Chemical Engineering Quarterly 29*(4), 291–298. https://doi.org/10.2298/CICEQ220511002R

Ramesh, B., Saravanan, A., Senthil Kumar, P., Yaashikaa, P. R., Thamarai, P., Shaji, A., and Rangasamy, G. (2023). A review on algae biosorption for the removal of hazardous pollutants from wastewater: Limiting factors, prospects and recommendations. *Environmental Pollution 327*, 121572. https://doi.org/10.1016/j.envpol.2023.121572

Reynoso-Cuevas, L, Torres-Castañón, L. A., Irigoyen-Campuzano, J. R., and Alarcón-Herrera, M. T. (2020). Contaminantes emergentes (CE), presencia en el agua, identificación y riesgo para la salud. In Santacruz de León, G., and Alarcón-Herrera, M. T. (Eds.) *Contaminantes emergentes en agua en México* (1–12). El Colegio de San Luis.

Ribeiro, A. C., Martins Moreira, W., Bruguer Ferri, B., dos Federici Santos, D., Neves Olsen Scaliante, M. H., de da Costa Neves Fernandes Almeida Duarte, E., and Bergamasco, R. (2024). Ibuprofen removal by modified natural zeolite: Characterization, modeling, and adsorption mechanisms. *Journal of Chemical Technology & Biotechnology 99*(11), 2407–2419. https://doi.org/10.1002/jctb.7729

Rios-Miguel, A. B., Smith, G. J., Cremers, G., van Alen, T., Jetten, M. S. M., Op den Camp, H. J. M., and Welte, C. U. (2022). Microbial paracetamol degradation involves a high diversity of novel amidase enzyme candidates. *Water Research X 16*, 100152. https://doi.org/10.1016/j.wroa.2022.100152

Rocheleau, H., Al-harthi, R., and Ouellet, T. (2019). Degradation of salicylic acid by *Fusarium graminearum*. *Fungal Biology 123*(1), 77–86. https://doi.org/10.1016/j.funbio.2018.11.002

Roshanfekr, L., Irani, M., Pourahmad, H., Sadegh, M., and Haririan, I. (2014). Simultaneous degradation of phenol and paracetamol during photo-Fenton process: Design and optimization. *Journal of the Taiwan Institute of Chemical Engineers 47*, 190–196. https://doi.org/10.1016/j.jtice.2014.10.014

Roy, D., Greenlaw, P. N., and Shane, B. S. (1993). Adsorption of heavy metals by green algae and ground rice hulls. *Journal of Environmental Science and Health, Part A 28*(1), 37–50. https://doi.org/10.1080/10934529309375861

Ryan, K. J. (2018). *Sherris Medical Microbiology*. McGraw-Hill Education LLC.

Sachu, M., Kynshi, B. L., and Syiem, M. B. (2023). Cyanobacterial degradation of herbicide 2,4-dichlorophenoxyacetic acid (2,4-D): Its response to the oxidative stress induced by the primary degradation product 2,4-dichlorophenol (2,4–DCP). *Comparative Biochemistry and Physiology Part C 273*, 109739. https://doi.org/10.1016/j.cbpc.2023.109739

Sandoval, M.A., Calzadilla, W., Vidal, J., Brillas, E., and Salazar-González, R. (2024). Contaminants of emerging concern: Occurrence, analytical techniques, and removal with electrochemical advanced oxidation processes with special emphasis in Latin America. *Environmental Pollution 345*, 123397. https://doi.org/10.1016/j.envpol.2024.123397.

Santaeufemia, S., Torres, E., and Abalde, J. (2018). Biosorption of ibuprofen from aqueous solution using living and dead biomass of the microalga *Phaeodactylum tricornutum*. *Journal of Applied Phycology 30*(1), 471–482. https://doi.org/10.1007/s10811-017-1273-5

Saravanan, A., Kumar, P. S., Varjani, S., Jeevanantham, S., Yaashikaa, P. R., Thamarai, P., Abirami, B., and George, C. S. (2021). A review on algal-bacterial symbiotic system for effective treatment of wastewater. *Chemosphere 271*, 129540. https://doi.org/10.1016/j.chemosphere.2021.129540

Scaria, J., Gopinath, A., and Nidheesh, P. V. (2021). A versatile strategy to eliminate emerging contaminants from the aqueous environment: Heterogeneous Fenton process. *Journal of Cleaner Production 278*, 124014. https://doi.org/10.1016/j.jclepro.2020.124014

Scott, C., Pandey, G., Hartley, C. J., Jackson, C. J., Cheesman, M. J., Taylor, M. C., Pandey, R., Khurana, J. L., Teese, M., Coppin, C. W., Weir, K. M., Jain, R. K., Lal, R., Russell, R. J., and Oakeshott, J. G. (2008). The enzymatic basis for pesticide bioremediation. *Indian Journal of Microbiology 48*(1), 65–79. https://doi.org/10.1007/s12088-008-0007-4

Shabana, E., Senousy, H., and Khourshid, E. (2019). Pharmaceutical wastewater treatment using free and immobilized cyanobacteria. *Egyptian Journal of Phycology 20*(1), 123–154.

Sharma, S., Mishra, A., Priyanka, and Singh, S. S. (2024). Redox cycle: Signaling and metabolic cross-talks in cyanobacteria. In Mishra, A K. and Singh, S. S. (Eds.) *Cyanobacteria Metabolisms to Molecules. Progress in Biochemistry and Biotechnology* (177–214). Elsevier. https://doi.org/10.1016/B978-0-443-13231-5.00011-8

Sharma, S., Singh, B., and Gupta, V. K. (2014). Assessment of imidacloprid degradation by soil-isolated *Bacillus alkalinitrilicus*. *Environmental Monitoring and Assessment 186*(11), 7183–7193.

Shi, X., Yeap, T. S., Huang, S., Chen, J., and Ng, H. Y. (2018). Pretreatment of saline antibiotic wastewater using marine microalga. *Bioresource Technology 258*, 240–246. https://doi.org/10.1016/j.biortech.2018.02.110

Shin, E. H., Choi, H. T., and Song, H. G. (2007). Biodegradation of endocrine-disrupting bisphenol A by white rot fungus *Irpex lacteus*. *Journal of Microbiology and Biotechnology 17*(7), 1147–1151. https://www.jmb.or.kr/journal/view.html?volume=17andnumber=7andspage=1147

Singh, B., Kaur, J., and Singh, K. (2012). Biodegradation of malathion by *Brevibacillus* sp. strain KB2 and *Bacillus cereus* strain PU. *World Journal of Microbiology and Biotechnology 28*(3), 1133–1141.

Singh, D. P., Khattar, J. I. S., Nadda, J., Singh, Y., Garg, A., Kaur, N., and Gulati, A. (2011). Chlorpyrifos degradation by the cyanobacterium *Synechocystis* sp. strain PUPCCC 64. *Environmental Science and Pollution Research 18*(8), 1351–1359. https://doi.org/10.1007/s11356-011-0472-x

Singh, S., Kant, C., Yadav, R. K., Reddy, Y. P., and Abraham, G. (2019). Cyanobacterial exopolysaccharides: Composition, biosynthesis, and biotechnological applications. In Mishra, A. K., Tiwari, D. N. and Rai, A. N. (Eds.) *Cyanobacteria. From Basic Science to Applications* (347–358). Elsevier. https://doi.org/10.1016/B978-0-12-814667-5.00017-9

Sirois, C., Couture, J., and Grégoire, J. P. (2012). Acetylsalicylic acid for primary prevention of cardiovascular diseases in older patients with diabetes: Do the benefits overcome the risks? *Therapeutic Advances in Drug Safety 3*(5), 213–226. https://doi.org/10.1177/2042098612451267

Smiljani, D., Gennaro, B. De, Izzo, F., Langella, A., Dakovi, A., Germinario, C., Rottinghaus, G. E., and Spasojevi, M. (2020). Removal of emerging contaminants from water by zeolite-rich composites: A first approach aiming at diclofenac and ketoprofen. *Microporous and Mesoporous Materials 298*, 110057298. https://doi.org/10.1016/j.micromeso.2020.110057

Soares, P. R. S., Birolli, W. G., Ferreira, I. M., and Porto, A. L. M. (2021). Biodegradation pathway of the organophosphate pesticides chlorpyrifos, methyl parathion and profenofos by the marine-derived fungus *Aspergillus sydowii* CBMAI 935 and its potential for methylation reactions of phenolic compounds. *Marine Pollution Bulletin 166*, 112185. https://doi.org/10.1016/j.marpolbul.2021.112185

Sonali, J. M. I., and Gayathri Krishnaswamy, V. (2023). Use of microalgae for the removal of emerging contaminants from wastewater. In Shah, M. P. and Boston, B. (Eds.) *Microbial Degradation and Detoxification of Pollutants* (189–204). De Gruyter. https://doi.org/10.1515/9783110743623-009

Stal, L. J. (2007). Cyanobacteria: Diversity and versatility, clues to life in extreme environments. In Seckbach, J. (ed). *Algae and Cyanobacteria in Extreme Environments* (661–680). Springer.

Streit, A. F. M., Collazzo, G. C., Druzian, S. P., Verdi, R. S., Foletto, E. L., Oliveira, L. F. S., and Dotto, G. L. (2021). Adsorption of ibuprofen, ketoprofen, and paracetamol onto activated carbon prepared from effluent treatment plant sludge of the beverage industry. *Chemosphere 262*, 128322. https://doi.org/10.1016/j.chemosphere.2020.128322

Suarez, S., Lema, J. M., and Omil, F. (2009). Technology pre-treatment of hospital wastewater by coagulation – flocculation and flotation. *Bioresource Technology 100*(7), 2138–2146. https://doi.org/10.1016/j.biortech.2008.11.015

Suárez-Martínez, D., Angulo-Mercado, E., Mercado-Martínez, I., Vacca-Jimeno, V., Tapia-Larios, C., and Cubillán, N. (2022). Enhanced tetracycline removal from highly concentrated aqueous media by lipid-free *Chlorella* sp. biomass. *ACS Omega 7*(16), 14128–14137. https://doi.org/10.1021/acsomega.2c00696

Sun, X.-L., Wang, Y., Xiong, H.-Q., Wang, S.-T., Fang, Y.-C., and Xiang, H. (2023). Removal of environmental estrogens from wastewater by microalgae under the influence of bacteria. *Journal of Cleaner Production 414*, 137635. https://doi.org/10.1016/j.jclepro.2023.137635

Sutherland, D. L., and Ralph, P. J. (2019). Microalgal bioremediation of emerging contaminants - Opportunities and challenges. *Water Research 164*, 114921. https://doi.org/10.1016/j.watres.2019.114921

Tamagnini, P., Axelsson, R., Lindberg, P., Oxelfelt, F., Wünschiers, R., and Lindblad, P. (2002). Hydrogenases and hydrogen metabolism of cyanobacteria. *Microbiology and Molecular Biology Reviews 66*(1), 1–20. https://doi.org/10.1128/MMBR.66.1.1-20.2002

Thakur, A., Sharma, N., and Mann, A. (2020). Removal of ofloxacin hydrochloride and paracetamol from aqueous solutions: Binary mixtures and competitive adsorption. *Materials Today: Proceedings 28*, 1514–1519. https://doi.org/10.1016/j.matpr.2020.04.833

Tiwari, B., Chakraborty, S., Srivastava, A. K., and Mishra, A. K. (2017). Biodegradation and rapid removal of methyl parathion by the paddy field cyanobacterium *Fischerella* sp. *Algal Research 25*, 285–296. https://doi.org/10.1016/j.algal.2017.05.024

Torán, J., Blánquez, P., and Caminal, G. (2017). Comparison between several reactors with *Trametes versicolor* immobilized on lignocellulosic support for the continuous treatments of hospital wastewater. *Bioresource Technology 243*, 966–974. https://doi.org/10.1016/j.biortech.2017.07.055

Touliabah, H. E. S., El-Sheekh, M. M., Ismail, M. M., and El-Kassas, H. (2022). A Review of microalgae- and cyanobacteria-based biodegradation of organic pollutants. *Molecules 27*(3), 1141. https://doi.org/10.3390/molecules27031141

Ulloa-Ovares, D., Rodríguez-Rodríguez, C. E., Masís-Mora, M., and Durán, J. E. (2021). Simultaneous degradation of pharmaceuticals in fixed and fluidized bed reactors using iron-modified diatomite as heterogeneous Fenton catalyst. 152, 97–107. *Process Safety and Environmental Protection|Journal 152*, 97–107 https://doi.org/10.1016/j.psep.2021.05.032

Vaishnav, P., and Demain, A. L. (2009). Industrial Biotechnology, (overview). In Schaechter, M. (Ed.) *Encyclopedia of Microbiology. Third Edition* (335–348). Academic Press. https://doi.org/10.1016/B978-012373944-5.00150-4

Vaksmaa, A., Guerrero-Cruz, S., Ghosh, P., Zeghal, E., Hernando-Morales, V., and Niemann, H. (2023). Role of fungi in bioremediation of emerging pollutants. *Frontiers in Marine Science 10*, 1070905.

Van Der Wal, A., Norde, W., Zehnder, A. J. B., and Lyklema, J. (1997). Determination of the total charge in the cell walls of Gram-positive bacteria. *Colloids and Surfaces B: Biointerfaces|Journal 9*(1–2), 81–100. https://doi.org/10.1016/S0927-7765(96)01340-9

Vargas-Berrones, K., Bernal-Jácome, L., Díaz de León-Martínez, L., and Flores-Ramírez, R. (2020). Emerging Pollutants (EPs) in Latin América: A critical review of under-studied EPs, case of study -nonylphenol. *Science of the Total Environment 726*, 138493. https://doi.org/10.1016/j.scitotenv.2020.138493.

Vasiliadou, I. A., Molina, R., Pariente, M. I., Christoforidis, K. C., Martinez, F., and Melero, J. A. (2019). Understanding the role of mediators in the efficiency of advanced oxidation processes using white-rot fungi. *Chemical Engineering Journal 359*, 1427–1435. https://doi.org/10.1016/j.cej.2018.11.035

Velichkova, F. A., Julcour-Lebigue, C., Delmas, H., Velichkova, F. A., Julcour-Lebigue, C., Koumanova, B., and Hetero -, H. D. (2022). Heterogeneous Fenton oxidation of paracetamol using iron oxide (nano) particles. *Journal of Environmental Chemical Engineering 1*(4), 1214–1222. https://doi.org/10.1016/j.jece.2013.09.011

Verma, S., and Kuila, A. (2019). Bioremediation of heavy metals by microbial process. *Environmental Technology & Innovation 14*, 100369. https://doi.org/10.1016/j.eti.2019.100369

Vieira, L. R., Soares, A. M. V. M., and Freitas, R. (2022). Caffeine as a contaminant of concern: A review on concentrations and impacts in marine coastal systems. *Chemosphere 286*, 131675. https://doi.org/10.1016/j.chemosphere.2021.131675

Vijaya Kumar, V. (2017). Mycoremediation: A step toward cleaner environment. In Prasad, R. (Ed.) *Mycoremediation and environmental sustainability. Fungal biology* (171–187) Springer. https://doi.org/10.1007/978-3-319-68957-9_10

Vijayaraghavan, K., and Yun, Y. S. (2008). Bacterial biosorbents and biosorption. *Biotechnology Advances 26*(3), 266–291. https://doi.org/10.1016/J.BIOTECHADV.2008.02.002

Volk, T. J. (2013). Fungi. In Levin, S. A. (Ed.) *Encyclopedia of Biodiversity* (624–640). Elsevier. https://doi.org/10.1016/B978-0-12-384719-5.00062-9

Vos, J. G., Dybing, E., Greim, H. A., Ladefoged, O., Lambré, C., Tarazona, J. V., Brandt, I., and Vethaak, A. D. (2000). Health effects of endocrine-disrupting chemicals on wildlife, with special reference to the European situation. *Critical Reviews in Toxicology 30*(1), 71–133. https://doi.org/10.1080/10408440091159176

Walker, D. H., and McGinnis, M. R. (2014). Diseases caused by fungi. In McManus, L. M. and Mitchell, R. N. (Eds.) *Pathobiology of Human Disease. A Dynamic Encyclopedia of Disease Mechanisms* (217–221). Elsevier. https://doi.org/10.1016/B978-0-12-386456-7.01710-X

Wang, C., Yu, L., Zhang, Z., Wang, B., and Sun, H. (2014). Tourmaline combined with *Phanerochaete chrysosporium* to remediate agricultural soil contaminated with PAHs and OCPs. *Journal of Hazardous Materials 264*, 439–448. https://doi.org/10.1016/j.jhazmat.2013.10.073

Wang, F., Wang, C., Du, X., Li, Y., Wang, F., and Wang, P. (2022). Efficient removal of emerging organic contaminants via photo-Fenton process over micron-sized Fe-MOF sheet. *Chemical Engineering Journal 429*, 132495. https://doi.org/10.1016/j.cej.2021.132495

Wang, S., and Peng, Y. (2010). Natural zeolites as effective adsorbents in water and wastewater treatment. *Chemical Engineering Journal 156*(1), 11–24. https://doi.org/10.1016/j.cej.2009.10.029

White, M. F. (2020). Salicylic acid for face (facial salicylic acid peel). In Costa, A. (Ed.) *Minimally Invasive Aesthetic Procedures* (121–126). Springer International Publishing. https://doi.org/10.1007/978-3-319-78265-2_18

Xiong, P., Zhang, H., Li, G., Liao, C., and Jiang, G. (2021). Adsorption removal of ibuprofen and naproxen from aqueous solution with Cu-doped Mil-101(Fe). *Science of the Total Environment 797*, 149179. https://doi.org/10.1016/j.scitotenv.2021.149179

Xu, A., Zhang, X., Wu, S., Xu, N., Huang, Y., Yan, X., Zhou, J., Cui, Z., and Dong, W. (2021). Pollutant degrading enzyme: Catalytic mechanisms and their expanded applications. *Molecules 26*(16), 4751. https://doi.org/10.3390/molecules26164751

Yang, F., Jacobsen, S., Jørgensen, H. J. L., Collinge, D. B., Svensson, B., and Finnie, C. (2013). *Fusarium graminearum* and its interactions with cereal heads: Studies in the proteomics era. *Frontiers in Plant Science 4*(37), 1–8. https://doi.org/10.3389/fpls.2013.00037

Yang, J., Cao, J., Xing, G., and Yuan, H. (2015). Lipid production combined with biosorption and bioaccumulation of cadmium, copper, manganese and zinc by oleaginous microalgae *Chlorella minutissima* UTEX2341. *Bioresource Technology 175*, 537–544. https://doi.org/10.1016/j.biortech.2014.10.124

Yannarell, A. C., and Kent, A. D. (2009). Bacteria, Distribution and community structure. In Likens G. E. (Ed.) *Encyclopedia of Inland Waters* (201–210). Elsevier. https://doi.org/10.1016/B978-012370626-3.00123-X

Zhang, H., Zhang, Y., Hou, Z., Wu, X., Gao, H., Sun, F., and Pan, H. (2014). Biodegradation of triazine herbicide metribuzin by the strain *Bacillus* sp. N1. *Journal of Environmental Science and Health Part B 49*(2), 79–86. https://doi.org/10.1080/03601234.2014.844610

Zhao, D. S., Farooq, M. A., Li, M., Chen, Y.-T., Xu, J.-M., Liu, X. L., Zhang, A., Yan, X., Zou, H. X., and Pang, Q. (2024). Acute toxicity of salicylic acid and its derivatives on the diatom *Phaeodactylum tricornutum*: Physico-Biochemical and transcriptomic insights. *Aquatic Toxicology 276*, 107116. https://doi.org/10.1016/j.aquatox.2024.107116

Zhao, Z., Shao, S., Liu, N., Liu, Q., Jacquemyn, H., and Xing, X. (2021). Extracellular enzyme activities and carbon/nitrogen utilization in mycorrhizal fungi isolated from epiphytic and terrestrial orchids. *Frontiers in Microbiology 12*, 787820.

Zhou, G.-J., Peng, F.-Q., Zhang, L.-J., and Ying, G.-G. (2012). Biosorption of zinc and copper from aqueous solutions by two freshwater green microalgae *Chlorella pyrenoidosa* and *Scenedesmus obliquus*. *Environmental Science and Pollution Research 19*(7), 2918–2929. https://doi.org/10.1007/s11356-012-0800-9

Zhou, X., and Li, Y. (2015). Basic Biology of Oral Microbes. In Zhou, X. and Li. Y. (Eds.) *Atlas of Oral Microbiology. From Healthy Microflora to Disease* (1–14). Academic Press. https://doi.org/10.1016/b978-0-12-802234-4.00001-x

3 Fungal biorefinery and bioprocessing
Advanced strategies for waste valorization

Damián Reyes-Jáquez, Itza Nallely Cordero-Soto, Sergio Valle-Cervantes, María Dolores Josefina Rodríguez-Rosales, and María Gorety Contreras-Hernández

3.1 INTRODUCTION

Fungal biotechnology has emerged as an essential tool for addressing global problems such as waste management, sustainable biomass production, and generating high-value-added compounds (Wikandari, Hasniah, and Taherzadeh 2022). These microorganisms, with their metabolic diversity and ability to grow in a wide range of conditions, are ideal for using agro-industrial waste as a substrate and transforming it into products such as enzymes, biofuels, pigments, single-cell proteins, and other secondary metabolites (Patel et al. 2023; Chavan et al. 2022; Melnichuk et al. 2020; Lin and Xu 2022; Behera 2020).

Among the cultivation strategies are solid fermentation (SSF) and liquid-state fermentation (SmF). SSF, which uses solid substrates with low water content, allows the efficient use of lignocellulosic residues and other agricultural waste (Lizardi-Jiménez and Hernández-Martínez 2017), while SmF is suitable to produce extracellular metabolites and soluble compounds (Iram et al. 2022). When combined with advanced bioreactors, these processes allow production to be scaled and conditions to be optimized to maximize performance and efficiency.

Scaling and process optimization are essential to guarantee the industrial viability of these systems (Palladino et al. 2024). This involves designing and implementing specialized bioreactors that allow control of critical parameters such as pH, temperature, dissolved oxygen, and agitation. Furthermore, integrating these technologies in biorefineries allows the conversion of renewable biomass into multiple products of industrial interest, promoting a circular economy model that minimizes waste and maximizes economic value (J.-J. Zhong 2011; Mitchell et al. 2006).

The valorization of agro-industrial waste as substrates not only addresses the problem of waste accumulation but also reduces production costs by using economic and abundant raw materials (Häder 2021; Ferrero et al. 2024; Melnichuk et al. 2020). This approach reinforces the sustainability of biotechnological processes by offering ecological alternatives for producing chemicals, bioenergy, and functional foods (Wikandari, Hasniah, and Taherzadeh 2022).

Information on the application of fungi in various industries, especially those derived from by-products, must be improved in certain aspects, particularly regarding their nutritional value and safety considerations. This context underlines the importance of delving into the capabilities of fungal-based biorefineries, which take advantage of different species to produce a wide range of valuable products. This analysis covers industrial applications and techno-economic evaluations, highlighting the viability and sustainability of processes that use fungi as crucial agents.

DOI: 10.1201/9781003500483-3
This chapter has been made available under a (CC-BY-NC-ND) 4.0 license

3.2 THE IMPORTANCE OF FUNGI IN NATURE

Fungi are eukaryotic organisms belonging to the fungi kingdom. They have a wide diversity of shapes, sizes, and habitats. The diversity of fungi is estimated at 13.2 million, but only between 3.5 and 5.1 million are documented worldwide (Hawksworth and Lücking 2017). Fungi are essential in global ecology since they play critical roles in the decomposition of organic matter (lignin, cellulose, and hemicellulose, among others), symbiosis with plants (mycorrhizae), production of bioactive compounds (secondary metabolites, enzymes, and bioactive compounds), degradation or transformation of toxic agents (bioaccumulation, biotransformation of heavy metals), and applications in biorefinery (enzymes) which currently makes them indispensable in industry and the biotechnological (Mokhtarian et al. 2020; Pushparaj et al. 2023; Ayangbenro and Babalola 2017; Prajapati et al. 2024; De Paula et al. 2022; Kijpornyongpan et al. 2022).

These microorganisms are peculiar and have specific characteristics that distinguish them from other organisms. In general, they tend to be eukaryotic heterotrophic; they have a cell wall made of chitin (a very resistant polysaccharide), their reproduction is by spores (asexual or sexual), and they usually reproduce in a multicellular way in the form of filamentous (molds or mushrooms) or unicellular (yeast) (Mueller and Schmit 2007).

Fungi can develop in diverse environments, from soil, plants, and decaying wood to extreme environments such as deserts, deep waters, or places contaminated with different toxic agents, such as heavy metals (Patel et al. 2023; De Paula et al. 2022; Kijpornyongpan et al. 2022). This is possible thanks to its ability to digest different types of organic matter and its tolerance to different pH levels, temperature, and humidity. The classification of fungi nowadays is extensive, thanks to the advances in molecular biology, allowing a better understanding of their evolutionary relationships. There are several main types, generally about their reproductive and genetic structure: *Chytridiomycota*, *Zygomycota* (*Rhizopus stolonifer*), *Ascomycota* (*Saccharomyces cerevisiae* and *Penicillium*), *Basidiomycota* (mushrooms), *Glomeromycota* (usually symbiotic) and *Deuteromycota*. This classification continues to evolve as new molecular techniques are investigated (Mattedi et al. 2023).

Fungi have an impact on the environment and the health of animals and humans, causing severe diseases to plant, animals, and human with pathogens such as *Puccinia gramini*, *Aspergillus fumigatus,* and *Candida albicans* (Bhabhra and Askew 2005; Aguirre-Acosta et al. 2014). On the other hand, other mushrooms have impacted society due to their culinary traditions, where diverse cultures highly appreciate some edible mushrooms (Royse, Baars, and Tan 2017). Research in mycology is constantly expanding, revealing new species, properties, and applications that underline the importance and complexity of these microorganisms (Mueller and Schmit 2007; Patel et al. 2023).

3.3 FUNGAL GROWTH STRATEGIES

The most common culture strategies for fungal propagation are solid-state fermentation (SSF) and liquid-state fermentation (SmF) utilizing specialized bioreactors. Depending on the target bioprocess and fungi's metabolic behavior, these systems present several advantages and limitations.

3.3.1 Liquid-state fermentation

The SmF is a cultivation technique characterized by using a growth medium for microorganisms with a humidity content of more than 95%, where nutrients and oxygen are dissolved, allowing greater control of the parameters. SmF is widely used to produce enzymes and pharmaceuticals with different microorganisms (El Enshasy 2022).

This technique is particularly valuable for propagating bacteria and yeasts and specifically for some filamentous fungal cultures since the culture conditions (pH, temperature, agitation, and oxygen concentration) can be precisely controlled, generating high production efficiency. Compared

TABLE 3.1
Comparative studies on solid-state and submerged fermentation using fungi

Microorganism	Fermentation	Substrate	Product	References
Trichoderma reesei	*SmF*	Sugarcane bagasse	Cellulases	Bischof, Ramoni, and Seiboth (2016)
Rhizopus oryzae		Coconut water	Organic acids	Skory (2004)
Fusarium oxysporum		Whey	Fungal biomass	Chavan et al. (2022)
Aspergillus terreus		Apple by-products	Itaconic acid	Teleky and Vodnar (2021)
Mucor circinelloides		Tomato pulp	Fatty acids	Tauk-Tornisielo et al. (2009)
Ganoderma lucidum		Rice bran	Exopolysaccharides	Feng et al. (2019)
Aspergillus fumigatus		Corn cob residues	Biofuels	García-Torreiro et al. (2016)
Aspergillus niger		Metal-contaminated soil	Cadmium and lead bioremediation	Qader, Muzhda and Shekha (2023)
Aspergillus niger	SSF	Citrus pulp	Pectinolytic enzymes	Bai et al. (2004)
Penicillium chrysogenum		Potato residues	Antibiotics	Devi et al. (2020)
Aspergillus oryzae		Rice husk	Citric acid	Behera (2020)
Pleurotus ostreatus		Corn stover	Ligninolytic enzymes	Olagunju et al. (2023)
Penicillium citrinum		Wheat bran	Alkaline proteases	Germano et al. (2003); Pawar, Singh, and Singh (2023)
Trichoderma harzianum		Sugarcane bagasse	Exopolysaccharides	F. Zhang et al. (2013)
Phanerochaete chrysosporium		Wood residues	Heavy metal bioremediation	Harms, Schlosser, and Wick (2011)

to SSF, higher yields are achieved in less time. Additionally, the process is simpler to scale for commercial applications (Iram et al. 2022).

One of the main applications of fungi with SmF is the production of organic acids used in the food and pharmaceutical industries. *Aspergillus niger* has produced considerable concentrations of citric acid, while *Aspergillus terreus* has stood out in the production of itaconic acid. Other products, such as bioethanol, have been obtained with *Aspergillus fumigatus* and Saccharomyces cerevisiae from agricultural waste (Khurshid et al. 2024; Yang, Lübeck, and Lübeck 2017; Ingale, Joshi, and Gupte 2014).

Despite its advantages, SmF leads to higher production costs, increased energy consumption, and lower productivity compared to SSF (El Enshasy 2022). Nonetheless, its capability to produce specific metabolites in large volumes makes this technique crucial for developing commercial fungal-based products (Iram et al. 2022) (Table 3.1).

3.3.2 Solid-state fermentation

SSF is an innovative bioprocessing technique that employs solid substrates to support fungal growth, offering numerous advantages over traditional submerged fermentation methods. One of the primary benefits of SSF is its ability to achieve higher product concentrations, which can significantly enhance the overall efficiency of the bioconversion process. This is largely due to the lower water content in the solid substrates, which reduces the need for large volumes of water typically required in liquid-state fermentation, thus lowering both energy consumption and downstream processing costs (J. Zhang and Zhang 2016; Pallín et al. 2024).

Furthermore, SSF presents a unique opportunity for the valorization of agricultural residues, such as apple pomace, sugarcane bagasse, and other lignocellulosic waste materials. These residues are typically abundant in cellulose, hemicellulose, and other complex organic compounds, making them ideal candidates for bioconversion into valuable products. By utilizing fungi in SSF, these agricultural by-products can be efficiently transformed into high-value metabolites, including enzymes, biofuels, antibiotics, aromas, pigments, biosurfactants, and organic acids, while simultaneously reducing waste and promoting sustainability (Pushparaj et al. 2023; Couder-García et al. 2024; Gómez Sánchez, Martínez-Trujillo, and Aguilar Osorio 2012).

Research has shown that SSF not only facilitates the breakdown of complex lignocellulosic materials but also contributes to improving the nutritional quality of agricultural residues. For example, fungal fermentation has been demonstrated to reduce the crude fiber content in these residues, making them more digestible and nutritionally beneficial for both animal feed and human consumption. Additionally, SSF enhances the bioavailability of certain nutrients, further improving the overall value of the processed material (Ben Hmad and Gargouri 2024; Gómez Sánchez, Martínez-Trujillo, and Aguilar Osorio 2012; Pallín et al. 2024; Upadhyay et al. 2023). This dual benefit waste valorization and nutritional enhancement highlights the potential of SSF as a sustainable and economically viable technology for the efficient processing of agricultural residues.

One of the most used fungal genera in SSF includes *Aspergillus* and *Trichoderma* due to their exceptional ability to thrive in adverse conditions such as low moisture levels and high substrate concentration (Ibarruri et al. 2021). However, other fungi have also demonstrated promising metabolic capabilities for producing valuable bioproducts (Table 3.1).

3.4 CHALLENGES IN FUNGAL BIOPROCESSES USING SUBMERGED AND SOLID-STATE FERMENTATIONS

Fungal bioprocesses harness the metabolic capabilities of fungi to efficiently convert lignocellulosic biomass and other organic residues into valuable products. The effectiveness of these processes is largely determined by the design of the bioreactor, which must be tailored to accommodate the unique growth characteristics of filamentous fungi. Unlike yeast or bacterial cultures, filamentous fungi exhibit complex growth patterns that can pose significant challenges for conventional reactor systems.

The growth of filamentous fungi has been evaluated using liquid-state fermentation and SSF to obtain sustainable products such as enzymes, pigments, and bioactive compounds from agro-industrial residues through biorefineries and circular bioeconomy strategies (Palladino et al. 2024; Couder-García et al. 2024).

Traditional submerged bioreactor designs, such as stirred-tank reactors (STRs), often struggle to optimize oxygen transfer and maintain suitable shear conditions for filamentous organisms. These challenges are particularly problematic due to the delicate balance required to support fungal growth without damaging the hyphal network, which is crucial for efficient bioconversion (Formenti et al. 2014; Cerrone et al. 2024; Supramani et al. 2023).

In response to these limitations, the development of specialized bioreactors has gained momentum. Airlift reactors, for instance, have been proposed as promising alternatives to traditional STRs. These systems offer significant advantages, including enhanced mass transfer and reduced shear stress, which are vital for optimizing fungal growth and metabolic activity. By promoting better aeration and minimizing mechanical forces that can damage delicate fungal filaments, these advanced bioreactor designs enable more efficient and scalable bioprocesses (Wei et al. 2017; Pallín et al. 2024; Ferreira, Lennartsson, and Taherzadeh 2015). Such innovations are crucial for overcoming the inherent challenges of scaling fungal bioprocesses for industrial applications and unlocking their full potential for sustainable bioconversion.

Conversely, reactors designed for SSF have overcome growth limitations caused by mechanical hyphae damage on submerged bioreactors. The most used bioreactors for SSF culture include fluidized bed bioreactor, rotating drum bioreactor, tray-based bioreactor, and packed-bed bioreactor (Gómez Sánchez, Martínez-Trujillo, and Aguilar Osorio 2012). Bioreactors for SSF have been developed for waste revalorization from the food industry, including bagasse, fruit peels and seeds, and lignocellulosic residues (Palladino et al. 2024; Couder-García et al. 2024).

Food residues considerably reduce the culture media cost since these residues are generally free or available at a low cost. Additionally, the configuration of solid bioreactors requires less water and energy consumption than STRs reactors. Nevertheless, one of the leading design challenges in these systems is related to heat transfer and aeration control since there are transition zones where these conditions cannot be controlled, causing heterogeneous fungal growth (Couder-García et al. 2024; Gómez Sánchez, Martínez-Trujillo, and Aguilar Osorio 2012). Other limitations include substrate sterilization, inoculum standardization, and the lack of information related to operational conditions and their influence on transport phenomena that impact fungal growth behavior (Palladino et al. 2024; Gómez-Ramos et al. 2025).

3.5 SCALE-UP TO OVERCOME FUNGAL GROWTH LIMITATIONS

Scaling up fungal bioprocesses from laboratory-scale experiments to industrial-scale operations presents a host of complex challenges, many of which stem from the need to maintain consistent process parameters and ensure uniformity in fungal growth throughout the larger system. As the scale of the bioreactor increases, the behavior of fungal cultures can undergo significant changes, particularly in terms of their morphology, growth patterns, and metabolic activity. These variations can have a profound impact on key factors such as mass transfer, nutrient availability, and overall process efficiency (Supramani et al. 2023; Wang et al. 2023).

For instance, filamentous fungi often display distinct growth characteristics in smaller-scale systems, such as shake flasks, compared to larger bioreactors. In small-scale setups, fungal hyphal networks tend to form more freely, while in larger reactors, the physical and hydrodynamic conditions can lead to altered growth patterns, including clumping, pellet formation, or reduced filamentous development. These morphological differences can result in significant discrepancies in biomass concentration, oxygen transfer, and the production of metabolites, thereby affecting both the yield and quality of the desired products (Thunuguntla et al. 2018; Wang et al. 2023).

To overcome these challenges and ensure successful scale-up, it is crucial to develop a comprehensive understanding of the bioprocess kinetics involved in fungal cultivation. This includes elucidating the relationships between fungal morphology, metabolic pathways, and environmental factors such as oxygen and nutrient levels. Additionally, the creation of predictive models is essential for optimizing reactor design and operational parameters across different scales. Such models can provide valuable insights into how the fungal culture will behave under varying conditions, enabling more accurate predictions of biomass growth and product formation. By integrating these predictive tools with advanced reactor design strategies, it becomes possible to achieve greater consistency and efficiency in large-scale fungal bioprocesses, ensuring that they meet the demands of industrial applications (Farinas 2015; Pallín et al. 2024).

Regarding large-scale SSF, operational control to improve fungal growth and intensification of bioproducts requires optimal temperature to avoid fungal enzyme denaturalization and to maintain adequate moisture in the solid substrate, preventing evaporation. Bioreactor design must consider several aspects, including controlling external contamination, substrate interaction with the fungi, and operational variables such as oxygen concentration and nutrients necessary to maintain the fungal metabolism process. Moreover, since kinetic models at different levels (intrinsic, apparent, and extrinsic) to relate transport phenomena resistances on the fungal growth behavior cannot be achieved on SFF, an approximation must be realized through a regime analysis (Gómez-Ramos et al. 2025).

3.6 REACTOR DESIGN CONSIDERATIONS

The design of bioreactors for fungal cultivation requires careful consideration of several critical factors, including aeration, mixing, and temperature control, all of which are essential for promoting optimal fungal growth and maximizing product yield. Aeration in particular plays a pivotal role, as filamentous fungi have high oxygen demands to sustain their metabolic activities. Adequate oxygen supply is crucial not only for supporting cellular respiration but also for influencing the production of secondary metabolites, such as enzymes and bioactive compounds. Research has consistently demonstrated that the amount and distribution of air supplied to the bioreactor can significantly impact both fungal growth and metabolite production (Aragão et al. 2020; Bonilla Loaiza et al. 2022; Tosun and Yaşar 2020). For example, airlift bioreactors have been shown to provide superior aeration and more effective mixing compared to traditional STRs, resulting in improved cultivation conditions for edible fungi and higher yields of desirable products (Pallín et al. 2024; Ferreira, Lennartsson, and Taherzadeh 2015).

In addition to aeration, maintaining appropriate temperature and relative humidity within the bioreactor is essential for optimizing fungal growth and ensuring high product output. Filamentous fungi are particularly sensitive to environmental fluctuations, and even minor deviations from the ideal conditions can hinder their metabolic processes and reduce overall efficiency. Thus, precise control of both temperature and humidity is required to create an environment that supports the fungal culture throughout the fermentation process (Sentís-Moré et al. 2023; Antunes et al. 2017). By fine-tuning these parameters, bioreactor systems can be optimized to enhance fungal growth, metabolic activity, and the production of target bioproducts, ultimately improving the efficiency and scalability of fungal bioprocesses.

3.7 INNOVATIVE BIOREACTOR DESIGNS

Recent advancements in bioreactor technology have led to the development of innovative reactor designs that are specifically tailored to meet the unique requirements of fungal cultivation. These innovations aim to address some of the key challenges associated with traditional bioreactor systems, ultimately enhancing both the efficiency and scalability of fungal bioprocesses. One such example is the Air-L-Shaped Bioreactor (ALSB), a novel design developed to minimize common issues such as wall growth and clumping of fungal mycelium, which frequently occur in conventional STRs. These problems can hinder mass transfer, reduce oxygen availability, and compromise overall fungal growth and metabolite production. The ALSB, by contrast, offers a more uniform and controlled environment for fungal growth, promoting better aeration and preventing the formation of mycelial aggregates that can obstruct nutrient and gas exchange (Ferreira, Lennartsson, and Taherzadeh 2015; Sharma, Sharma, and Arora 2018).

Another promising advancement is the integration of membrane bioreactors (MBRs) into fungal fermentation systems. MBRs, which combine biological treatment with membrane filtration, have demonstrated significant potential in improving the efficiency of fungal fermentation processes, especially in the treatment of complex liquid residues, such as expired milk and other organic waste streams. By employing membrane filtration, MBR facilitates the continuous removal of metabolic by-products, such as excess biomass or inhibitory compounds, which can otherwise accumulate and negatively impact the growth and productivity of fungal cultures. This continuous filtration system enhances process stability, reduces downtime, and ensures the sustained operation of bioreactors key factors for scaling up fungal bioprocesses for industrial applications (Antecka et al. 2019; Blibech et al. 2011).

A wall-cooled packed-bed bioreactor used for SSF with agro-industrial residues was proposed as an innovative system to obtain enzymes and bioactive compounds. The system configuration includes a solid phase (moist solid substrate) and a fluid phase (water vapor, oxygen, and carbon dioxide). This bioreactor maintains temperature control with a water jacket as an external cooling system, favoring heat transfer and homogenous fungal growth (Gómez-Ramos et al. 2025; Couder-García et al. 2024).

3.8 OPTIMIZATION OF OPERATIONAL PARAMETERS

The optimization of operational parameters is essential for maximizing the efficiency and productivity of fungal bioprocesses. Precise control over factors such as pH, temperature, and nutrient composition is vital to creating the ideal conditions for fungal growth and metabolic activity. Variations in these parameters can significantly influence both the growth rate of the fungi and the yield of the target products, making their careful regulation a critical aspect of process optimization (Germec et al. 2017; Supramani et al. 2019; Tosun and Yaşar 2020).

For instance, the implementation of fed-batch fermentation strategies has proven to be highly effective in enhancing the production of specific enzymes, such as β-mannanase, by maintaining a steady supply of nutrients throughout the fermentation process. This approach not only helps prevent nutrient depletion but also minimizes the risk of toxic metabolite accumulation, thereby ensuring that the fungal culture remains in an active and productive state for longer periods. By continuously providing the necessary nutrients, fed-batch systems facilitate higher enzyme production rates and improved overall process yields (Gimenez et al. 2014; Cai et al. 2014).

In addition to these strategies, the use of advanced statistical and computational techniques, such as response surface methodology (RSM), has emerged as an effective tool for optimizing multiple operational parameters simultaneously. RSM allows a systematic investigation of the interactions between different factors and their effects on product yield. By applying this method, researchers can identify the optimal conditions for fungal cultivation that result in the highest production of desired metabolites, while minimizing resource consumption and process inefficiencies. This approach has been successfully employed in a range of fungal bioprocesses, leading to significant improvements in product yields and overall process performance (Meyer et al. 2021).

3.9 DOWNSTREAM PROCESSING AND PRODUCT RECOVERY

Downstream processing is a crucial phase in the bioprocessing chain, responsible for the recovery, purification, and concentration of valuable products derived from fungal cultures. The selection of appropriate downstream processing methods is vital, as it can significantly influence the overall economic viability and efficiency of bioprocess. Effective recovery techniques are essential not only for ensuring high product yield but also for minimizing costs and resource consumption, ultimately affecting the profitability of the entire process. Commonly employed methods for the recovery and purification of enzymes, bioactive compounds, and other metabolites from fungal biomass include biosorption, enzymatic degradation, and membrane filtration. These techniques are particularly well-suited for isolating target products from complex fermentation broths, where contaminants and by-products can complicate the purification process (Germec et al. 2017; Supramani et al. 2019).

Biosorption, for example, is an effective technique for the recovery of bioactive compounds, as it leverages the ability of fungal biomass to bind and concentrate valuable metabolites. Similarly, enzymatic degradation processes can be employed to break down complex organic substrates into simpler forms, facilitating the extraction of bioactive compounds such as enzymes, peptides, or polysaccharides. Membrane filtration, including microfiltration, ultrafiltration, and nanofiltration, is another commonly used method that enables the separation of larger biomass particles from the liquid phase, thereby purifying the desired products and removing unwanted contaminants (Germec et al. 2017; Supramani et al. 2019).

One notable application of fungal bioprocesses in downstream processing is the use of immobilized fungal cells within bioreactors. This approach has been shown to enhance the efficiency of specific biotransformation processes, such as dye decolorization, by increasing the stability and reusability of fungal culture. Immobilized fungal cells can be repeatedly used in environmental applications, such as wastewater treatment, where they degrade pollutants like dyes and heavy metals. This not only improves the overall efficiency of the bioprocess but also makes it more sustainable by reducing the need for constant replenishment of the fungal culture (Germec et al. 2017).

In response to these limitations, the development of specialized bioreactors has gained momentum. Airlift reactors and SSF systems, for instance, have been proposed as promising alternatives to traditional STRs. These systems offer significant advantages, including enhanced mass transfer and reduced shear stress, which are vital for optimizing fungal growth and metabolic activity. By promoting better aeration and minimizing mechanical forces that can damage delicate fungal filaments, these advanced bioreactor designs enable more efficient and scalable bioprocesses (Pallín et al. 2024; Ferreira, Lennartsson, and Taherzadeh 2015; Wei, Tang, and Lu 2017). Such innovations are crucial for overcoming the inherent challenges of scaling fungal bioprocesses for industrial applications and unlocking their full potential for sustainable bioconversion.

3.10 WASTE VALORIZATION AND CIRCULAR ECONOMY

The valorization of agricultural, industrial, and organic residues through fungal bioprocesses offers a dual benefit contributing to waste reduction while simultaneously generating economic value by transforming low-cost feedstocks into high-value products. This approach not only helps address the growing issue of waste disposal but also creates opportunities to produce valuable metabolites, such as biofuels, biochemicals, enzymes, and other specialty products. By utilizing fungal fermentation, biorefineries can convert a wide range of biomass feedstocks, including lignocellulosic waste, into sustainable products that are in high demand across various industries, from energy to pharmaceuticals (Pallín et al. 2024; Antecka et al. 2019).

The integration of fungal fermentation into biorefineries holds significant promise for the sustainable production of biofuels and biochemicals, offering a more environmentally friendly alternative to traditional chemical production methods. Fungal bioprocesses are inherently more energy-efficient and can operate under milder conditions compared to conventional chemical processes, reducing the need for harmful reagents and extreme temperatures. This makes them particularly attractive for industries aiming to shift toward greener and more sustainable practices. By utilizing renewable biomass as a feedstock and producing valuable products through biological means, these biorefinery systems contribute to a circular economy model, where waste is transformed into resources, thereby minimizing environmental impact (Pallín et al. 2024; Antecka et al. 2019).

Moreover, the environmental footprint of fungal-based bioprocesses is significantly lower when compared to traditional chemical methods, particularly in terms of carbon emissions and energy consumption. The ability of fungi to degrade complex organic materials efficiently and at ambient temperatures, without the need for toxic solvents or high-energy inputs, makes these processes highly sustainable. As industries and governments increasingly focus on reducing their carbon footprint and mitigating climate change, fungal bioprocesses present an attractive and viable option for achieving these goals. By offering an eco-friendly, cost-effective, and scalable solution for waste valorization and the production of bio-based products, fungal biorefineries are well-positioned to play a key role in the transition toward a more sustainable and circular economy (Pallín et al. 2024; Antecka et al. 2019).

Biorefining agro-industrial waste using fungi reduces the waste's environmental impact and generates commercially valuable products. This approach is aligned with the principles of sustainability and circular economy, standing out as a key solution in the transition toward greener industrial processes (Wikandari, Hasniah, and Taherzadeh 2022) (Figure 3.1).

3.10.1 HIGH-VALUE PRODUCTS

Agricultural industrial waste, including cane bagasse, fruit peels, wheat straw, and coffee pulp, contains a high amount of nutrients that can be used as carbon and nitrogen sources for fungal growth

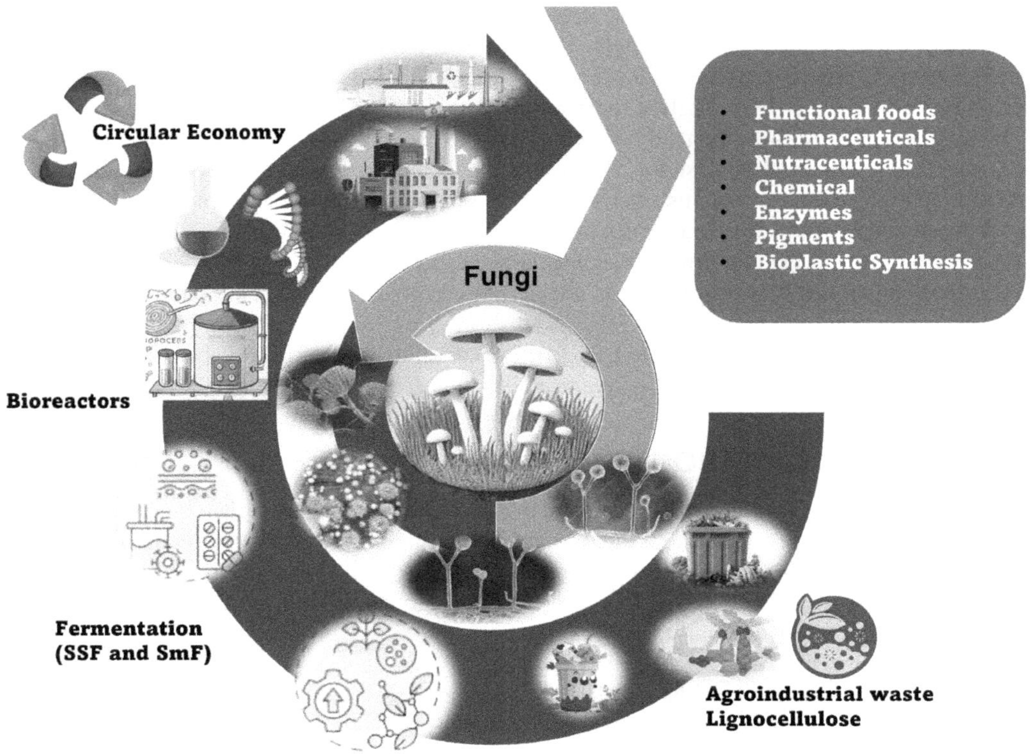

FIGURE 3.1 Fungi in industrial bioprocesses, highlighting their role in the conversion of agro-industrial waste into high-value-added products.

(Yafetto, Odamtten, and Wiafe-Kwagyan 2023). By utilizing SSF or SmF techniques, these wastes can be transformed into high-value products, as described below.

3.10.1.1 Enzymes

Fungal extracellular enzymes are essential biocatalysts because they break down complex compounds into simpler molecules, facilitating a wide range of industrial and environmental applications. In addition to their role in the production of bioethanol, food, textiles, and paper, these enzymes are critical in bioremediation, allowing the degradation of contaminants and reducing environmental impact (Verma, Kumar, and Bansal 2021; Arnau, Yaver, and Hjort 2020). Ongoing research in this field aims to enhance stability and activity, thereby broadening its applicability across various industries.

Among the most studied fungi and recognized for their ability to produce extracellular enzymes of great industrial interest (cellulases, amylases, proteases, and pectinases, among others) is *Trichoderma reesei*, used for the degradation of lignocellulosic biomass (obtaining fermentable sugars) to produce biofuels proposing bioenergy alternatives (Xiao et al. 2023). *Aspergillus niger* used in different agro-industrial waste, produces amylases used in the baking industry or fermented products such as yogurt and beer, improving efficiency and flavor (Melnichuk et al. 2020; Sahu et al. 2024).

Penicillium is utilized to obtain ligninolytic and cellulolytic enzymes for fiber treatment and bleaching, creating more sustainable processes by minimizing the use of harsh chemicals and water (Ayla, Golla, and Pallipati 2018). Other species studied in recent years are *Pleurotus ostreatus* and *Phanerochaete chrysosporium*, which produce laccase and peroxidase enzymes used in the bioremediation process (Dinakarkumar et al. 2024; Faraco et al. 2009).

3.10.1.2 Fungal protein

Throughout history, mushrooms have been a key source of protein, standing out for their environmental sustainability and cultural and medicinal relevance. Since 2000, edible mushrooms (*Agaricus bisporus*, *Lentinula edodes*, and *Pleurotus ostreatus*) have represented 54% of this industry (Ferrero et al. 2024). This is the case of obtaining mycoprotein rich in high-quality proteins, low in saturated fats, and with an amino acid profile suitable for food applications. This development has been fundamental to offering sustainable food options and reducing the environmental impact associated with meat production (Derbyshire et al. 2023).

Among the fungi studied to obtain single-cell protein or mycoprotein (SCP) is *Fusarium venenatum*, the most well-known species of fungus commercially used to obtain an alternative to meat, Quorn™ (Derbyshire et al. 2023). *Paecilomyces variotii* is used to produce protein for animal consumption (Voutilainen, Pihlajaniemi, and Parviainen 2021) and despite being marketed as animal feed, the product was also assessed as a supplement for meat-based foods, such as sausages and meatballs (Toledo Marante et al. 2012). *Rhizopus oryzae* was used in SmF and SSF to utilize residual fruit and vegetable waste to obtain SCP (Wikandari, Hasniah, and Taherzadeh 2022; Ibarruri et al. 2021). Other fungal species used for mycoprotein production in various substrates are *Aspergillus flavus, A. niger, A. ochraceus, A. oryzae, Cladosporium cladosporioides, Monascus ruber, Penicillium citrinum* and *Trichoderma viride* (Amara and El-Baky 2023).

However, the possibility of mycotoxin or allergen production associated with mycoproteins with certain fungal species (*Fusarium*, *Alternaria*, and *Aspergillus*) should be considered. Although data are limited, adverse reactions to mycoproteins have been reported in people with a history of mold allergies (Jacobson and DePorter 2018). Fungal SCP can improve the nutritional value and functional characteristics of foods, such as texture, emulsifying, and foaming capacity, and is an excellent source of protein-rich nutrients (Wikandari, Hasniah, and Taherzadeh 2022).

3.10.1.3 Pigments

Fungi can produce different pigments (carotenoids, melanins, anthocyanins, quinones, and azaphilones (polyketide derivatives) that have applications in the food, cosmetics, textiles, and pharmaceutical industries (Lin and Xu 2020). By using agro-industrial waste as a substrate, costs can be reduced, and low-value raw materials that would otherwise be discarded can be used (Durán et al. 2002).

Among the most studied fungi are those of the genus *Monascus* since they are well known for their ability to produce monascorubrin, rubropunctatin, and red and yellow pigments using waste such as rice bran, molasses, and sugarcane bagasse (Lin and Xu 2022). Its main application is natural food coloring. Other microorganisms, *Talaromyces*, *Penicillium*, *Trichoderma*, and *Aspergillus*, have also been reported for their ability to produce naphthoquinones, melanin, violacein, and carotenoids. These provide antioxidant and antimicrobial activities, making them ideal options in the pharmaceutical area (Elkhateeb and Daba 2023). *Blakeslea trispora* stands out as an important industrial fungus used to produce β-carotene as a food coloring, which was authorized by the EU Directorate-General for Health and Consumer Protection in 1995 (Lee and Schmidt-Dannert 2002; Lin and Xu 2022).

A recent analysis highlighted that environmental factors such as light exposure and nutrient limitation may play a crucial role in stimulating biosynthesis of pigments in fungi (Lin and Xu 2022; Elkhateeb and Daba 2023). These conditions optimize pigment production in solid and liquid fermentation systems by influencing microorganisms' metabolic pathways. Furthermore, pigments produced by fungi are competitive with synthetic ones due to their cost-effectiveness and sustainability, which is a promising alternative for reducing the environmental impact caused by chemical dyes (Ashok et al. 2021; Lin and Xu 2020).

13.10.1.4 Bioactive compounds

Medicinal plant extracts are widely recognized for containing hundreds or even thousands of individual biologically active compounds in variable quantities, which allow them to treat a wide range of conditions (antioxidant, anti-inflammatory, antidiabetic, antibacterial, and anticancer) (Ahmed, Fahim, and Abdelmohsen 2021), due to the combined action of multiple compounds with synergistic, additive, or antagonistic activity (Vaou et al. 2022).

However, in recent years, research has shown that fungi are a rich and reliable source of genetic variation, with the capacity to produce different bioactive compounds (secondary metabolites), which have been used in both agriculture and pharmacology, e.g., in drugs that fight cancer, fungi, viruses, and bacteria (Fontana et al. 2021).

Among the main types of fungal active bio-compounds are antibiotics produced by *Penicillium chrysogenum*, penicillin is one of the most essential products in the history of medicine (Fierro et al. 2022). Another antibiotic, griseofulvin, derived from *Penicillium griseofulvum*, is used to treat fungal infections (Kartsev et al. 2019; K1yoshi and Abe 1961). *Fusarium* and *Aspergillus* can synthesize compounds such as taxol and lovastatin, which have been studied for their antitumor properties (El-Sayed et al. 2019; Mulder et al. 2015).

Ganoderma lucidum produces phenolic compounds and polysaccharides that exhibit intense antioxidant activity, useful in preventing chronic diseases (Y. Zhong et al. 2024). β-glucans produced by *Saccharomyces cerevisiae* and *Pleurotus ostreatus* that strengthen the immune system and have applications as nutritional supplements (Vlassopoulou et al. 2021). *Beauveria bassiana* and *Metarhizium anisopliae* produce active compounds (beauvericin, tenelin, bassianolide, and oxalic acid used) for the biological control of agricultural pests (Shaalan et al. 2022; Lotfy and Moustafa 2021).

3.10.1.5 Other compounds

Due to the challenges of improving production processes at an industrial level, researchers have taken on the task of implementing more efficient development techniques. This has given rise to the use of genetic modifications in fungi to improve industrial processes, especially using agro-industrial waste. They have shown great potential to increase sustainability and efficiency. Such is the case of using genetically modified *Saccharomyces cerevisiae* to metabolize sugars in lignocellulosic hydrolysates, such as xylose, a key component in agricultural waste. These advances have allowed greater efficiency in the production of bioethanol from renewable biomass (Tiwari and Park 2024; Zou, Wei, and Ji 2023). *Aspergillus niger* and *Aspergillus terreus* were genetically optimized to improve the synthesis of citric and itaconic acid, using economical substrates derived from agro-industrial waste, reducing process costs and environmental impact (Li et al. 2012).

Fungi are also used as cellular factories to produce enzymes, bioplastics, and other valuable chemicals (Pilafidis et al. 2022). These technologies promote the reuse of waste and contribute to achieving sustainable development goals by reducing carbon emissions and using renewable raw materials (Gong et al. 2023; Zou, Nielsen, and Wei 2023). These new techniques have allowed fungi such as *Trichoderma* or *Fusarium* to optimize their ability to degrade toxic compounds in contaminated environments. Such advances promote a circular economy and open new opportunities for the development of economical and environmentally responsible bioprocesses. Notably, research in this field is rapidly expanding, with integrated approaches that combine biotechnology, genetic engineering, and materials science.

3.11 FUTURE DIRECTIONS AND BIOTECHNOLOGY EXPECTATIONS

Despite significant advancements in fungal bioprocesses and the design of bioreactor systems, several critical research gaps remain that must be addressed to further optimize the efficiency and scalability of these processes (Tiwari and Park 2024). Future research should prioritize the development of more robust and genetically modified fungal strains with enhanced metabolic capabilities, enabling them to better withstand industrial-scale conditions and more efficiently convert a wider range of substrates into high-value products (Häder 2021). By improving the resilience and productivity of fungal strains, it will be possible to enhance the overall performance of bioreactors and increase the yield of target metabolites (Derbyshire et al. 2023; Tiwari and Park 2024; Palladino et al. 2024).

Moreover, the optimization of bioreactor designs tailored to specific applications is an area that warrants further investigation. While current bioreactor systems, such as airlift and SSF, have shown promise for certain fungal applications, there remains considerable potential to refine and customize reactor configurations based on the unique requirements of different fungal species and production goals. This could involve the development of specialized reactors that better accommodate the specific growth patterns and metabolic needs of particular fungi, as well as improving aspects like mass transfer, oxygenation, and nutrient delivery for large-scale applications (Antecka et al. 2019).

In addition to strain improvement and reactor optimization, exploring novel and unconventional substrates for fungal fermentation represents another promising avenue for future research. The utilization of alternative feedstocks, such as agricultural waste, industrial by-products, and even food scraps, could significantly broaden the scope of fungal bioprocesses, offering new opportunities for waste valorization and the production of bio-based products. This could also help address the increasing demand for sustainable raw materials, reduce dependency on traditional crop-based feedstocks, and further contribute to circular economy models (Pallín et al. 2024; Antecka et al. 2019).

Furthermore, the integration of fungal bioprocesses with other waste treatment technologies holds great potential for enhancing both the sustainability and efficiency of these systems. By combining fungal fermentation with complementary processes, such as anaerobic digestion, membrane filtration, or bioremediation, it may be possible to create more holistic, multi-step biorefinery systems that address a wider range of waste streams while improving overall process stability and reducing operational costs. The synergistic effects of integrating fungal bioprocesses with other waste treatment and resource recovery technologies could pave the way for more sustainable, cost-effective, and scalable solutions in industrial biotechnology (Pallín et al. 2024; Antecka et al. 2019).

3.12 CONCLUSION

Integrating fungi into industrial bioprocesses marks a crucial step toward sustainability, addressing global challenges such as waste management, renewable energy production, and synthesizing valuable compounds. Thanks to their ability to degrade and transform agro-industrial and lignocellulosic waste, fungi emerge as key components in the circular economy, combining efficiency and sustainability. Strategies such as solid fermentation and submerged fermentation optimize the production of different compounds of industrial interest. Moreover, the scale-up and reactor design of fungal bioprocesses for the valorization of residues presents significant opportunities for sustainable development. The optimization of operational parameters, innovative bioreactor designs, and effective downstream processing strategies is crucial for enhancing the efficiency and economic viability of these processes. Continued research and development in this field will be essential for overcoming the challenges associated with scaling up fungal bioprocesses and realizing their full potential in industrial applications. Generally, these strategies consolidate fungi viability on an industrial scale. However, challenges such as mycotoxin mitigation and genetic improvement remain priorities to maximize the impact of biotechnology.

ACKNOWLEDGMENTS

We thank the National Council of Science and Technology (CONAHCyT-Mexico) for grant support for postdoctoral research stays funding (Cordero-Soto 344260 and Contreras-Hernández 489313).

REFERENCES

Aguirre-Acosta, E., Ulloa, M., Aguilar, S., Cifuentes, J., & Valenzuela, R. 2014. Biodiversidad de hongos en México. *Revista Mexicana de Biodiversidad, 85*, 76–81. https://doi.org/10.7550/rmb.33649

Ahmed, S., Fahim, J., & Abdelmohsen, U. 2021. Chemical and biological potential of *Ammi visnaga* (L) Lam. and *Apium graveolens* L.: A review (1963–2020). *Journal of Advanced Biomedical and Pharmaceutical Sciences, 4*(3), 160–176.

Amara, A. A., & El-Baky, N. A. 2023. Fungi as a source of edible proteins and animal feed. *Journal of Fungi, 9*(1), 73. https://doi.org/10.3390/jof9010073

Antecka, A., Blatkiewicz, M., Boruta, T., Górak, A., & Ledakowicz, S. 2019. Comparison of downstream processing methods in purification of highly active laccase. *Bioprocess and Biosystems Engineering, 42*(10), 1635–1645. https://doi.org/10.1007/s00449-019-02160-3

Antunes, F. A. F., Chandel, A. K., dos Santos, J. C., Milessi, T. S. S., Peres, G. F. D., & da Silva, S. S. 2017. Hemicellulosic ethanol production in fluidized bed reactor from sugar cane bagasse hydrolysate: Interplay among carrier concentration and aeration rate. *ACS Sustainable Chemistry & Engineering, 5*(9), 8250–8259. https://doi.org/10.1021/acssuschemeng.7b01916

Aragão, M. S., Menezes, D. B., Ramos, L. C., Oliveira, H. S., Bharagava, R. N., Romanholo Ferreira, L. F., Teixeira, J. A., Ruzene, D. S., & Silva, D. P. 2020. Mycoremediation of vinasse by surface response methodology and preliminary studies in air-lift bioreactors. *Chemosphere, 244*, 125432. https://doi.org/10.1016/j.chemosphere.2019.125432

Arnau, J., Yaver, D., & Hjort, C. M. 2020. Strategies and challenges for the development of industrial enzymes using fungal cell factories. In G. S. Gummadi (Ed.), *Fungal Applications in Sustainable Environmental Biotechnology* (pp. 179–210). Springer. https://doi.org/10.1007/978-3-030-29541-7_7

Ashok, G., Mohan, U., Boominathan, M., Ravichandiran, V., Viswanathan, C., & Senthilkumar, V. 2021. Natural pigments from filamentous fungi: Production and applications. In A. K. Chandel & R. da Silva Siqueira (Eds.), *Fungal Biotechnology and Bioengineering* (pp. 651–678). Springer. https://doi.org/10.1007/978-3-030-85603-8_19

Ayangbenro, A., & Babalola, O. 2017. A new strategy for heavy metal polluted environments: A review of microbial biosorbents. *International Journal of Environmental Research and Public Health, 14*(1), 94. https://doi.org/10.3390/ijerph14010094

Ayla, S., Golla, N., & Pallipati, S. 2018. Production of ligninolytic enzymes from *Penicillium* sp. and its efficiency to decolourise textile dyes. *The Open Biotechnology Journal, 12*(1), 112–122. https://doi.org/10.2174/1874070701812010112

Bai, Z., Zhang, H., Qi, H., Peng, X., & Li, B. 2004. Pectinase production by *Aspergillus niger* using wastewater in solid state fermentation for eliciting plant disease resistance. *Bioresource Technology, 95*(1), 49–52. https://doi.org/10.1016/j.biortech.2003.06.006

Behera, B. C. 2020. Citric acid from *Aspergillus niger*: A comprehensive overview. *Critical Reviews in Microbiology, 46*(6), 727–749. https://doi.org/10.1080/1040841X.2020.1828815

Ben Hmad, I., & Gargouri, A. 2024. Halophilic filamentous fungi and their enzymes: Potential biotechnological applications. *Journal of Biotechnology, 381*, 11–18. https://doi.org/10.1016/j.jbiotec.2023.12.008

Bhabhra, R., & Askew, D. S. 2005. Thermotolerance and virulence of *Aspergillus fumigatus*: Role of the fungal nucleolus. *Medical Mycology, 43*(Suppl 1), 87–93. https://doi.org/10.1080/13693780400029486

Bischof, R. H., Ramoni, J., & Seiboth, B. 2016. Cellulases and beyond: The first 70 years of the enzyme producer *Trichoderma reesei*. *Microbial Cell Factories, 15*(1), 106. https://doi.org/10.1186/s12934-016-0507-6

Blibech, M., Ellouz Ghorbel, R., Chaari, F., Dammak, I., Bhiri, F., Neifar, M., & Ellouz Chaabouni, S. 2011. Improved mannanase production from *Penicillium occitanis* by fed-batch fermentation using acacia seeds. *ISRN Microbiology, 2011*, 1–5. https://doi.org/10.5402/2011/938347

Bonilla Loaiza, A. M., Rodríguez-Jasso, R. M., Belmares, R., López-Badillo, C. M., Araújo, R. G., Aguilar, C. N., Chávez, M. L., Aguilar, M. A., & Ruiz, H. A. 2022. Fungal proteins from *Sargassum* spp. using solid-state fermentation as a green bioprocess strategy. *Molecules, 27*(12), 3887. https://doi.org/10.3390/molecules27123887

Cai, M., Zhang, Y., Hu, W., Shen, W., Yu, Z., Zhou, W., Jiang, T., Zhou, X., & Zhang, Y. 2014. Genetically shaping morphology of the filamentous fungus *Aspergillus glaucus* for production of antitumor polyketide aspergiolide A. *Microbial Cell Factories, 13*(1), 73. https://doi.org/10.1186/1475-2859-13-73

Cerrone, F., Lochlainn, C. Ó., Callaghan, T., McDonald, P., & O'Connor, K. E. 2024. Airlift bioreactor-based strategies for prolonged semi-continuous cultivation of edible *Agaricomycetes*. *Applied Microbiology and Biotechnology, 108*(1), 377. https://doi.org/10.1007/s00253-024-13220-4

Chavan, S., Yadav, B., Atmakuri, A., Tyagi, R. D., Wong, J. W. C., & Drogui, P. 2022. Bioconversion of organic wastes into value-added products: A review. *Bioresource Technology, 344*, 126398. https://doi.org/10.1016/j.biortech.2021.126398

Couder-García, M., Prado-Barragán, L. A., Huerta-Ochoa, S., & Castillo-Araiza, C. O. 2024. Assessing the impact of transport phenomena on modeling and optimization of solid-state fermentation for the revalorization of agro-industrial residues in a wall-cooled packed-bed bioreactor. *Chemical Engineering Research and Design, 210*, 365–381. https://doi.org/10.1016/j.cherd.2024.08.031

De Paula, N. M., da Silva, K., Brugnari, T., Haminiuk, C. W. I., & Maciel, G. M. 2022. Biotechnological potential of fungi from a mangrove ecosystem: Enzymes, salt tolerance and decolorization of a real textile effluent. *Microbiological Research, 254*, 126899. https://doi.org/10.1016/j.micres.2021.126899

Derbyshire, E. J., Theobald, H., Wall, B. T., & Stephens, F. 2023. Food for our future: The nutritional science behind the sustainable fungal protein – mycoprotein. A symposium review. *Journal of Nutritional Science, 12*, e44. https://doi.org/10.1017/jns.2023.29

Devi, R., Kaur, T., Guleria, G., Rana, K. L., Kour, D., Yadav, N., Yadav, A. N., & Saxena, A. K. 2020. Fungal secondary metabolites and their biotechnological applications for human health. In A. A. Rastegari, A. N. Yadav, & N. Yadav (Eds.), *New and Future Developments in Microbial Biotechnology and Bioengineering* (pp. 147–161). Elsevier. https://doi.org/10.1016/B978-0-12-820528-0.00010-7

Dinakarkumar, Y., Ramakrishnan, G., Gujjula, K. R., Vasu, V., Balamurugan, P., & Murali, G. 2024. Fungal bioremediation: An overview of the mechanisms, applications and future perspectives. *Environmental Chemistry and Ecotoxicology, 6*, 293–302. https://doi.org/10.1016/j.enceco.2024.07.002

Durán, N., Teixeira, M. F. S., De Conti, R., & Esposito, E. 2002. Ecological-friendly pigments from fungi. *Critical Reviews in Food Science and Nutrition, 42*(1), 53–66. https://doi.org/10.1080/10408690290825457

El-Sayed, A. S. A., El Sayed, M. T., Nada, H. S., Hassan, A. E., & Yousef, E. K. 2019. Production and characterization of Taxol as anticancer agent from *Aspergillus terreus*. *Journal of Pure and Applied Microbiology, 13*(4), 2055–2063. https://doi.org/10.22207/JPAM.13.4.17

El Enshasy, H. A. 2022. Fungal morphology: A challenge in bioprocess engineering industries for product development. *Current Opinion in Chemical Engineering, 35*, 100729. https://doi.org/10.1016/j.coche.2021.100729

Elkhateeb, W., & Daba, G. 2023. Fungal pigments: Their diversity, chemistry, food and non-food applications. *Applied Microbiology, 3*(3), 735–751. https://doi.org/10.3390/applmicrobiol3030051

Faraco, V., Pezzella, C., Miele, A., Giardina, P., & Sannia, G. 2009. Bio-remediation of colored industrial wastewaters by the white-rot fungi *Phanerochaete chrysosporium* and *Pleurotus ostreatus* and their enzymes. *Biodegradation, 20*(2), 209–220. https://doi.org/10.1007/s10532-008-9214-2

Farinas, C. S. 2015. Developments in solid-state fermentation for the production of biomass-degrading enzymes for the bioenergy sector. *Renewable and Sustainable Energy Reviews, 52*, 179–188. https://doi.org/10.1016/j.rser.2015.07.092

Feng, J., Feng, N., Tang, Q. J., Liu, Y. F., Yang, Y., Liu, F., Zhang, J. S., & Lin, C. C. 2019. Optimization of *Ganoderma lucidum* polysaccharides fermentation process for large-scale production. *Applied Biochemistry and Biotechnology, 189*(3), 972–986. https://doi.org/10.1007/s12010-019-02968-5

Ferreira, J. A., Lennartsson, P. R., & Taherzadeh, M. J. 2015. Production of ethanol and biomass from thin stillage by *Neurospora intermedia*: A pilot study for process diversification. *Engineering in Life Sciences, 15*(8), 751–759. https://doi.org/10.1002/elsc.201400213

Ferrero, D., Moscato, E., Spina, F., Cavalluzzi, M. M., Rotondo, N., Oddon, S. B., Gargano, M. L., Venturella, G., Lentini, G., Bertea, C. M., Gasco, L., & Varese, G. C. 2024. The fungal alternative: Insights on medicinal mushrooms-based protein-rich biomasses by submerged fermentation of agro-industrial by-products. *Innovative Food Science & Emerging Technologies, 95*, 103721. https://doi.org/10.1016/j.ifset.2024.103721

Fierro, F., Vaca, I., Castillo, N. I., García-Rico, R. O., & Chávez, R. 2022. *Penicillium chrysogenum*, a vintage model with a cutting-edge profile in biotechnology. *Microorganisms, 10*(3), 573. https://doi.org/10.3390/microorganisms10030573

Fontana, D. C., de Paula, S., Torres, A. G., de Souza, V. H. M., Pascholati, S. F., Schmidt, D., & Dourado Neto, D. 2021. Endophytic fungi: Biological control and induced resistance to phytopathogens and abiotic stresses. *Pathogens, 10*(5), 570. https://doi.org/10.3390/pathogens10050570

Formenti, L. R., Nørregaard, A., Bolic, A., Hernandez, D. Q., Hagemann, T., Heins, A., Larsson, H., Mears, L., Mauricio-Iglesias, M., Krühne, U., & Gernaey, K. V. 2014. Challenges in industrial fermentation technology research. *Biotechnology Journal, 9*(6), 727–738. https://doi.org/10.1002/biot.201300236

García-Torreiro, M., López-Abelairas, M., Lu-Chau, T. A., & Lema, J. M. 2016. Fungal pretreatment of agricultural residues for bioethanol production. *Industrial Crops and Products, 89*, 486–492. https://doi.org/10.1016/j.indcrop.2016.05.036

Germano, S., Pandey, A., Osaku, C. A., Rocha, S. N., & Soccol, C. R. 2003. Characterization and stability of proteases from *Penicillium* sp. produced by solid-state fermentation. *Enzyme and Microbial Technology, 32*(2), 246–251. https://doi.org/10.1016/S0141-0229(02)00283-1

Germec, M., Yatmaz, E., Karahalil, E., & Turhan, İ. 2017. Effect of different fermentation strategies on β-mannanase production in fed-batch bioreactor system. *3 Biotech, 7*(1), 77. https://doi.org/10.1007/s13205-017-0694-9

Gimenez, G. G., Ruiz, S. P., Caetano, W., Peralta, R. M., & Matioli, G. 2014. Biosorption potential of synthetic dyes by heat-inactivated and live *Lentinus edodes* CCB-42 immobilized in loofa sponges. *World Journal of Microbiology and Biotechnology, 30*(12), 3229–3244. https://doi.org/10.1007/s11274-014-1750-9

Gómez-Ramos, G. A., Prado-Barragán, L. A., Rivera, B. A., Huerta-Ochoa, S., Rivera, V. M., Couder-García, M., García-Hernández, R. de los Á., & Castillo-Araiza, C. O. 2025. Bioreactor engineering for circular economy: Bioactive compound production in solid-state fermentation Review. *Chemical Engineering & Technology, 48*(1), 1–28. https://doi.org/10.1002/ceat.202400289

Gómez Sánchez, C. E., Martínez-Trujillo, A., & Aguilar Osorio, G. 2012. Oxygen transfer coefficient and the kinetic parameters of exo-polygalacturonase production by *Aspergillus flavipes* FP-500 in shake flasks and bioreactor. *Letters in Applied Microbiology, 55*(6), 444–452. https://doi.org/10.1111/j.1472-765x.2012.03313.x

Gong, M., Wang, Y., Bao, D., Jiang, S., Chen, H., Shang, J., Wang, X., Hnin Yu, H., & Zou, G. 2023. Improving cold-adaptability of mesophilic cellulase complex with a novel mushroom cellobiohydrolase for efficient low-temperature ensiling. *Bioresource Technology, 376*, 128888. https://doi.org/10.1016/j.biortech.2023.128888

Häder, D. P. 2021. Biotechnological substances from fungi. In R. P. Sinha & D.-P. Häder (Eds.), *Natural Bioactive Compounds* (pp. 267–273). Academic Press. Elsevier. https://doi.org/10.1016/B978-0-12-820655-3.00013-6

Harms, H., Schlosser, D., & Wick, L. Y. 2011. Untapped potential: Exploiting fungi in bioremediation of hazardous chemicals. *Nature Reviews Microbiology, 9*(3), 177–192. https://doi.org/10.1038/nrmicro2519

Hawksworth, D. L., & Lücking, R. 2017. Fungal diversity revisited: 2.2 to 3.8 million species. *Microbiology Spectrum, 5*(4). https://doi.org/10.1128/microbiolspec.FUNK-0052-2016

Ibarruri, J., Goiri, I., Cebrián, M., & García-Rodríguez, A. 2021. Solid state fermentation as a tool to stabilize and improve nutritive value of fruit and vegetable discards: Effect on nutritional composition, in vitro ruminal fermentation and organic matter digestibility. *Animals, 11*(6), 1653. https://doi.org/10.3390/ani11061653

Ingale, S., Joshi, S. J., & Gupte, A. 2014. Production of bioethanol using agricultural waste: Banana pseudo stem. *Brazilian Journal of Microbiology, 45*(3), 885–892. https://doi.org/10.1590/S1517-83822014000300018

Iram, A., Özcan, A., Yatmaz, E., Turhan, İ., & Demirci, A. 2022. Effect of microparticles on fungal fermentation for fermentation-based product productions. *Processes, 10*(12), 2681. https://doi.org/10.3390/pr10122681

Jacobson, M. F., & DePorter, J. 2018. Self-reported adverse reactions associated with mycoprotein (Quorn-brand) containing foods. *Annals of Allergy, Asthma & Immunology, 120*(6), 626–630. https://doi.org/10.1016/j.anai.2018.03.020

Kiyoshi, U., & Abe, S. 1961. Production of griseofulvin by some strains of the genus *Penicillium*. *The Journal of Antibiotics, Series A, 14*(4), 215–220.

Kartsev, V., Geronikaki, A., Petrou, A., Lichitsky, B., Kostic, M., Smiljkovic, M., Soković, M., & Sirakanyan, S. 2019. Griseofulvin derivatives: Synthesis, molecular docking and biological evaluation. *Current Topics in Medicinal Chemistry, 19*(13), 1145–1161. https://doi.org/10.2174/1568026619666190523080136

Khurshid, S., Ashraf, H., Hussain, T., Iqbal, M., Qureshi, H., Anwar, T., Salmen, S. H., & Ansari, M. J. 2024. Enhanced citric acid production through *Aspergillus niger*: Insights from fermentation studies using sugarcane molasses. *Life, 14*(6), 756. https://doi.org/10.3390/life14060756

Kijpornyongpan, T., Schwartz, A., Yaguchi, A., & Salvachúa, D. 2022. Systems biology-guided understanding of white-rot fungi for biotechnological applications: A review. *iScience, 25*(7), 104640. https://doi.org/10.1016/j.isci.2022.104640

Lee, P., & Schmidt-Dannert, C. 2002. Metabolic engineering towards biotechnological production of carotenoids in microorganisms. *Applied Microbiology and Biotechnology, 60*(1–2), 1–11. https://doi.org/10.1007/s00253-002-1101-x

Li, A., Pfelzer, N., Zuijderwijk, R., & Punt, P. 2012. Enhanced itaconic acid production in *Aspergillus niger* using genetic modification and medium optimization. *BMC Biotechnology, 12*(1), 57. https://doi.org/10.1186/1472-6750-12-57

Lin, L., & Xu, J. 2020. Fungal pigments and their roles associated with human health. *Journal of Fungi, 6*(4), 280. https://doi.org/10.3390/jof6040280

Lin, L., & Xu, J. 2022. Production of fungal pigments: Molecular processes and their applications. *Journal of Fungi, 9*(1), 44. https://doi.org/10.3390/jof9010044

Lizardi-Jiménez, M. A., & Hernández-Martínez, R. 2017. Solid state fermentation (SSF): Diversity of applications to valorize waste and biomass. *3 Biotech, 7*(1), 44. https://doi.org/10.1007/s13205-017-0692-y

Lotfy, D. E. S., & Moustafa, H. Z. 2021. Field evaluation of two entomopathogenic fungi; *Beauveria bassiana* and *Metarhizium anisopliae* as a biocontrol agent against the spiny bollworm, *Earias insulana* Boisduval (Lepidoptera: Noctuidae) on cotton plants. *Egyptian Journal of Biological Pest Control, 31*(1), 78. https://doi.org/10.1186/s41938-021-00420-7

Mattedi, A., Sabbi, E., Farda, B., Djebaili, R., Mitra, D., Ercole, C., Cacchio, P., Del Gallo, M., & Pellegrini, M. 2023. Solid-state fermentation: Applications and future perspectives for biostimulant and biopesticides production. *Microorganisms, 11*(6), 1408. https://doi.org/10.3390/microorganisms11061408

Melnichuk, N., Braia, M. J., Anselmi, P. A., Meini, M.-R., & Romanini, D. 2020. Valorization of two agroindustrial wastes to produce alpha-amylase enzyme from *Aspergillus oryzae* by solid-state fermentation. *Waste Management, 106*, 155–161. https://doi.org/10.1016/j.wasman.2020.03.025

Meyer, V., Cairns, T., Barthel, L., King, R., Kunz, P., Schmideder, S., Müller, H., Briesen, H., Dinius, A., & Krull, R. 2021. Understanding and controlling filamentous growth of fungal cell factories: Novel tools and opportunities for targeted morphology engineering. *Fungal Biology and Biotechnology, 8*(1), 8. https://doi.org/10.1186/s40694-021-00115-6

Mitchell , D. A., Berovič, M., & Krieger, N. 2006. Solid-state fermentation bioreactor fundamentals: Introduction and overview. In D. A. Mitchell, N. Krieger, & M. Berovič (Eds.), *Solid-State Fermentation Bioreactors: Fundamentals of Design and Operation* (pp. 1–12). Springer.

Mokhtarian, M., Tavakolipour, H., Bagheri, F., Fernandes Oliveira, C. A., Corassin, C. H., & Khaneghah, A. M. 2020. Aflatoxin B1 in the Iranian pistachio nut and decontamination methods: A systematic review. *Quality Assurance and Safety of Crops & Foods, 12*(4), 15–25. https://doi.org/10.15586/qas.v12i4.784

Mueller, G. M., & Schmit, J. P. 2007. Fungal biodiversity: What do we know? What can we predict? *Biodiversity and Conservation, 16*(1), 1–5. https://doi.org/10.1007/s10531-006-9117-7

Mulder, K. C. L., Mulinari, F., Franco, O. L., Soares, M. S. F., Magalhães, B. S., & Parachin, N. S. 2015. Lovastatin production: From molecular basis to industrial process optimization. *Biotechnology Advances, 33*(6), 648–665. https://doi.org/10.1016/j.biotechadv.2015.04.001

Olagunju, L. K., Isikhuemhen, O. S., Dele, P. A., Anike, F. N., Ike, K. A., Shaw, Y., Brice, R. M., Orimaye, O. E., Wuaku, M., Essick, B. G., Holt, N., Udombang, N. S., Enemudo, J. O., Subedi, K., & Anele, U. Y. 2023. Effects of the incubation period of *Pleurotus ostreatus* on the chemical composition and nutrient availability of solid-state-fermented corn stover. *Animals, 13*(16), 2587. https://doi.org/10.3390/ani13162587

Palladino, F., Marcelino, P. R. F., Schlogl, A. E., José, Á. H. M., Rodrigues, R. de C. L. B., Fabrino, D. L., Santos, I. J. B., & Rosa, C. A. 2024. Bioreactors: Applications and innovations for a sustainable and healthy future—A critical review. *Applied Sciences, 14*(20), 9346. https://doi.org/10.3390/app14209346

Pallín, M. Á., González-Rodríguez, S., Eibes, G., López-Abelairas, M., Moreira, M. T., Lema, J. M., & Lú-Chau, T. A. 2024. Towards industrial application of fungal pretreatment in 2G biorefinery: Scale-up of solid-state fermentation of wheat straw. *Biomass Conversion and Biorefinery, 14*(1), 593–605. https://doi.org/10.1007/s13399-022-02319-1

Patel, A. K., Agrawal, R., Dong, C.-D., Chen, C.-W., Singhania, R. R., & Pandey, A. 2023. Filamentous fungal morphology in industrial aspects. In *Current Developments in Biotechnology and Bioengineering* Taherzadeh, M. J. (Ed.), (pp. 197–217). Elsevier. https://doi.org/10.1016/B978-0-323-91872-5.00015-6

Pawar, K. S., Singh, P. N., & Singh, S. K. 2023. Fungal alkaline proteases and their potential applications in different industries. *Frontiers in Microbiology, 14*. https://doi.org/10.3389/fmicb.2023.1138401

Pilafidis, S., Diamantopoulou, P., Gkatzionis, K., & Sarris, D. 2022. Valorization of agro-industrial wastes and residues through the production of bioactive compounds by macrofungi in liquid state cultures: Growing circular economy. *Applied Sciences, 12*(22), 11426. https://doi.org/10.3390/app122211426

Prajapati, J., Sheth, R., Bhatt, R., Chavda, K., Solanki, Z., Rawal, R., & Goswami, D. 2024. Biodiversity and biotechnological applications of host-specific endophytic fungi for sustainable agriculture and allied sector. In A. Kumar, J. F. White, & J. S. Panwar (Eds.), *Sustainable Agricultural Practices* (pp. 101–124). Academic Press. https://doi.org/10.1016/B978-0-443-19150-3.00003-5

Pushparaj, K., Meyyazhagan, A., Bhotla, H. K., Arumugam, V. A., Pappuswamy, M., Vadivalagan, C., Hakeem, K. R., Balasubramanian, B., Liu, W., & Mousavi Khaneghah, A. 2023. The crux of bioactive metabolites in endophytic and thermophilic fungi and their proximal prospects in biotechnological and industrial domains. *Toxicon, 223*, 107007. https://doi.org/10.1016/j.toxicon.2022.107007

Qader, M., & Shekha, Y. 2023. Bioremediation of heavy metals by using *Aspergillus niger* and *Candida albicans*. *Zanco Journal of Pure and Applied Sciences, 35*(3). https://doi.org/10.21271/ZJPAS.35.3.16

Royse, D. J., Baars, J., & Tan, Q. 2017. Current overview of mushroom production in the world. In Diego & A. Pardo-Giménez (Eds.), *Edible and Medicinal Mushrooms* (pp. 5–13). Wiley. https://doi.org/10.1002/9781119149446.ch2

Sahu, P. K., Singh, R., Shrivastava, M., Darjee, S., Mageshwaran, V., Phurailtpam, L., & Rohatgi, B. 2024. Microbial production of α-amylase from agro-waste: An approach towards biorefinery and bio-economy. *Energy Nexus, 14*, 100293. https://doi.org/10.1016/j.nexus.2024.100293

Sentís-Moré, P., Romero-Fabregat, M.-P., Rodríguez-Marca, C., Guerra-Sánchez, A.-J., & Ortega-Olivé, N. 2023. Design optimization of a tray bioreactor for solid-state fermentation: Study of process parameters through protein modification of by-products. *Fermentation, 9*(10), 921. https://doi.org/10.3390/fermentation9100921

Shaalan, R., Ibrahim, L., As-Sadi, F., & El Kayal, W. 2022. Impact of *Beauveria bassiana* and *Metarhizium anisopliae* on the metabolic interactions between cucumber (*Cucumis sativus* L.) and cucumber mosaic virus (CMV). *Horticulturae, 8*(12), 1182. https://doi.org/10.3390/horticulturae8121182

Sharma, R. K., Sharma, R., & Arora, D. S. 2018. Assessment of the efficiency of U-tube continuous bioreactor and immobilized enzyme beads for dye decolourization. *3 Biotech, 8*(5), 241. https://doi.org/10.1007/s13205-018-1275-2

Skory, C. D. 2004. Lactic acid production by *Rhizopus oryzae* transformants with modified lactate dehydrogenase activity. *Applied Microbiology and Biotechnology, 64*(2), 237–242. https://doi.org/10.1007/s00253-003-1480-7

Supramani, S., Ahmad, R., Ilham, Z., Suffian Mohamad Annuar, M., Klaus, A., & Abd Al Qadr Imad Wan-Mohtar, W. 2019. Optimisation of biomass, exopolysaccharide and intracellular polysaccharide production from the mycelium of an identified *Ganoderma lucidum* strain QRS 5120 using response surface methodology. *AIMS Microbiology, 5*(1), 19–38. https://doi.org/10.3934/microbiol.2019.1.19

Supramani, S., Rejab, N. A., Ilham, Z., Ahmad, R., Show, P.-L., Ibrahim, M. F., & Wan-Mohtar, W. A. A. Q. I. 2023. Performance of biomass and exopolysaccharide production from the medicinal mushroom *Ganoderma lucidum* in a new fabricated air-L-shaped bioreactor (ALSB). *Processes, 11*(3), 670. https://doi.org/10.3390/pr11030670

Tauk-Tornisielo, S. M., Arasato, L. S., Almeida, A. F. de, Govone, J. S., & Malagutti, E. N. 2009. Lipid formation and γ-linolenic acid production by *Mucor circinelloides* and *Rhizopus* sp., grown on vegetable oil. *Brazilian Journal of Microbiology, 40*(2), 342–345. https://doi.org/10.1590/S1517-83822009000200025

Teleky, B.-E., & Vodnar, D. C. 2021. Recent advances in biotechnological itaconic acid production, and application for a sustainable approach. *Polymers, 13*(20), 3574. https://doi.org/10.3390/polym13203574

Thunuguntla, R., Mahboubi, A., Ferreira, J. A., & Taherzadeh, M. J. 2018. Integration of membrane bioreactors with edible filamentous fungi for valorization of expired milk. *Sustainability, 10*(6), 1940. https://doi.org/10.3390/su10061940

Tiwari, P., & Park, K.-I. 2024. Advanced fungal biotechnologies in accomplishing Sustainable Development Goals (SDGs): What do we know and what comes next? *Journal of Fungi, 10*(7), 506. https://doi.org/10.3390/jof10070506

Toledo Marante, F. J., Mioso, R., Bermejo Barrera, J., González González, J. E., Santana Rodríguez, J. J., & Bravo de Laguna, I. H. 2012. Structural characterization and metabolite profiling of the facultative marine fungus *Paecilomyces variotii*. *Annals of Microbiology, 62*(4), 1601–1607. https://doi.org/10.1007/s13213-011-0416-1

Tosun, R., & Yaşar, S. 2020. Nutritional enrichment of apple pomace by fungal fermentations. *Kahramanmaraş Sütçü İmam Üniversitesi Tarım ve Doğa Dergisi, 23*(3), 781–787. https://doi.org/10.18016/ksutarimdoga.vi.629326

Upadhyay, S. K., Rani, N., Kumar, V., Mythili, R., & Jain, D. 2023. A review on simultaneous heavy metal removal and organo-contaminants degradation by potential microbes: Current findings and future outlook. *Microbiological Research, 273*, 127419. https://doi.org/10.1016/j.micres.2023.127419

Vaou, N., Stavropoulou, E., Voidarou, C. (Chrysa), Tsakris, Z., Rozos, G., Tsigalou, C., & Bezirtzoglou, E. 2022. Interactions between medical plant-derived bioactive compounds: Focus on antimicrobial combination effects. *Antibiotics, 11*(8), 1014. https://doi.org/10.3390/antibiotics11081014

Verma, N., Kumar, V., & Bansal, M. C. 2021. Valorization of waste biomass in fermentative production of cellulases: A review. *Waste and Biomass Valorization, 12*(2), 613–640. https://doi.org/10.1007/s12649-020-01048-8

Vlassopoulou, M., Yannakoulia, M., Pletsa, V., Zervakis, G. I., & Kyriacou, A. 2021. Effects of fungal beta-glucans on health – A systematic review of randomized controlled trials. *Food & Function, 12*(8), 3366–3380. https://doi.org/10.1039/D1FO00122A
Voutilainen, E., Pihlajaniemi, V., & Parviainen, T. 2021. Economic comparison of food protein production with single-cell organisms from lignocellulose side-streams. *Bioresource Technology Reports, 14*, 100683. https://doi.org/10.1016/j.biteb.2021.100683
Wang, J., Wang, S., Zhao, S., Sun, P., Zhang, Z., & Xu, Q. 2023. Productivity enhancement in L-lysine fermentation using oxygen-enhanced bioreactor and oxygen vector. *Frontiers in Bioengineering and Biotechnology, 11*. https://doi.org/10.3389/fbioe.2023.1181963
Wei, X., Tang, L., & Lu, Y. 2017. Dissolved oxygen control strategy for improvement of TL1-1 production in submerged fermentation by *Daldinia eschscholzii*. *Bioresources and Bioprocessing, 4*(1), 1. https://doi.org/10.1186/s40643-016-0134-4
Wikandari, R., Hasniah, N., & Taherzadeh, M. J. 2022. The role of filamentous fungi in advancing the development of a sustainable circular bioeconomy. *Bioresource Technology, 345*, 126531. https://doi.org/10.1016/j.biortech.2021.126531
Xiao, M., Wang, Y., Wang, Y., Yan, X., Zhu, Z., Tian, E., Yang, C., Ma, E., Zou, G., Zhou, Z., & Wang, P. 2023. Repurposing the cellulase workhorse *Trichoderma reesei* as a ROBUST chassis for efficient terpene production. *Green Chemistry, 25*(18), 7362–7371. https://doi.org/10.1039/D3GC01770B
Yafetto, L., Odamtten, G. T., & Wiafe-Kwagyan, M. 2023. Valorization of agro-industrial wastes into animal feed through microbial fermentation: A review of the global and Ghanaian case. *Heliyon, 9*(4), e14814. https://doi.org/10.1016/j.heliyon.2023.e14814
Yang, L., Lübeck, M., & Lübeck, P. S. 2017. *Aspergillus* as a versatile cell factory for organic acid production. *Fungal Biology Reviews, 31*(1), 33–49. https://doi.org/10.1016/j.fbr.2016.11.001
Zhang, F., Zhu, Z., Wang, B., Wang, P., Yu, G., Wu, M., Chen, W., Ran, W., & Shen, Q. 2013. Optimization of *Trichoderma harzianum* T-E5 biomass and determining the degradation sequence of biopolymers by FTIR in solid-state fermentation. *Industrial Crops and Products, 49*, 619–627. https://doi.org/10.1016/j.indcrop.2013.05.037
Zhang, J., & Zhang, J. 2016. The filamentous fungal pellet and forces driving its formation. *Critical Reviews in Biotechnology, 36*(6), 1066–1077. https://doi.org/10.3109/07388551.2015.1084262
Zhong, J.-J. 2011. Bioreactor engineering. In M. Moo-Young (Ed.), *Comprehensive Biotechnology* (2nd ed., Vol. 2, pp. 165–177). Elsevier. https://doi.org/10.1016/B978-0-08-088504-9.00097-0
Zhong, Y., Tan, P., Lin, H., Zhang, D., Chen, X., Pang, J., & Mu, R. 2024. A review of *Ganoderma lucidum* polysaccharide: Preparations, structures, physicochemical properties and application. *Foods, 13*(17), 2665. https://doi.org/10.3390/foods13172665
Zou, G., Nielsen, J. B., & Wei, Y. 2023. Harnessing synthetic biology for mushroom farming. *Trends in Biotechnology, 41*(4), 480–483. https://doi.org/10.1016/j.tibtech.2022.10.001
Zou, G., Wei, Y., & Ji, X.-J. 2023. Editorial: Fungal green biotechnology and biomanufacturing. *Frontiers in Microbiology, 14*. https://doi.org/10.3389/fmicb.2023.1334993

4 Novel materials for bioelectrodes

Abinash Kumararaj, Geetha Arunachalam, Rekha Pachaiappan, Divyadharshini Satheesh, Rathika Rajendran, Kovendhan Manavalan, and Tri Khoa Nguyen

4.1 INTRODUCTION AND HISTORY OF BIOELECTRODES

Bioelectrodes are derived from the electrodes that work both biologically and chemically on the interface. Electrodes are used as objects that transform ionic potential into electronic potential (Kumararaj, Kennedy, et al. 2025). A bioelectrode is a transducer that changes the body's natural ionic current into a conventional electronic current that flows through the electrode. Bioelectrodes are capable of conducting a modest current across the body's contact with the electronic measurement circuit (Figure 4.1). An interface between biological structures and electronic systems is provided by bioelectrodes. The biological structure is either sensitive to or stimulated by the electrical activity produced by the bioelectrodes. Two processes take place at the bioelectrodes, which are oxidation and reduction. When the current is flowing from electrode to electrolyte, oxidation predominates; when it is flowing the other way, reduction predominates. The net current, which travels across the contact from the electrode to the electrolyte, is composed of electrons and anions travelling against the direction of the electrode's current, whereas the cations travel along the same direction (Kumararaj, Perumal, et al. 2025). Bioelectrodes are not considered to be toxic because of various biological activities that they undergo. They are good conductors with minimum impedance, and they are also easy to clean. Bioelectrodes are considered to be mechanically rugged electrodes based on the materials they use. Gradually, the design of bioelectrodes changed from nonporous to contemporary porous designs, which depend on fibre, particles, or monoliths and a comparison of enactment qualities. Methods are meant to be effective when they make use of surface materials that facilitate effective electron transport and porous features that encourage microbial colonization (Xie, Criddle, and Cui 2015). A biological electrode that serves as a living "catalyst" for the transport of electrons. These micro-organisms pivot on the effective transmission of electrons from cells to the bioelectrode, the efficiency of reactant transportation, and product removal to maintain their performance. Biological structures and electronic systems. It has two functions: one is to sense and quantify the biological structure's internal electrical activity (passively) and the other one is to activate it by introducing an external electrical potential (actively). Electrical currents produced by various biological structures result in potential variations. Bioelectrodes can be used to measure these potential variations, which can provide information about how the biological structure works. On the other hand, bioelectrodes are used to apply current to a certain targeted biological structure in order to have the desired effect. The same bioelectrode may serve a passive or active role, depending on the need and situation. The electrode material can influence the immobilization and stability of the enzymes. The electrode material influences the conductivity and surface of the electrode, electrons' transmission between the surface of the electrode and the biocatalyst, and transport of fuel. The nanoparticles serve as a flexible tool for creating three-dimensional biomaterials intended to enhance the functionality of bioelectrodes. In order to cultivate the best electrode, it is inevitable

DOI: 10.1201/9781003500483-4
This chapter has been made available under a (CC-BY-NC-ND) 4.0 license

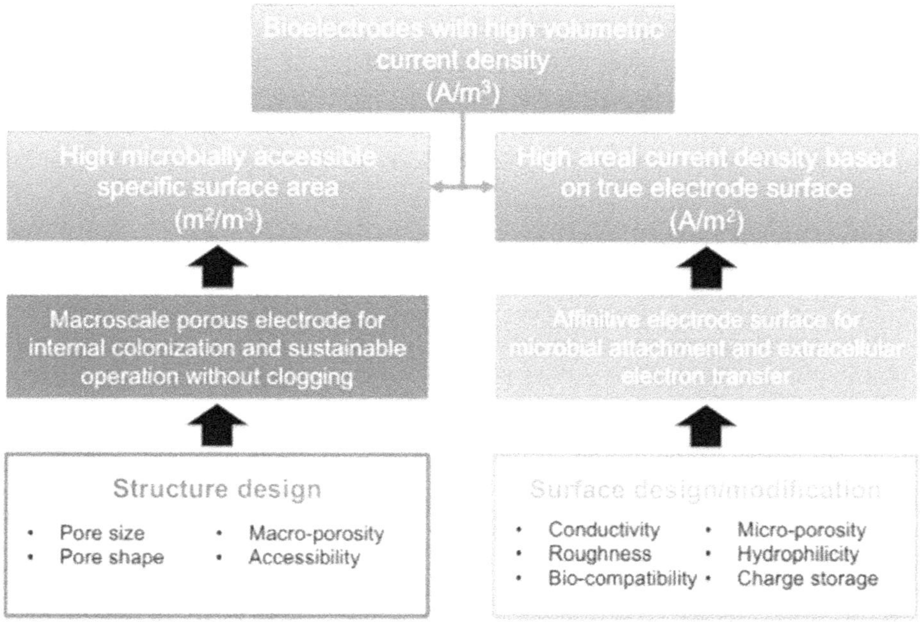

FIGURE 4.1 Strategy for preparing high-performance bioelectrodes.

Source: Adapted from Design and fabrication of bioelectrodes for microbial bioelectrochemical systems Xie, Criddle, and Cui (2015)

to depend on the mechanism of "charge-transfer" between current/charge carriers that occurs at the interface of the electrode. The need for a soft bioelectrode that can support implantable electronics in both rigid and flexible platforms is very important. Voltammetry and chronoamperometry were used to assess the bioelectrodes' sensing capabilities towards the various substrates. The enzyme presence in the interface can be examined using X-ray photon spectroscopy.

4.2 TYPES OF BIOELECTRODES

4.2.1 Surface or Transcutaneous Electrodes

Monitoring or recording electrodes are defined as transcutaneous/surface electrodes that are employed to quantify the electrical events that take place within the surface of the electrode's body (Venugopalan and Ideker 2013). Example: electrocardiography, electroencephalography, and electromyography.

4.2.2 Stimulator Electrodes

Stimulator electrodes are those that send information into the body and have an impact on particular physiological processes. Information is sent in a waveform of voltage or current to specific target sites of the body. This regulates a bioelectric event or indirectly affects the location of the target through the promotion of chemical change. Electrically excitable tissue can be stimulated by using electrodes to create electrical fields inside the tissue. By converting electrons to ions, these electrodes make it possible to inject electric charge into tissue. Stimulating electrodes function by creating brief electric fields in the area around them. The accuracy and homogeneity of these electrical fields, in turn, depend on the distribution of charge density by the stimulation electrode (Venugopalan and Ideker 2013).

4.2.3 Polarized and non-polarized electrodes

The electrodes in which the faradaic charge transfer doesn't occur then it is known as polarizable electrodes. Whereas in electrodes in which the charge transfer occurs without any disturbance are considered to be exactly faradaic or perfectly non-polarizable electrodes. Even though an electrode might act as a polarizable or nonpolarizable electrode depending on the circumstances at the interface (Venugopalan and Ideker 2013).

4.3 BIOELECTRODES

The target of bioelectrode development was to produce bioelectrodes of high volumetric current density. This characteristic feature of the electrode was obtained with its specific surface area and current density. It must be possible for microbes to colonies the electrode surface. Hence, both macroscale and microscale characteristics were considered for any high-performance bioelectrode (Xie, Criddle, and Cui 2015). Larger pores are necessary for the delivery of substrate and product removal in bioelectrodes. Also, the consideration of the thermodynamic properties is necessary. This includes making room for the microbial energy requirements (Xie, Criddle, and Cui 2015). The bio-electrodes consist of two major parts- bio-anodes and bio-cathodes. Figure 4.2 shows the enhanced biocatalysis in the anode and cathode. The organic substrates as a source of carbon provide the energy carrier molecule to microorganisms present in the anodic chamber by donating the charge carriers (here electrons). The electrons of these charge carriers are transferred from the cytoplasm (the citric acid cycle location) to the cell membrane. Then the electrons from the membrane cell are transported to the anode with the direct technique or the mediated method. Oxidation of organic substrates takes place due to the acceptance of an external electron by the anode (Watanabe 2008). Bucky papers are used to create a variety of catalytic bioelectrode interfaces. These interfaces are found to be excellent self-supporting frameworks. It supports guest molecules such as metals, redox compounds, polymers, etc., and also enzymes (Gross, Holzinger, and Cosnier 2018). Major

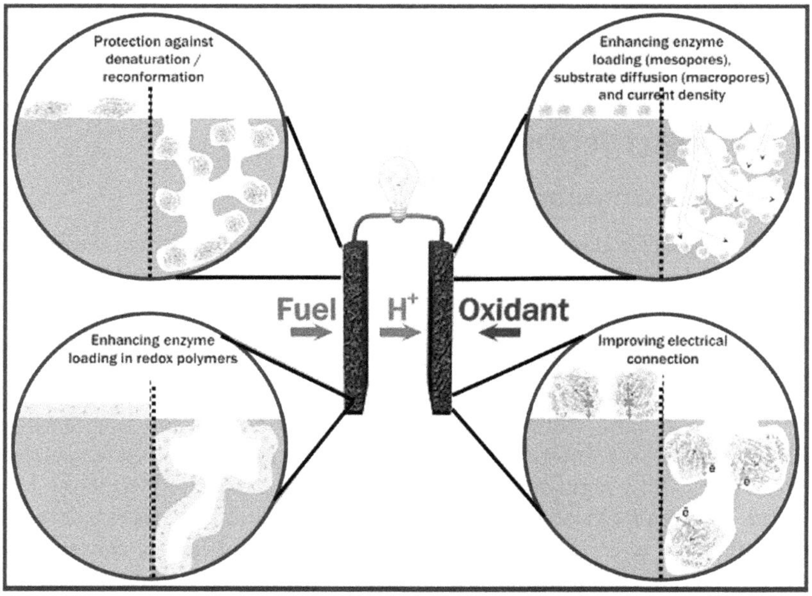

FIGURE 4.2 Schematic representation of enhanced bio-catalysis in anodes and cathodes of EFCs.

Source: Adapted from Recent developments in high surface area bioelectrodes for enzymatic fuel cells. Mazurenko, de Poulpiquet, and Lojou (2017a)

advancements in bioelectrode designs are necessary to enhance the operational stability of biofuel cells, output voltage, and power density. Improvements in electrical wiring techniques for enzymes are needed, as well as electrodes with good mechanical stability, conductivity, and high surface area (Gross, Holzinger, and Cosnier 2018). Biological or biochemical information can be transmitted into or out of the body using bioelectrodes, which are sensing devices. It is possible to cause reversible faradaic charge transfer using IrOx bioelectrodes (Cho et al. 2021). Metals with greater electrical conducting nature are utilized in the preparation of bioelectrodes. Due to its low response when it comes into contact with the body, stainless steel is a widely used metal. Sometimes, platinum, gold, or copper is used. The body must be covered because copper responds to the biochemical conditions in the body (M. Wang and Duan 2019).

4.3.1 Bioanode

At a bio-anode, dissolved organic material is oxidized (Bond et al. 2002). The surface of the bio-anode "competes" with electron acceptors, which are soluble as shown in Figure 4.3. After the transmission of electrons to the bio-anode, it can be moved to the cathode through an external circuit. This is possible only when the cathode potential is greater than the anode potential.

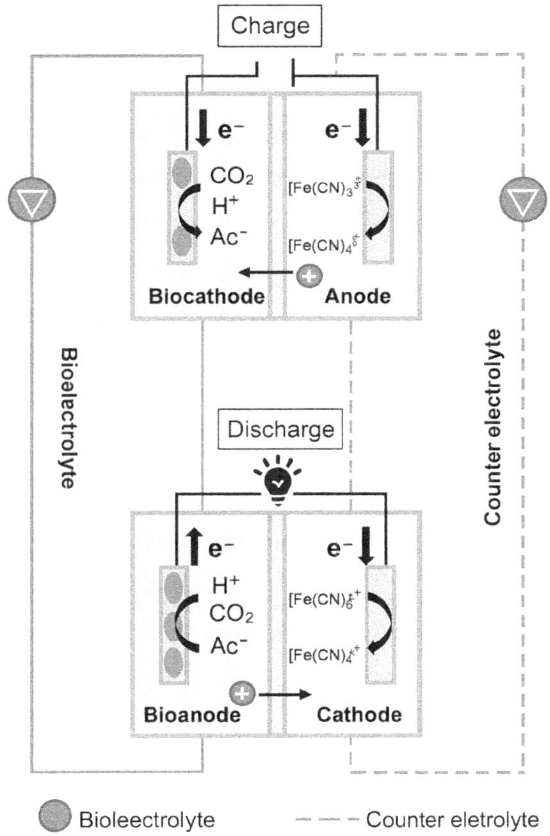

FIGURE 4.3 Simplified predominant reactions occurring at the bioanode, biocathode, and their respective counter electrodes; the movement of electrons (e–) across the external electrical circuits; and the transfer of cations (+) across the membranes.

Source: Adapted from Microbial Rechargeable Battery: Energy Storage and Recovery through Acetate Rusli et al. (2019)

Additionally, it must be lower than the cathode' s soluble electron acceptor potential (Xie, Criddle, and Cui 2015). Enzymatic bio-anodes possess at least one immobilized oxidoreductase enzyme that can oxidize one or more fuels (such as sugars and alcohols) to release electrons (Cho et al. 2021). Microorganisms present in the bio-anode, like algae, bacteria, fungi, etc., play as biocatalysts, which oxidize organic materials and transfer electrons to the bio-electrode either directly or indirectly (Strik, Hamelers, and Buisman 2010). The organic or biodegradable substance is added to the bio-anode, where it engages in a biocatalytic reaction to split into protons and electrons (Yaqoob et al. 2020). A bioanode that could move extracellular electrons from a bacterium to an electrode was used to produce electricity. The key advancements for the bio-anode were to improve the biofilm growth and bacterial adhesion through surface treatment. Significant efforts were taken to raise the specific surface area of the material to obtain greater anodic biofilm densities (Peckham, Ackermann, and Moss 2013a).

4.3.2 Biocathode

At the cathode, the oxidant O_2 is reduced (Chaudhuri and Lovley 2003; Tender et al. 2002). Applications for biosensors that benefit from the linear correlation between analyte concentration and current can use bio-cathodes (Kumlanghan et al. 2007; Liang et al. 2011). The design and selection of the materials, which can range from carbon to metal base materials, are the most challenging parts of making a biocathode. Stainless steel, carbon/graphite, and carbon are employed as the biocathodes in microbial fuel cells (MFCs; Rusli et al. 2019). A biocathode, which transfers extracellular electrons from an electrode to a microbe, was utilized to generate electricity. Oxygen reduction reaction was the preferred reaction for the electron-accepting mechanism on the cathode side. The efforts are taken to create electrodes with non-platinum group metals as catalysts (Peckham, Ackermann, and Moss 2013a).

4.3.3 Electrochemically active bacteria

The microorganisms that facilitate these electron exchanges are known to be electro-generators, anode- or cathode-respiring bacteria, exoelectrogens, and electrochemically active bacteria. These microorganisms possess the capacity to generate biofilms on different surfaces with various topographies. The topographies include both two-dimensional surface (carbon paper) and three-dimensional media, which shows the range from nanometres to millimetres. In a variety of natural habitats (soils, aquifers, lakes, thermal vents, and ocean sediment), under a wide range of physicochemical conditions, electrochemically active microorganisms mediate electron exchanges between solids and dissolved molecules (pH, ionic strength, pressure, temperature). Growing atop bio-anodes, electrochemically active bacteria steal electrons from soluble organic materials, which is a valuable source of electrons. These electrons are then transmitted to the bio-anode's surface, which may or may not form a coating on it (Xie, Criddle, and Cui 2015).

4.3.4 Extracellular electron transfer

In order to receive continuous reduction of an oxidized bio-anode by its connected cells depend upon the delivery of electrons (Figure 4.4). Whereas the removal of electrons produces the prolonged oxidation of a reduced bio-cathode by its connected cells. Slow electron transfer restricts the intrinsic rates of substrate usage. However, the restrictions are overcome with the usage of conductive coatings, progress in electrode topography, and current collectors made of stainless steel that promote adhesion (Liang et al. 2011; Rusli et al. 2019). It was observed that the diffusion rate of soluble substrates and products is rate-limiting when rapid transfer of electrons takes place. This includes both the waste products removal and the delivery of reactants.

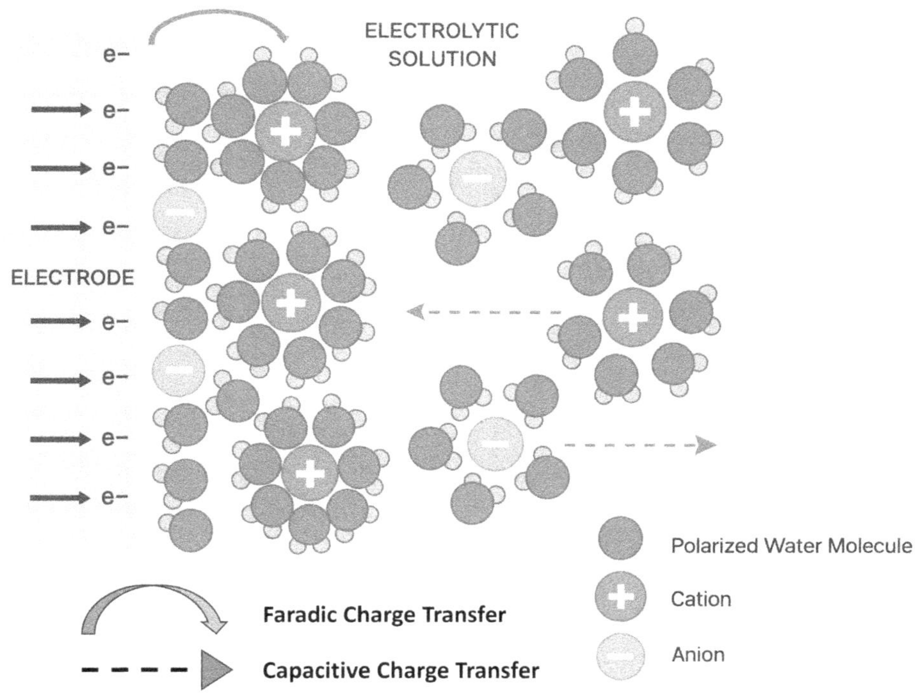

FIGURE 4.4 Representation of the electrode–electrolyte interface.

Source: Adapted from Role of Biomaterials in stimulating bioelectrodes Peckham, Ackermann, and Moss (2013a)

4.3.4.1 Direct electron transfer (DET)

Direct electron transfer (DET) is a direct interaction between the electrode surface and the bacterial enzyme, as shown in Figure 4.5. These enzymes are from the central cell membrane (c-type cytochrome, periplasmic, and inner membrane) found to be active (Huang, Regan, and Quan 2011). These microorganisms have an electron transport protein that is membrane-bound that relays electrons from the interior of the cell to the exterior (the electrode) or vice versa (Schröder 2007). Because the enzyme's active region is located inside the protein environment, DET occurs at a relatively slow rate. The active sites of some exoelectrogens species redox enzymes are directly facing the electrodes or media because they are embedded in the membrane of the microorganism.

However, this DET technique necessitates direct physical contact among the electrode, cytochrome, and bacterial cell. Therefore, the initial monolayer of bacteria on the electrode is the only one that is electrochemically active (Du, Li, and Gu 2007). Typically, the Geobacter, Rhodoferax, and Shewanella species were used in DET processes. In this process, an enzyme from the active centre of the cell membrane comes into direct contact with the electrode surface. However, the only biofilm monolayer that is electrochemically active is the first one on the surface of the electrode (Mook et al. 2013). The electrode material and the enzyme can exchange electrons directly during the power-producing redox reactions. DET, which benefits from the enzyme's catalytic centre's optimum overpotential and raises cell voltages, is one sort of electron transfer (Milton and Minteer 2017). HSM functionalization and enzyme engineering are the two main avenues that have been heavily researched to optimize enzyme orientation. When the spherical pore's radius is close to the enzyme's radius, DET is feasible (Mazurenko et al., 2017). Since there are no shuttle molecules

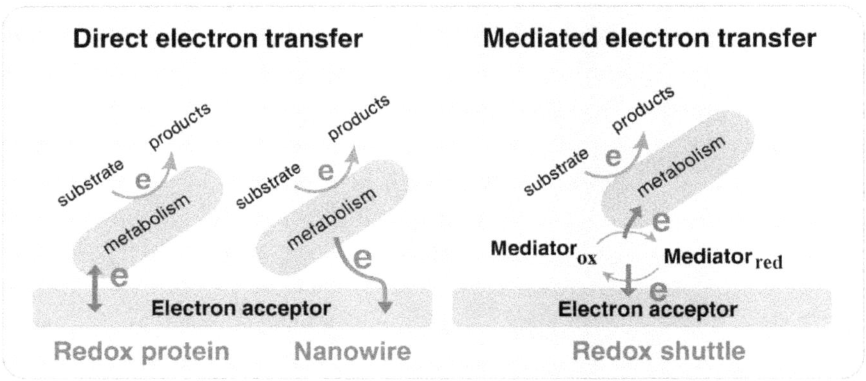

FIGURE 4.5 A comparison between DET and MET mechanisms in BFCs.

Source: Adapted from Electron Transfer in Gram-Positive Electroactive Bacteria and Its Application

in between the biocatalyst and electrode during DET operations, several problems associated with mediator use are eliminated. Several issues related to mediator use are removed since, during DET operations, there are no shuttle molecules between the biocatalyst and the electrode. Since most redox mediators might hinder the biological activity of enzymes and the kinetic mechanism of electrochemical processes, DET between the biocatalyst and the electrode surface is preferred as shown in Figure 4.5 (Navaee and Salimi 2015).

4.3.4.2 Mediated electron transfer (MET)

The majority of microorganisms' outer layers are made up of peptidoglycans, lipopolysaccharides, and nonconductive lipid membranes. They are unable to transfer electrons directly to the electrodes. To move electrons between bacteria and electrodes, mediators are needed. These redox mediators can be retrieved at the electrode and are not eaten by microbes (Du, Li, and Gu 2007; Rosenbaum et al. 2011). Another sort of MET (mediated electron transfer) will produce on its own and doesn't require artificial redox mediators. Some microbes can produce redox mediators through primary metabolites and secondary metabolites, which leads to a transfer of an electron which was not dependent on foreign redox shuttles. The mediator acts as a reversible donor or acceptor of electrons. This was carried out by moving from the anode to the cathode or vice versa (Pham, Aelterman, and Verstraete 2009). Most of the microorganisms can't carry electrons straight to the electrodes. So, mediators are needed to transfer the electrons between microorganisms and electrodes. The essential alternative is MET, which uses a redox mediator to act as an electron shuttle between the enzyme and the electrode (Prévoteau, Courjean, and Mano 2010; Kavanagh and Leech 2013). A diffusible redox molecule or redox polymer collects electrons from the biocatalyst. Then transfers these electrons to the electrode or the biocatalyst itself. MET is the term for this. In fuel cell applications, the MET mechanism is used to attain effective electron transport between the enzyme active centre and the electrode. A link was established between electrochemical surfaces and enzymes by a redox molecule, which acts as a shuttle of electrons. Immobilized glucose oxidase (Gox), an enzyme based on flavin adenine dinucleotide, is one of the examples (Wooten et al. 2014; Luong et al. 2017).

4.3.5 2D Bioelectrodes

The 2D carbon structure of graphene has gained interest because of its unusual layered structure, outstanding conductivity, incredibly huge surface area, and electro-optical capabilities. The next generation of flexible and transparent (opto)electronics is expected to be made of 2D materials with outstanding flexibility and atomic thickness (Xie, Criddle, and Cui 2015).

4.3.6 3D Bioelectrodes

Porous structure of 3D macroscale that optimizes the removal of waste materials, reduces clogging, and allows for advective delivery of substrates. In 3D porous electrodes (open or closed), their pore size and shape, accessibility, and macro-porosity are included. Examples of 3D porous bioelectrodes are carbon felt, carbon brush, packed bed electrodes, stainless steel mesh, CNT-textile, and monolithic porous electrodes (Xie, Criddle, and Cui 2015). 3D bioelectrodes are receiving a lot of attention due to their access to the deep regions of different 3D regions and tissues (Cho et al. 2021). Many research studies were carried out on the manufacture of bio-electrodes and probes of a three-dimensional micro- and nanoscale range. These electrodes and probes were utilized to detect signals or administer biochemicals within the cellular membrane, due to the rapid advancements in microfabrication technologies with 3D structures over the past several decades. There are still efforts to use nanofabrication techniques like lithographic patterning or 3D printing to accomplish intracellular-like recording of many neurons concurrently in a live-cell condition. Electroporation or electropermeabilization has been frequently employed to open cell membranes. Initially, the cell's electrical activities are recorded with 3D bioelectrodes. Inserting electrodes inside tissue is necessary for activating a particular area of multifunctional 3D tissue or for recording local electrophysiological signals. Numerous 3D bioelectrodes have been created for this reason. On consideration of electrochemical inertness, electrical conductivity, mechanical flexibility, and strength, the carbon materials like carbon nanotubes (CNTs), graphite, and graphene were used as neural interface (Keefer et al. 2008). Noble metals such as platinum, iridium, and gold are used for bioelectrodes because of their chemical unresponsiveness, biocompatibility, and high electrical conductivity (Wellman et al. 2018). Very tiny, three-dimensional carbon fibre or nanotube structures can be created synthetically and employed as bioelectrodes. Surface coatings of CNTs and carbon fibre can maximize the potential of 3D bioelectrodes. To enable non-faradaic charge transmission, oxide bioelectrodes function as a capacitive layer because no chemical species are produced or consumed during the stimulation process. Capacitive and non-faradaic charge transfer is preferable as a stimulation of electrode. For example, Tantalum oxide (Ta_2O_5) or titanium oxide (TiO_2) acts for electrochemical double layer formation (X. Yuan et al. 2020). Titanium nitride (TiN) is used as a bioelectrode in medical devices such as cardiac pacemakers and is used for dental implants since it is an electrically conductive oxide (Mezger and Creugers 1992).

4.4 BIOELECTRODES BASED ON POROUS NATURE

For effective electron transfer, the bioelectrode should possess a porous structure with ample surface area and an affinity electrode surface with enhanced binding capability. Bioelectrodes with significant current outputs have been created by scientists; however, extensive research and substantial capital costs are needed for BES usage on a large scale. The majority of high-performance bioelectrodes now on the market either involve time- and energy-consuming synthesis processes or pricey components. The creation of reliable and affordable porous electrodes is still a top focus because they have a larger contact area and provide better contact for microorganisms and the electrode surface. Porous electrodes often function better than nonporous electrodes. As of this date, carbonaceous materials like graphene, carbon black, CNTs, and mesoporous carbons are used in the preparation of bio-electrodes (Gross, Holzinger, and Cosnier 2018).

4.4.1 Nonporous bulk electrodes

Bioelectrodes with nm to mm-sized pores only resemble nonporous bulk electrodes. The current generation of nonporous bulk electrodes is only practical up close to the electrode surface. The interfacial is constrained towards the electrode's specified exposed area as a result of the exoelectrogens, which only grow on the exterior surface. A nonporous electrode consists of carbon electrodes (graphite rods, graphite disks, or graphite plates) and metal electrodes (gold, platinum, and titanium).

4.4.2 Particle-based porous electrode

For conventional electrochemical systems (fuel cells or batteries), 3D porous electrodes are developed with the particle "piling" method. Bioelectrodes are routinely made using this method as well. Example: graphite assorted with PTFE (polytetrafluoroethylene) (Zhang et al. 2006). Anodic microorganisms combined with carbon nanoparticles and PTFE, the resulting product is spread on a carbon cloth collector (Y. Yuan et al. 2011).

4.4.3 Monolithic porous electrodes

A monolithically structured porous electrode is porous but made of a single, intrinsically connected piece of material. Reticulated vitreous carbon (RVC), usually referred as carbon form, is the most widely utilized monolithic porous electrode material. Because of their open 3D linked architecture, robust mechanical support, possibility for evenly spread and customizable microbially accessible pores, and conductive electron routes, monolithic porous electrodes hold the most promise for the practical implementation of BESs. Amidst many electrodes, monolithic porous electrodes have shown an increased rate of current density. The monolithic porous electrodes that have been described so far either involve pricey components like CNTs or call for labour-intensive synthesis processes like carbonization or freezing (Xie, Criddle, and Cui 2015).

4.5 FACTORS INFLUENCING MATERIAL SELECTION FOR ELECTRODES

4.5.1 Potential of hydrogen

The ideal pH range for microbial activity is 6.0 to 7.0. A pH gradient across the membrane leads to decrease in the cell's power and voltage output. The underlying reasons of this problem include acid generation at the anode, alkaline synthesis at the cathode, and non-specific proton exchange over the membrane. The creation of a reversible bioelectrode, which is the cause of the bio-catalysed anodic and cathodic electron transfer, can also correct this (Strik, Hamelers, and Buisman 2010).

4.5.2 Surface area of Bio-anode material

Greater surface areas allow for more microbial adhesion, which boosts the rate of electron transfer. This suggests that the biofilm adhered to the electrode surface affects power output and electricity production (Liu and Li 2007). The anodic surface area was increased by utilizing carbon or graphite in different forms, such as nanotubes, fibres, granules, and foam (Zou et al. 2008; Catal et al. 2008; Biffinger et al. 2007; Cheng, Dempsey, and Logan 2007; Cheng, Liu, and Logan 2006).

4.5.3 Effect of spacing of electrode

One of the main restrictions is internal resistance, commonly referred to as ohmic losses (Behera et al. 2010). Additionally, lost potentials during the electron and proton transfer procedures must be taken into account. Decreased electrode spacing can lower internal resistance (W.-W. Li et al. 2011). However, the oxygen in the cathodic chamber might permeate onto the anodic chamber in single-chambered MFCs, too tight, where the electrode spacing can reduce the performance. In contrast, since MECs primarily operate in anaerobic circumstances, the electrode separation can be very tiny (Martin et al. 2010; Puig et al. 2010).

4.5.4 Concentration of organic substance

The amount of organic matter influences the coulombic efficiency and power density in addition to bacterial size and biofilm morphology. Higher initial organic matter concentrations cause more organic matter to be removed, but they also cause coulombic efficiency to decline. This occurs due to other microbial processes, processes like fermentation and methanogenesis utilize organic matter, resulting in the formation of different byproducts (Sukkasem et al. 2008; Virdis et al. 2008).

4.6 ELECTRODE MATERIALS

It has been proposed that the incorporation of nanomaterials into bioelectrodes may enhance certain functional properties, including electron conduction, resistance to thermal and mechanical changes, and conversion rate (Tawalbeh et al. 2022). Aimed at long-term MFC operation, it is essential for electrode material to be extremely steady in challenging wastewater conditions. To prevent clogging-related problems for use in wastewater remediation applications, 3D electrode materials in particular ought to have the ideal pore size. Currently, scaling up MFCs for real-world use is primarily hampered by the cost of the materials and surface modification techniques. Therefore, to expand the use of MFCs on a large scale, more affordable and stable materials, as well as effective methods for creating composite metal- or carbon-based electrodes, should be developed. Upscaling of the effective electrodes for MFCs must be tested in the future, and creative combining both anode and cathode membranes must be a perfect membrane electrode assembly (Kalathil, Patil, and Pant 2018).

4.6.1 Noble materials

Glomerella cingulate's glucose dehydrogenase (GDH) was coupled using an Os-complex-modified hydrogel that was placed on nano-porous gold electrodes with various porosities (9–60 nm) (Siepenkoetter, Salaj-Kosla, et al. 2017). Gold or silver bioelectrodes were deposited on the underside of the PVP-based microneedle patch using the thermal evaporation technique to optimize the effective drug release. For the biocompatibility SU8 adhesion layer is used instead of chromium on gold-coated glass substrate bioelectrode for microelectronics applications (Matarèse et al. 2018).

4.6.2 Non-noble materials

When anodic polarization occurs, tantalum and titanium can create insulating oxide layers that can be employed to make capacitive electrodes (charge-injecting electrodes that don't undergo faradaic reactions at the electrode-electrolyte contact). Although titanium oxide has a substantially higher dielectric strength than tantalum oxide, its usage in electrode applications is constrained by severe DC leakage. Tantalum-tantalum pentoxide-based capacitive electrodes have a limited capacity to store charge (100–150 $\mu C/cm^2$) and can only be employed in applications above a specific geometric size (0.05 cm^2) for various purposes (Rose, Kelliher, and Robblee 1985).

4.6.3 Oxides and nitrite

Iridium oxide is considered as a predominant material for the implanted bio-electrodes because of the excellent biocompatibility, corrosion resistance, high charge density, and low impedance. The stability of neural signal transmission can be ensured by good surface morphological properties. It can be used for the modification of the implantable electrodes. Because of this effect, the bio-electrode modifying coatings can enhance charge transfer at the electrode interface, which increases the efficiency of electrical stimulus by decreasing the inflammatory response and fibre cyst formation. And, it is also increasing the life of the bio-electrodes (Qin et al. 2014).

4.6.4 Carbon-based materials (BFCs)

Substantial improvements on designing bioelectrodes are important factors to enhance the power density, voltage output, and operational stability. Improvements in electrical wiring techniques for enzymes are needed, as well as electrodes with high surface areas, high conductivities, and mechanical stability. CNTs have been widely utilizing in creating enzymatic biofuel cells (EBFCs) suitable for delivering adequate power densities, ranging from microwatts to milliwatts, to operate low power bioelectronic devices using renewable substrate (Gross, Holzinger, and Cosnier 2018).

4.6.4.1 Graphene

Graphene is considered as a promising candidate for application such as enzymatic bioelectrodes and biofuel cells. Graphene has great electrical conductivity and is simple to functionalize. Numerous functional characteristics of graphene can be exploited to immobilize enzymes on electrode surfaces and facilitates DET from enzyme's redox centre to the surface (Karimi et al. 2015).

4.7 APPLICATION OF BIO-ELECTRODES

4.7.1 Supercapacitor

The charging and storing properties of the supercapacitor were significantly influenced by the level of porosity and exposed surface area of the bioelectrodes as shown in Table 4.1. It will be simpler for electrolytes to diffuse through connected channels and raise ion transport rates thanks to the bioelectrode carbon's large specific surface area and porous structure, which will significantly enhance the bioelectrode's capacity to store energy. TTO exhibits significant potential as a bioelectrode material for long-term supercapacitor applications (Rafieerad et al. 2021a). It was discovered that a specified capacitance could be reached 136 F/g at 0.5 A/g using a commercially procured activated carbon-based electrode that was fabricated through bioelectrolyte. Supercapacitor devices made with bioelectrodes and bioelectrolytes showed specific capacitance of 640 F/g, specific energy of 22.2 Wh/kg, and specific power of 948 F/g at a current density of 0.5 A/g takes place under

TABLE 4.1
Various bioelectrode materials with their specific capacitance and surface area

Electrode materials	Specific capacitance (F/g)	Surface area	References
Banana peel	206	1650 m^2/g	Lv et al. (2012)
Coconut husk	184	1033.20 m^2/g	Taer, Taslim, Putri, et al. (2018)
Cellulose acetate	241	241.4 m^2/g	Cai et al. (2016)
Bamboo powder	268	2352 m^2/g	J. Li and Wu (2015)
Durian shell	103	456.63	Ong et al. (2012)
Rubber wood	138	1704	Farma et al. (2013)
Rice husk	147	2696	Teo et al. (2016)
Tea leaves	330	2841	Peng et al. (2013)
Apricot shell	339	2335	Xu et al. (2010)
Sunflower seed shell	244	2584	X. Li et al. (2011)
Coconut fibres	155	2898	He et al. (2013)
Peanut shell	199	1634	Taer, Taslim, Mustika, et al. (2018)
Banana stem	170	835.939	Rufford et al. (2010a)
TTO	640	51.06	Rafieerad et al. (2021b)
Sugarcane	300	–	Rufford et al. (2010b)
Corn grains	257	–	Balathanigaimani et al. (2008)
Casava peel waste	368	–	Ismanto et al. (2010)

the same testing conditions (Dhar et al. 2020). $Ta_4C_3T_x$ MXene-tantalum oxide (TTO) has great promise for usage in long-term supercapacitor applications as a bioelectrode material (Rafieerad et al. 2021a). The TTO hybrid supercapacitor structure outperformed nearly every other type of bioelectrode material (Rafieerad et al. 2021a). A trihybrid bioelectrode consisting of lignin, poly (3,4-ethylenedioxythiophene) (PEDOT), and poly (aminoanthraquinone) (PAAQ) is synthesized through a two-step galvanostatic electro polymerization process and characterized for supercapacitor applications. The hybrid electrode PEDOT/Lignin/PAAQ was constructed using PEDOT/Lignin as a base layer and subsequently deposited with PAAQ, which has a high specific capacitance of 418 F/g with minimal self-discharge (Dhar et al. 2020).

4.7.2 Fuel cells

Emerging energy sources known as "biological fuel cells" use enzymes or microorganisms as catalysts to generate electric energy obtained from chemically made substrates found in biological fluids (Cosnier, Le Goff, and Holzinger 2014; Bandodkar 2017; Taghavi et al. 2015; Han, Yu, and Liu 2010; Dong et al. 2013). Biofuel cells operate on the principle of bioelectrocatalytic oxidation of a "fuel" (e.g., glucose) at the anode, producing electrons that are transmitted to the cathode, where bioelectrocatalytic reduction of the oxidant (e.g., O_2) occurs. The anode oxidizes the fuel through bioelectrocatalysis, generating electrons that flow to the cathode, where they are used in the bioelectrocatalytic reduction of the oxidant, which is the basis for how biofuel cells function. Glucose oxidase and GDH are the two most prevalent enzymes for oxidizing glucose (Gross, Holzinger, and Cosnier 2018). The cofactors for each GDH enzyme, flavin adenine dinucleotide, nicotine adenine dinucleotide, and pyrroloquinoline quinone, are used to identify them. Enzymes such as laccase or bilirubin oxidase, which act as multicopper oxidases, catalyse the reduction of oxygen to water at the cathode (Christenson et al. 2006; Sakai et al. 2009; Le Goff, Holzinger, and Cosnier 2015).

4.7.1.1 Microbial fuel cell

For purposes like self-sustaining wastewater treatment, microbial biofuel cells are more appropriate for large-scale, eco-friendly electricity generation over extended periods. However, there have been some reports using MFCs to supply energy for implantable and wearable power generation. The use of buck paper-based bioelectrodes with biofuel cells has led to among the leading current and power densities reported so far for EBFCs (Gross, Holzinger, and Cosnier 2018). The bioelectrode used to construct the first rechargeable MFC was able to carry electrons out of the cell in both directions (Chu et al. 2021). MFCs consist of both anodic chamber and cathodic chamber, which are separated by proton exchange membrane (Rusli et al. 2019). A separator is employed to transmit a proton from the anode to the cathode and stop oxygen from diffusing into the cathode chamber from the cathode site (Rahimnejad et al. 2014). Due to the tremendous availability of bacteria from different sources, it was considered for MFCs. In MFCs, energy is processed by the degradation of organic matter and waste by catalytic reaction at the anode. Paper-based CNT bioelectrodes were prepared for MFCs, which produce a power output of 192 $\mu W/cm^2$ with a high current density of 1.3 mA/cm^2 (Gamella, Koushanpour, and Katz 2018; Cinquin et al. 2010).

4.7.1.2 Enzymatic fuel cell

EBFCs are measured using more advantageous option than MFCs for supplying power to implantable and wearable devices, due to their higher power density capabilities (Katz and MacVittie 2013). Finding an effective transfer of electrons from the enzyme to the electrode (at the anode) and from the electrode to the enzyme is one of the ongoing issues in EBFC development (at the cathode) (Courjean, Gao, and Mano 2009). Enzymes, rather than noble metals, serve as catalysts for the fuel and oxidant transformation in enzymatic fuel cells (EFCs), which operate similarly to low-temperature proton exchange membrane fuel cells (PEMFC) (Mazurenko, de Poulpiquet, and Lojou 2017b). EBFCs operate at a low-temperature and rely on enzymes as a catalyst in place of traditional materials like standard metal catalysts used in conventional fuel cells to catalyse chemical processes (Karimi et al. 2015). EFCs use enzymes as catalysts for a fuel and oxidant transformation. For enhanced power delivery, enzymes with high surface ratio conducting materials were considered. Enzymes are used in EFCs as a catalyst for the conversion of fuel and oxidant. Enzymes with high surface ratio conducting materials were taken into consideration for improved power delivery (Mazurenko, de Poulpiquet, and Lojou 2017b). Because the combination of enzymes and nanomaterials in EFCs shows greater electrical combinations. Most widely used nanomaterials are high surface area nanomaterials (HSM), which are commonly carbon. This includes carbon black, graphene, CNTs, and buckypaper (Pereira et al. 2016; de Poulpiquet et al. 2014). The EFCs use enzymes as a catalyst in the oxidation and reduction process, which takes place in the cathode and anode of the fuel cells. For enzyme considerations, nanomaterials with a high surface area are taken. Enhanced surface area leads to higher catalytic currents, which creates issues related to porosity, wiring, and stability (Xie, Criddle, and Cui 2015). In EFC's chemical energy is converted to electrical energy by redox reactions that take place in the fuel cell. The electrons move from the anode and reach the cathode, which is an electron acceptor due to the catalysis process. Fuel flows in the anode, and oxygen flows freely in the cathode for excellent performance. A separator is developed between the cathode and the anode to make different devices. Enzymes, which act as a catalyst, are mixed with a certain medium that is used as an electrolyte. For the preparation of electrode materials, it is important to reduce the resistance produced by those materials. The CNT-higher surface area, compatibility in fabrication techniques, excellent conductivity, and biocompatibility (Mazurenko, de Poulpiquet, and Lojou 2017a).

4.7.3 Energy Storage and Conversion

It can be utilized to convert solar energy by increasing the stability of photosystem I-based bioelectrodes. Neem tree gum, which is produced naturally, can serve as a versatile energy storage system. The biodegradable electrodes and electrolytes made from renewable sources can be efficiently utilized in high-energy and power storage systems (Dhar et al. 2020).

4.8 PROBLEMS, LIMITATIONS, AND CHALLENGES

The bioelectrodes continue to have serious limitations due to their slow response times. The response time is often slow due to the extended diffusion distance at the interface of the test solution and detector's inner surface. The response times ranged between 10 and 20 min, and it was reduced to 3 min by removing the extra support membranes (Joseph. Wang and Lin 1988). Increasing the current density of the bioelectrodes and improving their stability are just two of the numerous problems that still need to be solved. Nanostructured materials have been created and changed in the field of bioelectrocatalysis to increase current densities for a range of enzyme electrocatalysis. Given that the electroactive region of most redox enzymes is located deep within the protein's three-dimensional (3D) architecture, efficient electron transfer between the electrode and the immobilized enzyme must be guaranteed. The electron transfer rate and current flow are the two essential parameters for maintaining the efficiency of biofuel cells, which determine the power output of EBFCs. To properly connect and maintain the enzyme in its steric functional form, better materials and enzyme immobilization techniques are needed. In general, multienzyme co-immobilization techniques offer effective ways to enhance the bioelectrode's characteristics in bioelectrochemistry. Co-immobilization procedures must take into account simplicity, reproducibility, cost-effectiveness, and processing duration. An innovation in multi-enzyme bioelectrode-based devices will significantly rely on the complexity of co-immobilizing different enzymes with distinct properties (such as size, optimal pH, stability), the comprehensive investigation of the relationships between the catalytic efficacy of multienzyme systems and the conformations of various enzymes, and the utilization of superior electrode materials. The inherent rates of substrate utilization may be limited if the electron transfer rates are sluggish. To overcome this issue, conductive coatings, stainless steel current collectors, and the development of electrode topography that promotes adhesion can all be used to overcome these restrictions.

4.8.1 Long-term stability

Enzymes are constantly being replaced in vivo; thus, there is no problem with their intrinsic stability (Siepenkoetter, Salaj-Kosla, et al. 2017). The solvent employed as electrolyte or protein solubilizer profoundly influences the structure of the enzyme restrained on CNTs and, therefore, its stability (Wu et al. 2017). Comparatively, H_2 oxidation by two homologous O_2-tolerant hydrogenases illustrated the protective function of the detergent employed in the purification process against enzyme denaturation upon immobilization on negatively charged CNTs (Monsalve et al. 2016). Pore size influences enzyme stability, evident by the enhanced thermal stability of fructose dehydrogenase encapsulated in MgO-templated carbon when the pore size dimension approximates the enzyme (Funabashi, Murata, and Tsujimura 2015).

4.8.2 Biocompatibility and integration of devices

It is crucial to evaluate and improve the bioacceptability of bioelectrodes for implanted and wearable biofuel cells to reduce unforeseen dangers to people and the environment. Strict rules that adhere to safety standards must be followed for implanted devices to receive accreditation. Numerous aspects of biocompatibility, such as cytotoxicity, sensitization and irritability, systemic toxicity, genotoxicity, carcinogenicity, and hemocompatibility, must be carefully taken into account. The chemical biocompatibility of an electrode depends on the implant's ability to endure the environment it is exposed to inside the body as well as the tissue's capacity to withstand the passive chemical interaction with the electrode. Successful materials historically utilized in implanted devices are inert and interact chemically with their surroundings as little as possible (Peckham, Ackermann, and Moss 2013b).

4.8.3 Design and miniaturization

The size of implanted devices is generally a concern because large implants necessitate invasive surgery. The use of an alternate energy source in place of batteries can significantly reduce the size of implantable power devices. Additionally, implantable BFCs may in the future change medical technology because the use of rechargeable devices in place of batteries can eliminate the need for additional procedures to replace power sources, dramatically lowering the danger of infection (Sedenho et al. 2018).

4.9 SUMMARY AND FUTURE SCOPE

Recent advances in novel materials for bioelectrodes have not only improved their electrical and mechanical properties but also extended their functional versatility for wearable applications. The use of CNTs-based materials offers high conductivity, flexibility, and large surface area making them a suitable for constructing high-performance enzymatic electrodes in biofuel cells and other energy harvesting biodevices. Similarly, the development of graphene-based conductive hydrogel with injectability and tunable degradability allows for minimally invasive implantation and control over device lifespan, addressing major limitations of conventional hydrogel electrodes. When it comes to wearable technology, single-wall CNTs with stretchable nanosheets have yielding bioelectrodes that are not only highly flexible and comfortable to the skin but also comfort during prolonged use. Furthermore, the emergence of bio-inspired and programmable materials, including engineered living materials, points to a future where bioelectrodes can self-assemble, adapt or even repair themselves, bringing up new possibilities for responsive biomedical interface. Overall, the continued exploration and integration of these novel materials are expected to drive the next generation of bioelectrodes, enabling more reliable, patient-friendly, and multifunctional devices for diverse application in healthcare, energy harvesting, and beyond.

ACKNOWLEDGMENT

The author RP thanks the Solar Energy Research Center, SERC-Chile (ANID/FONDAP/15110019), FONDECYT 1201314.

REFERENCES

Balathanigaimani, M.S., Wang-Geun Shim, Min-Joo Lee, Chan Kim, Jae-Wook Lee, and Hee Moon. 2008. "Highly Porous Electrodes from Novel Corn Grains-Based Activated Carbons for Electrical Double Layer Capacitors." *Electrochemistry Communications* 10 (6): 868–871. https://doi.org/10.1016/j.elecom.2008.04.003.

Bandodkar, Amay J. 2017. "Review—Wearable Biofuel Cells: Past, Present and Future." *Journal of The Electrochemical Society* 164 (3): H3007–H3014. https://doi.org/10.1149/2.0031703jes.

Behera, Manaswini, Partha S. Jana, Tanaji T. More, and M.M. Ghangrekar. 2010. "Rice Mill Wastewater Treatment in Microbial Fuel Cells Fabricated Using Proton Exchange Membrane and Earthen Pot at Different PH." *Bioelectrochemistry* 79 (2): 228–233. https://doi.org/10.1016/j.bioelechem.2010.06.002.

Biffinger, Justin C., Jeremy Pietron, Ricky Ray, Brenda Little, and Bradley R. Ringeisen. 2007. "A Biofilm Enhanced Miniature Microbial Fuel Cell Using Shewanella Oneidensis DSP10 and Oxygen Reduction Cathodes." *Biosensors and Bioelectronics* 22 (8): 1672–1679. https://doi.org/10.1016/j.bios.2006.07.027.

Bond, Daniel R., Dawn E. Holmes, Leonard M. Tender, and Derek R. Lovley. 2002. "Electrode-Reducing Microorganisms That Harvest Energy from Marine Sediments." *Science* 295 (5554): 483–485. https://doi.org/10.1126/science.1066771.

Cai, Jie, Haitao Niu, Hongxia Wang, Hao Shao, Jian Fang, Jingren He, Hanguo Xiong, Chengjie Ma, and Tong Lin. 2016. "High-Performance Supercapacitor Electrode from Cellulose-Derived, Inter-Bonded Carbon Nanofibers." *Journal of Power Sources* 324 (August): 302–308. https://doi.org/10.1016/j.jpowsour.2016.05.070.

Catal, Tunc, Kaichang Li, Hakan Bermek, and Hong Liu. 2008. "Electricity Production from Twelve Monosaccharides Using Microbial Fuel Cells." *Journal of Power Sources* 175 (1): 196–200. https://doi.org/10.1016/j.jpowsour.2007.09.083.

Chaudhuri, Swades K., and Derek R. Lovley. 2003. "Electricity Generation by Direct Oxidation of Glucose in Mediatorless Microbial Fuel Cells." *Nature Biotechnology* 21 (10): 1229–1232. https://doi.org/10.1038/nbt867.

Cheng, Shaoan, Brian A. Dempsey, and Bruce E. Logan. 2007. "Electricity Generation from Synthetic Acid-Mine Drainage (AMD) Water Using Fuel Cell Technologies." *Environmental Science & Technology* 41 (23): 8149–8153. https://doi.org/10.1021/es0712221.

Cheng, Shaoan, Hong Liu, and Bruce E. Logan. 2006. "Increased Performance of Single-Chamber Microbial Fuel Cells Using an Improved Cathode Structure." *Electrochemistry Communications* 8 (3): 489–494. https://doi.org/10.1016/j.elecom.2006.01.010.

Cho, Yo Han, Young-Geun Park, Sumin Kim, and Jang-Ung Park. 2021. "3D Electrodes for Bioelectronics." *Advanced Materials* 33 (47). https://doi.org/10.1002/adma.202005805.

Christenson, Andreas, Sergey Shleev, Nicolas Mano, Adam Heller, and Lo Gorton. 2006. "Redox Potentials of the Blue Copper Sites of Bilirubin Oxidases." *Biochimica et Biophysica Acta (BBA) - Bioenergetics* 1757 (12): 1634–1641. https://doi.org/10.1016/j.bbabio.2006.08.008.

Chu, Na, Lixia Zhang, Wen Hao, Qinjun Liang, Yong Jiang, and Raymond Jianxiong Zeng. 2021. "Rechargeable Microbial Fuel Cell Based on Bidirectional Extracellular Electron Transfer." *Bioresource Technology* 329 (June): 124887. https://doi.org/10.1016/j.biortech.2021.124887.

Cinquin, Philippe, Chantal Gondran, Fabien Giroud, Simon Mazabrard, Aymeric Pellissier, François Boucher, Jean-Pierre Alcaraz, et al. 2010. "A Glucose BioFuel Cell Implanted in Rats." *PLoS ONE* 5 (5): e10476. https://doi.org/10.1371/journal.pone.0010476.

Cosnier, Serge, Alan Le Goff, and Michael Holzinger. 2014. "Towards Glucose Biofuel Cells Implanted in Human Body for Powering Artificial Organs: Review." *Electrochemistry Communications* 38 (January): 19–23. https://doi.org/10.1016/j.elecom.2013.09.021.

Courjean, Olivier, Feng Gao, and Nicolas Mano. 2009. "Deglycosylation of Glucose Oxidase for Direct and Efficient Glucose Electrooxidation on a Glassy Carbon Electrode." *Angewandte Chemie International Edition* 48 (32): 5897–5899. https://doi.org/10.1002/anie.200902191.

Dhar, Abhishek, Nadavala Siva Kumar, Mehul Khimani, Ahmed S. Al-Fatesh, Ahmed A. Ibrahim, Anish H. Fakeeha, Poonam Bhadja, and Rohit L. Vekariya. 2020. "Naturally Occurring Neem Gum: An Unprecedented Green Resource for Bioelectrochemical Flexible Energy Storage Device." *International Journal of Energy Research* 44 (2): 913–924. https://doi.org/10.1002/er.4949.

Dong, Kun, Boyang Jia, Chaoling Yu, Wenbo Dong, Fangzhou Du, and Hong Liu. 2013. "Microbial Fuel Cell as Power Supply for Implantable Medical Devices: A Novel Configuration Design for Simulating Colonic Environment." *Biosensors and Bioelectronics* 41 (March): 916–919. https://doi.org/10.1016/j.bios.2012.10.028.

Du, Zhuwei, Haoran Li, and Tingyue Gu. 2007. "A State of the Art Review on Microbial Fuel Cells: A Promising Technology for Wastewater Treatment and Bioenergy." *Biotechnology Advances* 25 (5): 464–482. https://doi.org/10.1016/j.biotechadv.2007.05.004.

Farma, Rakhmawati, Mohamad B. Deraman, Awitdrus. Awitdrus, Ibrahim Abu Talib, Erman Taer, NurHamizah. Basri, J.G. Manjunatha, Maria Muhammad Ishak, B.N.M. Dollah, and Safir Ahmad Hashmi. 2013. "Preparation of Highly Porous Binderless Activated Carbon Electrodes from Fibres of Oil Palm Empty Fruit Bunches for Application in Supercapacitors." *Bioresource Technology* 132 (March): 254–261. https://doi.org/10.1016/j.biortech.2013.01.044.

Funabashi, Hiroto, Kazuki Murata, and Seiya Tsujimura. 2015. "Effect of Pore Size of MgO-Templated Carbon on the Direct Electrochemistry of D-Fructose Dehydrogenase." *Electrochemical Society of Japan* 83 (5): 372–375. https://doi.org/10.5796/ELECTROCHEMISTRY.83.372.

Gamella, Maria, Ashkan Koushanpour, and Evgeny Katz. 2018. "Biofuel Cells – Activation of Micro- and Macro-Electronic Devices." *Bioelectrochemistry* 119 (February): 33–42. https://doi.org/10.1016/j.bioelechem.2017.09.002.

Goff, Alan Le, Michael Holzinger, and Serge Cosnier. 2015. "Recent Progress in Oxygen-Reducing Laccase Biocathodes for Enzymatic Biofuel Cells." *Cellular and Molecular Life Sciences* 72 (5): 941–952. https://doi.org/10.1007/s00018-014-1828-4.

Gross, Andrew James, Michael Holzinger, and Serge Cosnier. 2018. "Buckypaper Bioelectrodes: Emerging Materials for Implantable and Wearable Biofuel Cells." *Energy & Environmental Science* 11 (7): 1670–1687. https://doi.org/10.1039/C8EE00330K.

Han, Yufeng, Chaoling Yu, and Hong Liu. 2010. "A Microbial Fuel Cell as Power Supply for Implantable Medical Devices." *Biosensors and Bioelectronics* 25 (9): 2156–2160. https://doi.org/10.1016/j.bios.2010.02.014.

He, Xiaojun, Pinghua Ling, Jieshan Qiu, Moxin Yu, Xiaoyong Zhang, Chang Yu, and Mingdong Zheng. 2013. "Efficient Preparation of Biomass-Based Mesoporous Carbons for Supercapacitors with Both High Energy Density and High Power Density." *Journal of Power Sources* 240 (October): 109–113. https://doi.org/10.1016/j.jpowsour.2013.03.174.

Huang, Liping, John M. Regan, and Xie Quan. 2011. "Electron Transfer Mechanisms, New Applications, and Performance of Biocathode Microbial Fuel Cells." *Bioresource Technology* 102 (1): 316–323. https://doi.org/10.1016/j.biortech.2010.06.096.

Ismanto, Andrian Evan, Steven Wang, Felycia Edi Soetaredjo, and Suryadi Ismadji. 2010. "Preparation of Capacitor's Electrode from Cassava Peel Waste." *Bioresource Technology* 101 (10): 3534–3540. https://doi.org/10.1016/j.biortech.2009.12.123.

Kalathil Shafeer, Sunil A. Patil, and Deepak Pant. 2018. "Microbial Fuel Cells: Electrode Materials." In *Encyclopedia of Interfacial Chemistry*, 309–318. Elsevier. https://doi.org/10.1016/B978-0-12-409547-2.13459-6.

Karimi, Anahita, Ali Othman, Aytekin Uzunoglu, Lia Stanciu, and Silvana Andreescu. 2015. "Graphene Based Enzymatic Bioelectrodes and Biofuel Cells." *Nanoscale* 7 (16): 6909–6923. https://doi.org/10.1039/C4NR07586B.

Katz, Evgeny, and Kevin MacVittie. 2013. "Implanted Biofuel Cells Operating in Vivo – Methods, Applications and Perspectives – Feature Article." *Energy & Environmental Science* 6 (10): 2791. https://doi.org/10.1039/c3ee42126k.

Kavanagh, Paul, and Dónal Leech. 2013. "Mediated Electron Transfer in Glucose Oxidising Enzyme Electrodes for Application to Biofuel Cells: Recent Progress and Perspectives." *Physical Chemistry Chemical Physics* 15 (14): 4859. https://doi.org/10.1039/c3cp44617d.

Keefer, Edward W., Barry R. Botterman, Mario I. Romero, Andrew F. Rossi, and Guenter W. Gross. 2008. "Carbon Nanotube Coating Improves Neuronal Recordings." *Nature Nanotechnology* 3 (7): 434–439. https://doi.org/10.1038/nnano.2008.174.

Kumararaj, Abinash, Milan Joseph Kennedy, Leena Baskar, Geetha Arunachalam, Rekha Pachaiappan, Shailendra K. Saxena, Rathika Rajendran, and Kovendhan Manavalan. 2025. "Exploring the Electronic Characteristics of Metal Oxides for Diverse Energy Applications." *Electric and Electronic Applications of Metal Oxides*, January. Elsevier, 127–169. https://doi.org/10.1016/B978-0-443-26554-9.00005-5.

Kumararaj, Abinash, Suresh Perumal, Kamala Bharathi Karuppanan, and Geetha Arunachalam. 2025. "Electrochemical Performance of TiO2/Mn2O3 Nanocomposite in Different Electrolyte Environments." *ChemNanoMat*. John Wiley and Sons Inc, 2500207. https://doi.org/10.1002/CNMA.202500207.

Kumlanghan, Ampai, Jing Liu, Panote Thavarungkul, Proespichaya Kanatharana, and Bo Mattiasson. 2007. "Microbial Fuel Cell-Based Biosensor for Fast Analysis of Biodegradable Organic Matter." *Biosensors and Bioelectronics* 22 (12): 2939–2944. https://doi.org/10.1016/j.bios.2006.12.014.

Li, Jiangfeng, and Qingsheng Wu. 2015. "Water Bamboo-Derived Porous Carbons as Electrode Materials for Supercapacitors." *New Journal of Chemistry* 39 (5): 3859–3864. https://doi.org/10.1039/C4NJ01853B.

Li, Wen-Wei, Guo-Ping Sheng, Xian-Wei Liu, and Han-Qing Yu. 2011. "Recent Advances in the Separators for Microbial Fuel Cells." *Bioresource Technology* 102 (1): 244–252. https://doi.org/10.1016/j.biortech.2010.03.090.

Li, Xiao, Wei Xing, Shuping Zhuo, Jin Zhou, Feng Li, Shi-Zhang Qiao, and Gao-Qing Lu. 2011. "Preparation of Capacitor's Electrode from Sunflower Seed Shell." *Bioresource Technology* 102 (2): 1118–1123. https://doi.org/10.1016/j.biortech.2010.08.110.

Liang, Peng, Huiyong Wang, Xue Xia, Xia Huang, Yinghui Mo, Xiaoxin Cao, and Mingzhi Fan. 2011. "Carbon Nanotube Powders as Electrode Modifier to Enhance the Activity of Anodic Biofilm in Microbial Fuel Cells." *Biosensors and Bioelectronics* 26 (6): 3000–3004. https://doi.org/10.1016/j.bios.2010.12.002.

Liu, Zhi-Dan, and Hao-Ran Li. 2007. "Effects of Bio- and Abio-Factors on Electricity Production in a Mediatorless Microbial Fuel Cell." *Biochemical Engineering Journal* 36 (3): 209–214. https://doi.org/10.1016/j.bej.2007.02.021.

Luong, John H.T., Jeremy D. Glennon, Aharon Gedanken, and Sandeep K. Vashist. 2017. "Achievement and Assessment of Direct Electron Transfer of Glucose Oxidase in Electrochemical Biosensing Using Carbon Nanotubes, Graphene, and Their Nanocomposites." *Microchimica Acta* 184 (2): 369–388. https://doi.org/10.1007/s00604-016-2049-3.

Lv, Yaokang, Lihua Gan, Mingxian Liu, Wei Xiong, Zijie Xu, Dazhang Zhu, and Dominic S. Wright. 2012. "A Self-Template Synthesis of Hierarchical Porous Carbon Foams Based on Banana Peel for Supercapacitor Electrodes." *Journal of Power Sources* 209 (July): 152–157. https://doi.org/10.1016/j.jpowsour.2012.02.089.

Martin, E., O. Savadogo, S.R. Guiot, and B. Tartakovsky. 2010. "The Influence of Operational Conditions on the Performance of a Microbial Fuel Cell Seeded with Mesophilic Anaerobic Sludge." *Biochemical Engineering Journal* 51 (3): 132–139. https://doi.org/10.1016/j.bej.2010.06.006.

Matarèse, Bruno F. E., Paul L. C. Feyen, Aniello Falco, Fabio Benfenati, Paolo Lugli, and John C. deMello. 2018. "Use of SU8 as a Stable and Biocompatible Adhesion Layer for Gold Bioelectrodes." *Scientific Reports* 8 (1): 5560. https://doi.org/10.1038/s41598-018-21755-6.

Mazurenko Ievgen., Anne de Poulpiquet, and Elisabeth Lojou. 2017a. "Recent Developments in High Surface Area Bioelectrodes for Enzymatic Fuel Cells." *Current Opinion in Electrochemistry* 5 (1): 74–84. https://doi.org/10.1016/j.coelec.2017.07.001.

Mazurenko, I., A. de Poulpiquet, and E. Lojou. 2017b. "Recent Developments in High Surface Area Bioelectrodes for Enzymatic Fuel Cells." *Current Opinion in Electrochemistry* 5 (1): 74–84. https://doi.org/10.1016/j.coelec.2017.07.001.

Mezger P.R., and Nico H.J. Creugers. 1992. "Titanium Nitride Coatings in Clinical Dentistry." *Journal of Dentistry* 20 (6): 342–344. https://doi.org/10.1016/0300-5712(92)90021-4.

Milton, Ross D., and Shelley D. Minteer. 2017. "Direct Enzymatic Bioelectrocatalysis: Differentiating between Myth and Reality." *Journal of The Royal Society Interface* 14 (131): 20170253. https://doi.org/10.1098/rsif.2017.0253.

Monsalve, Karen, Ievgen Mazurenko, Cristina Gutierrez-Sanchez, Marianne Ilbert, Pascale Infossi, Stefan Frielingsdorf, Marie Thérèse Giudici-Orticoni, Oliver Lenz, and Elisabeth Lojou. 2016. "Impact of Carbon Nanotube Surface Chemistry on Hydrogen Oxidation by Membrane-Bound Oxygen-Tolerant Hydrogenases." *ChemElectroChem* 3 (12): 2179–2788. https://doi.org/10.1002/CELC.201600460.

Mook, Wei Tze, Mohamed Kheireddine Taeib Aroua, Mohammed Harun Chakrabarti, Ishenny Muhammad Noor, Muhammad Faisal Irfan, and Chee Tong John Low. 2013. "A Review on the Effect of Bio-Electrodes on Denitrification and Organic Matter Removal Processes in Bio-Electrochemical Systems." *Journal of Industrial and Engineering Chemistry* 19 (1): 1–13. https://doi.org/10.1016/j.jiec.2012.07.004.

Navaee, Aso, and Abdollah Salimi. 2015. "Graphene-Supported Pyrene-Functionalized Amino-Carbon Nanotube: A Novel Hybrid Architecture of Laccase Immobilization as Effective Bioelectrocatalyst for Oxygen Reduction Reaction." *Journal of Materials Chemistry A* 3 (14): 7623–7630. https://doi.org/10.1039/C4TA06867J.

Ong Lu Ki, Alfin Kurniawan, Anita Carolina Suwandi, Chunxiang. Lin, X.S. Zhao, and Suryadi Ismadji. 2012. "A Facile and Green Preparation of Durian Shell-Derived Carbon Electrodes for Electrochemical Double-Layer Capacitors." *Progress in Natural Science: Materials International* 22 (6): 624–630. https://doi.org/10.1016/j.pnsc.2012.11.001.

Peckham, P. Hunter, D. Michael Ackermann, and Christa W. Moss. 2013a. "The Role of Biomaterials in Stimulating Bioelectrodes." In *Biomaterials Science*, 981–996. Elsevier. https://doi.org/10.1016/B978-0-08-087780-8.00084-X.

Peckham, P. Hunter, D. Michael Ackermann, and Christa W. Moss. 2013b. "The Role of Biomaterials in Stimulating Bioelectrodes." *Biomaterials Science: An Introduction to Materials: Third Edition*, January, 981–996. https://doi.org/10.1016/B978-0-08-087780-8.00084-X.

Peng, Chao, Xing-bin Yan, Ru-tao Wang, Jun-wei Lang, Yu-jing Ou, and Qun-ji Xue. 2013. "Promising Activated Carbons Derived from Waste Tea-Leaves and Their Application in High Performance Supercapacitors Electrodes." *Electrochimica Acta* 87 (January): 401–408. https://doi.org/10.1016/j.electacta.2012.09.082.

Pereira, Andressa R., João C.P. de Souza, Rodrigo M. Iost, Fernanda C.P.F. Sales, and Frank N. Crespilho. 2016. "Application of Carbon Fibers to Flexible Enzyme Electrodes." *Journal of Electroanalytical Chemistry* 780 (November): 396–406. https://doi.org/10.1016/j.jelechem.2016.01.004.

Pham, The Hai, Peter Aelterman, and Willy Verstraete. 2009. "Bioanode Performance in Bioelectrochemical Systems: Recent Improvements and Prospects." *Trends in Biotechnology* 27 (3): 168–178. https://doi.org/10.1016/j.tibtech.2008.11.005.

Poulpiquet, A. de, A. Ciaccafava, R. Gadiou, S. Gounel, M.T. Giudici-Orticoni, N. Mano, and E. Lojou. 2014. "Design of a H2/O2 Biofuel Cell Based on Thermostable Enzymes." *Electrochemistry Communications* 42 (May): 72–74. https://doi.org/10.1016/j.elecom.2014.02.012.

Prévoteau, Antonin, Olivier Courjean, and Nicolas Mano. 2010. "Deglycosylation of Glucose Oxidase to Improve Biosensors and Biofuel Cells." *Electrochemistry Communications* 12 (2): 213–215. https://doi.org/10.1016/j.elecom.2009.11.027.

Puig, Sebastià, Marc Serra, Marta Coma, Marina Cabré, M. Dolors Balaguer, and Jesús Colprim. 2010. "Effect of PH on Nutrient Dynamics and Electricity Production Using Microbial Fuel Cells." *Bioresource Technology* 101 (24): 9594–9599. https://doi.org/10.1016/j.biortech.2010.07.082.

Qin, Ge, Ya Fei Deng, Hong Mei Zhou, and Juan Juan Li. 2014. "Review of Iridium Oxide Surface Modification on Bio-Electrodes." *Advanced Materials Research* 1027 (October): 191–194. https://doi.org/10.4028/www.scientific.net/AMR.1027.191.

Rafieerad, Alireza, Ahmad Amiri, Glen Lester Sequiera, Weiang Yan, Yijun Chen, Andreas A. Polycarpou, and Sanjiv Dhingra. 2021a. "Development of Fluorine-Free Tantalum Carbide MXene Hybrid Structure as a Biocompatible Material for Supercapacitor Electrodes." *Advanced Functional Materials* 31 (30). https://doi.org/10.1002/adfm.202100015.

Rafieerad, Alireza, Ahmad Amiri, Glen Lester Sequiera, Weiang Yan, Yijun Chen, Andreas A. Polycarpou, and Sanjiv Dhingra. 2021b. "Development of Fluorine-Free Tantalum Carbide MXene Hybrid Structure as a Biocompatible Material for Supercapacitor Electrodes." *Advanced Functional Materials* 31 (30). https://doi.org/10.1002/adfm.202100015.

Rahimnejad, Mostafa, Gholamreza Bakeri, Ghasem Najafpour, Mostafa Ghasemi, and Sang-Eun Oh. 2014. "A Review on the Effect of Proton Exchange Membranes in Microbial Fuel Cells." *Biofuel Research Journal* 1 (1): 7–15.

Rose, T.L., E.M. Kelliher, and L.S. Robblee. 1985. "Assessment of Capacitor Electrodes for Intracortical Neural Stimulation." *Journal of Neuroscience Methods* 12 (3): 181–193. https://doi.org/10.1016/0165-0270(85)90001-9.

Rosenbaum, Miriam, Federico Aulenta, Marianna Villano, and Largus T. Angenent. 2011. "Cathodes as Electron Donors for Microbial Metabolism: Which Extracellular Electron Transfer Mechanisms Are Involved?" *Bioresource Technology* 102 (1): 324–333. https://doi.org/10.1016/j.biortech.2010.07.008.

Rufford, Thomas E., Denisa Hulicova-Jurcakova, Kiran Khosla, Zhonghua Zhu, and Gao Qing Lu. 2010a. "Microstructure and Electrochemical Double-Layer Capacitance of Carbon Electrodes Prepared by Zinc Chloride Activation of Sugar Cane Bagasse." *Journal of Power Sources* 195 (3): 912–918. https://doi.org/10.1016/j.jpowsour.2009.08.048.

Rufford, Thomas E., Denisa Hulicova-Jurcakova, Kiran Khosla, Zhonghua Zhu, and Gao Qing Lu. 2010b. "Microstructure and Electrochemical Double-Layer Capacitance of Carbon Electrodes Prepared by Zinc Chloride Activation of Sugar Cane Bagasse." *Journal of Power Sources* 195 (3): 912–918. https://doi.org/10.1016/j.jpowsour.2009.08.048.

Rusli, Siti Farah Nadiah, Mimi Hani Abu Bakar, Kee Shyuan Loh, and Mohd Shahbudin Mastar. 2019. "Review of High-Performance Biocathode Using Stainless Steel and Carbon-Based Materials in Microbial Fuel Cell for Electricity and Water Treatment." *International Journal of Hydrogen Energy* 44 (58): 30772–30787. https://doi.org/10.1016/j.ijhydene.2018.11.145.

Sakai, Hideki, Takaaki Nakagawa, Yuichi Tokita, Tsuyonobu Hatazawa, Tokuji Ikeda, Seiya Tsujimura, and Kenji Kano. 2009. "A High-Power Glucose/Oxygen Biofuel Cell Operating under Quiescent Conditions." *Energy Environment Science* 2 (1): 133–138. https://doi.org/10.1039/B809841G.

Schröder, Uwe. 2007. "Anodic Electron Transfer Mechanisms in Microbial Fuel Cells and Their Energy Efficiency." *Physical Chemistry Chemical Physics.* 9 (21): 2619–2629. https://doi.org/10.1039/B703627M.

Sedenho Graziela Cristina., Andressa Riberio Pereira, Kamala Cassia Pagnoncelli, J. C.P. De Souza, and Frank Nelson Crespilho. 2018. "Implantable Enzyme-Based Biofuel Cells." January, 248–60. https://doi.org/10.1016/B978-0-12-409547-2.13709-6.

Siepenkoetter, Till, Urszula Salaj-Kosla, Xinxin Xiao, Peter Ó Conghaile, Marcos Pita, Roland Ludwig, and Edmond Magner. 2017. "Immobilization of Redox Enzymes on Nanoporous Gold Electrodes: Applications in Biofuel Cells." *ChemPlusChem* 82 (4): 553–560. https://doi.org/10.1002/cplu.201600455.

Siepenkoetter, Till, Urszula Salaj-Kosla, Xinxin Xiao, Peter Conghaile, Marcos Pita, Roland Ludwig, and Edmond Magner. 2017. "Immobilization of Redox Enzymes on Nanoporous Gold Electrodes: Applications in Biofuel Cells." *ChemPlusChem* 82 (4): 553–560. https://doi.org/10.1002/CPLU.201600455.

Strik, David P.B.T.B., Hubertus V.M. Hamelers, and Cees J.N. Buisman. 2010. "Solar Energy Powered Microbial Fuel Cell with a Reversible Bioelectrode." *Environmental Science & Technology* 44 (1): 532–537. https://doi.org/10.1021/es902435v.

Sukkasem, Chontisa, Shoutao Xu, Sunhwa Park, Piyarat Boonsawang, and Hong Liu. 2008. "Effect of Nitrate on the Performance of Single Chamber Air Cathode Microbial Fuel Cells." *Water Research* 42 (19): 4743–4750. https://doi.org/10.1016/j.watres.2008.08.029.

Taer Erman, R. Taslim, W.S. Mustika, B. Kurniasih, Agustino, A. Afrianda, and Apriwandi. 2018. "Production of an Activated Carbon from a Banana Stem and Its Application as Electrode Materials for Supercapacitors." *International Journal of Electrochemical Science* 13 (9): 8428–8439. https://doi.org/10.20964/2018.09.55.

Taer, E., R. Taslim, A.W. Putri, A. Apriwandi, and A. Agustino. 2018. "Activated Carbon Electrode Made From Coconut Husk Waste For Supercapacitor Application." *International Journal of Electrochemical Science* 13 (12): 12072–12084. https://doi.org/10.20964/2018.12.19.

Taghavi, M, A Stinchcombe, J Greenman, V Mattoli, L Beccai, B Mazzolai, C Melhuish, and I A Ieropoulos. 2015. "Self Sufficient Wireless Transmitter Powered by Foot-Pumped Urine Operating Wearable MFC." *Bioinspiration & Biomimetics* 11 (1): 016001. https://doi.org/10.1088/1748-3190/11/1/016001.

Tawalbeh, Muhammad, Rana Muhammad Nauman Javed, Amani Al-Othman, and Fares Almomani. 2022. "The Novel Advancements of Nanomaterials in Biofuel Cells with a Focus on Electrodes' Applications." *Fuel* 322 (August): 124237. https://doi.org/10.1016/j.fuel.2022.124237.

Tender, Leonard M., Clare E. Reimers, Hilmar A. Stecher, Dawn E. Holmes, Daniel R. Bond, Daniel A. Lowy, Kanoelani Pilobello, Stephanie J. Fertig, and Derek R. Lovley. 2002. "Harnessing Microbially Generated Power on the Seafloor." *Nature Biotechnology* 20 (8): 821–825. https://doi.org/10.1038/nbt716.

Teo, Ellie Yi Lih, Lingeswarran Muniandy, Eng-Poh Ng, Farook Adam, Abdul Rahman Mohamed, Rajan Jose, and Kwok Feng Chong. 2016. "High Surface Area Activated Carbon from Rice Husk as a High Performance Supercapacitor Electrode." *Electrochimica Acta* 192 (February): 110–119. https://doi.org/10.1016/j.electacta.2016.01.140.

Venugopalan, Ramakrishna, and Ray Ideker. 2013. "Bioelectrodes." In *Biomaterials Science*, 957–966. Elsevier. https://doi.org/10.1016/B978-0-08-087780-8.00082-6.

Virdis, Bernardino, Korneel Rabaey, Zhiguo Yuan, and Jürg Keller. 2008. "Microbial Fuel Cells for Simultaneous Carbon and Nitrogen Removal." *Water Research* 42 (12): 3013–3024. https://doi.org/10.1016/j.watres.2008.03.017.

Wang, Joseph, and Meng Shan Lin. 1988. "Mixed Plant Tissue Carbon Paste Bioelectrode." *Analytical Chemistry* 60 (15): 1545–1548. https://doi.org/10.1021/ac00166a014.

Wang,Min, and Bin Duan. 2019. "Materials and Their Biomedical Applications." In *Encyclopedia of Biomedical Engineering*, 135–152. Elsevier. https://doi.org/10.1016/B978-0-12-801238-3.99860-X.

Watanabe, Kazuya. 2008. "Recent Developments in Microbial Fuel Cell Technologies for Sustainable Bioenergy." *Journal of Bioscience and Bioengineering* 106 (6): 528–536. https://doi.org/10.1263/jbb.106.528.

Wellman, Steven M., James R. Eles, Kip A. Ludwig, John P. Seymour, Nicholas J. Michelson, William E. McFadden, Alberto L. Vazquez, and Takashi D. Y. Kozai. 2018. "A Materials Roadmap to Functional Neural Interface Design." *Advanced Functional Materials* 28 (12). https://doi.org/10.1002/adfm.201701269.

Wooten, Marilyn, Sushma Karra, Maogen Zhang, and Waldemar Gorski. 2014. "On the Direct Electron Transfer, Sensing, and Enzyme Activity in the Glucose Oxidase/Carbon Nanotubes System." *Analytical Chemistry* 86 (1): 752–757. https://doi.org/10.1021/ac403250w.

Wu, Fei, Lei Su, Ping Yu, and Lanqun Mao. 2017. "Role of Organic Solvents in Immobilizing Fungus Laccase on Single-Walled Carbon Nanotubes for Improved Current Response in Direct Bioelectrocatalysis." *Journal of the American Chemical Society* 139 (4): 1565–1574. American Chemical Society.

Xie, Xing, Craig Criddle, and Yi Cui. 2015. "Design and Fabrication of Bioelectrodes for Microbial Bioelectrochemical Systems." *Energy & Environmental Science* 8 (12): 3418–3441. https://doi.org/10.1039/C5EE01862E.

Xu, Bin, Yufeng Chen, Gang Wei, Gaoping Cao, Hao Zhang, and Yusheng Yang. 2010. "Activated Carbon with High Capacitance Prepared by NaOH Activation for Supercapacitors." *Materials Chemistry and Physics* 124 (1): 504–509. https://doi.org/10.1016/j.matchemphys.2010.07.002.

Yaqoob, Asim Ali, Asma Khatoon, Siti Hamidah Mohd Setapar, Khalid Umar, Tabassum Parveen, Mohamad Nasir Mohamad Ibrahim, Akil Ahmad, and Mohd Rafatullah. 2020. "Outlook on the Role of Microbial Fuel Cells in Remediation of Environmental Pollutants with Electricity Generation." *Catalysts* 10 (8): 819. https://doi.org/10.3390/catal10080819.

Yuan, Xiaobo, Nikolaus Wolf, Timm J. J. Hondrich, Pegah Shokoohimehr, Frano Milos, Manuel Glass, Dirk Mayer, et al. 2020. "Engineering Biocompatible Interfaces via Combinations of Oxide Films and Organic Self-Assembled Monolayers." *ACS Applied Materials & Interfaces* 12 (14): 17121–17129. https://doi.org/10.1021/acsami.0c02141.

Yuan, Yong, Shungui Zhou, Nan Xu, and Li Zhuang. 2011. "Microorganism-Immobilized Carbon Nanoparticle Anode for Microbial Fuel Cells Based on Direct Electron Transfer." *Applied Microbiology and Biotechnology* 89 (5): 1629–1635. https://doi.org/10.1007/s00253-010-3013-5.

Zhang, Tian, Changzheng Cui, Shengli Chen, Xinping Ai, Hanxi Yang, Ping Shen, and Zhenrong Peng. 2006. "A Novel Mediatorless Microbial Fuel Cell Based on Direct Biocatalysis of Escherichia Coli." *Chemical Communications* (21): 2257. https://doi.org/10.1039/b600876c.

Zou, Yongjin, Cuili Xiang, Lini Yang, Li-Xian Sun, Fen Xu, and Zhong Cao. 2008. "A Mediatorless Microbial Fuel Cell Using Polypyrrole Coated Carbon Nanotubes Composite as Anode Material." *International Journal of Hydrogen Energy* 33 (18): 4856–4862. https://doi.org/10.1016/j.ijhydene.2008.06.061.

5 Napier grass grown in arid and saline water conditions for biochar production and its applications

Ramachandran Subramanian, Souvik Kumar Paul, and Prakash Kumar B G

5.1 INTRODUCTION

A surge in carbon emissions dispersed in our atmosphere in 2019 has sparked an interest and created an urgent demand for sustainable biomass resources to produce renewable energies. Energy reservoirs of biomaterials augment fuel diversification and alleviate current environmental pollution as there are no hazardous air pollutants emitted such as heavy metals in its production. Addressing this, an attempt to explore and produce biochar as an alternative in a fossil fuel-dependent region was undertaken. Biochar is a carbon-rich solid material derived through the thermo-chemical conversion of wood and agro-forestry residues in an oxygen-limited environment (Zhang et al., 2019). Most of the biochar production through thermal pyrolysis processes have been optimized for batch and continuous methods. It is categorized as a sustainable carbon-neutral energy and it reduces consumption of fossil fuels. By incorporating the biochar for co-firing with coal, approximately 12% of carbon dioxide emissions can be reduced (Narzari et al., 2015).

Biochar is a smokeless fuel, and it has been reported to be used as biocoal and bio-composite fuel. These fuels meet the criteria set by the regulatory agencies for biomass-based fuels (Bis et al., 2018) and will assist developed and developing countries in adhering to the Paris Agreement of 2015. Among the agro-forestry-derived materials, date palm (Khalifa and Yousef, 2015), miscanthus, switchgrass, and Napier grass are reported for biochar and bioenergy production (Brassard et al., 2018). The major drawback related to these materials is the necessity to use fertile lands, fresh water, appropriate climate conditions, and extensive growth time. In the United Arab Emirates where an arid climate is ubiquitous, the arable forest and agricultural lands have dwindled for biomass production. In this regard, wastelands and the use of poor-quality water for cultivation of biomass are being explored.

Napier grass (*Pennisetum purpureum*) is a channel for carbon sequestration and has been found to be an energy crop in all three states of matter in the form of biochar, bio-oil, and biogas (Mohammed et al., 2015). The objective of this study is to successfully establish Napier grass growth for biochar production under arid climate conditions utilizing fresh water and saline irrigation. Napier grass biomass grown using fresh water and saline irrigations was harvested and processed. Efforts to grow Napier grass in other countries such as the United States and Thailand under saline conditions have shown that canopy temperature was higher compared to non-saline control plants under infra-red measurement (Wang et al., 2002). Salinity also reduced plant height, total plant chlorophyll, and leaf area index (AL-Shoaibi, 2008). Despite the unfavorable conditions, the high rate of biomass production makes it a viable energy crop that can reduce the dependency of imports. Napier grass can yield 40–80 dry ton biomass/ha/yr that is higher than that of eucalyptus and sugarcane

DOI: 10.1201/9781003500483-5
This chapter has been made available under a (CC-BY-NC-ND) 4.0 license

(Scholl et al., 2015; Rocha et al., 2017). It can grow in conditions of low water requirements and possesses tolerance to arid environments (Campbell et al., 2008).

Physicochemical properties and yield of biochar are mainly controlled by the feedstock species and thermochemical conditions. The influence of pyrolysis temperatures with various environmental conditions on the yield and calorific value (CV) of the produced biochar is also studied in this work.

5.2 MATERIALS AND METHODS

5.2.1 Biomass feedstocks

We sourced two Napier grass varieties CO(CN)4, (N1) and CO(BN)5, (N2) from Tamil Nadu Agricultural University (TNAU), Coimbatore, India, and their growth was monitored at the International Center for Biosaline Agriculture (ICBA), Dubai, United Arab Emirates (Coordinates 25.09445, 55.38968). The experiment was carried out in an arid desert climate where the seedlings were subjected to high temperatures and negligible rainfall. Trials were conducted using fresh water 0.4 dS/m (FW), saline water 7 dS/m, (S1), and 14 dS/m (S2) without any exposure to fertilizers. Biomass was harvested after eight months. Random samples were collected from each treatment and composited to form a representation of the harvested biomass. The samples were dried in a hot air oven at 60°C for 72 h, and the biomass was powdered to a particle size of 1–2 mm using a pulverizer for biochar production and further analyses.

5.2.2 Biochar production

The biomass feed stocks were pyrolyzed in a tubular furnace (Protherm PC442), which involved a thermochemical method wherein the biomass undergoes partial combustion under conditions of restricted oxygen supply. Five grams of the samples were loaded in the crucibles and placed inside the tubular furnace with the heating rate of 2°C/min with a holding time of 30 min. Experimental set-up for the production of biochar is shown in Figure 5.1. Experiments were carried out under three different environmental conditions for pyrolysis, (a) open crucible/air (OC), (b) open crucible/nitrogen (OCN), and (c) closed crucible/self-generated (CC).

5.2.3 Characterization techniques

5.2.3.1 Biomass analysis

The samples were characterized for proximate (moisture, volatile, ash, and fixed carbon content), ultimate analysis (C, H, N, S, and O), biochar yield, CV, and Thermogravimetric analysis (TGA). Moisture content was determined using Shimadzu moisture analyzer (MOC63u). Volatile matter and ash content were measured according to ASTM E872 – 82 (2013) and ASTM D1102 – 84

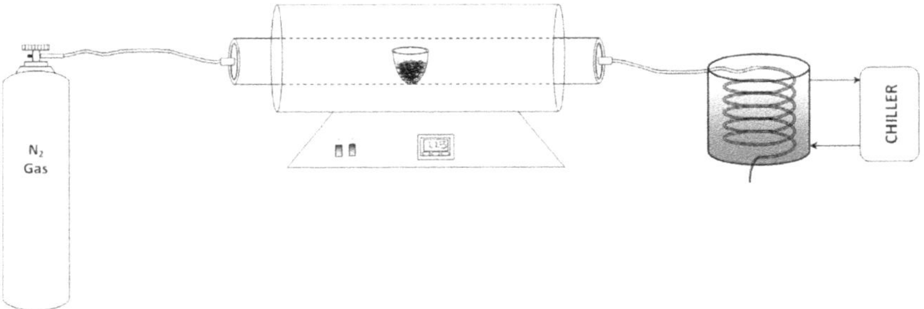

FIGURE 5.1 Schematic of laboratory batch pyrolysis set-up for the production of biochar.

(2013) standards and fixed carbon by the difference. Ultimate composition analysis (CHNS) was performed on a dry weight basis with Thermo Finnigan, Italy (FLASH EA 1112 series). CVs were determined using the bomb calorimeter (Parr 6050). Thermogravimetric analysis of the samples was performed with a heating rate of 10°C/min in nitrogen atmosphere (Perkin Elmer, TGA-4000).

Biomass samples were digested in 3% HNO_3 in a microwave reaction system at 180°C, 1500W (Anton Parr Multiwave PRO). Minor element composition such as magnesium (Mg), calcium (Ca), sodium (Na), and potassium (K) were estimated using Inductively Coupled Plasma – Optical Emission Spectrometer (ICP-OES), Perkin Elmer Optima 7000 DV.

5.3 RESULTS AND DISCUSSIONS

5.3.1 Proximate and ultimate analysis

The proximate, ultimate analysis of harvested Napier grasses N1, N2 under irrigation with FW, salinity S1, and S2 are summarized in Table 5.1. Residual moisture content of the leaves and stems ranges from 3.47 to 7.88 wt % and 7.25 to 9.45 wt %, respectively. Volatile matter varies from 77.42 to 88 wt %. The volatile content does not follow any trend however less volatile matter content in the sample implies that the method produces a better quality of biochar, which can serve as an ideal solid fuel. Ash content varies from 4.1 to 9.8 wt %, and it was found that fresh water (FW) grown plant biomass had less ash content compared to saline water grown biomass. Fixed carbon (FC) varies from 0.11 to 8.35 wt % with a similar observation on the biomass of FW with higher values than salinity-treated samples. FC content was comparatively higher in the leaves than stem parts. The biomass is composed of cellulose, hemicellulose, and lignin. Energy obtained from sunlight is stored in the chemical bonds of carbon, hydrogen, and oxygen molecules and is released when they are broken through any chemical oxidation process. CV is a key indicator to ensure the capacity of biomass to serve as an energy source. CV of the biomass samples analyzed varied from 15 to 16.91 MJ/kg under freshwater and salinity conditions. Salinity had minimum effect on energy content of the samples undertaken in this study (Table 5.1).

Higher hydrogen and carbon percentages are critical factors in determining combustion properties of any material. The data derived from the ultimate analysis of Napier grass showed that samples had low sulfur and nitrogen contents. The presence of higher amounts of sulfur and nitrogen in any fuel may result in the formation of undesirable oxides. The results confirmed that the Napier grass was free from sulfur and not in the detectable range. A minimal amount of nitrogen under the reported growing conditions was detected (Yadav et al., 2016). With respect to oxygen/carbon (O/C) and hydrogen/carbon (H/C), ratios of the samples were 0.98 to 1.09 and 1.69 to 1.81, respectively. All of the biomass samples showed consistent results irrespective of the salinity treatment. The molar ratios of H/C and O/C indicate the degree of aromaticity, maturation, and bonding arrangement of C atoms typical of the saturated form prevalent in cellulose material (Ghani et al., 2013).

5.3.2 Thermogravimetric analysis

The thermal stability of the Napier grass samples was analyzed using TGA. It was observed that three major phases such as moisture loss (room temperature to 150°C), thermal degradation of cellulose, and hemicelluloses occurred at higher rates in reaction temperatures ranging from 150 to 375°C, thermal degradation of lignin at a slower rate forms the biochar (375 to 700°C) (Yang et al., 2007). Figure 5.2 shows the TGA decomposition data of the biochar produced from the FW and salinity-treated biomass. It was observed that similar thermal decomposition patterns have emerged irrespective of the saline water used for the biomass production. The samples, N2FW(L), N1S1(S), and N2FW(S) where the second phase extended up to 450°C, beyond which the reaction rate is negligible. From the analysis, salinity treatment for the growth of biomass has no impact on thermal conversion to biochar.

TABLE 5.1
Proximate and ultimate analysis of air-dried biomass (dry basis)

			Proximate analysis (wt %)					Ultimate analysis (wt %)						
S. no.	Air-dried biomass	References	Moisture Content	Volatile Matter	Ash Content	Fixed carbon	CV (MJ/kg)	C	H	N	O	S	O/C molar ratio	H/C molar ratio
1	N1 FW (L)	Present work	7.73	77.42	6.49	8.35	16.78	40.32	6.05	0.48	53.16	–	0.99	1.79
2	N1 S1 (L)		7.46	81.50	7.70	3.34	16.91	38.38	5.58	0.50	55.54	–	1.09	1.73
3	N1 S2 (L)		6.73	82.10	8.90	2.27	15.44	38.91	5.72	0.51	54.87	–	1.06	1.75
4	N2 FW (L)		7.88	82.00	6.00	4.12	16.2	40.03	6.00	0.50	53.48	–	1.00	1.79
5	N2 S1 (L)		4.5	83.10	8.40	4.00	16.4	39.52	5.95	0.97	53.57	–	1.02	1.79
6	N2 S2 (L)		3.47	83.80	9.80	2.93	15.0	39.63	5.71	0.56	54.10	–	1.02	1.72
7	N1 FW (S)		8.29	86.80	4.80	0.11	15.55	40.90	5.90	0.00	53.20	–	0.98	1.72
8	N1 S1 (S)		7.58	88.00	4.10	0.32	16.74	39.62	6.03	0.00	54.35	–	1.03	1.81
9	N1 S2 (S)		7.3	84.86	7.50	0.33	15.96	38.25	5.65	0.56	55.54	–	1.09	1.76
10	N2 FW (S)		9.45	82.60	4.80	3.15	16.4	40.22	5.87	0.36	53.55	–	1.00	1.74
11	N2 S1 (S)		8.42	83.98	4.68	2.95	16.2	38.42	5.70	0.45	55.42	–	1.08	1.77
12	N2 S2 (S)		7.25	85.20	5.70	1.85	15.93	40.30	5.73	0.43	53.54	–	1.00	1.69
13	Napier Grass	Mythili et al. (2013); Suntivarakorn et al. (2018); Yadav et al.(2016); Mohammed et al. (2017); Strezov et al. (2008b); Braga et al. (2014); De Conto et al. (2016)	7.07–12.40	65.00–81.51	1.75–8.26	7.33–19.20	15.23–24.79	39.63–58.30	2.60–6.77	0.45–2.80	3.90–52.16	0–48.64	0.09–0.96	0.12–1.79

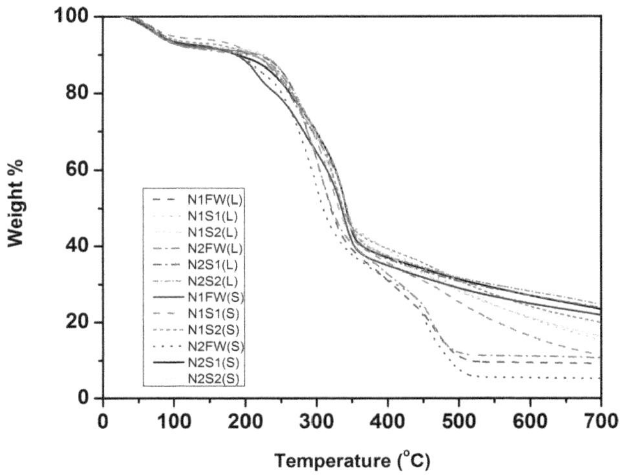

FIGURE 5.2 TGA of Napier grass samples.

TABLE 5.2
ICP – OES analysis of biomass samples

S. no	Air-dried biomass	Mg (mg/kg)	Ca (mg/kg)	Na (mg/kg)	K (mg/kg)
1	N1 FW (L)	19.6	62.19	2.57	60.42
2	N1 S1 (L)	33.37	111.5	21.13	107.5
3	N1 S2 (L)	101.1	215.6	58.05	268
4	N2 FW (L)	27.7	24.44	11.37	109.9
5	N2 S1 (L)	31.37	82.62	14.74	141.2
6	N2 S2 (L)	36.43	88.02	14.85	195.3
7	N1 FW (S)	16.21	9.74	5.74	138
8	N1 S1 (S)	38.07	32.5	54.51	235
9	N1 S2 (S)	66.46	67.28	128.9	404.4
10	N2 FW (S)	22.01	23.52	5.334	141.2
11	N2 S1 (S)	26.27	25.45	23.94	160.8
12	N2 S2 (S)	36.15	33.96	65.04	233.4

5.3.3 Biomass elemental composition

The effect of saline irrigation on biomass elemental composition was analyzed by ICP-OES. Table 5.2 shows the distribution of minor elements under different irrigation conditions on biomass of Napier grass stems and leaves. In all the samples, the minor element composition varied and was found to be in the range of Mg 16.21–101.1 mg/kg, Ca from 9.74 to 215.6 mg/kg, Na from 2.57 to 128.9 mg/kg and K from 60 to 404.4 mg/kg. It was observed that in all the samples, the elemental composition increased with salinity for stalks and leaves portion of the Napier grass. The salinity-treated N1S2 had relatively higher concentrations of minor elements compared to other biomass.

The permissible limits of minor elements for coal/biocoal mineral matter for magnesium, calcium, potassium, and sodium are 100–1000 ppm (Xu et al., 2003). It was concluded that the salinity had no significant impact on the mineral composition of the biomass and does not pose any detrimental environmental effects with respect to metal pollution from biochar.

5.3.4 Pyrolysis of Salinity-Grown Napier Biomass

Pyrolysis is an efficient thermochemical process to convert organic matter to energy. Saline water-grown N1S1(L) based on CV and yield (Table 5.1) was pyrolyzed for biochar production. The yield and CV results of OC, OCN, and CC processes with the function of temperature are shown in Figure 5.3. In all the above three methods tested, the yield decreases as temperature increases (Mullen and Boateng, 2008). In the open crucible (OC) method, the biomass sample was heated without any sweeping gas. The oxygen present in the tube furnace burnt off the biomass samples after 250°C. The CV value increased from 16.16 to 16.80 MJ/kg due to bone dry material and aerial oxidation of oxidizing groups and yielded light brown partially formed char with an overall yield of 92.84% (Figure 5.3a). Further increase of temperature to 275°C led to complete ash and total loss of biomass.

In the OC under nitrogen environment (OCN), nitrogen gas was used as sweeping gas at a flow rate of 1 L/min. Due to the inert environment, the pyrolysis could be continued at higher temperatures up to 600°C. The biochar CV has increased up to 16.61 MJ/kg until 325°C. With temperature more than 325°C, the yield of biochar steadily decreased due to burn-off the biomass although the CV increased up to 16.77 MJ/kg (Figure 5.3b). Biochar yield in the current study was found to be 33.86%, whereas reported results reached a level of 29.3% (Lee et al., 2010) and 31% of Napier grass, respectively (Strezov et al., 2008).

In the case of closed crucible (CC), a self-generated atmosphere with inert environment prevents the oxidation of biomass. Biochar yield of 61.34–49.41% with CV 18.51–19.74 MJ/kg was observed in the temperature range 350–425°C. The self-generated atmosphere resulted in an increase in carbonization of the biomass and contributed higher biochar yield and CV of the Napier grass. It was observed that a containment of volatile matter produced in the CC method helps in the effective thermal conversion of biomass into biochar. Thermal decay of the biomass was prevented in such conditions as an anoxic environment was created.

Comparing the above three different conditions for the production of biochar, two common trends were observed: (a) increasing the pyrolysis process temperature led to a gradual decrease in yield of biochar produced and (b) CV rises to a threshold temperature and then falls due to ashing. Overall, the CC self-generated atmosphere has achieved higher CV and at a lower temperature (425°C). Biomass pyrolysis at higher temperatures in the range 400–700°C has been reported with the biochar yields of 28.3 to 52% (Mythili et al., 2013; Saikia et al., 2015; Irfan et al., 2016; Yadav et al., 2016). Under optimum conditions, the CVs 19.74 MJ/kg of the biochar produced are comparable as reported values between 18 and 24.8 MJ/kg (Mythili et al., 2013; Yadav et al., 2016).

5.4 CONCLUSION

Arid environments that prevail in UAE limit the total species that can be exploited for the growing demand of renewable energy. Napier is known for its high biomass production and ability to tolerate higher temperature conditions. Salinity tolerance was reported for the Napier grass by AL-Shoaibi (2008) and Wang et al. (2002). Biochar produced from Napier grass grown under saline conditions and their characteristics applicable in energy or soil amendments have not been reported. It is an established fact that salinity affects the plant growth due to salt accumulation in the shoot system of plants. Physiochemical characterization of biochar produced from such biomass is of significance. Current study was undertaken to assess the hybrid Napier grass for biomass production under saline irrigation for biochar production.

Under the three different water irrigation conditions (FW, S1, and S2) with Napier grass varieties (N1 and N2), N1S1 both stems and leaves showed comparatively higher CV and yield and lower sodicity and ash content. Although the biomass was grown in the higher salinity condition S2, the biochar physiochemical data does not significantly differ from that of the biochar produced with salinity S1. Biochar from S1 gave an output of the CV (MJ/kg) values of the stem 16.74 (N1S1),

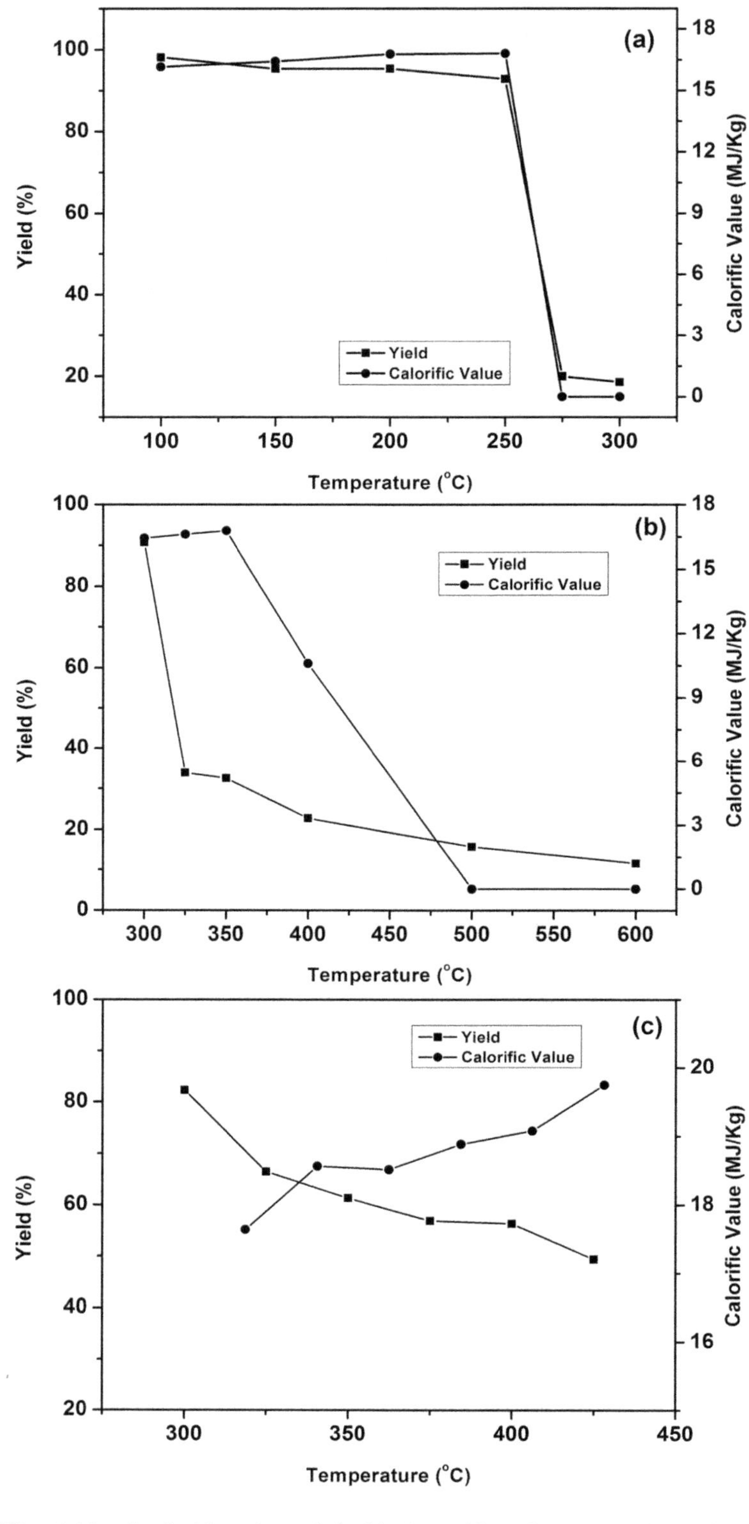

FIGURE 5.3 The yield and calorific values of the biochar with various atmospheres for N1S1(L) (a) open crucible/air (OC), (b) open crucible/nitrogen (OCN), and (c) closed crucible/self-generated (CC).

16.2 (N2S1) and leaves 16.91 (N1S1), 16.4 (N2S1) as listed whereas biochar from S2, the CV values obtained of the stem 15.96 (N1S2), 15.93 (N2S2) and the leaves 15.44 (N1S2), 16.4 (N2S1) are as mentioned. In the case of fresh water grown biochar, CV values of the stem for the samples are 15.55 (N1FW), 16.4 (N2FW) and the leaves 16.78 (N1FW), 16.2 (N2FW) (Table 5.1). Similar trend was observed with respect to sodicity (Table 5.2). It shows that Napier grass grown in S2 also does not accumulate much salt in its biomass.

From the TGA analysis, the thermal decomposition also did not significantly vary for the biomass samples exposed to different conditions. This may be due to negligible impact on the inorganic composition of the biomass properties irrespective of the salinity treatment and further confers no effects on the thermal conversion to biochar. The ICP-OES analyses gave an insight of the overall elemental composition of the biomass including bivalent ions (Mg^{2+} and Ca^{2+}) and monovalent ions (Na^+ and K^+). This did not increase above current prescribed threshold levels for use as biochar, and it meets the requisite environmental criteria.

This study provides the first concrete data reported for Napier grass growth under saline conditions for biochar production. Among the tested methods with various pyrolysis conditions, the CC method gave a promising yield of 49.41% with CV 19.74 MJ/kg at 425°C. The biochar produced from Napier grass with saline conditions can be made into pellets and be used as a direct combustible form of energy thereby proposing it to be a suitable alternate for coal combustion.

ACKNOWLEDGMENT

This collaborative research work was supported by the seed grant of BITS Pilani, Dubai Campus and International Center for Biosaline Agriculture (ICBA) (ICBA/DRI/2017/02-1). The authors acknowledge Prof. C Babu, Professor, Dept. of Forage Crops, TNAU, India, for the germplasm. We thank Dr Suresh Gupta, Associate Professor, Dept. of Chemical Engg., BITS Pilani, Pilani Campus, India, for thermal decomposition analysis. We also thank Mr Bala Gurusamy, Agronomy Assistant, ICBA, Dubai, UAE, for field studies and Ms. Safiya Aafreen for technical support in the preparation of this manuscript.

REFERENCES

AL- Shoaibi, A. (2008). Photosynthetic response of elephant grass (Pennisetum purpureum) to NaCl salinity. *Journal of Biological Sciences*, 8 (3), 610–615. https://doi.org/10.3923/jbs.2008.610.615

Bis, Z., Kobyłecki, R., Ścisłowska, M., & Zarzycki, R. (2018). Biochar – Potential tool to combat climate change and drought. *Ecohydrology & Hydrobiology*, 18(4), 441–453. https://doi.org/10.1016/j.ecohyd.2018.11.005

Brassard, P., Godbout, S., Pelletier, F., Raghavan, V., & Palacios, J.H. (2018). Pyrolysis of switchgrass in an auger reactor for biochar production: A greenhouse gas and energy impacts assessment. *Biomass and Bioenergy*, 116, 99–105. https://doi.org/10.1016/j.biombioe.2018.06.007

Campbell, J.E., Lobell, D.B., Genova, R.C., & Field, C.B. (2008). The global potential of bioenergy on abandoned agriculture lands. *Environmental Science & Technology*, 42(15), 5791–5794. https://doi.org/10.1021/es800052w

de Carvalho Rocha, J.R.d .A.S., Machado, J.C., Carneiro, P.C.S., da Costa Carneiro, J., Resende, M.D.V., Pereira, A.V., & de Souza Carneiro, J.E. (2017). Elephant grass ecotypes for bioenergy production via direct combustion of biomass. *Industrial Crops and Products*, 95, 27–32. https://doi.org/10.1016/j.indcrop.2016.10.014

Ghani, W.A.W.A.K., Mohd, A., da Silva, G., Bachmann, R.T., Taufiq-Yap, Y.H., Rashid, U., & Al-Muhtaseb, A.H. (2013). Biochar production from waste rubber-wood-sawdust and its potential use in C sequestration: Chemical and physical characterization. *Industrial Crops and Products*, 44, 18–24. https://doi.org/10.1016/j.indcrop.2012.10.017

Irfan, M., Chen, Q., Yue, Y., Pang, R., Lin, Q., Zhao, X., & Chen, H. (2016). Co-production of biochar, bio-oil and syngas from halophyte grass (*Achnatherum splendens L.*) under three different pyrolysis temperatures. *Bioresource Technology*, 211, 457–463. https://doi.org/10.1016/j.biortech.2016.03.077

Khalifa, N., & Yousef, L.F. (2015). A short report on changes of quality indicators for a sandy textured soil after treatment with biochar produced from fronds of date palm. *Energy Procedia*, 74, 960–965. https://doi.org/10.1016/j.egypro.2015.07.729

Lee, M-K., Tsai, W-T., Tsai, Y-L., & Lin, S-H. (2010). Pyrolysis of Napier grass in an induction-heating reactor. *Journal of Analytical and Applied Pyrolysis*, 88(2), 110–116. https://doi.org/10.1016/j.jaap.2010.03.003

Mohammed, I.Y., Abakr, Y.A., Kazi, F.K., Yusuf, S., Alshareef, I., & Chin, S.A. (2015). Pyrolysis of Napier grass in a fixed bed reactor: Effect of operating conditions on product yields and characteristics. *Bio Resources*, 10 (4), 6457–6478. https://doi.org/10.15376/biores.10.4.6457-6478

Mullen, C.A., & Boateng, A.A. (2008). Chemical composition of bio-oils produced by fast pyrolysis of two energy crops. *Energy & Fuels*, 22(3), 2104–2109. https://doi.org/10.1021/ef700776w

Mythili, R., Venkatachalam, P., Subramanian, P., & Uma, D. (2013). Characterization of bioresidues for biooil production through pyrolysis. *Bioresource Technology*, 138, 71–78. https://doi.org/10.1016/j.biortech.2013.03.161.

Narzari, R., Bordoloi, N., Chutia, R.S., Borkotoki, B., Gogoi, N., Bora, A., & Kataki, R. (2015). An overview on its production, properties and potential benefits. In *book: Biology, Biotechnology and Sustainable Development* (pp.13–40). Research India Publications.

Rocha, J. R. do. A. S. de. C., Machado, J.C., Carneiro, P.C. S., Carneiro, J. da. C., Resende, M.D.V., Pereira, A.V., & Carneiro, J. E. de. S (2017). Elephant grass ecotypes for bioenergy production *via* direct combustion of biomass. *Industrial Crops and Products*, 95, 27–32. https://doi.org/10.1016/j.indcrop.2016.10.014

Saikia, R., Chutia, R.S., Kataki, R., & Pant, K.K. (2015). Perennial grass (*Arundo donax L.*) as a feedstock for thermo-chemical conversion to energy and materials. *Bioresource Technology*, 188, 265–272. https://doi.org/10.1016/j.biortech.2015.01.089

Scholl, A.L., Menegol, D., Pitarelo, A.P., Fontana, R.C., Filho, A.Z., Ramos, L.P., Dillon, A.J.P., & Camassola, M. (2015). Elephant grass (*Pennisetum purpureum Schum.*) pretreated via steam explosion as a carbon source for cellulases and xylanases in submerged cultivation. *Industrial Crops and Products*, 70, 280–291. https://doi.org/10.1016/j.indcrop.2015.03.056

Strezov, V., Evans, T.J., & Hayman, C. (2008). Thermal conversion of elephant grass (*Pennisetum purpureum Schum*) to bio-gas, bio-oil and charcoal. *Bioresource Technology*, 99(17), 8394–8399. https://doi.org/10.1016/j.biortech.2008.02.039

Wang, D., Poss, J., Donovan, T.J., Shannon, M.C., & Lesch, S.M. (2002). Biophysical properties and biomass production of elephant grass under saline conditions. *Journal of Arid Environments*, 52 (4), 447–456. https://doi.org/10.1006/jare.2002.1016

Xu, M., Yan, R., Zheng, C., Qiao, Y., Han, J., & Sheng, C. (2003). Status of trace element emission in a coal combustion process: A review. *Fuel Processing Technology*, 85(2–3), 215–237. https://doi.org/10.1016/S0378-3820(03)00174-7

Yadav, A., Ansari, K.B., Simha, P., Gaikar, V.G., & Pandit, A.B. (2016). Vacuum pyrolysed biochar for soil amendment. *Resource-Efficient Technologies*, 2, S177–S185. https://doi.org/10.1016/j.reffit.2016.11.004

Yang, H., Yan, R., Chen, H., Lee, D.H., & Zheng, C. (2007). Characteristics of hemicellulose, cellulose and lignin pyrolysis. *Fuel*, 86(12–13), 1781–1788. https://doi.org/10.1016/j.fuel.2006.12.013

Zhang, Z., Zhu, Z., Shen, B., & Liu, L. (2019). Insights into biochar and hydrochar production and applications: A review. *Fuel*, 171, 581–598. https://doi.org/10.1016/j.energy.2019.01.035

6 Natural biopolymer-derived porous materials as super adsorbents for wastewater treatment

Akhtar Alam, Atikur Hassan, and Neeladri Das

6.1 INTRODUCTION

Due to the rapidly growth in population and continuous improvement of living standard, the massive number of industries and technologies are developed day by day. As a consequence, a wide range of waste pollutants is dumped from different sources such as mining, industrial wastes of electronic devices, production of chemicals, pharmaceuticals, cosmetics, production of dyes, textiles, oil refining, petrochemicals, fertilizers, pesticides, paints, and paper printing. However, most of these wastes are toxic in nature and even carcinogenic to microbial populations and also difficult to degrade. Therefore, the water resources are getting worse day by day globally due to the contamination of such huge quantities of hazardous wastes particularly heavy metal ions/minerals, toxic dyes, organic impurities, and pharmaceutical poisons, which is become a serious concern for being healthy and natural environment as water is the most essential for lives. For instance, numerous toxic metal ions especially Cu^{2+} (copper), As (arsenic), Co^{2+} (cobalt), Ni^{2+} (nickel), Cd^{2+} (cadmium), Zn^{2+} (zinc), Hg^{2+} (mercury), Pb^{2+} (lead), and Cr^{4+}/Cr^{6+} (chromium) can produce a harmful effect to our environment (Baby et al., 2019; Chen et al., 2022). These toxic metal ions may be stored in our body through the food/water and could damage several organs/tissues such as kidney, liver, eyes, skins, gastrointestinal, and central nervous system (Zamora-Ledezma et al., 2021). On the other hand, the presence of toxic dyes like methylene blue (MB), congo red (CR), methyl orange dye (MO), Rhodamine B (RB), malachite green (MG), crystal violet (CV), and so on in water might possess serious risks to the mankind and aquatic communities (Robinson et al., 2001). Whereas, organic micropollutants containing cyanides, phosphates, phenols, petroleum oils, and pharmaceutical wastes in water have been recognized as hazardous pollutants to the ecosystem (Hojjati-Najafabadi et al., 2022). Thus, it is necessary to remove these toxic pollutants (before discharging) from contaminated water to avoid the negative effects on environment and human health (Saravanan et al., 2021). To date, a variety of conventional methods such as precipitation, coagulation, evaporation, distillation, oxidation, electrolysis, reverse osmosis, ion exchange, filtration, and adsorption have been established for removing of aforesaid toxic pollutants from wastewaters (Bolisetty et al., 2019; Ghafoori et al., 2022; Phoon et al., 2020). However, above these various approaches, adsorption by using a solid adsorbent is believed as a supreme because it is a simple, efficient, and inexpensive technique (Gupta et al., 2009; Sahoo & Prelot, 2020; Zhou & Haynes, 2010). Importantly, it is a conventional one that is associated with the ability for regeneration and facilitating large-scale applications. Indeed, varieties of inorganic adsorbents such as activated carbon, silica, zeolites, metal oxides, and clay minerals have been used for the removal of toxic contaminants from wastewaters (Ali, 2010; Han et al., 2019).

DOI: 10.1201/9781003500483-6

This chapter has been made available under a (CC-BY-NC-ND) 4.0 license

However, the use of these traditional adsorbents has several disadvantages including low adsorption capacities (Crini, 2006). Thus, exploring of novel adsorbent materials for the effective and efficient adsorption toward toxic pollutants from wastewater is still of great research interest (Chai et al., 2021; Chowdhury & Balasubramanian, 2014). For the same perspective, several of solid porous adsorbents including synthetic polymers, porous organic polymers (POPs), organic-inorganic hybrid polymers, polymeric composites, metal organic frameworks (MOFs), graphene-based nanomaterials, and many more have been reported for the wastewater treatment, but are limited to the laboratory level owing to many drawbacks such as high cost, time-consuming treatment, lower adsorption capacity, difficult to synthesis in large scale, non-selectivity, lack of selectivity, and reusability (Han et al., 2021; Huang et al., 2021; Samiey et al., 2014; Yu et al., 2021). As promising adsorbents for removal of water contaminants should not only have good adsorption capacity and feasibility but should also have the ability to easily desorb the adsorbed molecules/ions, to be efficiently recyclable and reusable for several time. Thus, for cost-effective and efficient treatment of industrial wastewater, choosing an appropriate adsorbent is very important to fulfill the desired requirements including high adsorption capacity, selectivity, fast adsorption kinetics, multiple absorbability, and productivity (Han et al., 2021; Qiu et al., 2022).

Over the last few decades, natural biopolymer-based materials have received significant attention due to their distinctive characteristics such as physicochemical stability, large specific surface area, biodegradability, cost-effectiveness, non-toxicity, and eco-friendly (Das et al., 2023; Udayakumar et al., 2021). Hence, the development of eco-friendly functionalized biopolymer-based materials could be a great choice for removal of various toxic pollutants especially heavy metals or inorganic ions, toxic dyes, hazardous organic and pharmaceutical compounds (Russo et al., 2021). Among several biopolymers, naturally occurring cellulose, chitosan, alginate, gelatin, starch, and carrageenan have been recognized as highly attractive adsorbents for the removal of aqueous pollutants (Khademian et al., 2020). These biopolymers are widely available and present a remarkable structural diversity, favoring to be super adsorbents for water remediation. In contemporary research, several biopolymer-based adsorbents have been developed in various forms of composites, blends, aerogels, hydrogels, foams, fibers, films, and membranes through the incorporation of activated carbon, carbon nanotubes, silica, clay, zeolite, graphene, metal nanoparticles, and other synthetic polymers or natural polymers. This chapter summarizes the latest synthesis and development of various advanced biopolymer-based materials for the treatment of toxic industrial wastes such as metal ions, textile dyes, organic micropollutants, and pharmaceutical impurities with their advantages and significant adsorption performances. Apart from that, the theoretical equations, adsorption isotherms, adsorption kinetic models, and adsorption thermodynamics are equally important parameters to be considered while evaluating an efficient adsorbent in applications related to the same. Hence, it is essential to understand the adsorption process first.

6.2 ADSORPTION

Adsorption techniques are broadly used for all kinds of water treatment, capture/storage of small gases (especially CO_2, H_2, and CH_4), evaluation of surface area and pore size of a variety of porous materials (e.g., industrial adsorbents, catalysts, and building materials), and so on (Fu et al., 2021; Gür, 2022). Adsorption refers to the enrichment of adsorbates (molecules/ions) at the surface or interface of an adsorbent. Adsorption can be termed as physisorption or chemisorption process depending on their interactions between adsorbate and adsorbent (Dąbrowski, 2001). In physisorption, adsorbed molecules/ions can be attached via weak and reversible Van der Waals forces, while chemisorption occurs mostly through the binding of irreversible covalent or electrostatic bonds. The most essential requirements of an effective and efficient adsorbent are inexpensive, non-toxic, biocompatibility, good physiochemical stability, large specific surface area, high adsorption capacity with a high rate, high selectivity, and reusability. The adsorption capability might be influenced by several factors like initial concentration of adsorbate, adsorbent dosage, temperature, contact time, and pH of the solution.

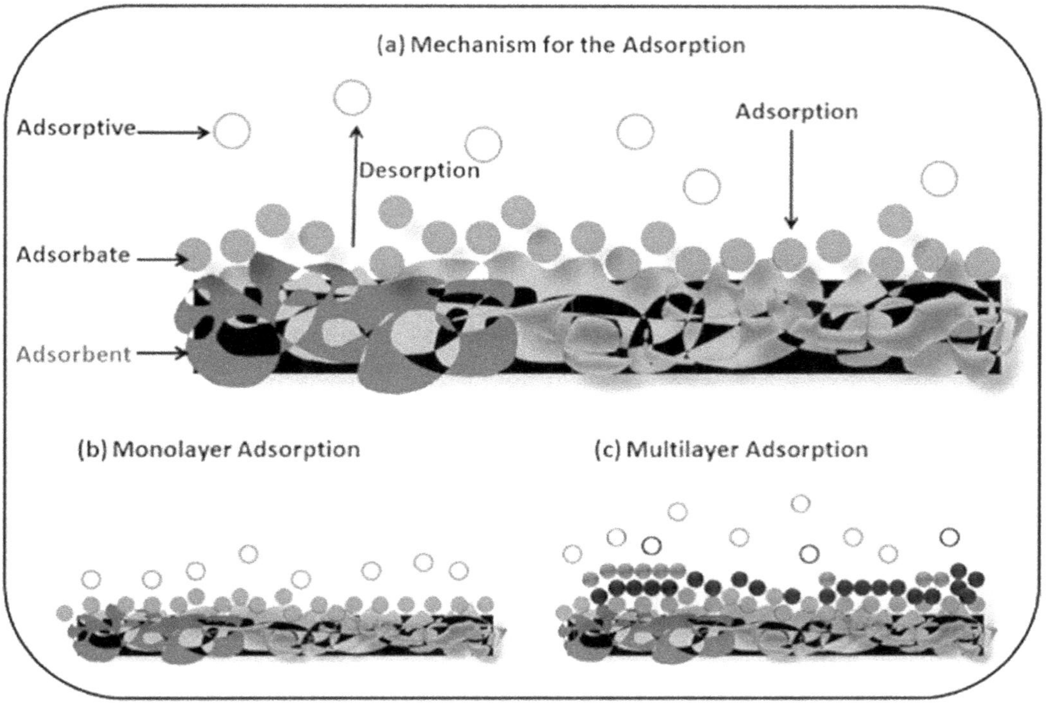

FIGURE 6.1 General adsorption mechanism (a), monolayer adsorption (b), and multilayer adsorption (c).

Source: Reproduced from Gupta et al. (2021) with permission.

6.2.1 Adsorption Mechanism

To evaluate the mechanism of adsorption using solid adsorbents, many approaches and theoretical models in terms of isotherms, kinetics, and thermodynamics were frequently performed. The adsorption of water pollutants takes place in two different states such as at surface and interstitial of the adsorbents. General mechanism of adsorption is depicted in Figure 6.1 (Gupta et al., 2021). In surface adsorption, adsorbate molecules/ions are attracted to the solid surface from the aqueous medium via Van der Waals forces, dipole interactions, or hydrogen bonding. On the other hand, in case of interstitial adsorption, the adsorbate molecules/ions diffuse into the adsorbents, entering the pores (micro/meso/macro) of the materials (Gupta et al., 2021). In this context, the use of natural bioadsorbents having electron-rich active functional groups (e.g., amino, hydroxyl, carboxyl, thiol, etc.) and high surface area facilitating the efficient capturing/adsorbing/binding of positively charged molecules/ions from wastewater systems (Alsawy et al., 2022). To understand the adsorption mechanism, some theoretical equations/parameters, adsorption isotherms, kinetic models, and adsorption thermodynamics are described concisely.

6.2.2 Adsorption Isotherms

The adsorption isotherm defines the relation between the amount of adsorbate adsorbed by the adsorbent at equilibrium as a function of its concentration (if adsorbate in the liquid phase) or pressure (if gas) at constant temperature. In the past few decades, several mathematical models such as Langmuir, Freundlich, Tempkin, Brunauer-Emmett-Teller, Dubinin-Radushkevich, and Flory-Huggins to name a few equilibrium adsorption isotherms have been developed for evaluating adsorption capacity (Kyzas et al., 2018). The equilibrium adsorption capacity (Q_e) and the removal efficiency (% R) can be considered according to equations (1) and (2) for different concentrations of the adsorbate solution.

$$Q_e = \frac{(C_0 - C_e) \times V}{M} \tag{1}$$

$$\text{Removal efficiency } (\%R) = \frac{C_0 - C_e}{C_e} \times 100\% \tag{2}$$

Herein, C_0 denotes initial concentration of adsorbate solution, C_e signifies the equilibrium concentration of adsorbate solution, V represents volume of adsorbate solution taken, and M is weight of adsorbent charged. In order to estimate the adsorption mechanism (for liquid phase solutes) by solid adsorbent, the Langmuir and Freundlich adsorption isotherm models are frequently employed. The Langmuir isotherm model is defined by equation (3) and implies the homogeneous formation of monolayer of adsorbates (dye molecules) since it is anticipated that all non-interacting adsorption sites are energetically identical. Whereas, the Freundlich isotherm model is described by the equation (4) and assumes non-ideal and multilayer sorption wherein all adsorption sites are non-identical, and therefore these sites have diverse affinities for the adsorbate molecules.

$$\frac{C_e}{Q_e} = \frac{C_e}{Q_m} + \frac{1}{Q_m K_L} \tag{3}$$

$$\ln Q_e = \ln K_F + \frac{1}{n} \ln C_e \tag{4}$$

where Q_e (mg/g) is the equilibrium adsorption capacity, C_e (mg/L) is the equilibrium concentration, Q_m (mg/g) is the maximum adsorption capacity of the Langmuir isotherm, K_L (L/mg) is the Langmuir adsorption coefficient, K_F (L/mg) is the Freundlich constant, and 1/n is an indicator that describes the nonlinear degree of adsorption.

6.2.3 Adsorptions kinetics

The adsorption kinetic modeling gives valuable evidence on the mechanism of the adsorption reaction and the reaction pathway related to the possible rate-controlling steps. However, several kinetic models have been developed, but it should be mentioned that two most established models such as the pseudo-first order and pseudo-second order equations are regularly employed to study the adsorption kinetics. The pseudo-first order and pseudo-second order kinetic models are defined by equations (5) and (6), respectively.

$$\ln (Q_e - Q_t) = \ln Q_e - k_1 t \tag{5}$$

$$\frac{t}{Q_t} = \frac{1}{k_2 Q_e^2} + \frac{t}{Q_e} \tag{6}$$

where Q_e is the equilibrium adsorption capacity (mg/g), Q_t is adsorption capacity at the *t* (min) contact time, and k_1 (min^{-1}) and k_2 (g/mg/min) are the corresponding adsorption rate constants. The activation energy is also an important parameter of the adsorption process as it suggests either the adsorption proceeds via a physical or chemical process. The activation energy can be calculated by using the Arrhenius equation (7).

$$\ln k = \ln A - \frac{E_a}{RT} \tag{7}$$

where *k* is the adsorption rate constant, *A* is the Arrhenius constant, E_a (kJ/mol) is the activation energy, R (8.314 J/mol·K) is the ideal gas constant, and T (K) denotes absolute temperature.

6.2.4 Adsorption Thermodynamic Studies

The thermodynamic studies are also concerned as the temperature plays a key role in adsorption process. These studies provide the information regarding spontaneity of the adsorption process. The thermodynamic studies are usually evaluated by increasing or decreasing the temperature during the adsorption process. In order to study the adsorption thermodynamic, the magnitude of the free Gibbs energy ($\Delta G°$) is obtained from the Gibbs-Helmholtz relation (8).

$$K_d = \frac{Q_e}{C_e} \tag{8}$$

where $\Delta H°$ is the standard enthalpy change and $\Delta S°$ is the standard entropy change. The $\Delta H°$ and $\Delta S°$ can be estimated from Van't Hoff equation (9).

$$K_d = \frac{\Delta S^{\circ}}{R} - \frac{\Delta H^{\circ}}{RT} \tag{9}$$

where R is the ideal gas constant, T *is* the absolute temperature, and K_d is the equilibrium constant, which can be described by the equation (10).

$$K_d = \frac{Q_e}{C_e} \tag{10}$$

where Q_e is the equilibrium adsorption capacity and C_e is the equilibrium concentration.

6.3 NATURAL BIOPOLYMER-BASED ADSORBENTS

Naturally occurring polymeric materials or biomolecules are mostly formed by living organisms during their life cycle, and these raw materials are often known as natural biopolymers. As adsorption by using biopolymer-based materials is the most promising approach for the treatment of water pollutants due to the low-cost of bioadsorbents, environmental friendly, high effectiveness, and good regeneration opportunities (Yaashikaa et al., 2022). Thus, the new challenges of developing alternative natural biopolymer-based adsorbents have revealed avenues for researchers to remove toxic pollutants for water treatments. In this concern, the most common natural biopolymers like cellulose, chitosan, gelatin, alginate, starch, and carrageenan have been widely researched and developed for wastewater treatment for decades. These biopolymers decorated with multiple functional groups (such as amino, hydroxyl, carboxyl, carbonyl, thiol, and sulfate) are the major ingredients of bioadsorbents, responsible for the significant interaction between adsorbents and contaminants. These types of interactions usually may take place through complexation/chelation, ion exchange, electrostatic interaction, aggregation, microprecipitation, oxidation, and reduction during the adsorption process (Figure 6.2) (Elwakeel et al., 2020). In this chapter, our main focuses to discuss a variety of

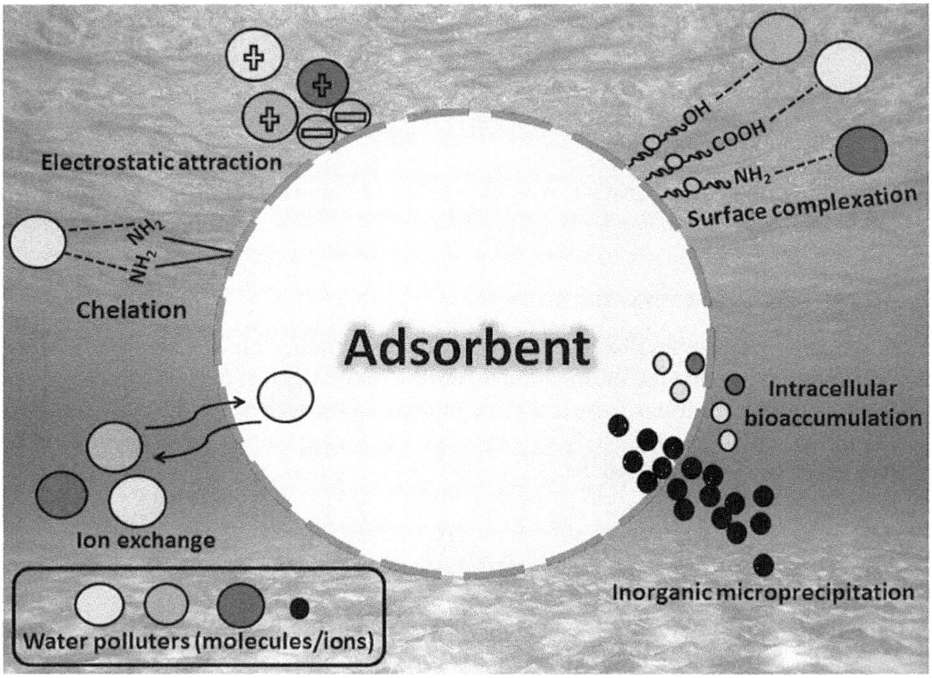

FIGURE 6.2 Various interactions take place during the adsorption process.

Source: Reproduced from Elwakeel et al. (2020) with permission.

naturally occurring biopolymer-based materials as super adsorbents and to summarize their potential application for removal of various wastewater contaminants.

6.3.1 Cellulose-based adsorbents

Cellulose is a polysaccharide with the chemical formula $(C_6H_{10}O_5)_n$, a natural biopolymer consisting of a linear chain of anhydroglucose units linked through of β(C1→C4) positions. Among the naturally occurring polymers, cellulose is the most abundant natural raw material. However, it is observed that natural cellulose exhibits a poor adsorption capacity as compared to modified/functionalized cellulose (Suhas et al., 2016). Thus, the compact and inactive molecular structure of cellulose needs to be modified or functionalized to improve its adsorption properties. In the past decade, a wide range of possible modification or functionalization of natural cellulose has been established by researchers, and several exciting results have been disclosed. Functionalized cellulose-based bioadsorbents have several favorable features including natural availability, cost-effective, nontoxicity, high specific surface area, micro/nano-size, physicochemical stability, biocompatibility, biodegradability, and so on. Consequently, cellulose-based bioadsorbents have been proven as promising candidates for removal of a wide variety of water pollutants including heavy metal ions, dyes, petroleum wastes, and pesticides (Zhou et al., 2013). In this section, we summarize the development and utilization of functionalized cellulose-based biomaterials as illustrative examples of super adsorbents. The adsorption capacity of several reported functionalized cellulose-based bioadsorbents toward hazardous pollutants is shown in Table 6.1. Currently, natural cellulose has been mostly used as a cost-effective precursor for fabrication of activated carbon with considerably high surface area (upto 1300 m^2/g) and large pore volumes, which facilitate the higher adsorption capacities for wastewater treatment (Suhas et al., 2016). For the same perspective, Athanasia *et al.* have developed a promising approach for functionalization of nanocellulose (EFB-NCP) with activated carbon obtained from

TABLE 6.1
Cellulose-based biomaterials as super adsorbents toward hazardous pollutant

Cellulose-based adsorbents	Adsorbate (hazardous pollutants)		Adsorption capacity (mg/g)	References
EFB-NCP	Pb(II)	Metal ions	24.94	Septevani et al. (2020)
ZIF-8@CA	Cr(VI)		41.84	Bo et al. (2018)
Cellulose-graft-poly (acrylic acid)	Cu^{2+}, Mn^{2+}		201, 175	J. Wang et al. (2016)
In situ TEMPO functionalized nanocellulose-based membranes	Cu^{+2}, Fe^{+2}/Fe^{+3}		374, 456	Karim et al. (2017)
PCA@AC	Cr(VI)		507.61	Hu et al. (2019)
NCNB	Cr, Co, Cu		2749.685, 916.65, 1937.49	Shahnaz et al. (2020)
Cellulose-based porous spherical/cotton	Cu^{2+}		110	Wittmar et al. (2021)
Magnetic chitosan/cellulose	Cu^{2+}, Pb^{2+}, Cd^{2+}		88.21, 61.12, 45.86	Luo et al. (2015)
Magnetic TZFNC	Pb(II)		554.4	Alipour et al. (2020)
CGD	MG, BF	Dyes	458.72, 1155.76	Zhou et al. (2013)
Cellulose citrate (CC)	MB		96.2	Olivito et al. (2021)
Cellulose/chitosan aerogels (CE/CS)	CR		381.7 (303 K), 580.8 (323 K)	Yixi Wang et al. (2018)
Cellulose acetate/chitosan blend films	orange seven, brilliant yellow		9.98, 9.38	Gopi et al. (2019)
Cellulose/biochar cryogels	Petroleum, SAE20W50 oil	Others	73, 54	Kunz Lazzari et al. (2021)
PCC	CO_2		2.31 mmol/g	Wang and Okubayashi (2019)

the empty oil palm fruit bunches before being modified with activated carbon (Suhas et al., 2016). The modified nanocellulose-based bioadsorbent showed a selective and outstanding performance for removal of Pb(II) with 86% efficiency and the maximum adsorption capacity of 24.94 mg/g. whereas, Yao and coworkers have successfully developed a facile method for hybrid cellulose aerogels/Zeolitic Imidazolate Framework (termed as ZIF-8@CA) by combining organic cellulose aerogels and inorganic ZIF-8 particles for elimination of heavy metal ions from wastewater (Bo et al., 2018). The adsorption capacity of porous hybrid ZIF-8@CA for Cr(VI) was significantly improved, and the maximum adsorption capacity (calculated from the Langmuir isotherm model) extended up to 41.84 mg/g. The adsorption experiments showed that adsorption capacity of ZIF-8@CA for Cr(VI) ions has significantly improved when compared with either cellulose aerogels or ZIF-8. Wang *et al.* synthesized cellulose-graft-poly (acrylic acid) microporous spheres as efficient adsorbents for Cu^{2+} and Mn^{2+} metal ions. The resulting cellulose and acrylic acid-based biopolymers showed the maximum adsorption capacity of 201 and 175 mg/g for Cu^{2+} and Mn^{2+} ions, respectively (J. Wang et al., 2016). Mathew and coworkers have developed the unique nanocellulose-based membranes via altering the composition of sludge microfibers/cellulose nanofibers and *in situ* TEMPO surface modification to enhance the removal efficiencies for heavy metal ions (Karim et al., 2017). The *in situ* TEMPO functionalized nanocellulose-based membranes with high mechanical stability and water permeability showed the adsorption capacity upto 374 mg/g for Cu^{+2} and 456 mg/g for Fe^{+2}/Fe^{+3} ions, and these values were higher (around 1.2–1.3 times) as compared to that of unfunctionalized cellulose nanofibers and cellulose nanocrystals. A cellulose-based composite (PCA@AC) was fabricated via catechol-amine polymer (copolymer of catechol tetraethylenepentamine and p-phenylenediamine) adhering onto cellulose substrate (Hu et al., 2019). The resulting biocomposite exhibited a significant performance for adsorbing of Cr(VI) ions with an adsorption capacity of 507.61 mg/g, derived from the Langmuir isotherm model at 30°C. The obtained value was also greater than that of the pure cellulose substrate, which is attributed to the electrostatic interaction as well as reduction of Cr(VI) to Cr(III) ions during the adsorption experiments. Senthilmurugan and coworkers have also successfully synthesized nanobentonite-incorporated nanocellulose/chitosan aerogel (NCNB) that displayed potential application for removal of metals from simulated wastewater (Shahnaz et al., 2020). The maximum adsorption capacities of NCNB were found to be 2749.685, 916.65, and 1937.49 mg/g for Cr, Co, and Cu, respectively, while the corresponding removal efficiencies were obtained as 98.90, 97.45, and 99.01% under the optimum conditions. Recently, Wittmar et al. have developed a promising method for synthesis of cellulose-based porous spherical adsorbers by using natural cotton as precursor (Wittmar et al., 2021). The resulting natural bioadsorbers showed the maximum adsorption capacity of 110 mg/g Cu^{2+} ions.

From the economical perspective, magnetic adsorbents have attracted researchers because it offers the recovery of applied adsorbent materials from aqueous medium without using filter or centrifugation (Luo et al., 2016; Zhu et al., 2011). In this regard, a new class of efficient reusable cellulose-based magnetic bioadsorbents for water purification has received much attention in recent decades. The advantage of this approach is the functionalized bioadsorbents can be separated out easily from the aqueous medium by using external magnetic force and could be applied again for the next cycle after acid treatment. The illustrative examples are amino-functionalized magnetic cellulose composite (Sun et al., 2014), porous magnetic cellulose beads (Yu et al., 2014), and magnetic carboxylated cellulose nanocrystal-based composite (CCN-Fe_3O_4). Figure 6.3 shows a representative example of the adsorption of Pb (II) ions by magnetic CCN-Fe_3O_4 that could be easily collected by applying an external magnetic force. The applied bioadsorbent can be regenerated upon the treatment of dilute acid. However, the adsorption capacity of the CCN-Fe_3O_4 was slowly reduced after using several cycles, but the performance of the bioadsorbent was quiet good with the removal ratio of more than 80%. Using same strategy, the cost-effective magnetic chitosan/cellulose microspheres as an effective and recyclable adsorbent were prepared from polymeric blend of chitosan/

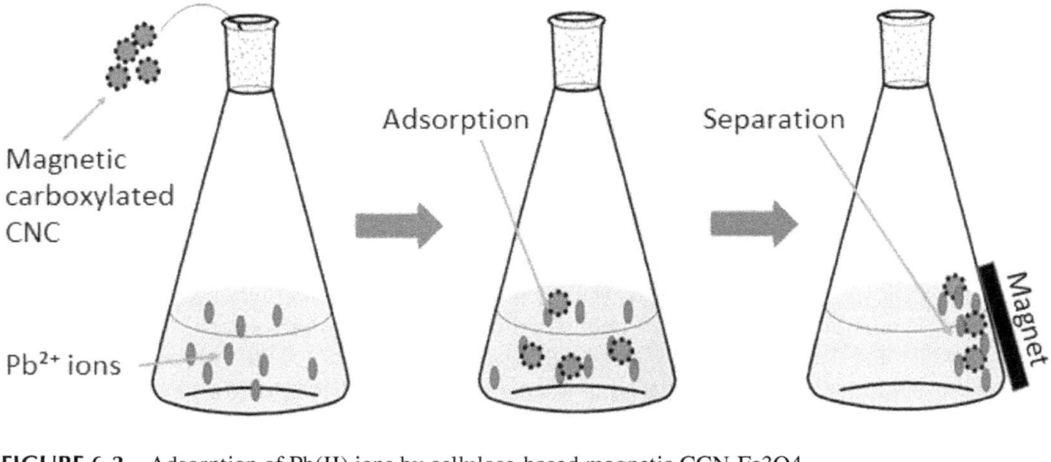

FIGURE 6.3 Adsorption of Pb(II) ions by cellulose-based magnetic CCN-Fe3O4.

Source: Reproduced from Faiz Norrahim et al. (2021) with permission.

cellulose and evaluated for the removal of heavy metal ions of Cu^{2+}, Pb^{2+}, and Cd^{2+} (Luo et al., 2015). Moreover, novel magnetic thiourea-modified ZnO/nanocellulose composite (TZFNC) was fabricated by Alipour *et al.* with high adsorption capacity and removal efficiency toward Pb(II) ions (Alipour et al., 2020). The experimental studies showed that the removal efficiency of Pb(II) ions was found upto 99.99% (at the amount of adsorbent = 40 mg, concentration of Pb(II) = 60 mg/L, at pH = 6.5 and contact time = 14.5 min). The designed bioadsorbent (TZFNC) demonstrated excellent potential for removal of Pb(II) ions due to their easy magnetic separation ability and recyclability.

Cellulose-based bioadsorbents have also been applied for removal of toxic dye molecules for water treatments. For example, Zhou et al. reported a cost-effective cellulose-based bioadsorbent (CGD) obtained from naturally occurring cellulose adapting with glycidyl methacrylate and diethylenetriamine pentaacetic acid for adsorption of cationic dyes such as MG and basic fuchsine (BF) (Zhou et al., 2013). The dye adsorption studies suggested that the adsorption (CGD) for MG was fitted well with the Langmuir isotherm model, while basic fuchsine was fitted with the Freundlich isotherm model. The calculated adsorption capacity was found to be 1155.76 mg/g for BF and 458.72 mg/g for MG at internal concentration of 2000 mg/L. Interestingly, the recyclability experiments demonstrated that CGD was retained their adsorption efficiency around 85 and 90% for BF and MG dye, respectively, after four or five cycles. Recently, Nino and coworkers have developed cellulose citrate (CC) as a reusable bioadsorbent via a green and convenient reaction of two natural products such as cellulose and citric acid (Olivito et al., 2021). The synthesized cellulose citrate (CC) displayed the significant efficiency for elimination of cationic methylene blue (MB) from contaminated water due to the substantial interaction between carboxylic groups of cellulose citrate and cationic dye molecules. The adsorption studied showed that the maximum adsorption capacity for MB was found to be 96.2 mg/g, and the adsorption process was followed monolayer adsorption, which indicated the Langmuir model, while the adsorption kinetics followed a pseudo-second order model. Cellulose-based bioadsorbents can also be applied as efficient adsorbents toward anionic dyes for the same purposes. For example, Liu and coworkers prepared eco-friendly cellulose/chitosan porous aerogels (CE/CS) using sol-gel and freeze-drying techniques by varying the mass ratios of CE and CS (Yixi Wang et al., 2018). The CE/CS composite showed remarkable adsorption capacity for anionic congo red (CR) with capacity of 381.7 mg/g at 303 K, and 580.8 mg/g at 323 K. The increase in adsorption capacity at higher temperature clearly indicated that the adsorption of CR dye via endothermic process, which might attribute to the electrostatic interaction and hydrogen bonding. The CE/CS aerogel also demonstrated that the maximum removal efficiency for CR was observed under the optimum conditions of composite ratio of 1:3, adsorbent dosage of 2.5 g/L and at a pH range of 3–11. Moreover, Thomas and coworkers fabricated cellulose acetate/chitosan blend films via a convenient solvent casting process and further modified the resultant films by deacetylation method (Gopi et al., 2019). The adsorption behavior of both unmodified and modified cellulose acetate/chitosan composite films was investigated for anionic dyes like acid orange 7 and brilliant yellow. The experimental data revealed that modified cellulose acetate/chitosan composite films showed improved adsorption capacity and dye removal efficiency and were found to be 9.98 mg/g and 99.8% for acid orange 7, while 9.38 mg/g and 99.7% for brilliant yellow. Attractively, Lazzari *et al.* synthesized cellulose/biochar cryogels from *Pinus elliotti* cellulose and biochar using freeze-drying techniques and studied the adsorption behavior toward organic liquids such as petroleum and SAE20W50 oil through adsorption isotherm and kinetic models (Kunz Lazzari et al., 2021). The synthesized cellulose/biochar cryogels demonstrated their potential to be a promising bioadsorbent for petroleum and SAE20W50 oil with the high magnitude of heterogeneous sorption capacity of 73 and 54 g/g, respectively.

Moreover, carbon dioxide capture and separation by solid porous biomaterials is a frontier research area to reduce global CO_2 (greenhouse gas) emissions. A large number of POPs and metal organic frameworks (MOFs) are well established for selectively carbon dioxide capture and separation. However, Okubayashi and coworkers successfully developed a unique polyethyleneimine-crosslinked cellulose (PCC) porous bioadsorbent with significantly high specific surface area of 234.2 m^2/g by using a cost-effective sol-gel method (Wang & Okubayashi, 2019). The resulting PCC aerogel showed remarkably high CO_2 uptake capacity upto 2.31 mmol/g at 25°C and under dry CO_2 atmosphere. Furthermore, the PCC aerogel with three-dimensional irregularly shaped exhibited superb CO_2 adsorption/desorption recyclability even after ten cycles, suggesting a probable solid bioadsorbent for efficient CO_2 capture. The current research trends witness that cellulose-based bioadsorbents would play an important role for the practical application related to the environmental remediation.

6.3.2 Chitosan-based adsorbents

As the biodegradable natural polymers are significantly important in various aspects of implementations, among them, chitosan could be the most promising candidate as super adsorbent for wastewater treatment. Chitosan is another polysaccharide produced from the deacetylation of chitin, which is the second most abundant natural biopolymer after cellulose, and it is mostly obtained from insect cuticles and sea crustacean shells. Although chitosan has owned various promising characteristics such as non-toxicity, low cost, biodegradability, rich in active functional sites, it cannot be applied directly for adsorption purposes due to its poor mechanical strength, high crystallinity, low surface area, and solubility in acidic medium. Hence, chitosan needs to be functionalized or modified to use as potential adsorbents, and therefore it has been frequently modified into various forms including nanofibers, composites, films, foams, blends, and hydrogel beads. The major advantage of chitosan over other polysaccharides (i.e., cellulose or starch) is their unique chemical structure that permits to tune definite modifications needed for designing biomaterials for desired applications. Chitosan and its derivatives are being widely researched and exhibit attractive adsorption performances due to the presence of amine (or protonated NH_3^+) and hydroxyl (-OH) functioning groups in its backbone. Additionally, the unique property of chitosan's polycationic nature offers to be a flocculating agent and that can facilitate to chelate with metal/organic molecules and adsorbing them via abundant electrostatic interactions. To date, several studies have modified raw chitosan by crosslinking it with other precursors, by combining it with porous materials/polymers, and by grafting functional groups onto it. Few examples of chitosan/chitin-based biopolymers as super adsorbents are reviewed and summarized in Table 6.2.

Hameed and coworkers prepared crosslinked chitosan/sepiolite composites from low cost and environmental friendly materials like chitosan and sepiolite clay and were crosslinked using epichlorohydrin as an additive (Marrakchi et al., 2016). The synthesized chitosan/sepiolite composite was explored as a potential bioadsorbent for toxic dyes such as methylene blue (MB) and reactive

TABLE 6.2
Chitosan-based biomaterials as super adsorbents toward hazardous pollutants

Chitosan-based adsorbents	Adsorbate (hazardous pollutants)		Adsorption capacity (mg/g)	References
CS-PDA	Cr(VI),	Metal ions	374.4,	Guo et al. (2018)
	Pb(II)		441.2	
Chitosan/CDTA/GO	Cr(VI)		166.98	Ali (2018)
Fe_3O_4@Zr-chitosan	Cr(VI)		280.97	X. Chen et al. (2017)
Chitosan/sepiolite composite	MB,		40.98,	Marrakchi et al. (2016)
	RO16	Dyes	190.96	
Chitosan-grafted-polyethyleneimine	Reactive Black 5		707.27	Chatterjee et al. (2011)
Chitosan–$Fe(OH)_3$	MO,		314.45,	Li et al. (2018)
	CR		445.32	
Chitosan/PVA	nitrate ions	Acid radicals	35.03	A. Rajeswari et al. (2016)
Chitosan/PEG	nitrate ions		50.68	A. Rajeswari et al. (2016)

orange 16 (RO16), and the monolayer adsorption capacities were recorded as 40.98 and 190.96 mg/g, respectively, at 30°C. Chitosan can also be blended with other polymers to enrich the adsorption properties. For example, Rajeswari *et al.* developed chitosan/PVA and chitosan/PEG composites and studied the adsorption of nitrate ions from aqueous solutions (Rajeswari et al., 2016). The adsorption capacities of nitrate ions were found to be 35.03 and 50.68 mg/g by using chitosan/PVA and chitosan/PEG, respectively. Chitosan was also grafted with other polymers to improve the dye adsorption capacity like the adsorption capacity of chitosan-grafted-polyethyleneimine for reactive black 5 (RB5), which was reported as 707.27 mg/g, while in case of non-grafted chitosan, it was 209.90 mg/g only (Chatterjee et al., 2011), whereas Guo *et al.* prepared polydopamine-modified chitosan aerogels (CS-PDA) via dopamine self-polymerization and glutaraldehyde crosslinking reactions to improve the adsorption properties and acid resistance of chitosan (Guo et al., 2018). The metal adsorption studies of the resultant CS-PDA aerogels suggested that the adsorption isotherms and kinetic data were advocated to the Langmuir isotherm and pseudo-second-order kinetic models. The CS-PDA aerogels displayed superb adsorption performances toward removal of Cr(VI) and Pb(II) metal ions with the maximum capacities of 374.4 and 441.2 mg/g, respectively. While Yang *et al.* fabricated Chitosan–$Fe(OH)_3$ beads as efficient adsorbents for anionic dye removal from contaminated water (Li et al., 2018). The removal efficiencies for anionic dyes like methyl orange (MO) and congo red (CR) by using the chitosan–$Fe(OH)_3$ beads surpassed the pure chitosan beads. The maximum adsorption capacities were determined from the Langmuir isotherm equation and were obtained as 314.45 and 445.32 mg/g for CR and MO, respectively. The recyclability studies suggested that the chitosan–$Fe(OH)_3$ beads displayed good reusability and the removal efficiencies for the removal of both dyes, and surpassed upto 95% after being used five cycles. Ali and coworkers developed a unique chitosan-based bioadsorbents termed as chitosan/CDTA/GO (chitosan/1,2-Cyclohexylenedinitrilotetraacetic acid/graphene oxide) using glutaraldehyde as a cross-linker. The removal efficiency of the synthesized chitosan/CDTA/GO nanoparticles toward Cr(VI) ions were evaluated at various adsorption conditions such as adsorbent dose, the effects of the chemical composition of the adsorbent (CDTA/GO concentration), temperature, time of contact, pH of the solution, and initial concentration Cr(VI) metal ion (Ali, 2018). The adsorption data showed that the adsorption capacity of the chitosan/CDTA/GO nanoparticles toward Cr(VI) ions was 166.98 mg/g under the optimal adsorbent dose of 2 g/L, at an equilibrium time of 60 min, and a pH value of 3.5. Besides, the results suggested that the adsorption capacity can be influenced by the temperature and pH immensely, and the adsorption processes were followed via the pseudo-second-order kinetic model and the adsorption isotherm fitted with the Langmuir model. For the perspective of easy and simple reusability, Chen et al. synthesized magnetic zirconium(IV) cross-linked chitosan microspheres (Fe_3O_4@Zr-chitosan) as a reusable bioadsorbent through the coordination reaction between chitosan biopolymeric matrix and zirconiumoxychloride for effective removal and simultaneous detoxification of Cr(VI) ions in aqueous medium (Chen et al., 2017). The synthesized Fe3O4@Zr-chitosan bioadsorbent demonstrated preferential adsorption for Cr(VI) ions with the coexistence of several other ions such as Na^+, K^+, Ca^{2+}, Mg^{2+}, Cu^{2+}, Zn^{2+}, Cl^-, SO_4^{-2}, CO_3^{-2}, and NO_3^-.The batch adsorption studies of Cr(VI) ions showed the adsorption capacity of the synthesized Fe3O4@Zr-chitosan microspheres was found to be 280.97 mg/g at pH of 4.0, and at the temperature of 298 K. Importantly, the resultant bioadsorbent retained outstanding reusability for water purification and dropped the contents of effluent Cr(VI) metal ions down to the ppb (parts per billion) level, reaching the drinking water standard recommended by the WHO (World Health Organization).

6.3.3 Alginate-based adsorbents

Sodium alginate (SA) is a renewable anionic biopolymer that consists of a natural polysaccharide and α–1, 4-L-glucuronic acid. It is a low-cost water-soluble biomaterial containing abundant hydroxyl (–OH) and carboxyl (–COOH) functional groups, which have the high adsorption affinity

TABLE 6.3
Alginate-based biomaterials as super adsorbents toward hazardous pollutants

Alginate-based adsorbents	Adsorbate (hazardous pollutants)		Adsorption capacity (mg/g)	References
Cu–PVA–SA	Cu(II)	Metal ions	79.3	Chen et al. (2011)
Phosphate-embedded calcium alginate beads	Cd(II)		82.6	Y.-y. Wang et al. (2016)
Alginate@PEI	Cr(VI)		431.6	Yan et al. (2017)
Alginate-based attapulgite foams	Cu(II), Cd(II)		119.0, 160.0	Yaquan Wang et al. (2018)
Sodium alginate-based crosslinked beads	Pb(II)		2042	Shao et al. (2018)
MPA	Cr(VI)		538.97	Feng et al. (2021)
Sodium alginate-based crosslinked beads	MB	Dyes	2977	Shao et al. (2018)
MPA	CR		3568	Feng et al. (2021)
N-doped carbon monoliths	CO_2	Others	8.99 mmol/g	Ma et al. (2014)

toward heavy metal ions. However, the stability, heat resistance, and mechanical strength of sodium alginate are moderately low. Thus, chemical or physical modifications are commonly applied to use it as green bioadsorbents in wastewater remediation. Therefore, the alginate-based bioadsorbents have received considerable attention for the decontamination of numerous pollutants from polluted water. The recent works have focused on improving the raw alginate materials by incorporating various functional groups via grafting or crosslinking polymerization reaction (Table 6.3). For example, Chen *et al.* prepared alginate-based Cu(II)-imprinted porous films (Cu–PVA–SA) and explored them for removal of Cu(II) ions from aqueous medium (Chen et al., 2011). They investigated the effects of various parameters on adsorption behaviors by changing the concentration of Cu(II) in the Cu–PVA–SA, adsorbent dosage, pH of the solution, ionic strength, contact time, and initial concentration of Cu(II) solution. The resulting Cu–PVA–SA demonstrated the adsorption capacity of 79.3 mg/g for Cu(II) ions. Wang *et al.* developed phosphate-embedded calcium alginate aerogel beads for removal of metal ions of Cd(II) ions with the maximum adsorption capacity of 82.6 mg/g (Y.-y. Wang et al., 2016), whereas Zhai and coworkers designed and synthesized flexible core-shell/bead-like alginate@PEI biosorbent by cross-linking reaction of polyethylenimine (PEI) used as a modification reagent (Yan et al., 2017). The maximum adsorption capacity of the alginate@PEI for Cr(VI) was found to be 431.6 mg/g, and this value was superior than that of unmodified sodium alginate (24.2 mg/g). To reduce the cost and improve the mechanical strength of alginate-based adsorbents, a typical phyllosilicate like attapulgite (ATP) was introduced into them. For instance, Wang *et al.* constructed alginate-based attapulgite foams by encapsulating ATP in sodium alginate using a freeze-drying and post-cross-linking technique. The fabricated floatable porous foam showed excellent adsorption capacity of 119.0 and 160.0 mg/g for Cu(II) and Cd(II), respectively (Yaquan Wang et al., 2018). In addition, the resulting alginate-based bioadsorbents exhibited good chemical stability and mechanical stability, and were easily recyclable due to their floatability nature in water. Shao *et al.* have revealed a facile method for the synthesis of engineering sodium alginate-based crosslinked beads having a remarkable removal capability for both organic dyes and toxic metal ions (Shao et al., 2018). The synthesized sodium alginate beads showed the maximum adsorption capacities of methylene blue (MB) and Pb(II) metal ions were observed as 2977 and 2042 mg/g, respectively. Moreover, the alginate-based beads also exhibited outstanding performances for absorbing methylene violet dye and other heavy metal ions such as Cu^{2+}, Ni^{2+}, and Cd^{2+}. Recently, Wang and coworkers fabricated MXene/PEI-functionalized sodium alginate composite aerogels (MPA) by incorporating amino-functionalized $Ti_3C_2T_x$ and polyethylenimine

(PEI) into sodium alginate aerogel matrix via cross-linking reactions (Feng et al., 2021). The fabricated MPA bioadsorbents exhibited an ultrahigh adsorption performance toward Congo Red (CR) dye and Cr(VI) metal ions due to the abundant active sites of PEI coupled and MXene, attributing to the significant electrostatic attraction force. The observed adsorption capacities were calculated as 3568 and 538.97 mg/g for CR and Cr(VI) ions, respectively, whereas Ma *et al.* developed a novel N-doped carbon monoliths using binary mixed acid (H_3PO_4–HNO_3) as co-activating agent and natural sodium alginate as carbon precursor (Ma et al., 2014). The resultant N-doped carbon monoliths displayed high surface area (1740 m^2/g) with a narrow pore size distribution. The N-doped carbon monoliths recorded the highest CO_2 uptake capacities of 8.99 mmol/g at 273 K, and 4.57 mmol/g at 298 K. Hence, the CO_2 gas adsorption studies have admitted that alginate-based bioadsorbents could be the encouraging materials for carbon dioxide capture and separation (CCS).

6.3.4 Starch-based adsorbents

Starch is also a well-known naturally occurring biodegradable polymer that is found in roots, stalks, and crop seeds of various plants. Functionalized starch-based biopolymers have also been utilized as super adsorbents for water remediation due to their low cost, easy availability, non-toxicity, biocompatibility, high surface area, and renewability (Gholinejad et al., 2016; Nasrollahzadeh et al., 2021). Here, the potential applications of starch-based bioadsorbents for the elimination of various pollutants from wastewater have been highlighted and summarized in Table 6.4. For example, Guo *et al.* prepared crosslinked porous starch (CPS) via crosslinking of native starch with epichlorohydrin and then by hydrolyzation of the crosslinked starch with α-amylase (Guo et al., 2013). The resulting safe and biodegradable adsorbent CPS was investigated to remove methylene blue dye, and the adsorption studies suggested that the adsorption data were well-fitted with Langmuir model with the capacity of 9.46 mg/g. Moreover, the dye adsorption data indicated that the removal efficiency of CPS is greater than that of native starch or porous starch. While Singh et al. fabricated starch-functionalized iron oxide nanoparticles (SIONPs) and iron oxide nanoparticles (IONPs) and evaluated their adsorption capability for Cr(VI) ions (Singh et al., 2014). The experimental data disclosed that the adsorption capacity of SIONPs was significantly improved as compared to IONPs, and the monolayer adsorption capacity of SIONPs for Cr(VI) ions was obtained as 9.02 mg/g. The negatively charged starch has demonstrated to be an efficient bioadsorbent for removal of cationic dye molecules (Ihsanullah et al., 2022; Nasrollahzadeh et al., 2021). Pourjavadi et al. prepared a magnetic nanocomposite nanoparticle@starch-*g*-poly (vinyl sulfate) for effectively adsorption of cationic dye molecules like MG and methylene blue with high reusability

TABLE 6.4
Starch-based biomaterials as super adsorbents toward hazardous pollutants

Starch-based adsorbents	Adsorbate (hazardous pollutants)		Adsorption capacity (mg/g)	References
SIONPs	Cr(VI)	Metal ions	9.02	Guo et al. (2013)
HIPS/SA	Cu(II)		25.81	Dai et al. (2019)
Crosslinked porous starch	MB	Dyes	9.46	Guo et al. (2013)
Nanoparticle@starch-*g*-poly(vinyl sulfate)	MB, MG		621, 567	Pourjavadi et al. (2016)
Starch/GO/PAM	MG		297	Hosseinzadeh and Ramin, (2018)
TiO_2/CCMS	golden yellow		208.77	Guo et al. (2019)
CMS-g-PMAA	NH_3, phenol	Others	31, 250.1	Haq et al. (2020)

(Pourjavadi et al., 2016). The synthesized nanoparticle@starch-*g*-poly (vinyl sulfate) exhibited a significant removal efficiency with the capacity of 621 mg/g for MB and 567 mg/g for MG, and these values were comparable or superior to most of the other adsorbents. Latterly, Ramin and coworkers fabricated a nanocomposite hydrogel of starch grafted poly(acrylamide)/graphene oxide/hydroxypatite (Starch/GO/PAM) for adsorbing cationic MG dye from wastewater (Hosseinzadeh & Ramin, 2018). Additionally, the temperature dependence results for MG dye suggested that the adsorption take place via endothermic, feasible, and spontaneous, and the dye adsorption kinetics were followed by the pseudo-second-order model. The adsorption experiments also showed that isotherm data were well-fitted with the Langmuir isotherm model with the capacity of 297 mg/g for cationic MG dye. While Guo et al. synthesized and explored the TiO_2/crosslinked carboxymethyl starch (TiO_2/CCMS) for adsorption of golden yellow dye from aqueous medium with the maximum adsorption capacity of 208.77 mg/g at the temperature of 308 K (Guo et al., 2019). Furthermore, Dai *et al.* developed a novel starch-based thermoresponsive hydrogel (HIPS/SA) from 2-hydroxy-3-isopropoxypropyl starch (HIPS) and sodium alginate (SA) for adsorbing Cu(II) metal ions from aqueous medium (Dai et al., 2019). The HIPS/SA hydrogel with porous network structure disclosed good adsorption capacity of 25.81 mg/g for Cu(II) metal ions, ascribing to the sufficient binding sites (carboxy groups) inside the hydrogel. Interestingly, the porous HIPS/SA hydrogel also showed the high feasibility of regeneration as it could be easily desorb the metal ions upon treatment with dilute acid (hydrochloric acid) in a very short time due to its thermoresponsive nature. Whereas, Haq *et al.* also disclosed a new bioadsorbent CMS-g-PMAA by grafting carboxymethyl starch (CMS) and polymethacrylic acid (PMAA) for adsorption of ammonia (NH_3) and phenol (Haq et al., 2020). The adsorption capacities of NH_3 and phenol were found in the range of 20–31 mg/g and 244.5–250.1 mg/g, respectively. The CMS-g-PMAA owing immense "O" centers might be responsible for improving the adsorption performances toward NH_3 and phenol via the formation of H-bond between ammonia/phenol and –OH or –COOH groups of the adsorbents.

6.3.5 Gelatin-based adsorbents

Gelatin, a high molecular weight polypeptide, is a natural biopolymer with multiple characteristic features including water solubility, biodegradability, non-toxicity, abundant surface area, and non-expensive. Gelatin has been mostly used in various sectors like foods, cosmetics, and biomedical-related applications. However, gelatin is also applied as promising bioadsorbents for elimination of contaminants from wastewater because its incorporation in other compounds/materials offers network structures decorated with various functional groups such as NH_2, OH, and COOH. A variety of gelatin-based bioadsorbents have been developed in the form of composites, nanoparticles, blends, hydrogels, aerogels, sphere beads, membranes, films and so on. These gelatin-based biomaterials have been proven as effective and efficient adsorbent for removing of water contaminants especially organic dyes, oil and toxic metal ions. Herein, we summarize some important gelatin-based bioadsorbents and their potential applications for water remediation with adsorption capacity (Table 6.5). A ecofriendly and inexpensive gelatin/activated carbon composite bead (GE/AC) was prepared by Hayeeye et al. via a drip emulsification process for Pb^{+2} ions from aqueous solutions (Hayeeye et al., 2018). The adsorption studies disclosed that the maximum adsorption capacity of these bioadsorbent beads (GE/AC) for Pb^{+2} ions was found to be 370.37 mg/g, and this value was comparable or better than that of natural zeolites and commercial ion exchange resins. Moreover, the influence of pH on the adsorption was also explored, and the results showed that the maximum adsorption of Pb^{+2} ions was reached at a pH of about 5, while low adsorption value was observed at a pH of 2.0. It is noted that the adsorption studies of metal ions were mostly conducted in ranges close to neutrality (i.e., pH values around 6.0 and 7.0) because at lower pH, the surface of the adsorbents becomes positive, avoiding the adsorption of the targeted metal ions (Meng et al., 2019; Wang et al., 2018), whereas Jing and coworkers synthesized a sponge of polyethylenimine (PEI)-grafted gelatin for effectively adsorbing heavy metals from wastewater (Li et al.,

TABLE 6.5
Gelatin-based biomaterials as super adsorbents toward hazardous pollutants

Gelatin-based adsorbents	Adsorbate (hazardous pollutants)		Adsorption capacity (mg/g)	References
Gelatin/activated carbon composite bead	Pb^{+2}	Metalions	370.37	Hayeeye et al. (2018)
PEI-grafted gelatin sponge	Pb(II), Cd(II)		66, 65	Li et al. (2016)
Silica-gelatin hybrid mesoporous aerogels	Hg(II)		209	Herman et al. (2020)
SPIONs/gel/PVA nanoparticles	Cu(II), Zn(II),		56.051, 40.865	Dolgormaa et al. (2018)
Sepiolite/gelatin nanocomposites	MB	Dyes	684.8	Sabzi et al. (2019)
Gelatin/TiO2/PEI composites	CV, MO, CR,		64.31, 85.21, 86.67	Jiang et al. (2019)
Gelatin templated hierarchically porous calcium oxide composites	organophosphate pesticides	Others	3895	Nagpal and Kakkar (2020a)

2016). The absorption capacity of the PEI-grafted gelatin sponge for Pb(II) and Cd(II) ions was 66 and 65 mg/g, which were superior than that of the gelatin sponge (9.75 and 9.35 mg/g). The reason behind the increasing adsorption capacity was the sufficient interaction between heavy metals with the adsorbents, as wastewater could remain onto the spongy PEI-grafted gelatin for a long time. Recently, Herman *et al.* developed supercritically dried silica-gelatin hybrid mesoporous aerogels and evaluated their removal efficiency via batch adsorption methods for Hg(II) in simultaneous presence of several other metal ions like Cu(II), Co(II), Ni(II), Cd(II), Pb(II), Ag(I), and Zn(II) (Herman et al., 2020). The maximum adsorption capacity of silica-gelatin hybrid adsorbent was estimated by using the Langmuir model and was observed to be 209 mg/g for Hg(II) at 24 wt % of gelatin content. In addition, the silica-gelatin aerogel demonstrated significant reusability without significant loss of adsorption capacity at the end of five cycles. Moreover, Huang *et al.* designed and successfully synthesized novel SPIONs/gel/PVA nanoparticles from super-paramagnetic iron oxide nanoparticles (SPIONs), gelatin (gel), and polyvinyl alcohol (PVA) for adsorbing Cu(II) and Zn(II) ions from polluted water (Dolgormaa et al., 2018). The resulting SPIONs/gel/PVA materials exhibited the maximum capacities of 56.051 and 40.865 mg/g for Cu(II) and Zn(II), respectively. To date, a variety of gelatin-based adsorbents have been evaluated for adsorbing toxic organic dyes, such as chitosan-gelatin-based hydrogels (Kaur & Jindal, 2019), gelatin/calcium alginate nanofiber membranes (Che et al., 2019), gelatin-CNT-iron oxide nanocomposite beads (Saber-Samandari et al., 2017), and gelatin/HPET/chitosan nanocomposites (Haroun et al., 2013). For the same perspective, Mohammadi and coworkers fabricated sepiolite/gelatin nanocomposites from naturally available sepiolite clay and gelatin for cost-effective and efficient dye removal application from wastewater (Sabzi et al., 2019). The synthesized sepiolite/gelatin nanocomposites showed effective and excellent dye removal efficiency for cationic methylene blue (MB) with the adsorption capacity of 684.8 mg/g at an equilibrium time of 30 min, whereas Jiang *et al.* developed a multifunctional gelatin/TiO_2/PEI (GTP) composite aerogels with hierarchical porous structure from natural gelatin, branched polyethyleneimine, and TiO_2 nanoparticles (Jiang et al., 2019). The synthesized gelatin/TiO2/PEI composites exhibited excellent potential for practical applications in wastewater treatment and demonstrated combined performances including copper (Cu) ions removal, organic dyes adsorption, oil/water separation, and photocatalytic property. The gelatin/TiO_2/PEI aerogels could remove cationic dyes (such as methylene blue (MB) and CV) as well as anionic dyes (i.e. congo red (CR) and methyl orange (MO)) and showed the maximum adsorption capacity of 64.31, 85.21,

86.67 mg/g for CV, MO, and CR, respectively at an initial concentration of 500 mg/L. Additionally, gelatin-based adsorbents have also been reported for removals of organophosphate pesticides (phosmet) (Nagpal & Kakkar, 2020b). For example, Kakkar and coworkers (2020) prepared a gelatin-templated hierarchical porous calcium oxide composite (Hr–CaO) via a precipitation technique by using water/glycerol solvent mixture and gelatin as a template (Nagpal & Kakkar, 2020a). The obtained gelatin-based composites displayed a remarkable adsorption capacity of 3895 mg/g for the organophosphate pesticides at an adsorbent dosage of 0.1 g/L.

6.3.6 Carrageenan-based adsorbents

Carrageenan is unique class of linear-sulfated polysaccharides that consist of linear 1,3 glycosidic-linked β-D-galactopyransose moiety and 1,4 glycosidic-linked 3,6-anhydro-α-D-galactopyranose or 1,4 glycosidic-linked α-D-galactopyranose units. It has an anionic charge across the polymer backbone and can be extracted from red seaweeds. Based on the degree of sulfation, the common forms of carrageenan are kappa-carrageenan, lambda-carrageenan, and iota-carrageenan and are widely used for the preparation of polymeric nanocomposites, gels, beads, membranes, etc. It is also used as an attractive bioadsorbent for the removal of toxic heavy metal ions and cationic dye molecules due to its highly negatively charged structure that can easily attract the species having positive charges. In literature, numerous carrageenan-based bioadsorbents were prepared in the form of composites or hybrid materials such as κ-carrageenan/poly(glycidyl methacrylate) composite (Lapwanit et al., 2018), cellulose/carrageenan/TiO2 composite (Jo et al., 2017), κ-carrageenan/poly(acrylic acid)/CdS hydrogel (Dargahi et al., 2019), κ-carrageenan/silver composite (Singh & Poluri, 2023), κ-carrageenan/graphene oxide composite gel beads (κ-Car/GO GBs) (Yang et al., 2017), carrageenan/reduced GO/Ag composite (Zheng et al., 2015), lambda carrageenan/hydroxyapatite composite (Agougui et al., 2017), chitosan/κ-carrageenan magnetic composite (Karimi et al., 2018), κ-carrageenan/silica hybrid magnetic shells (Soares et al., 2017), chitosan/kappa-carrageenan magnetic nanocomposite (Mahdavinia & Mosallanezhad, 2016), carrageenan/carbon nanotube composite (Hosseinzadeh, 2015), and κ-carrageenan-gpoly (acrylamide)/sepiolite hydrogel (Mahdavinia & Asgari, 2013). Few illustrative examples of carrageenan-based materials as super bioadsorbents are summarized in Table 6.6 and discussed concisely. For example, Doroudian and coworkers synthesized a novel aminosilica-functionalized and TiO_2-immobilized carrageenan hydrogel (κC-g-PAA/TiO_2–NH_2) that showed outstanding adsorption capacity of 833 mg/g for cationic MG dye, ascribed to its high specific surface area and active functionality (Pourjavadi et al., 2014). While Men and coworkers developed a series of eco-friendly bioadsorbents, κ-Car/GO gel beads from κ-carrageenan and graphene oxide (Yang et al., 2017). The adsorption capacity of the κ-Car/GO GBs for methylene blue dye was observed as 658.4 mg/g, and the dye removal efficiency was scarcely dropped at the end of five cycles, whereas Liang *et al.* fabricated chitosan/carrageenan/Fe_2O_3 magnetic composite for removal of both cationic and anionic dyes, and heavy metal ions from wastewater (Liang et al., 2017). The synthesized nanocomposite exhibited good adsorption capacities of 190 and 118 mg/g for toxic dyes such as Congo red and methylene blue, respectively. Additionally, the adsorption capacities toward metal ions like Cu(II) and Cr(III) were found to be 17.9 and 10.8 mg/g, respectively. Furthermore, Choudhury *et al.* developed a novel adsorbent of poly (N-vinylpyrrolidoneco-acrylic acid)/carrageenan biocomposite via mixing κ-carrageenan and poly (N-vinylpyrrolidone-co-acrylic acid) (Choudhury & Ray, 2018). The resulting carrageena-based bioadsorbents displayed good adsorption capacities of 362.5 and 398 mg/g for organic dyes like Safranine T (ST) and brilliant cresyl blue (BCB), respectively, while the binary mixture of each dye solution containing 100 mg/L at the adsorbent dose of 0.25 g/L. Recently, Abdellatif *et al.* synthesized a new bio-based i-carrageenan magnetic aerogels via crosslinking of iota-carrageenan and PAMAM (polyamidoamine hyperbranched polymer generation 1) (Abdellatif & Abdellatif, 2020). The synthesized aerogel owing active sites like –COOH, –OH (from acrylic acid) and sulfate group (of carrageenan) demonstrated a superb adsorption capacity toward hazardous metal ions due to the

TABLE 6.6
Carrageenan-based biomaterials as super adsorbents toward hazardous pollutants

Carrageenan-based adsorbents	Adsorbate (hazardous pollutants)		Adsorption capacity (mg/g)	References
K-carrageenan/poly (glycidyl methacrylate) composite	MB	Dyes	166.62	Lapwanit et al. (2018)
κ-carrageenan/ poly(N-vinylpyrrolidone-co-acrylic acid) composite	ST, BCB		362.5, 398	Choudhury and Ray (2018)
κ-Car/GO GBs	MB		658.4	Yang et al. (2017)
κ-carrageenan/silica magnetic shells	MB		350	Soares et al. (2017)
κC-g-PAA/TiO_2–NH_2	MG		833	Pourjavadi et al. (2014)
Chitosan/carrageenan/Fe_2O_3	CR, MB		190, 118	Liang et al. (2017)
Agar/κ-carrageenan hydrogel	MB		242.3	Duman et al. (2020)
Bio-based i-carrageenan aerogels	Cr(VI), Co(II), Mn(II), Cu(II), Cd(II)	Metalions	105, 144.9, 133, 158.7, 128	Abdellatif and Abdellatif (2020)
Chitosan/carrageenan/Fe_2O_3	Cu(II), Cr(III)		17.9, 10.8	Abdellatif and Abdellatif (2020)

abundant electrostatic interaction between adsorbent and metal ions. Moreover, the terminal amine functional groups due to the presence of polydopamine enhanced the adsorption capacity due to the formation of a coordination complex with metal ions. The carrageenan-based aerogel exhibited the adsorption capacity of 105 mg/g for Cr(VI), 144.9 mg/g for Co(II), 133 mg/g for Mn(II), 158.7 mg/g for Cu(II), and 128 mg/g for Cd(II). Duman *et al.* prepared agar/κ-carrageenan composite hydrogel via a free radical reaction using tri(ethylene glycol) divinyl ether as a crosslinker (Duman et al., 2020). The agar/κ-carrageenan hydrogel was explored to adsorb methylene blue dye from aqueous solution, and the adsorption capacity was obtained as 242.3 mg/g at 35°C and pH 7.

6.3.7 Other biopolymer-based adsorbents

Apart from them, other biopolymers like collagen, agar, and lignin are also developed as efficient adsorbents toward various hazardous pollutants, as summarized in Table 6.7. Collagen is a naturally occurring polymer matrix that consists of amino acids. The hyperbranched structure of collagen has many beneficial properties which lead to be good bioadsorbents in the areas of wastewater treatments. For example, Wang et al. synthesized carboxylated collagen fiber (CCF) via functionalization with collagen fiber with glyoxylic acid (Qiang et al., 2014). The resultant CCF demonstrated an effective bioadsorbent for elimination of Cr(III) ions from contaminated water. The adsorption capacity toward Cr(III) ions increased by 74.13% after modification, and the maximum adsorption capacity was obtaining as 106.88 mg/g, whereas Qiang et al. synthesized hyperbranched aminated collagen fibers by altering collagen fibers with ethylenediamine and cyanuric chloride as a crosslinking agent. The modified collagen-based fibers were recognized as effective bioadsorbents for the elimination of the acid black dye NT from wastewater (Qiang et al., 2012). For the stabilization of collagen, Thanikaivelan et al. incorporated IONPs to obtain collagen/IONP composites for oil-water separation. From the oil adsorption studies, the maximum adsorption capacity of

TABLE 6.7
Other biopolymer-based biomaterials as super adsorbents toward hazardous pollutants

Other biopolymer-based adsorbents	Adsorbate (hazardous pollutants)		Adsorption capacity (mg/g)	Refs
Carboxylated collagen fiber	Cr(III)	Inorganic	106.88	Qiang et al. (2014)
Fe_3O_4@Agarose	U(VI), Eu(III)		1.15, 1.27 (mmol/g)	Li et al. (2011)
Lignin-based hybrid magnetic nanoparticles	Pb^{2+}, Cu^{2+}		150.33, 70.69	Zhang et al. (2019)
ECLNPs	Pb(II), Cu(II)		126, 54.4	Xie et al. (2021)
Agar@Fe/Pd	MB, RB	Organic	875, 780	Patra et al. (2016)
agarose/rGO	RB, aspirin		321.7, 196.4	Cheng et al. (2018)
Agar/graphene oxide aerogel	MB		578	L. Chen et al. (2017)
Collagen/iron oxide nanoparticles	Motor oil		2 g/g	Thanikaivelan et al. (2012)

collagen-based bioadsorbent for motor oil was found to be 2 g/g. Additionally, the magnetic property of IONPs provided the advantage of easy separation of the adsorbent from the aqueous medium (Thanikaivelan et al., 2012), whereas agar is a hydrophilic polysaccharide composed of neutral agarose and fraction agaropectin (a composition similar to starch) and extracted from certain red algae. It is one of the eldest dynamic phycocolloid which is soluble in hot water and primarily employed for the preparation of solid microbiological culture media. Various agar/agarose-based bioadsorbents were developed for water treatment applications. For example, Li and coworkers developed magnetic agarose-based microspheres (Fe_3O_4@Agarose) for the removal of radionuclides from aqueous medium (Li et al., 2011). The synthesized Fe_3O_4@Agarose composite exhibited high adsorption capacities of 1.15 and 1.27 mmol/g for U(VI) and Eu(III) radionuclides and could be easily separated from aqueous medium by using external magnetic forces. Patra et al. prepared hybrid agar-based bioadsorbents via altering monometallic or bimetallic nanoparticles (like Fe, Cu, Pd, Fe/Pd, and Fe/Cu) for adsorbing toxic cationic dyes such as methylene blue (MB) and rhodamine B (RB) (Patra et al., 2016). The synthesized agar@Fe/Pd nanoparticle aerogel showed the maximum adsorption capacity of 875 mg/g for MB and 780 mg/g for RB dye. Interestingly, the recyclability studies demonstrated that the agar-based bioadsorbents could be recycled for more than 20 cycles with excellent removal efficiency upto 90%. Wang et al. synthesized a hybrid agarose/rGO hydrophobic hydrogel beads with microchannels for selective adsorption of organic compounds from water (Cheng et al., 2018). Importantly, the fabricated rGO-incorporated agarose hydrogels demonstrated a superb adsorption of water-soluble organic compounds, including dyes and pharmaceutical drugs, ascribed to the π–π interaction with the rGO. The agarose/rGO hydrogel beads displayed a remarkable adsorption capacity of 321.7 mg/g for RB dye and 196.4 mg/g for aspirin. While Chen et al. fabricated the agar/graphene oxide aerogel via a vacuum freeze-drying technique and evaluated its adsorption capacity toward methylene blue (MB) dye (L. Chen et al., 2017). The adsorption capacity of agar/graphene oxide aerogel for MB dye was determined by applying the Langmuir isotherm models and was found to be 578 mg/g. Lignin is also a natural biopolymers derived from black liquor and is considered as a cheap bioadsorbent compared to activated carbon for removal of toxic metal ions (Gupta et al., 2021). The key factor which responsible for the high adsorption capability of lignin is the presence of polyhydric phenols and other active functional groups in it. For example, Fatehi and coworkers fabricated lignin-based hybrid magnetic nanoparticles as bioadsorbents via a simple method by using epichlorohydrin as a crosslinker of carboxymethylated lignin and amino-functionalized magnetic nanoparticles for elimination of heavy metal ions (Zhang et al., 2019). The resulting hybrid nanoparticles showed good adsorption capacity of 150.33 69 mg/g for $Pb^{2+}$and 70.69 mg/g for Cu^{2+} ions. The adsorption equilibriums for these metal ions onto the lignin-based hybrid adsorbent were achieved within 30 s, and this equilibrium time indicated that it could be the promising lignin-based functional bioadsorbents for removal of Pb^{2+} and Cu^{2+} metal ions. Recently, Xie et al. synthesized modified eucalyptus lignin nanospheres (ECLNPs) and studied the adsorption behavior of lead and copper metal ions for wastewater treatments (Xie et al., 2021). The maximum adsorption capacities of ECLNPs for Pb(II) and Cu(II) ions were found to be 126 and 54.4 mg/g, respectively.

6.4 CONCLUSIONS AND FUTURE SCOPES

In conclusion, a wide range of natural biopolymers (of cellulose, chitosan, alginate, gelatin, starch, carrageenan, etc.) have been established (in the form of composites, blends, aerogels, hydrogels, foams, fibers, films, membranes, and so on) as super adsorbents for the cost-effective and efficient adsorption of various hazardous water pollutants. The major advantages of natural biopolymers over other porous adsorbent materials (such as activated carbon, zeolite, POPs, MOFs, etc.) are their diverse chemical structure owing active functional groups that permits to tune definite modifications that are essentially needed for designing biomaterials for desired water treatment-related applications. These biopolymers decorated with multiple functional groups like –OH of cellulose, -OH and $–NH_2$ of chitosan, -OH and –COOH of alginate, sulfate of carrageenan are the major ingredients that are responsible for the significant interaction between adsorbents and contaminants of metal ions or dye molecules. Moreover, biopolymers having anionic charges across the polymer backbone of alginate and carrageenan have been used as attractive bioadsorbents for the removal of toxic heavy metal ions and cationic dye molecules due to their highly negatively charged structures that can easily attract the species having positive charges. Fascinatingly, biopolymer-based magnetic composites could be a new class of efficient and reusable super adsorbent for wastewater treatment due to the beneficial advantages in particular, easily separation of applied adsorbents from the aqueous medium by using external magnetic force.

Nevertheless, natural biopolymers and their derivatives still have a lot of scope with enormous opportunities for exploring novel bioadsorbents toward industrial waste pollutants. Ultimately, future perspectives for the development of natural biopolymers as advanced adsorbents might be applied for the purification of industrial wastewater and move toward a new technological aspect. We are fully confident that this chapter will not only provide the library of biopolymer-based adsorbents in general, but it will also deliver valuable understanding on designing of efficient adsorbents and benefit budding researchers globally to further explore novel natural biopolymer-based super adsorbents for industrial wastewater treatments.

ACKNOWLEDGMENT

A.A. expresses gratitude to the DST INSPIRE Faculty Fellowship Program and the Bose Institute under the Department of Science and Technology of the Government of India for their financial support and research facilities. A.H. would like to thank IIT Patna for the research fellowship. N.D. acknowledges IIT Patna for providing research facilities.

REFERENCES

Abdellatif, F. H. H., & Abdellatif, M. M. (2020). Bio-based i-carrageenan aerogels as efficient adsorbents for heavy metal ions and acid dye from aqueous solution. *Cellulose*, *27*, 441–453.

Agougui, H., Jabli, M., & Majdoub, H. (2017). Synthesis, characterization of hydroxyapatite-lambda carrageenan, and evaluation of its performance for the adsorption of methylene blue from aqueous suspension. *Journal of Applied Polymer Science*, *134*(40), 45385.

Ali, I. (2010). The Quest for Active Carbon Adsorbent Substitutes: Inexpensive Adsorbents for Toxic Metal Ions Removal from Wastewater. *Separation & Purification Reviews*, *39*(3–4), 95–171. https://doi.org/10.1080/15422119.2010.527802

Ali, M. E. A. (2018). Synthesis and adsorption properties of chitosan-CDTA-GO nanocomposite for removal of hexavalent chromium from aqueous solutions. *Arabian Journal of Chemistry*, *11*(7), 1107–1116. https://doi.org/10.1016/j.arabjc.2016.09.010

Alipour, A., Zarinabadi, S., Azimi, A., & Mirzaei, M. (2020). Adsorptive removal of Pb (II) ions from aqueous solutions by thiourea-functionalized magnetic ZnO/nanocellulose composite: Optimization by response surface methodology (RSM). *International journal of biological macromolecules*, *151*, 124–135.

Alsawy, T., Rashad, E., El-Qelish, M., & Mohammed, R. H. (2022). A comprehensive review on the chemical regeneration of biochar adsorbent for sustainable wastewater treatment. *npj Clean Water*, *5*(1), 29. https://doi.org/10.1038/s41545-022-00172-3

Baby, R., Saifullah, B., & Hussein, M. Z. (2019). Carbon nanomaterials for the treatment of heavy metal-contaminated water and environmental remediation. *Nanoscale Research Letters*, *14*(1), 341. https://doi.org/10.1186/s11671-019-3167-8

Bo, S., Ren, W., Lei, C., Xie, Y., Cai, Y., Wang, S.,...Yao, J. (2018). Flexible and porous cellulose aerogels/zeolitic imidazolate framework (ZIF-8) hybrids for adsorption removal of Cr (IV) from water. *Journal of Solid State Chemistry*, *262*, 135–141.

Bolisetty, S., Peydayesh, M., & Mezzenga, R. (2019). Sustainable technologies for water purification from heavy metals: Review and analysis. *Chemical Society Reviews*, *48*(2), 463–487. https://doi.org/10.1039/C8CS00493E

Chai, W. S., Cheun, J. Y., Kumar, P. S., Mubashir, M., Majeed, Z., Banat, F.,...Show, P. L. (2021). A review on conventional and novel materials towards heavy metal adsorption in wastewater treatment application. *Journal of Cleaner Production*, *296*, 126589. https://doi.org/10.1016/j.jclepro.2021.126589

Chatterjee, S., Chatterjee, T., & Woo, S. H. (2011). Influence of the polyethyleneimine grafting on the adsorption capacity of chitosan beads for Reactive Black 5 from aqueous solutions. *Chemical Engineering Journal*, *166*(1), 168–175.

Che, B., Li, H., Zhou, D., Zhang, Y., Zeng, Z., Zhao, C.,...Lu, X. (2019). Porous polyaniline/carbon nanotube composite electrode for supercapacitors with outstanding rate capability and cyclic stability. *Composites Part B: Engineering*, *165*, 671–678. https://doi.org/10.1016/j.compositesb.2019.02.026

Chen, J. H., Lin, H., Luo, Z. H., He, Y. S., & Li, G. P. (2011). Cu (II)-imprinted porous film adsorbent Cu–PVA–SA has high uptake capacity for removal of Cu (II) ions from aqueous solution. *Desalination*, *277*(1–3), 265–273.

Chen, L., Li, Y., Du, Q., Wang, Z., Xia, Y., Yedinak, E.,...Ci, L. (2017). High performance agar/graphene oxide composite aerogel for methylene blue removal. *Carbohydrate Polymers*, *155*, 345–353.

Chen, W.-H., Hoang, A. T., Nižetić, S., Pandey, A., Cheng, C. K., Luque, R.,...Nguyen, X. P. (2022). Biomass-derived biochar: From production to application in removing heavy metal-contaminated water. *Process Safety and Environmental Protection*, *160*, 704–733. https://doi.org/10.1016/j.psep.2022.02.061

Chen, X., Zhang, W., Luo, X., Zhao, F., Li, Y., Li, R., & Li, Z. (2017). Efficient removal and environmentally benign detoxification of Cr (VI) in aqueous solutions by Zr (IV) cross-linking chitosan magnetic microspheres. *Chemosphere*, *185*, 991–1000.

Cheng, C., Cai, Y., Guan, G., Yeo, L., & Wang, D. (2018). Hydrophobic-force-driven removal of organic compounds from water by reduced graphene oxides generated in agarose hydrogels. *Angewandte Chemie International Edition*, *57*(35), 11177–11181.

Choudhury, S., & Ray, S. K. (2018). Efficient removal of cationic dye mixtures from water using a bio-composite adsorbent optimized with response surface methodology. *Carbohydrate Polymers*, *200*, 305–320.

Chowdhury, S., & Balasubramanian, R. (2014). Recent advances in the use of graphene-family nanoadsorbents for removal of toxic pollutants from wastewater. *Advances in Colloid and Interface Science*, *204*, 35–56. https://doi.org/10.1016/j.cis.2013.12.005

Crini, G. (2006). Non-conventional low-cost adsorbents for dye removal: A review. *Bioresource Technology*, *97*(9), 1061–1085. https://doi.org/10.1016/j.biortech.2005.05.001

Dąbrowski, A. (2001). Adsorption — from theory to practice. *Advances in Colloid and Interface Science*, *93*(1), 135–224. https://doi.org/10.1016/S0001-8686(00)00082-8

Dai, M., Liu, Y., Ju, B., & Tian, Y. (2019). Preparation of thermoresponsive alginate/starch ether composite hydrogel and its application to the removal of Cu (II) from aqueous solution. *Bioresource Technology*, *294*, 122192.

Dargahi, M., Ghasemzadeh, H., & Torkaman, A. (2019). CdS quantum dot nanocomposite hydrogels based on κ-carrageenan and poly (acrylic acid), photocatalytic activity and dye adsorption behavior. *Polymer Bulletin*, *76*, 5039–5058.

Das, A., Ringu, T., Ghosh, S., & Pramanik, N. (2023). A comprehensive review on recent advances in preparation, physicochemical characterization, and bioengineering applications of biopolymers. *Polymer Bulletin*, *80*(7), 7247–7312. https://doi.org/10.1007/s00289-022-04443-4

Dolgormaa, A., Lv, C.-j., Li, Y., Yang, J., Yang, J.-x., Chen, P.,…Huang, J. (2018). Adsorption of Cu(II) and Zn(II) Ions from Aqueous Solution by Gel/PVA-Modified Super-Paramagnetic Iron Oxide Nanoparticles. *Molecules*, *23*(11), 2982.

Duman, O., Polat, T. G., Diker, C. Ö., & Tunç, S. (2020). Agar/κ-carrageenan composite hydrogel adsorbent for the removal of Methylene Blue from water. *International journal of biological macromolecules*, *160*, 823–835.

Elwakeel, K. Z., Elgarahy, A. M., Khan, Z. A., Almughamisi, M. S., & Al-Bogami, A. S. (2020). Perspectives regarding metal/mineral-incorporating materials for water purification: With special focus on Cr(vi) remova. *Materials Advances*, *1*(6), 1546–1574. https://doi.org/10.1039/D0MA00153H

Faiz Norrrahim, M. N., Mohd Kasim, N. A., Knight, V. F., Mohamad Misenan, M. S., Janudin, N., Ahmad Shah, N. A.,…Zin Wan Yunus, W. M. (2021). Nanocellulose: A bioadsorbent for chemical contaminant remediation [10.1039/D0RA08005E]. *RSC Advances*, *11*(13), 7347–7368. https://doi.org/10.1039/D0RA08005E

Feng, Y., Wang, H., Xu, J., Du, X., Cheng, X., Du, Z., & Wang, H. (2021). Fabrication of MXene/PEI functionalized sodium alginate aerogel and its excellent adsorption behavior for Cr (VI) and Congo Red from aqueous solution. *Journal of Hazardous Materials*, *416*, 125777.

Fu, L., Li, J., Wang, G., Luan, Y., & Dai, W. (2021). Adsorption behavior of organic pollutants on microplastics. *Ecotoxicology and Environmental Safety*, *217*, 112207. https://doi.org/10.1016/j.ecoenv.2021.112207

Ghafoori, S., Omar, M., Koutahzadeh, N., Zendehboudi, S., Malhas, R. N., Mohamed, M.,…Mehrvar, M. (2022). New advancements, challenges, and future needs on treatment of oilfield produced water: A state-of-the-art review. *Separation and Purification Technology*, *289*, 120652. https://doi.org/10.1016/j.seppur.2022.120652

Gholinejad, M., Saadati, F., Shaybanizadeh, S., & Pullithadathil, B. (2016). Copper nanoparticles supported on starch micro particles as a degradable heterogeneous catalyst for three-component coupling synthesis of propargylamines [10.1039/C5RA22292C]. *RSC Advances*, *6*(6), 4983–4991. https://doi.org/10.1039/C5RA22292C

Gopi, S., Pius, A., Kargl, R., Kleinschek, K. S., & Thomas, S. (2019). Fabrication of cellulose acetate/chitosan blend films as efficient adsorbent for anionic water pollutants. *Polymer Bulletin*, *76*, 1557–1571.

Guo, D.-M., An, Q.-D., Xiao, Z.-Y., Zhai, S.-R., & Yang, D.-J. (2018). Efficient removal of Pb(II), Cr(VI) and organic dyes by polydopamine modified chitosan aerogels. *Carbohydrate Polymers*, *202*, 306–314. https://doi.org/10.1016/j.carbpol.2018.08.140

Guo, J., Wang, J., Zheng, G., & Jiang, X. (2019). A TiO 2/crosslinked carboxymethyl starch composite for high-efficiency adsorption and photodegradation of cationic golden yellow X-GL dye. *Environmental Science and Pollution Research*, *26*, 24395–24406.

Guo, L., Li, G., Liu, J., Meng, Y., & Tang, Y. (2013). Adsorptive decolorization of methylene blue by crosslinked porous starch. *Carbohydrate Polymers*, *93*(2), 374–379. https://doi.org/10.1016/j.carbpol.2012.12.019

Gupta, A., Sharma, V., Sharma, K., Kumar, V., Choudhary, S., Mankotia, P.,…Ekielski, A. (2021). A review of adsorbents for heavy metal decontamination: Growing approach to wastewater treatment. *Materials*, *14*(16), 4702.

Gupta, A., Sharma, V., Sharma, K., Kumar, V., Choudhary, S., Mankotia, P.,…Mishra, P. K. (2021). A review of adsorbents for heavy metal decontamination: Growing approach to wastewater treatment. *Materials*, *14*(16), 4702.

Gupta, V. K., Carrott, P. J. M., Ribeiro Carrott, M. M. L., & Suhas. (2009). Low-cost adsorbents: growing approach to wastewater treatment—a review. *Critical Reviews in Environmental Science and Technology*, *39*(10), 783–842. https://doi.org/10.1080/10643380801977610

Gür, T. M. (2022). Carbon dioxide emissions, capture, storage and utilization: Review of materials, processes and technologies. *Progress in Energy and Combustion Science*, *89*, 100965. https://doi.org/10.1016/j.pecs.2021.100965

Han, H., Rafiq, M. K., Zhou, T., Xu, R., Mašek, O., & Li, X. (2019). A critical review of clay-based composites with enhanced adsorption performance for metal and organic pollutants. *Journal of Hazardous Materials*, *369*, 780–796. https://doi.org/10.1016/j.jhazmat.2019.02.003

Han, Z.-y., Huang, L.-j., Qu, H.-j., Wang, Y.-x., Zhang, Z.-j., Rong, Q.-l.,…Tang, J.-g. (2021). A review of performance improvement strategies for graphene oxide-based and graphene-based membranes in water treatment. *Journal of Materials Science*, *56*, 9545–9574.

Haq, F., Yu, H., Wang, Y., Wang, L., Haroon, M., Khan, A.,…Lin, T. (2020). Synthesis of carboxymethyl starch grafted poly (methacrylic acids)(CMS-g-PMAAs) and their application as an adsorbent for the removal of ammonia and phenol. *Journal of Molecular Structure*, *1207*, 127752.

Haroun, A. A., Mashaly, H. M., & El-Sayed, N. H. (2013). Novel nanocomposites based on gelatin/HPET/chitosan with high performance acid red 150 dye adsorption. *Clean Technologies and Environmental Policy*, *15*, 367–374.

Hayeeye, F., Yu, Q. J., Sattar, M., Chinpa, W., & Sirichote, O. (2018). Adsorption of Pb2+ ions from aqueous solutions by gelatin/activated carbon composite bead form. *Adsorption Science & Technology*, *36*(1–2), 355–371.

Herman, P., Fábián, I., & Kalmár, J. (2020). Mesoporous silica–gelatin aerogels for the selective adsorption of aqueous Hg(II). *ACS Applied Nano Materials*, *3*(1), 195–206. https://doi.org/10.1021/acsanm.9b01903

Hojjati-Najafabadi, A., Mansoorianfar, M., Liang, T., Shahin, K., & Karimi-Maleh, H. (2022). A review on magnetic sensors for monitoring of hazardous pollutants in water resources. *Science of The Total Environment*, *824*, 153844. https://doi.org/10.1016/j.scitotenv.2022.153844

Hosseinzadeh, H. (2015). Synthesis of carrageenan/multi-walled carbon nanotube hybrid hydrogel nanocomposite for adsorption of crystal violet from aqueous solution. *Polish Journal of Chemical Technology*, *17*(2), 70–76.

Hosseinzadeh, H., & Ramin, S. (2018). Fabrication of starch-graft-poly (acrylamide)/graphene oxide/hydroxyapatite nanocomposite hydrogel adsorbent for removal of malachite green dye from aqueous solution. *International Journal of Biological Macromolecules*, *106*, 101–115.

Hu, T., Liu, Q., Liu, Q., Wu, Y., Qiao, C., & Yao, J. (2019). Toxic Cr removal from aqueous media using catechol-amine copolymer coating onto as-prepared cellulose. *Carbohydrate Polymers*, *209*, 291–298. https://doi.org/10.1016/j.carbpol.2019.01.046

Huang, L., Liu, R., Yang, J., Shuai, Q., Yuliarto, B., Kaneti, Y. V., & Yamauchi, Y. (2021). Nanoarchitectured porous organic polymers and their environmental applications for removal of toxic metal ions. *Chemical Engineering Journal*, *408*, 127991. https://doi.org/10.1016/j.cej.2020.127991

Ihsanullah, I., Bilal, M., & Jamal, A. (2022). Recent developments in the removal of dyes from water by starch-based adsorbents. *The Chemical Record*, *22*(7), e202100312.

Jiang, J., Zhang, Q., Zhan, X., & Chen, F. (2019). A multifunctional gelatin-based aerogel with superior pollutants adsorption, oil/water separation and photocatalytic properties. *Chemical Engineering Journal*, *358*, 1539–1551.

Jo, S., Oh, Y., Park, S., Kan, E., & Lee, S. H. (2017). Cellulose/carrageenan/TiO2 nanocomposite for adsorption and photodegradation of cationic dye. *Biotechnology and Bioprocess Engineering*, *22*(6), 734–738. https://doi.org/10.1007/s12257-017-0267-0

Karim, Z., Hakalahti, M., Tammelin, T., & Mathew, A. P. (2017). In situ TEMPO surface functionalization of nanocellulose membranes for enhanced adsorption of metal ions from aqueous medium. *RSC Advances*, *7*(9), 5232–5241. https://doi.org/10.1039/C6RA25707K

Karimi, M. H., Mahdavinia, G. R., Massoumi, B., Baghban, A., & Saraei, M. (2018). Ionically crosslinked magnetic chitosan/κ-carrageenan bioadsorbents for removal of anionic eriochrome black-T. *International Journal of Biological Macromolecules*, *113*, 361–375.

Kaur, K., & Jindal, R. (2019). Comparative study on the behaviour of Chitosan-Gelatin based Hydrogel and nanocomposite ion exchanger synthesized under microwave conditions towards photocatalytic removal of cationic dyes. *Carbohydrate Polymers*, *207*, 398–410. https://doi.org/10.1016/j.carbpol.2018.12.002

Khademian, E., Salehi, E., Sanaeepur, H., Galiano, F., & Figoli, A. (2020). A systematic review on carbohydrate biopolymers for adsorptive remediation of copper ions from aqueous environments-part A: Classification and modification strategies. *Science of The Total Environment*, *738*, 139829. https://doi.org/10.1016/j.scitotenv.2020.139829

Kunz Lazzari, L. d., Perondi, D., Zattera, A. J., & Campomanes Santana, R. M. (2021). Cellulose/biochar cryogels: A study of adsorption kinetics and isotherms. *Langmuir*, *37*(10), 3180–3188.

Kyzas, G. Z., Deliyanni, E. A., Matis, K. A., Lazaridis, N. K., Bikiaris, D. N., & Mitropoulos, A. C. (2018). Emerging nanocomposite biomaterials as biomedical adsorbents: An overview. *Composite Interfaces*, *25*(5–7), 415–454. https://doi.org/10.1080/09276440.2017.1361716

Lapwanit, S., Sooksimuang, T., & Trakulsujaritchok, T. (2018). Adsorptive removal of cationic methylene blue dye by kappa-carrageenan/poly(glycidyl methacrylate) hydrogel beads: Preparation and characterization. *Journal of Environmental Chemical Engineering*, *6*(5), 6221–6230. https://doi.org/10.1016/j.jece.2018.09.050

Li, B., Zhou, F., Huang, K., Wang, Y., Mei, S., Zhou, Y., & Jing, T. (2016). Highly efficient removal of lead and cadmium during wastewater irrigation using a polyethylenimine-grafted gelatin sponge. *Scientific Reports*, *6*(1), 33573. https://doi.org/10.1038/srep33573

Li, J., Guo, Z., Zhang, S., & Wang, X. (2011). Enrich and seal radionuclides in magnetic agarose microspheres. *Chemical Engineering Journal*, *172*(2–3), 892–897.

Li, Y., Gao, H., Wang, C., Zhang, X., & Zhou, H. (2018). One-step fabrication of chitosan-Fe (OH) 3 beads for efficient adsorption of anionic dyes. *International Journal of Biological Macromolecules*, *117*, 30–41.

Liang, X., Duan, J., Xu, Q., Wei, X., Lu, A., & Zhang, L. (2017). Ampholytic microspheres constructed from chitosan and carrageenan in alkali/urea aqueous solution for purification of various wastewater. *Chemical Engineering Journal*, *317*, 766–776.

Luo, X., Lei, X., Cai, N., Xie, X., Xue, Y., & Yu, F. (2016). Removal of heavy metal Ions from water by magnetic cellulose-based beads with embedded chemically modified magnetite nanoparticles and activated carbon. *ACS Sustainable Chemistry & Engineering*, *4*(7), 3960–3969. https://doi.org/10.1021/acssuschemeng.6b00790

Luo, X., Zeng, J., Liu, S., & Zhang, L. (2015). An effective and recyclable adsorbent for the removal of heavy metal ions from aqueous system: Magnetic chitosan/cellulose microspheres. *Bioresource Technology*, *194*, 403–406. https://doi.org/10.1016/j.biortech.2015.07.044

Ma, X., Li, Y., Cao, M., & Hu, C. (2014). A novel activating strategy to achieve highly porous carbon monoliths for CO 2 capture. *Journal of Materials Chemistry A*, *2*(13), 4819–4826.

Mahdavinia, G. R., & Asgari, A. (2013). Synthesis of kappa-carrageenan-g-poly (acrylamide)/sepiolite nanocomposite hydrogels and adsorption of cationic dye. *Polymer Bulletin*, *70*, 2451–2470.

Mahdavinia, G. R., & Mosallanezhad, A. (2016). Facile and green rout to prepare magnetic and chitosan-crosslinked κ-carrageenan bionanocomposites for removal of methylene blue. *Journal of Water Process Engineering*, *10*, 143–155.

Marrakchi, F., Khanday, W., Asif, M., & Hameed, B. (2016). Cross-linked chitosan/sepiolite composite for the adsorption of methylene blue and reactive orange 16. *International Journal of Biological Macromolecules*, *93*, 1231–1239.

Meng, J., Lin, X., Li, H., Zhang, Y., Zhou, J., Chen, Y.,...Luo, X. (2019). Adsorption capacity of kelp-like electrospun nanofibers immobilized with bayberry tannin for uranium(vi) extraction from seawater [10.1039/C8RA09297D]. *RSC Advances*, *9*(14), 8091–8103. https://doi.org/10.1039/C8RA09297D

Nagpal, M., & Kakkar, R. (2020a). Adsorptive Degradation of Phosmet Using Hierarchically Porous Calcium Oxide : An Experimental and Theoretical Study. *ChemistrySelect*, *5*(3), 1235–1246. https://doi.org/10.1002/slct.201904740

Nagpal, M., & Kakkar, R. (2020b). Facile synthesis of mesoporous magnesium oxide–graphene oxide composite for efficient and highly selective adsorption of hazardous anionic dyes. *Research on Chemical Intermediates*, *46*(5), 2497–2521.

Nasrollahzadeh, M., Sajjadi, M., Iravani, S., & Varma, R. S. (2021). Starch, cellulose, pectin, gum, alginate, chitin and chitosan derived (nano) materials for sustainable water treatment: A review. *Carbohydrate Polymers*, *251*, 116986.

Olivito, F., Algieri, V., Jiritano, A., Tallarida, M. A., Tursi, A., Costanzo, P.,...De Nino, A. (2021). Cellulose citrate: A convenient and reusable bio-adsorbent for effective removal of methylene blue dye from artificially contaminated water [10.1039/D1RA05464C]. *RSC Advances*, *11*(54), 34309–34318. https://doi.org/10.1039/D1RA05464C

Patra, S., Roy, E., Madhuri, R., & Sharma, P. K. (2016). Agar based bimetallic nanoparticles as high-performance renewable adsorbent for removal and degradation of cationic organic dyes. *Journal of Industrial and Engineering Chemistry*, *33*, 226–238.

Phoon, B. L., Ong, C. C., Mohamed Saheed, M. S., Show, P.-L., Chang, J.-S., Ling, T. C.,...Juan, J. C. (2020). Conventional and emerging technologies for removal of antibiotics from wastewater. *Journal of Hazardous Materials*, *400*, 122961. https://doi.org/10.1016/j.jhazmat.2020.122961

Pourjavadi, A., Abedin-Moghanaki, A., & Tavakoli, A. (2016). Efficient removal of cationic dyes using a new magnetic nanocomposite based on starch-g-poly(vinylalcohol) and functionalized with sulfate groups [10.1039/C6RA02517J]. *RSC Advances*, *6*(44), 38042–38051. https://doi.org/10.1039/C6RA02517J

Pourjavadi, A., Doulabi, M., & Doroudian, M. (2014). Adsorption characteristics of malachite green dye onto novel kappa-carrageenan-g-polyacrylic acid/TiO 2–NH 2 hydrogel nanocomposite. *Journal of the Iranian Chemical Society*, *11*, 1057–1065.

Qiang, T., Bu, Q., Ren, L., & Wang, X. (2014). Adsorption behaviors of Cr (III) on carboxylated collagen fiber. *Journal of Applied Polymer Science*, *131*(11), 40285.

Qiang, T., Luo, M., Bu, Q., & Wang, X. (2012). Adsorption of an acid dye on hyperbranched aminated collagen fibers. *Chemical Engineering Journal*, *197*, 343–349.

Qiu, B., Shao, Q., Shi, J., Yang, C., & Chu, H. (2022). Application of biochar for the adsorption of organic pollutants from wastewater: Modification strategies, mechanisms and challenges. *Separation and Purification Technology*, *300*, 121925. https://doi.org/10.1016/j.seppur.2022.121925

Rajeswari, A., Amalraj, A., & Pius, A. (2016). Adsorption studies for the removal of nitrate using chitosan/PEG and chitosan/PVA polymer composites. *Journal of Water Process Engineering*, *9*, 123–134. https://doi.org/10.1016/j.jwpe.2015.12.002

Rajeswari, M., Seenivasagan, R., Prabhakaran, P., Rajakumar, S., & Ayyasamy, P. M. (2016). Lab scale process on the removal of nitrate in ground water enriched with denitrifying bacterium and starch as a sole carbon source. *Journal of Water Process Engineering*, *13*, 189–195. https://doi.org/10.1016/j.jwpe.2016.09.003

Robinson, T., McMullan, G., Marchant, R., & Nigam, P. (2001). Remediation of dyes in textile effluent: a critical review on current treatment technologies with a proposed alternative. *Bioresource Technology*, *77*(3), 247–255. https://doi.org/10.1016/S0960-8524(00)00080-8

Russo, T., Fucile, P., Giacometti, R., & Sannino, F. (2021). Sustainable removal of contaminants by biopolymers: A novel approach for wastewater treatment: Current state and future perspectives. *Processes*, *9*(4), 719.

Saber-Samandari, S., Saber-Samandari, S., Joneidi-Yekta, H., & Mohseni, M. (2017). Adsorption of anionic and cationic dyes from aqueous solution using gelatin-based magnetic nanocomposite beads comprising carboxylic acid functionalized carbon nanotube. *Chemical Engineering Journal*, *308*, 1133–1144.

Sabzi, M., Shafagh, N., & Mohammadi, M. (2019). Assembly of gelatin biopolymer to fibrous sepiolite clay for efficient dye removal from wastewater. *Journal of Applied Polymer Science*, *136*(48), 48266.

Sahoo, T. R., & Prelot, B. (2020). Chapter 7- Adsorption processes for the removal of contaminants from wastewater: the perspective role of nanomaterials and nanotechnology. In B. Bonelli, F. S. Freyria, I. Rossetti, & R. Sethi (Eds.), *Nanomaterials for the Detection and Removal of Wastewater Pollutants* (pp. 161–222). Elsevier. https://doi.org/10.1016/B978-0-12-818489-9.00007-4

Samiey, B., Cheng, C.-H., & Wu, J. (2014). Organic-inorganic hybrid polymers as adsorbents for removal of heavy metal ions from solutions: A review. *Materials*, *7*(2), 673–726.

Saravanan, A., Senthil Kumar, P., Jeevanantham, S., Karishma, S., Tajsabreen, B., Yaashikaa, P. R., & Reshma, B. (2021). Effective water/wastewater treatment methodologies for toxic pollutants removal: Processes and applications towards sustainable development. *Chemosphere*, *280*, 130595. https://doi.org/10.1016/j.chemosphere.2021.130595

Septevani, A. A., Rifathin, A., Sari, A. A., Sampora, Y., Ariani, G. N., Sudiyarmanto, & Sondari, D. (2020). Oil palm empty fruit bunch-based nanocellulose as a super-adsorbent for water remediation. *Carbohydrate Polymers*, *229*, 115433. https://doi.org/10.1016/j.carbpol.2019.115433

Shahnaz, T., Sharma, V., Subbiah, S., & Narayanasamy, S. (2020). Multivariate optimisation of Cr (VI), Co (III) and Cu (II) adsorption onto nanobentonite incorporated nanocellulose/chitosan aerogel using response surface methodology. *Journal of Water Process Engineering*, *36*, 101283. https://doi.org/10.1016/j.jwpe.2020.101283

Shao, Z.-j., Huang, X.-l., Yang, F., Zhao, W.-f., Zhou, X.-z., & Zhao, C.-s. (2018). Engineering sodium alginate-based cross-linked beads with high removal ability of toxic metal ions and cationic dyes. *Carbohydrate polymers*, *187*, 85–93.

Singh, K. R., & Poluri, K. M. (2023). Facile synthesis and physicochemical characterization of κ-Carrageenan-silver-bentonite based nanocatalytic platform for efficient degradation of anionic azo dyes. *Environmental Research*, *231*, 116145. https://doi.org/10.1016/j.envres.2023.116145

Singh, P. N., Tiwary, D., & Sinha, I. (2014). Improved removal of Cr(VI) by starch functionalized iron oxide nanoparticles. *Journal of Environmental Chemical Engineering*, *2*(4), 2252–2258. https://doi.org/10.1016/j.jece.2014.10.003

Soares, S. F., Simoes, T. R., Trindade, T., & Daniel-da-Silva, A. L. (2017). Highly efficient removal of dye from water using magnetic carrageenan/silica hybrid nano-adsorbents. *Water, Air, & Soil Pollution*, *228*, 1–11.

Suhas, Gupta, V. K., Carrott, P. J. M., Singh, R., Chaudhary, M., & Kushwaha, S. (2016). Cellulose: A review as natural, modified and activated carbon adsorbent. *Bioresource Technology*, *216*, 1066–1076. https://doi.org/10.1016/j.biortech.2016.05.106

Sun, X., Yang, L., Li, Q., Zhao, J., Li, X., Wang, X., & Liu, H. (2014). Amino-functionalized magnetic cellulose nanocomposite as adsorbent for removal of Cr(VI): Synthesis and adsorption studies. *Chemical Engineering Journal*, *241*, 175–183. https://doi.org/10.1016/j.cej.2013.12.051

Thanikaivelan, P., Narayanan, N. T., Pradhan, B. K., & Ajayan, P. M. (2012). Collagen based magnetic nanocomposites for oil removal applications. *Scientific reports*, *2*(1), 230.

Udayakumar, G. P., Muthusamy, S., Selvaganesh, B., Sivarajasekar, N., Rambabu, K., Sivamani, S.,… Hosseini-Bandegharaei, A. (2021). Ecofriendly biopolymers and composites: Preparation and their applications in water-treatment. *Biotechnology advances*, *52*, 107815.

Wang, C., & Okubayashi, S. (2019). Polyethyleneimine-crosslinked cellulose aerogel for combustion CO2 capture. *Carbohydrate Polymers*, *225*, 115248.

Wang, J., Dai, L., Cheng, J., Deng, L.-H., & He, J. (2016). Characterization of adsorbent microspheres of cellulose and acrylic acid and its adsorption behaviors for metal ions. *Desalination and Water Treatment*, *57*(13), 5821–5827. https://doi.org/10.1080/19443994.2015.1004593

Wang, X., Huang, K., Chen, Y., Liu, J., Chen, S., Cao, J.,…Jing, T. (2018). Preparation of dumbbell manganese dioxide/gelatin composites and their application in the removal of lead and cadmium ions. *Journal of Hazardous Materials*, *350*, 46–54.

Wang, Y.-y., Yao, W.-b., Wang, Q.-w., Yang, Z.-h., Liang, L.-f., & Chai, L.-y. (2016). Synthesis of phosphate-embedded calcium alginate beads for Pb (II) and Cd (II) sorption and immobilization in aqueous solutions. *Transactions of Nonferrous Metals Society of China*, *26*(8), 2230–2237.

Wang, Y., Feng, Y., Zhang, X.-F., Zhang, X., Jiang, J., & Yao, J. (2018). Alginate-based attapulgite foams as efficient and recyclable adsorbents for the removal of heavy metals. *Journal of Colloid and Interface Science*, *514*, 190–198.

Wang, Y., Wang, H., Peng, H., Wang, Z., Wu, J., & Liu, Z. (2018). Dye adsorption from aqueous solution by cellulose/chitosan composite: Equilibrium, kinetics, and thermodynamics. *Fibers and Polymers*, *19*(2), 340–349. https://doi.org/10.1007/s12221-018-7520-9

Wittmar, A. S. M., Baumert, D., & Ulbricht, M. (2021). Cotton as precursor for the preparation of porous cellulose adsorbers. *Macromolecular Materials and Engineering*, *306*(5), 2000778. https://doi.org/10.1002/mame.202000778

Xie, B., Hou, Y., & Li, Y. (2021). Modified lignin nanosphere adsorbent for lead and copper ions. *BioResources*, *16*(1), 249.

Yaashikaa, P. R., Senthil Kumar, P., & Karishma, S. (2022). Review on biopolymers and composites – Evolving material as adsorbents in removal of environmental pollutants. *Environmental Research*, *212*, 113114. https://doi.org/10.1016/j.envres.2022.113114

Yan, Y., An, Q., Xiao, Z., Zheng, W., & Zhai, S. (2017). Flexible core-shell/bead-like alginate@ PEI with exceptional adsorption capacity, recycling performance toward batch and column sorption of Cr (VI). *Chemical Engineering Journal*, *313*, 475–486.

Yang, M., Liu, X., Qi, Y., Sun, W., & Men, Y. (2017). Preparation of κ-carrageenan/graphene oxide gel beads and their efficient adsorption for methylene blue. *Journal of Colloid and Interface Science*, *506*, 669–677. https://doi.org/10.1016/j.jcis.2017.07.093

Yu, S., Pang, H., Huang, S., Tang, H., Wang, S., Qiu, M.,…Wang, X. (2021). Recent advances in metal-organic framework membranes for water treatment: A review. *Science of The Total Environment*, *800*, 149662. https://doi.org/10.1016/j.scitotenv.2021.149662

Yu, X., Kang, D., Hu, Y., Tong, S., Ge, M., Cao, C., & Song, W. (2014). One-pot synthesis of porous magnetic cellulose beads for the removal of metal ions [10.1039/C4RA05601A]. *RSC Advances*, *4*(59), 31362–31369. https://doi.org/10.1039/C4RA05601A

Zamora-Ledezma, C., Negrete-Bolagay, D., Figueroa, F., Zamora-Ledezma, E., Ni, M., Alexis, F., & Guerrero, V. H. (2021). Heavy metal water pollution: A fresh look about hazards, novel and conventional remediation methods. *Environmental technology & innovation*, *22*, 101504. https://doi.org/10.1016/j.eti.2021.101504

Zhang, Y., Ni, S., Wang, X., Zhang, W., Lagerquist, L., Qin, M.,…Fatehi, P. (2019). Ultrafast adsorption of heavy metal ions onto functionalized lignin-based hybrid magnetic nanoparticles. *Chemical Engineering Journal*, *372*, 82–91.

Zheng, Y., Yang, J., Yang, R., Wang, A., Deng, B., Peng, F., …Fu, L. (2015). Novel carrageenan/reduced graphene oxide/ag composite as adsorbent for removal methylene blue from aqueous solution. *Digest Journal of Nanomaterials & Biostructures (DJNB)*, *10*(2), 349.

Zhou, Y.-F., & Haynes, R. J. (2010). Sorption of heavy metals by inorganic and organic components of solid wastes: Significance to use of wastes as low-cost adsorbents and immobilizing agents. *Critical Reviews in Environmental Science and Technology*, *40*(11), 909–977. https://doi.org/10.1080/10643380802586857

Zhou, Y., Zhang, M., Hu, X., Wang, X., Niu, J., & Ma, T. (2013). Adsorption of cationic dyes on a cellulose-based multicarboxyl adsorbent. *Journal of Chemical & Engineering Data*, *58*(2), 413–421. https://doi.org/10.1021/je301140c

Zhu, H. Y., Fu, Y. Q., Jiang, R., Jiang, J. H., Xiao, L., Zeng, G. M.,…Wang, Y. (2011). Adsorption removal of congo red onto magnetic cellulose/Fe3O4/activated carbon composite: Equilibrium, kinetic and thermodynamic studies. *Chemical Engineering Journal*, *173*(2), 494–502. https://doi.org/10.1016/j.cej.2011.08.020

7 Separation processes in valorization of biomass for circular bioeconomy

Anju Tomy, Sree Priya S, and Rakesh K Yasarla

7.1 INTRODUCTION

The concept of circular bioeconomy is based on renewable, biological materials and aims at enhancing the core value of economy by utilizing the resources completely in a loop, maximizing the secondary biomass utilization and resources or new materials produced without depleting the existing natural resources. A sustainable, low-carbon bioeconomy with maximum product recovery from biological resources is one of the key principles of a circular bioeconomy. Although in a circular bioeconomy, virgin resources are fed with the waste streams in the production cycle, the circular flow is infinite and mimics the natural circle of life. Biomass from agriculture, forest, and industrial wastes is the major raw material. The majority of biomass is processed into feed and food products, and smaller portions are converted to bioproducts and biofuels like bioethanol and bioplastics. Biobased products and energy are expected to grow stronger compared to food and feed for the circular bioeconomy. In chemical processing industries, bio-based chemicals often provide a vital precursor that takes a crucial role in circular bioeconomy.

It is anticipated that biomass will be crucial to achieving the global climate goals outlined in the Paris Agreement. The European Union and almost 50 countries across the globe have agreed upon sustainability and have proposed the idea of bioeconomy. Creating value added item including food, feed, biobased products, and bioenergy through the generation of renewable bioresources and the conversion of the resources and waste streams is known as bioeconomy (European Commission 2012). The United Nations in 2015 have adopted sustainable developmental goals (SDGs) as a step toward no poverty, to conserve planet and to make all people globally free from hunger and to enjoy peace and prosperity. 17 SDGs are integrated in order to achieve the goal and recognize that an action for the outcome toward the development of the balance in social, economic, and environmental sustainability, and goal 12 is one of the utmost importance in the context of circular bioeconomy, and the goal focuses on responsible consumption and production. With an aim to reduce the ecological footprint while we produce and consume products. The SDG goal also sheds light on support to developing countries to strengthen the scientific and technological capability to move toward more sustainable pattern of production and consumption.

7.2 SUSTAINABLE BIOMASS RESOURCES

Biorefinery is the concept of converting the renewable biomass mostly non-edible also referred to as lignocellulosic biomass by various bioprocessing unit operations, which involves multiple steps starting from biomass selection, pretreatment, detoxification, enzymatic hydrolysis, separation, and purification of fermentable sugars, which can be further converted into various bioproducts including biofuels and bioproducts (Biochemicals) [1–5]. Biomass is considered as a renewable resource, and it offers multifaceted benefits of carbon sequestration and helps in bioenergy generation. With

DOI: 10.1201/9781003500483-7

This chapter has been made available under a (CC-BY-NC-ND) 4.0 license

the ever-rising demand for energy, the climatic change driven by fossil fuels and greenhouse gas emissions, biomass holds a potential role in meeting current and future needs of mankind. Cherubini et all introduced the biorefinery concept as a way to optimize biomass consumption while reducing waste and emissions related to the production bioenergy and sustainable products. To ensure sustainability and to reduce environmental impacts, urban waste, agro-industrial or agricultural waste, can be used as a feedstock for renewable bioenergy production [6–8].

A zero-waste biorefinery and zero-waste discharge in industrial applications to reuse, recycle, and produce a range of products from the waste streams also shows a potential development in industries like paper and pulp, food processing, dairy, and textile. Waste is an essential component of biorefineries in the circular economy, where opportunities for reuse and recycling and reproduction should be pragmatic. Biorefineries with zero discharge have grown to be a desirable substitute for producing sustainable biofuels, energy, and additional biobased goods like biopolymers and biochemical.

Pretreatment process is primarily applied to solubilize the pentose and hexose sugars in the lignocellulosic substrate by treating at high temperatures, usually performed by water, mild mineral acids, and alkaline solutions [9–13]. The degradation of biomass depends on the severity of the pretreatment and reaction conditions. The hydrolyzate solutions produced during the pretreatment process contain particulates, colloidal substances, dissolved and undissolved polymers of lignin, and monomeric oligomeric forms of carbohydrates [13–15]. Most of the components degraded from the cellulosic material are potent fermentation inhibitors, and undissolved colloidal particulates can interfere with the enzyme activity and foul the membrane used for purification process [10,16,15].

The degradation of the polymers present in the biomass results in the formation of various components when pretreated in low pH and high temperature conditions [17–29]. The primary inhibitors generated in the process of pretreatment are from the acetyl groups in hemicellulose, which form acetic acid. Furans are formed from the degradation of the monosaccharides, formic acid, and levulinic acid are formed due to the degradation of furan, and phenolic compounds are formed as a result of lignin degradation [30–40].

The paper and pulp industry is one specific industry distinguished by a high degree of capital intensity, demanding high natural resources and generates huge amount wastewater with components like lignin and cellulose and paper and pulp rejects with high moisture content, which takes longer time to dry. The rejects and the waste stream from the industry release foul odor and contaminate ground water. The Paper and pulp industry is a potential bioresources industry in circular economy by utilizing the waste streams by co-producing lignin and its derivatives, recycle water stream with advanced technologies, and converting the rejects from paper and pulp into bioproducts like cellulosic sugars, which can further be treated to biochemicals and bioenergy [33,35].

Based on the technological level, pulp and paper grades and wood quality different quantities of energy-rich biomass are generated from pulp and paper mills. Paper mill fines rejects, pulp rejects (ash), and fiber rejects are the three main waste streams from the paper industry. Cellulose is observed to be found in higher quantities from paper rejects and is seen as an important source of sugars that can be fermented for bioplastics, biofuels, and other bioproducts [41]. An economically viable process that can convert paper rejects into fermentable sugars and also bring profits to the paper mills by valorization of waste products and also reduces the adverse environmental impacts caused by them [42].

Paper and pulp industry is one of the largest industries utilizing the wood as the raw material for the production of the paper, lignin, and also production of wood-based chemicals including nano-cellulose, cellulose fibers, and electricity by using the by productions. Paper industry is considered one of the recycled process industries for recycling of the paper, wastewater, and wood components. In the concept of integrated paper and biofuel industry, wood can also be utilized for the production of the second-generation biofuels along with the production of the paper. In recycled paper industry especially old cardboard containers, produce huge quantity of fiber fragments, which segregated through waste streams. The fines are composed of the cellulose and hemicellulose short chains of the hexose and pentose and take long time to degrade in the environment.

Several experimental results and published literatures tend to agree with the above pattern of the findings [42]. On the other hand, the price of enzymes being high, slow rate of enzyme reaction, and an efficient reactor system to accommodate various complex catalysis are lacking; this has generally discouraged the commercial implementation of enzymatic cellulose hydrolysis [43]. In bench-scale batch reactions, the optimum reaction time, quality of substrate, structure, product yield, or conversion of substrate is observed to be satisfactory, which could be further studied for scale-up. Cost-effective technology can be developed by improving the cellulase machinery as well as by rendering the cellulosic substrates more susceptible to hydrolysis. A better knowledge of enzyme-substrate interactions and the hydrolysis process is pivotal in achieving a cost-efficient process [42].

With the constant increase of carbon emissions and greenhouse gases, it becomes increasingly important to reduce humanity's carbon footprint. Decades of fossil fuel use and environmentally unfriendly waste management practices have caused irreversible damage to our planet's atmosphere. Leading climate scientists predict that even if we cease all carbon emissions immediately, there would still be permanent changes to earth's climate, including sea level rise, extreme temperatures, and melting of glacial areas such as the West Antarctica Glacier [44]. Fortunately, biomasses provide a convenient way to provide both of these materials, as it is easily obtainable and can be made and recycled from waste products [45]. It can be directly utilized for production of various alternative transportation fuels, ethanol (C_6H_5OH) in particular. Previously, the primary source for bioplastics and biofuels has been edible sources such as starch, sugar, and oil [46]. However, conversion of waste biomasses such as waste paper fines from paper mills into usable sugars is becoming a more environmentally friendly and cost-effective way to produce transportation fuels and biodegradable materials. A cost-effective and environmentally friendly way to achieve this is by an enzymatic hydrolysis process for cellulosic waste. The abundancy and disposal methods of waste paper fines make it an even more obvious choice for biofuel and bioplastic sources.

The key to the production of biofuels and bioplastics from cellulose-based materials is the production of useful sugars. The sugars are then fermented to be used as biofuel and other useful products. There are many ways to accomplish this, including many biological or chemical routes to convert the cellulose into sugar. These processes range in economic friendliness and cost effectiveness, making some processes more effective than others. One process that is relatively cheap and environmentally friendly is enzymatic hydrolysis, where enzymes are used to hydrolyze cellulose. Usually, the cellulosic material needs to be pretreated to remove inhibiting materials such as lignin and hemicellulose, which cannot be converted into sugars. However, one of the advantages of using waste pulp from paper mills as a biomass source is its relatively low lignin content. This practically eliminates the need for pretreatment steps, providing an environmental and economic benefit [46]. There are two broad categories for the conversion technologies: hydrolysis and thermochemical conversion [47]. In thermochemical treatments, the biomass is exposed to gas to produce syngas, a mixture of carbon monoxide (CO), hydrogen (H_2), carbon dioxide (CO_2), methane (CH_4), and nitrogen (N_2). Ethanol (C_6H_5OH) is generated by fermentation or catalytic conversion of syngas. Biomass contains polysaccharides, which are complex carbohydrate polymers consisting of more than two monosaccharides linked together covalently by glycosidic linkages and are broken down into their monosaccharide components during hydrolysis. There are several forms of hydrolysis, including acid hydrolysis, base hydrolysis, and enzymatic hydrolysis. In enzymatic hydrolysis, the enzyme cellulase is used to break down the cellulose in the cell wall into monosaccharides. This can be achieved by breaking the molecular bonds of the cellulose [48]. Cellulase can be produced by both bacteria and fungi. Factors that affect the enzymatic hydrolysis of cellulose include substrates, cellulase activity, and reaction conditions (such as consistency, surfactant dosage, reaction time, enzyme dosage, reaction temperature, and pH) [49]. Paper mills generate rejects that can be enzymatically hydrolyzed for releasing sugar, which can be used for the production of biofuels and bioplastics or into platform chemicals such as succinic acid, lactic acid, levulinic acid, and furfurals. Min et al. have established the enzymatic hydrolysis of fines from old corrugated paper mill, consisting of 40% carbohydrates (34% cellulose and 6% hemi-cellulose) and 60% ash content to produce fermentable sugars using commercial cellulases. Main inhibitors of enzymatic hydrolysis fines are fillers, such as $CaCO_3$ and Kaolin, which reduce the activity of enzyme by increasing the pH and by enzyme adsorption.

With a dry weight of roughly 15 to 40%, the most prevalent aromatic biopolymer in nature is lignin and is found in terrestrial plants. The lignin market was projected to be worth over 700 million USD in 2021 and is anticipated to expand at a compound annual growth rate (CAGR) of 6% in the years to come. Among 50 million tons of lignin was estimated to be produced annually worldwide as a waste product of paper and pulp industry. Currently, it is used as a fuel for cogeneration power production and releases huge amount of carbon gases and ashes. Only small percentage of lignin is converted to commercial utilization. Due to different feedstock and industrial lignin extraction processes, the characteristics of the lignin change in chemical structure, molecular weight, and thermal properties. In search of novel materials for circular and sustainable bioeconomy lignin represents as a potential feedstock for value-added production. In this regard, the paper and pulp industry provides lignin as a by-product; therefore, studies in this arena are highly promising and paves a way for innovative applications. Recently, different lignin valorization methods like production of carbon fibers, plastics, and biopolymers were investigated.

Bioprocessing is an essential part of many food, pharmaceutical, and chemical industries. Biomass bioprocessing is an advanced alternative method to produce various eco-friendly and alternative to petroleum products and fossil fuels. Bioprocessing of biomass involves multiple steps starting from biomass selection, its pretreatment, separation of inhibitors, enzymatic hydrolysis, separation and purification of products to retrieval of final product in the pure form [50–53]. To achieve the final product in the purest form, a lot of scientific methodologies, quantitative and qualitative analysis are required throughout the entire processing steps [5,6,10,11,54,55]. The first step is to choose a perfect biomass that has all the qualities required to produce the end product [9,50,56]. Biomass can be agricultural leftovers or residues, industrial wastes or forest wood resources; this selection has to be done keeping in mind about the components in them required to produce the end product [16,57,58]. The next step is the pretreatment process where the biomass is pretreated either with water, acid, or alkali. Pretreatment is expected to release sugars in monomeric or oligomeric form thereby improving the accessibility of enzymes to these oligomers present in the polymeric form in the lignocelluloses [10,54,59]. However, numerous other chemicals are also released as a result of pretreatment of biomass; most of the chemicals released tend to be inhibitory to the bioprocessing or fermentation step. These inhibitory compounds are formed from the three primary biopolymers that make up the lignocellulosic biomass [12,14,60–62].

7.3 SEPARATION PROCESSES FOR BIOPROCESSING

Bioprocessing of biomass involves multiple steps starting from biomass selection, like agricultural and industrial biomass corn, corn fiber, wheat straw, rice straw; paper and pulp industry waste, sugar cane bagasse and sugar cane trash are widely used for the production of the fermentable sugars for by pretreatment and enzymatic hydrolysis process. To achieve the final product in the purest form, many scientific methodologies, quantitative and qualitative analysis are required throughout the entire processing steps [61,63–65]. Detoxification is essential when fermentation of strongly inhibiting hydrolysates is performed, recirculation of streams results in high concentrations of inhibitors in the fermentation unit, or when an organism with low inhibitory tolerance is used for fermentation [65–72]. An ideal detoxification method should be able to remove inhibitors selectively, should be economic, and easy to integrate into the process [73–86]. The main approaches for mitigating the deleterious influence of inhibitors are inhibitor removal prior to enzyme hydrolysis and inhibitor removal after the enzyme hydrolysis [69,87–92].

7.4 SEPARATION BY ADSORPTION MECHANISM

Adsorption process is a surface phenomenon; various types of adsorption processes have reported based on the type of adsorbents. Physical properties of adsorbents are responsible for the selective adsorption process; the important properties include pore volume (ml/g), mean surface area (m^2/g), mean pore diameter (Å), and particle size (mm) [93–96].

The detoxification of the lignocellulosic hydrolyzates by adsorptive purification was investigated with activated charcoal, cationic resins, neutral polymer adsorbents, granulated activated carbon, and zeolites [93,95,97]. Pure carbon is hydrophobic in nature therefore the selective adsorption happens in the presence furfurals, which are hydrophobic compounds. While considering the length of the entire process cycle, the productivity of the process should be the basis for choosing the optimum adsorbent. The hydrophobic properties of fermentation inhibitors such as phenolic compounds, furfural, and HMF are responsible for easy removal by adsorption process, whereas acetic acid and formic acid removal efficiency is very low [97–100].

Activated carbon is well-established and low-cost detoxification process for the separation of the inhibitory components from the wood extracts. The inhibitors removal is related with the hydrophobic nature of the activated charcoal and hydrophobic nature of the phenolic and components and furans extracted during the pretreatment and the nature of the pretreatment and biomass type [100–103].

The adsorption capacity of the inhibitory component was calculated by using the following equation.

$$q_e = \frac{C_0 - C_e V}{m} \tag{1}$$

where

q_e= sorption capacity at equilibrium (mg/g)
V = Volume of the inhibitory solution (L)
C_0 = initial concentration of the inhibitory component (mg/L)
C_e = concentration of inhibitory component at equilibrium (mg/L)
m = mass of the adsorbent (g)

7.4.1 ADSORPTION KINETICS

The adsorption process of the inhibitory components to the adsorbent was controlled by different parameters, i.e., mass transfer, temperature, reaction mechanism, and particle diffusion.

Pseudo-first order:

$$log(q_e - q_t) = logq_e - \frac{1}{2.303} k_1 t \tag{2}$$

Pseudo-second order

$$\frac{t}{q_t} = \frac{1}{k_{2q_e^2}} + \frac{1}{q_e} t \tag{3}$$

where

q_e = concentration at equilibrium (mg/g)
t = adsorption time (s)
q_t = adsorption capacity at t (s)
k_1 = adsorption constants (1/s)
k_2 = adsorption constants (g/mg/s)

For interparticle diffusion equilibrium, the behavior of the adsorption

$$q_t = k_{in} t^{\frac{1}{2}} \tag{4}$$

k_{in} – constant for intraparticle diffusion velocity (mg/g/$s^{-1/2}$)

7.4.2 Adsorption isotherms

The thermodynamics between the solid and liquid phase for the adsorption process at equilibrium condition is characterized by the isotherm. For the monolayer adsorption, Langmuir adsorption isotherm is considered and is given by the equation

$$q_e = \frac{q_{max} b_L C_e}{1 + b_L Ce} \tag{5}$$

where

q_{max} = maximum capacity in the monolayer
b_L = affinity between the adsorbate and adsorbent
q_e = concentration of solute in solid at equilibrium
c_e = concentration of liquid phase at equilibrium

For the heterogeneous and multi-layered adsorption and for a constant temperature, Freundlich model was considered and is given by the equation

$$q_e = k_F C_e^{\frac{1}{n}} \tag{6}$$

The equilibrium data is used to establish the time at which the inhibitory component will break through the column and is compared with the experimental results.

Adsorption isotherms and thermodynamics of the inhibitory components generated during the pretreatment of the agricultural residues were studied with the adsorbents, i.e., activated carbon, activated charcoal, zeolites [103–108]. The hydrolyzates treated with activated carbon showed a significant impact in the removal of formic acid, acetic acid, and hydroxymethylfurfural [109–115]. Several studies have shown the importance of inhibitor removal from pretreatment liquid to obtain the highest enzyme activity and optimum fermentation results [116–120]. When the activated carbon was used in a batch adsorption procedure, it was found that the components furfural, acetic acid, sulfuric acid, vanillic acid, and 4-hydroxybenzoic acid had the highest affinity for adsorption toward activated carbon [101,121–123]. Activated charcoal has a higher affinity toward furan and phenolic compounds. Activated charcoal adsorption was effective for the removal of acetic acid, furfural, and phenolic compounds, about 90.4% of phenolics were removed for the hydrolyzates of eucalyptus wood acid hydrolyzates [123–125]. Activated carbon dosage, temperature, and pH. The adsorptive removal of the main inhibitors such as phenols and acetic acid from the concentrated hydrolysate of oat hull hemicellulose was dependent on the activated carbon dosage, temperature, and pH [101–103,116,122]. Zeolites are capable of improving the ethanol yield from the fermentation process by adsorbing inhibitors such as five-hydroxymethylfurfural (HMF), furfural, and vanillin from biomass hydrolyzates with minimal loss of sugars [125–128]. The detoxification method for spruce dust biomass pretreated with dilute acid for the production of polyhydroxyalkanates (PHA) by microbial fermentation was adsorbed with activated carbon and lignite. Lignite improved the inhibitors removal efficiency and increased the yields of PHA [128–130].

7.5 FLOCCULATION PROCESS FOR SEPARATING COLLOIDAL PARTICLES

Flocculation is the process widely used for the separation of the colloidal range particles, which cannot be sedimented by gravity. Lignocellulosic hydrolytes generated during the pretreatment process contain the particulates and colloidal suspended particles mostly of lignin derivates and hydrolyzed solution after the enzymatic hydrolysis contains the unhydrolyzed cellulosic materials of both lignin and carbohydrate complexes [131–134].

In order to improve the fermentability of the sugars, the separation of colloidal materials is highly essential. Smaller colloidal particles are made to form large aggregates and are settled by flocculation or are filtered. Separation of colloidal particles from wood extracts can be efficiently performed using polymer-induced flocculation method [132–136]. Cationic polymers can be used to flocculate the colloidal particles; at certain conditions, these polyelectrolyte residues can inhibit the enzymes or microbes and can sometimes be toxic to different microorganisms.

In polymer induced flocculation process, polymers aggregate the colloidal particles in the suspension through the mechanisms of bridging, charge neutralization, and patching. The aggregation process depends on the size of the polymer molecule, its concentration and charge density, shear forces during the aggregation, pH of the suspension, temperature of the system, copolymers, and presence of electrolytes [137–140]. Polymers of both cationic, anionic and non-ionic are applied for the separation of the lignin-derived inhibitory components and phenolic components of the biomass hydrolyzates.

Polymers pDADMAC and polyethylene imine (PEI) have lower molecular weight, and high charge density polymers attach to the particles and form cationic patches resulting in attractive interactions between the particles [132,136,140].

Tween 20 and PEG 4000 are surfactants with high hydrophilic-lipophilic balance and gave promising results in extraction of hydrophobic lignin degradation products into soluble phase. Tween 20 was tested on the separation of the phenols from the lignocellulosic hydrolysates and the pre-hydrolysates of steam-treated residues of the biomass the tool soluble phenols were found to be removed [137,140–143].

Biomass hydrolysates extracted during pretreatment contain colloidal particles mostly of lignin and chemical components from hemicellulose. The particles not only foul the membranes used for the downstream processing but also inhibit the fermentation process [133,144–146]. The polymers of cationic, anionic and non-ionic were studied by Yasarla et al., and the separation mechanism, efficiency and parameters affecting the separation efficiency. The study was conducted on the sugar maple wood hydrolysates. The hydrolysates were extracted by autohydrolysis, water has the liquid medium, and the process is at high pressure and temperature conditions. The extraction process optimizes the release of maximum pentose sugars and prevents the conversion of the pentose sugars to furans as they are toxic for the fermentation process [132–134,146,147].

7.6 MEMBRANE FILTRATION METHODS FOR SEPARATION & PURIFICATION

In biorefinery, membrane filtration received a great importance because of its low cost environmentally friendly and high efficiency in recovery of the product and energy utilization. Membrane-based filtration was extensively applied for the research activities by both academic and industry for the analysis of the product recovery and system development [148–150]. Bio-energy and bio-refining production involves a wide array of several membrane processes, of which microfiltration, nanofiltration, reverse osmosis, membrane distillation, and pervaporation are a few. Application of the membrane separation technology in detoxification has been extensively investigated in last decade. In biorefinery various lignocellulosic feedstocks various pretreatment procedures and process parameters extract not only hemicellulose sugars but also polysaccharides, monosaccharides, acetic acid, soluble and insoluble lignin, phenols of aliphatic, alicyclic ash, etc., the existence of non-monomeric sugars will inhibit the conversion process, but some of these products can have a value addition hence can be separated and purified [150–155]. For the separation of the specific selective molecules for the delignified and lignocellulosic hydrolyzates, membrane separation is a promising application and has an advantage as most of the lignin separation is based on molecular weight [147,150,156]. In the context of biorefineries and biofuels through green process, membrane-based separation is a potential unit operation to estimate the characteristics of operational flexibility, process conditions and integrating into the systems already existing, cost to performance indicators, energy consumption and industrial scalability [149,156–158]. It also has the advantage of enabling selective product purification and concentration and recovery of value-added co-products from complex lignocellulosic hydrolyzates. Figure 7.1 illustrates the typical membrane filtration system applied for the separation and concentration of biomolecules in bioprocessing operations.

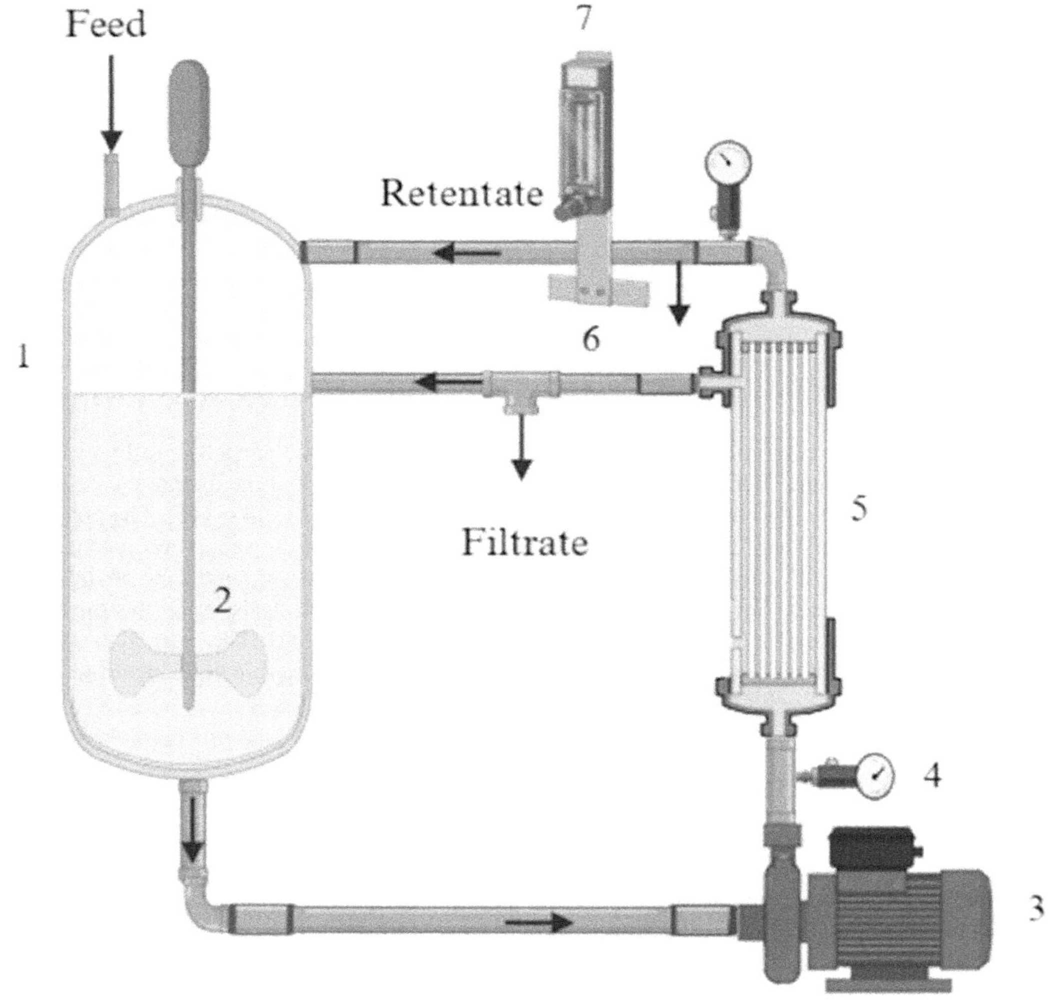

FIGURE 7.1 Crossflow microfiltration system set-up. 1-Feed Tank; 2-Stirrer; 3-Centrifugal Pump; 4-Pressure gauge; 5-Membrane casing with membrane; 6-Sample port; 7-Doppler flow meter.

For a membrane separation process, the quality of the membranes, membrane characteristics including membrane material, stability separation efficiency, challenges deriving from engineering aspects such as membrane fouling, module design, process optimization were highly considered [158–160].

A wide range of membrane materials was investigated for the separation of the inhibitory components for detoxification of the lignocellulosic hydrolyzates and also for the purification of the fermentative products. Membrane materials like ceramic membranes of Al_2O_3, ZrO_2, TiO_2, cellulose acetate, polyether sulfone, microfiber, polysulfone, polyvinylidene fluoride, and also the composite membranes and also layered membranes [160–163]. The membranes were also tested for the operating parameters of pH, temperature, cross-flow velocity, fouling characteristics, and transmembrane pressure.

Microfiltration was widely for the separation processes associated with pretreatment and hydrolysis of biomass extracts, where ultrafiltration, nano filtration, and reverse osmosis are applied for the molecular level separation for the recovery of the products with value addition and concentration of the products facilitating toward bioproducts conversion [149,156,159,161]. Microfiltration by tangential flow filtration and dead-end filtration has been widely studied on different membranes, materials, and different pore sizes. Ceramic, tubular membranes were studied to understand the behavior of the colloidal particles, concentration polymerization of the carbohydrates, and separation efficiency of the inhibitors and fouling characteristics over the membranes [164–167].

Colloidal lignin was found to be fouling material and reduced the separation efficiency of the ceramic membranes of the pore sizes 0.2, 0.01 μm. Fouled lignin also acted as the secondary membrane and reduced the efficiency of the hemicellulose sugar concentration [149,163,166].

Ultrafiltration membrane of 0.1-to-0.001-μmrange removes typically colloidal material, organic, and inorganic components. Hemicellulose sugars, mostly xylose, C5 sugars are concentrated by separating organic acids like acetic acid, phenolics like furfural, and 5-HMF, which are considered as toxic components for enzymatic hydrolysis and fermentation [168–171].

Filtration was considered as a separation step for the acetic acid and furfural from a hemi cellulose rich hydrolyzates, and reverse osmosis membranes were applied, and acetic acid is separated as the permeate. For the recovery of the lignin from delignified and pretreated biomass liquors, ceramic membranes were chosen as the material of the membranes is non-reactive and can stand against high transmembrane pressure, pH, temperature, and cross-flow velocity [162,166,168,172]. The lignin was recovered in the retentate streams, and the lignin recovered had a particle size range of 300nm, and it has a cationic charge. The lignin also fouled the membranes and acted as secondary membrane, which reduces the permeate velocity and also loss in sugar recovery [166–170].

In nano-filtration and reverse osmosis, membrane fouling is the serious issue because of the decline in permeate flux and high expensive at large scale. Hasan et al. applied microfiltration by ceramic filters for hot water extracted wood hydrolyzates, at high transmembrane pressures, flux was reduced, and fouling was rapid and continuous [173–176].

Nanofiltration and reverse osmosis have successfully applied for the sugar fractionation, concentration, and removal of organic contaminants from water and recovery of solvents. Nanofiltration is considered as an important unit in the down-stream processing and classified in between ultrafiltration and reverse osmosis [160–162,170–172]. Nanofiltration has a wide range of applications for the separation of substances with molar masses higher than ~300g/mol and multivalent ions and considered for size exclusion with a molecular weight cut-off (MWCO) range of 0.01–1kDa. In biorefinery and biomaterials research, nanofiltration applications were studied in wide range for the separation and purification of carbohydrates and acids [170–173]. For detoxification of biomass hydrolyzates, specifically furfural and acetic acid having molecular weights of 96.09 and 60.05 g/mol nanofiltration was able to separate the two components. Recovery of acetic acid and furfural from hydrolyzates is a value addition as acetic acid can be used for the production of monomers like vinyl acetate and furfural for the conversion of biofuels and other industrial applications including plastics and biochemicals [175–178]. Retention characteristics of membranes depend on molecular weight of solutes and in case of bioproducts like carbohydrates and amino acids properties like charge and hydrophobicity also affect the retention [160,166,176].

Membrane fouling is important to determine the feasibility of the separation process. Fouling of the membranes in ultrafiltration and nanofiltrations occurs due to the deposition of the organics, which can be reversible and also irreversible and is depends on the interaction between the membrane surface and the fouling materials [170–173]. In order to understand the mechanism of the flux decline and fouling behavior of the membranes, membrane filtration models were adopted. The total resistance from the filtrate flow results from blocking of the membrane pores by the suspended particles here insoluble lignin particles, ash, and concentration polarization by the molecular scale components including carbohydrates, acetic acid. The suspended particles also block the membrane pores completely or partially [168,171–174]. The blocking of the membranes reduced the permeate flow and recovery of the chemicals.

Darcy's law describes the permeate flux and the total resistance of the membrane.

$$J = \frac{\Delta P}{\mu(R_m + R_p + R_c)} \tag{7}$$

The resistances acting in the series are as follows.

R_m = clean membrane resistance
R_p = blocking resistance by particles deposited in the pores of the membranes
R_c = cake resistance caused by the particles deposited on the membrane surface

The kinetics of the permeate flux decay and the mechanism of the blocking was studied by the following expressions.

For membrane resistance limitations

$$\frac{1}{J} = \frac{1}{J_0} + K_m \tag{8}$$

Pore blocking resistance

$$lnJ = -K_p t + lnJ_o \tag{9}$$

Cake resistance.

$$\frac{1}{J^2} = \frac{1}{J_0^2} + K_c t \tag{10}$$

By fitting the filtration data to linearized models, the mechanism of the fouling can be identified [47].

7.7 CONCLUSION

Circular bioeconomy aims to utilize renewable, biological resources and maximize secondary biomass from industrial and agricultural residues which are rich in cellulosic carbohydrates. Biorefinery, the concept of industrial operations integrating with the existing facilities for the valorization of the secondary biomass toward the conversion of the biochemicals and biofuels, requires a several thermochemical and biological conversion technologies including pretreatment, hydrolysis, fermentation, and downstream unit operations like centrifugation, membrane filtration, and adsorptive-based chromatographic and membrane separations. Separation and purification involve multiple steps in biorefinery and bioethanol processes at the industrial scale, which involves in separation of colloidal and microbial biomass from upstream and downstream processes, which are processes by microfiltration, centrifugation. Concentration and purification of the specific biological components require a specific unit operation either by filtration or adsorption processes with charged resins or membranes. This chapter emphasizes in detail the separation processes toward the valorization of the biomass from industrial and agricultural residues for circular bioeconomy and the mechanism of the separation processes of membrane filtration and adsorption-based purification for the sustainable production of biochemicals and bioenergy.

REFERENCES

1. McKendry, P. (2002). Energy production from biomass (part 1): Overview of biomass. *Bioresource Technology*, 83(1), 37–46.
2. Faaij, A. (2006). Modern biomass conversion technologies. *Mitigation and Adaptation Strategies for Global Change*, 11, 343–375.
3. Agbor, V. B., Cicek, N., Sparling, R., Berlin, A., & Levin, D. B. (2011). Biomass pretreatment: Fundamentals toward application. *Biotechnology Advances*, 29(6), 675–685.
4. Grewal, J., Sadaf, A., Yadav, N., & Khare, S. K. (2020). Agroindustrial waste based biorefineries for sustainable production of lactic acid. In *Waste biorefinery*, 125–153.
5. Siqueira, J. G. W., Rodrigues, C., de Souza Vandenberghe, L. P., Woiciechowski, A. L., & Soccol, C. R. (2020). Current advances in on-site cellulase production and application on lignocellulosic biomass conversion to biofuels: A review. *Biomass and Bioenergy*, 132, 105419.
6. Demirbaş, A. (2001). Biomass resource facilities and biomass conversion processing for fuels and chemicals. *Energy conversion and Management*, 42(11), 1357–1378.
7. Saha, B. C. (2003). Hemicellulose bioconversion. *Journal of Industrial Microbiology and Biotechnology*, 30(5), 279–291.
8. Detroy, R. W., & St Julian, G. (1982). Biomass conversion: Fermentation chemicals and fuels. *CRC Critical Reviews in Microbiology*, 10(3), 203–228.
9. Leonard, R. H., & Hajny, G. J. (1945). Fermentation of wood sugars to ethyl alcohol. *Industrial & Engineering Chemistry*, 37(4), 390–395.
10. Jae, J., Tompsett, G. A., Foster, A. J., Hammond, K. D., Auerbach, S. M., Lobo, R. F., & Huber, G. W. (2011). Investigation into the shape selectivity of zeolite catalysts for biomass conversion. *Journal of Catalysis*, 279(2), 257–268.
11. Klinke, H. B., Thomsen, A. B., & Ahring, B. K. (2004). Inhibition of ethanol-producing yeast and bacteria by degradation products produced during pre-treatment of biomass. *Applied Microbiology and Biotechnology*, 66, 10–26.
12. Qi, X., Yan, L., Shen, F., & Qiu, M. (2019). Mechanochemical-assisted hydrolysis of pretreated rice straw into glucose and xylose in water by weakly acidic solid catalyst. *Bioresource Technology*, 273, 687–691.
13. Xu, J. K., Sun, Y. C., & Sun, R. C. (2014). Ionic liquid pretreatment of woody biomass to facilitate biorefinery: Structural elucidation of alkali-soluble hemicelluloses. *ACS Sustainable Chemistry & Engineering*, 2(4), 1035–1042.
14. Kim, S. M., Dien, B. S., & Singh, V. (2016). Promise of combined hydrothermal/chemical and mechanical refining for pretreatment of woody and herbaceous biomass. *Biotechnology for Biofuels*, 9, 1–15.
15. Zakaria, M. R., Hirata, S., & Hassan, M. A. (2014). Combined pretreatment using alkaline hydrothermal and ball milling to enhance enzymatic hydrolysis of oil palm mesocarp fiber. *Bioresource Technology*, 169, 236–243.
16. Modig, T., Liden, G., & Taherzadeh, M. J. (2002). Inhibition effects of furfural on alcohol dehydrogenase, aldehyde dehydrogenase and pyruvate dehydrogenase. *Biochemical Journal*, 363(3), 769–776.
17. Scordia, D., Cosentino, S. L., & Jeffries, T. W. (2013). Effectiveness of dilute oxalic acid pretreatment of Miscanthus× giganteus biomass for ethanol production. *Biomass and Bioenergy*, 59, 540–548.
18. Geng, X., & Henderson, W. A. (2012). Pretreatment of corn stover by combining ionic liquid dissolution with alkali extraction. *Biotechnology and Bioengineering*, 109(1), 84–91.
19. Moxley, G., Gaspar, A. R., Higgins, D., & Xu, H. (2012). Structural changes of corn stover lignin during acid pretreatment. *Journal of Industrial Microbiology and Biotechnology*, 39(9), 1289–1299.

20. Li, C., Knierim, B., Manisseri, C., Arora, R., Scheller, H. V., Auer, M., & Singh, S. (2010). Comparison of dilute acid and ionic liquid pretreatment of switchgrass: Biomass recalcitrance, delignification and enzymatic saccharification. *Bioresource Technology*, 101(13), 4900–4906.
21. Lenihan, P., Orozco, A., O'Neill, E., Ahmad, M. N. M., Rooney, D. W., & Walker, G. M. (2010). Dilute acid hydrolysis of lignocellulosic biomass. *Chemical Engineering Journal*, 156(2), 395–403.
22. Guo, G. L., Chen, W. H., Chen, W. H., Men, L. C., & Hwang, W. S. (2008). Characterization of dilute acid pretreatment of silvergrass for ethanol production. *Bioresource Technology*, 99(14), 6046–6053.
23. Sannigrahi, P., Ragauskas, A. J., & Miller, S. J. (2008). Effects of two-stage dilute acid pretreatment on the structure and composition of lignin and cellulose in loblolly pine. *BioEnergy Research*, 1, 205–214.
24. Rogalinski, T., Ingram, T., & Brunner, G. (2008). Hydrolysis of lignocellulosic biomass in water under elevated temperatures and pressures. *The Journal of Supercritical Fluids*, 47(1), 54–63.
25. Öhgren, K., Bura, R., Saddler, J., & Zacchi, G. (2007). Effect of hemicellulose and lignin removal on enzymatic hydrolysis of steam pretreated corn stover. *Bioresource Technology*, 98(13), 2503–2510.
26. Tu, M., Chandra, R. P., & Saddler, J. N. (2007). Evaluating the distribution of cellulases and the recycling of free cellulases during the hydrolysis of lignocellulosic substrates. *Biotechnology Progress*, 23(2), 398–406.
27. Gámez, S., González-Cabriales, J. J., Ramírez, J. A., Garrote, G., & Vázquez, M. (2006). Study of the hydrolysis of sugar cane bagasse using phosphoric acid. *Journal of Food Engineering*, 74(1), 78–88.
28. Dien, B. S., Jung, H. J. G., Vogel, K. P., Casler, M. D., Lamb, J. F., Iten, L., & Sarath, G. (2006). Chemical composition and response to dilute-acid pretreatment and enzymatic saccharification of alfalfa, reed canarygrass, and switchgrass. *Biomass and Bioenergy*, 30(10), 880–891.
29. Rahman, S. H. A., Choudhury, J. P., & Ahmad, A. L. (2006). Production of xylose from oil palm empty fruit bunch fiber using sulfuric acid. *Biochemical Engineering Journal*, 30(1), 97–103.
30. Roberto, I. C., Mussatto, S. I., & Rodrigues, R. C. (2003). Dilute-acid hydrolysis for optimization of xylose recovery from rice straw in a semi-pilot reactor. *Industrial Crops and Products*, 17(3), 171–176.
31. Chang, V. S., Nagwani, M., & Holtzapple, M. T. (1998). Lime pretreatment of crop residues bagasse and wheat straw. *Applied Biochemistry and Biotechnology*, 74, 135–159.
32. Torget, R., Werdene, P., Himmel, M., & Grohmann, K. (1990). Dilute acid pretreatment of short rotation woody and herbaceous crops. *Applied Biochemistry and Biotechnology*, 24, 115–126.
33. Maloney, M. T., Chapman, T. W., & Baker, A. J. (1985). Dilute acid hydrolysis of paper birch: Kinetics studies of xylan and acetyl-group hydrolysis. *Biotechnology and Bioengineering*, 27(3), 355–361.
34. Zheng, Y., Pan, Z., & Zhang, R. (2009). Overview of biomass pretreatment for cellulosic ethanol production. *International Journal of Agricultural and Biological Engineering*, 2(3), 51–68.
35. Zhu, J. Y., & Pan, X. J. (2010). Woody biomass pretreatment for cellulosic ethanol production: Technology and energy consumption evaluation. *Bioresource Technology*, 101(13), 4992–5002.
36. Palmqvist, E., Grage, H., Meinander, N. Q., & Hahn-Hägerdal, B. (1999). Main and interaction effects of acetic acid, furfural, and p-hydroxybenzoic acid on growth and ethanol productivity of yeasts. *Biotechnology and Bioengineering*, 63(1), 46–55.
37. Alves, L. A, Felipe, M. G. a, Silva, J. B. A. E, Silva, S. S, and Prata, A. M. R. (1998) Pretreatment of sugarcane bagasse hemicellulose hydrolysate for xylitol production by *Candida guilliermondi, vol. 70, Applied Biochemistry and Biotechnology*, 89–98.
38. Bhatia, S. K., Jagtap, S. S., Bedekar, A. A., Bhatia, R. K., Patel, A. K., Pant, D., ... & Yang, Y. H. (2020). Recent developments in pretreatment technologies on lignocellulosic biomass: Effect of key parameters, technological improvements, and challenges. *Bioresource Technology*, 300, 122724.
39. Rabelo, S. C., Filho, R. M., & Costa, A. C. (2008). A comparison between lime and alkaline hydrogen peroxide pretreatments of sugarcane bagasse for ethanol production. In *Biotechnology for Fuels and Chemicals: Proceedings of the Twenty-Ninth Symposium on Biotechnology for Fuels and Chemicals Held April 29–May 2, 2007, in Denver, Colorado*, 63–576.
40. Mesa, L., González, E., Ruiz, E., Romero, I., Cara, C., Felissia, F., & Castro, E. (2010). Preliminary evaluation of organosolv pre-treatment of sugar cane bagasse for glucose production: Application of 23 experimental design. *Applied Energy*, 87(1), 109–114.
41. Dwivedi, P., Alavalapati, J. R., & Lal, P. (2009). Cellulosic ethanol production in the United States: Conversion technologies, current production status, economics, and emerging developments. *Energy for Sustainable Development*, 13(3), 174–182.
42. Min, B. C., Bhayani, B. V., Jampana, V. S., & Ramarao, B. V. (2015). Enhancement of the enzymatic hydrolysis of fines from recycled paper mill waste rejects. *Bioresources and Bioprocessing*, 2, 1–10.

43. Gan, Q., Allen, S. J., & Taylor, G. (2003). Kinetic dynamics in heterogeneous enzymatic hydrolysis of cellulose: An overview, an experimental study and mathematical modelling. *Process Biochemistry*, 38(7), 1003–1018.
44. Collins, M., Knutti, R., Arblaster, J., Dufresne, J. L., Fichefet, T., Friedlingstein, P., & Wehner, M. (2013). Long-term climate change: Projections, commitments and irreversibility. In T. F. Stocker, et al. (Eds.), *Climate Change 2013: The Physical Science Basis. Contribution of Working Group I to the Fifth Assessment Report of the Intergovernmental Panel on Climate Change* (pp. 1029–1136). Cambridge University
45. Salam, M. A., Pondith, P. C., Islam, A., Khan, M. R., Uddin, M. R., & Islam, M. A. (2013). Conversion of cellulosic waste into fermentable sugar: Process optimization. *Journal of Chemical Engineering*, 28(1), 27–31.
46. Binder, J. B., & Raines, R. T. (2009). Simple chemical transformation of lignocellulosic biomass into furans for fuels and chemicals. *Journal of the American Chemical Society*, 131(5), 1979–1985.
47. Lim, A. L., & Bai, R. (2003). Membrane fouling and cleaning in microfiltration of activated sludge wastewater. *Journal of Membrane Science*, 216(1–2), 279–290.
48. Wyman, C. E., Decker, S. R., Himmel, M. E., Brady, J. W., Skopec, C. E., & Viikari, L. (2005). Hydrolysis of cellulose and hemicellulose. *Polysaccharides: Structural Diversity and Functional Versatility*, 1, 1023–1062.
49. Sun, Y., & Cheng, J. (2002). Hydrolysis of lignocellulosic materials for ethanol production: A review. *Bioresource Technology*, 83(1), 1–11.
50. Harun, R., Danquah, M. K., & Forde, G. M. (2010). Microalgal biomass as a fermentation feedstock for bioethanol production. *Journal of Chemical Technology & Biotechnology*, 85(2), 199–203.
51. Bridgwater, A. V. (1994). Catalysis in thermal biomass conversion. *Applied Catalysis A:* General, 116(1–2), 5–47.
52. Demirbaş, A. (2001). Biomass resource facilities and biomass conversion processing for fuels and chemicals. *Energy Conversion and Management*, 42(11), 1357–1378.
53. Taarning, E., Osmundsen, C. M., Yang, X., Voss, B., Andersen, S. I., & Christensen, C. H. (2011). Zeolite-catalyzed biomass conversion to fuels and chemicals. *Energy & Environmental Science*, 4(3), 793–804.
54. Yasarla, L. R. K., Ramarao, B. V., & Amidon, T. (2017). *U.S. Patent No.* 9,751,781. U.S. Patent and Trademark Office.
55. Berlin, A., Balakshin, M., Gilkes, N., Kadla, J., Maximenko, V., Kubo, S., & Saddler, J. (2006). Inhibition of cellulase, xylanase and β-glucosidase activities by softwood lignin preparations. *Journal of Biotechnology*, 125(2), 198–209.
56. Zaldivar, J., Martinez, A., & Ingram, L. O. (1999). Effect of selected aldehydes on the growth and fermentation of ethanologenic Escherichia coli. *Biotechnology and Bioengineering*, 65(1), 24–33.
57. Luo, C., Brink, D. L., & Blanch, H. W. (2002). Identification of potential fermentation inhibitors in conversion of hybrid poplar hydrolyzate to ethanol. *Biomass and Bioenergy*, 22(2), 125–138.
58. Barakat, A., Monlau, F., Steyer, J. P., & Carrere, H. (2012). Effect of lignin-derived and furan compounds found in lignocellulosic hydrolysates on biomethane production. *Bioresource Technology*, 104, 90–99.
59. Zeng, Y., Zhao, S., Yang, S., & Ding, S. Y. (2014). Lignin plays a negative role in the biochemical process for producing lignocellulosic biofuels. *Current Opinion in Biotechnology*, 27, 38–45.
60. Świątek, K., Gaag, S., Klier, A., Kruse, A., Sauer, J., & Steinbach, D. (2020). Acid hydrolysis of lignocellulosic biomass: Sugars and furfurals formation. *Catalysts*, 10(4), 437.
61. Kobayashi, H., Kaiki, H., Shrotri, A., Techikawara, K., & Fukuoka, A. (2016). Hydrolysis of woody biomass by a biomass-derived reusable heterogeneous catalyst. *Chemical Science*, 7(1), 692–696.
62. Loow, Y. L., Wu, T. Y., Md. Jahim, J., Mohammad, A. W., & Teoh, W. H. (2016). Typical conversion of lignocellulosic biomass into reducing sugars using dilute acid hydrolysis and alkaline pretreatment. *Cellulose*, 23, 1491–1520.
63. Persson, P., Larsson, S., Jönsson, L. J., Nilvebrant, N. O., Sivik, B., Munteanu, F., & Gorton, L. (2002). Supercritical fluid extraction of a lignocellulosic hydrolysate of spruce for detoxification and to facilitate analysis of inhibitors. *Biotechnology and Bioengineering*, 79(6), 694–700.
64. Lee, J. M., Venditti, R. A., Jameel, H., & Kenealy, W. R. (2011). Detoxification of woody hydrolyzates with activated carbon for bioconversion to ethanol by the thermophilic anaerobic bacterium *Thermoanaerobacterium saccharolyticum*. *Biomass and Bioenergy*, 35(1), 626–636.

65. Monlau, F., Sambusiti, C., Antoniou, N., Zabaniotou, A., Solhy, A., & Barakat, A. (2015). Pyrochars from bioenergy residue as novel bio-adsorbents for lignocellulosic hydrolysate detoxification. *Bioresource Technology*, 187, 379–386.
66. Taherzadeh, M. J., Eklund, R., Gustafsson, L., Niklasson, C., & Lidén, G. (1997). Characterization and fermentation of dilute-acid hydrolyzates from wood. *Industrial & Engineering Chemistry Research*, 36(11), 4659–4665.
67. Mithra, M. G., & Padmaja, G. (2016). Phenolic inhibitors of saccharification and fermentation in lignocellulo-starch prehydrolysates and comparative efficacy of detoxification treatments. *Journal of Biomass to Biofuel*, 3, 1–15.
68. Berlin, A., Balakshin, M., Gilkes, N., Kadla, J., Maximenko, V., Kubo, S., & Saddler, J. (2006). Inhibition of cellulase, xylanase and β-glucosidase activities by softwood lignin preparations. *Journal of Biotechnology*, 125(2), 198–209.
69. Mussatto, S. I., & Roberto, I. C. (2004). Alternatives for detoxification of diluted-acid lignocellulosic hydrolyzates for use in fermentative processes: A review. *Bioresource Technology*, 93(1), 1–10.
70. Wang, Z., Jiang, J., Wang, X., Fu, Y., Li, Z., Zhang, F., & Qin, M. (2014). Selective removal of phenolic lignin derivatives enables sugars recovery from wood prehydrolysis liquor with remarkable yield. *Bioresource Technology*, 174, 198–203.
71. Yu, Y., & Christopher, L. P. (2017). Detoxification of hemicellulose-rich poplar hydrolysate by polymeric resins for improved ethanol fermentability. *Fuel*, 203, 187–196.
72. Orozco, R. L., Redwood, M. D., Leeke, G. A., Bahari, A., Santos, R. C. D., & Macaskie, L. E. (2012). Hydrothermal hydrolysis of starch with CO2 and detoxification of the hydrolysates with activated carbon for bio-hydrogen fermentation. *International Journal of Hydrogen Energy*, 37(8), 6545–6553.
73. Kim, D. (2018). Physico-chemical conversion of lignocellulose: Inhibitor effects and detoxification strategies: A mini review. *Molecules*, 23(2), 309.
74. Rivard, C. J., Engel, R. E., Hayward, T. K., Nagle, N. J., Hatzis, C., & Philippidis, G. P. (1996). Measurement of the inhibitory potential and detoxification of biomass pretreatment hydrolysate for ethanol production. *Applied Biochemistry and Biotechnology*, 57, 183–191.
75. Martinez, A., Rodriguez, M. E., Wells, M. L., York, S. W., Preston, J. F., & Ingram, L. O. (2001). Detoxification of dilute acid hydrolysates of lignocellulose with lime. *Biotechnology Progress*, 17(2), 287–293.
76. Vallejos, M. E., Chade, M., Mereles, E. B., Bengoechea, D. I., Brizuela, J. G., Felissia, F. E., & Area, M. C. (2016). Strategies of detoxification and fermentation for biotechnological production of xylitol from sugarcane bagasse. *Industrial Crops and Products*, 91, 161–169.
77. Meinita, M. D. N., Hong, Y. K., & Jeong, G. T. (2012). Detoxification of acidic catalyzed hydrolysate of Kappaphycus alvarezii (cottonii). *Bioprocess and Biosystems Engineering*, 35, 93–98.
78. Chandel, A. K., Da Silva, S. S., & Singh, O. V. (2013). Detoxification of lignocellulose hydrolysates: Biochemical and metabolic engineering toward white biotechnology. *BioEnergy Research*, 6, 388–401.
79. Huang, C. F., Lin, T. H., Guo, G. L., & Hwang, W. S. (2009). Enhanced ethanol production by fermentation of rice straw hydrolysate without detoxification using a newly adapted strain of *Pichia stipitis*. *Bioresource technology*, 100(17), 3914–3920.
80. Hu, B. B., Li, M. Y., Wang, Y. T., & Zhu, M. J. (2018). Enhanced biohydrogen production from dilute acid pretreated sugarcane bagasse by detoxification and fermentation strategy. *International Journal of Hydrogen Energy*, 43(42), 19366–19374.
81. Lewis Liu, Z., Ma, M., & Song, M. (2009). Evolutionarily engineered ethanologenic yeast detoxifies lignocellulosic biomass conversion inhibitors by reprogrammed pathways. *Molecular Genetics and Genomics*, 282, 233–244.
82. Chandel, A. K., Kapoor, R. K., Singh, A., & Kuhad, R. C. (2007). Detoxification of sugarcane bagasse hydrolysate improves ethanol production by *Candida shehatae NCIM 3501. Bioresource Technology, 98*(10), 1947–1950.
83. López, M. J., Nichols, N. N., Dien, B. S., Moreno, J., & Bothast, R. J. (2004). Isolation of microorganisms for biological detoxification of lignocellulosic hydrolysates. *Applied Microbiology and Biotechnology*, 64, 125–131.
84. Villarreal, M. L. M., Prata, A. M. R., Felipe, M. G. A., & Silva, J. A. E. (2006). Detoxification procedures of eucalyptus hemicellulose hydrolysate for xylitol production by *Candida guilliermondii*. *Enzyme and Microbial Technology*, 40(1), 17–24.

85. Hodge, D. B., Andersson, C., Berglund, K. A., & Rova, U. (2009). Detoxification requirements for bioconversion of softwood dilute acid hydrolyzates to succinic acid. *Enzyme and Microbial Technology*, 44(5), 309–316.
86. Li, H., & Chen, H. (2008). Detoxification of steam-exploded corn straw produced by an industrial-scale reactor. *Process Biochemistry*, 43(12), 1447–1451.
87. Nilvebrant, N. O., Reimann, A., Larsson, S., & Jönsson, L. J. (2001). Detoxification of lignocellulose hydrolysates with ion-exchange resins. *Applied Biochemistry and Biotechnology*, 91, 35–49.
88. Larsson, S., Reimann, A., Nilvebrant, N. O., & Jönsson, L. J. (1999). Comparison of different methods for the detoxification of lignocellulose hydrolyzates of spruce. *Applied Biochemistry and Biotechnology*, 77, 91–103.
89. Martinez, A., Rodriguez, M. E., Wells, M. L., York, S. W., Preston, J. F., & Ingram, L. O. (2001). Detoxification of dilute acid hydrolysates of lignocellulose with lime. *Biotechnology Progress*, 17(2), 287–293.
90. Millati, R., Niklasson, C., & Taherzadeh, M. J. (2002). Effect of pH, time and temperature of overliming on detoxification of dilute-acid hydrolyzates for fermentation by Saccharomyces cerevisiae. *Process Biochemistry*, 38(4), 515–522.
91. Lee, S. C., & Park, S. (2016). Removal of furan and phenolic compounds from simulated biomass hydrolysates by batch adsorption and continuous fixed-bed column adsorption methods. *Bioresource Technology*, 216, 661–668.
92. Mithra, M. G., & Padmaja, G. (2016). Phenolic inhibitors of saccharification and fermentation in lignocellulo-starch prehydrolysates and comparative efficacy of detoxification treatments. *Journal of Biomass to Biofuel*, 3, 1–15.
93. Parajó, J. C., Domínguez, H., & Domínguez, J. M. (1996). Charcoal adsorption of wood hydrolysates for improving their fermentability: Influence of the operational conditions. *Bioresource Technology*, 57(2), 179–185.
94. Wang, L., & Chen, H. (2011). Increased fermentability of enzymatically hydrolyzed steam-exploded corn stover for butanol production by removal of fermentation inhibitors. *Process Biochemistry*, 46(2), 604–607.
95. Ranjan, R., Thust, S., Gounaris, C. E., Woo, M., Floudas, C. A., von Keitz, M., & Tsapatsis, M. (2009). Adsorption of fermentation inhibitors from lignocellulosic biomass hydrolyzates for improved ethanol yield and value-added product recovery. *Microporous and Mesoporous Materials*, 122(1–3), 143–148.
96. Kim, Y., Kreke, T., Hendrickson, R., Parenti, J., & Ladisch, M. R. (2013). Fractionation of cellulase and fermentation inhibitors from steam pretreated mixed hardwood. *Bioresource Technology*, 135, 30–38.
97. Zhang, K., Agrawal, M., Harper, J., Chen, R., & Koros, W. J. (2011). Removal of the fermentation inhibitor, furfural, using activated carbon in cellulosic-ethanol production. *Industrial & Engineering Chemistry Research*, 50(24), 14055–14060.
98. Weil, J. R., Dien, B., Bothast, R., Hendrickson, R., Mosier, N. S., & Ladisch, M. R. (2002). Removal of fermentation inhibitors formed during pretreatment of biomass by polymeric adsorbents. *Industrial & Engineering Chemistry Research*, 41(24), 6132–6138.
99. Gurram, R. N., Datta, S., Lin, Y. J., Snyder, S. W., & Menkhaus, T. J. (2011). Removal of enzymatic and fermentation inhibitory compounds from biomass slurries for enhanced biorefinery process efficiencies. *Bioresource Technology*, 102(17), 7850–7859.
100. Heinonen, J., Tamminen, A., Uusitalo, J., & Sainio, T. (2012). Ethanol production from wood via concentrated acid hydrolysis, chromatographic separation, and fermentation. *Journal of Chemical Technology & Biotechnology*, 87(5), 689–696.
101. Trinh, L. T. P., Kundu, C., Lee, J. W., & Lee, H. J. (2014). An integrated detoxification process with electrodialysis and adsorption from the hemicellulose hydrolysates of yellow poplars. *Bioresource Technology*, 161, 280–287.
102. Sainio, T., Turku, I., & Heinonen, J. (2011). Adsorptive removal of fermentation inhibitors from concentrated acid hydrolyzates of lignocellulosic biomass. *Bioresource Technology*, 102(10), 6048–6057.
103. Kim, Y., Ximenes, E., Mosier, N. S., & Ladisch, M. R. (2011). Soluble inhibitors/deactivators of cellulase enzymes from lignocellulosic biomass. *Enzyme and Microbial Technology*, *48*(4–5), 408–415.
104. Jeong, S. Y., Trinh, L. T. P., Lee, H. J., & Lee, J. W. (2014). Improvement of the fermentability of oxalic acid hydrolysates by detoxification using electrodialysis and adsorption. *Bioresource Technology*, 152, 444–449.

105. Zhang, Y., Li, M., Wang, Y., Ji, X., Zhang, L., & Hou, L. (2015). Simultaneous concentration and detoxification of lignocellulosic hydrolyzates by vacuum membrane distillation coupled with adsorption. *Bioresource Technology*, 197, 276–283.
106. Soleimani, M., Tabil, L., & Niu, C. (2015). Adsorptive isotherms and removal of microbial inhibitors in a bio-based hydrolysate for xylitol production. *Chemical Engineering Communications*, 202(6), 787–798.
107. Li, Y., Qi, B., & Wan, Y. (2020). Separation of monosaccharides from pretreatment inhibitors by nanofiltration in lignocellulosic hydrolysate: Fouling mitigation by activated carbon adsorption. *Biomass and Bioenergy*, 136, 105527.
108. Candido, J. P., Claro, E. M. T., de Paula, C. B. C., Shimizu, F. L., de Oliveria Leite, D. A. N., Brienzo, M., & de Angelis, D. D. F. (2020). Detoxification of sugarcane bagasse hydrolysate with different adsorbents to improve the fermentative process. *World Journal of Microbiology and Biotechnology*, 36, 1–12.
109. Yu, Y., & Christopher, L. P. (2017). Detoxification of hemicellulose-rich poplar hydrolysate by polymeric resins for improved ethanol fermentability. *Fuel*, 203, 187–196.
110. Wang, X., Zhuang, J., Fu, Y., Tian, G., Wang, Z., & Qin, M. (2016). Separation of hemicellulose-derived saccharides from wood hydrolysate by lime and ion exchange resin. *Bioresource Technology*, 206, 225–230.
111. Lodi, G., Pellegrini, L. A., Aliverti, A., Torres, B. R., Bernardi, M., Morbidelli, M., & Storti, G. (2017). Recovery of monosaccharides from lignocellulosic hydrolysates by ion exclusion chromatography. *Journal of Chromatography A*, *1496*, 25–36.
112. Lee, J. M., Venditti, R. A., Jameel, H., & Kenealy, W. R. (2011). Detoxification of woody hydrolyzates with activated carbon for bioconversion to ethanol by the thermophilic anaerobic bacterium *Thermoanaerobacterium saccharolyticum*. *Biomass and Bioenergy*, 35(1), 626–636.
113. Jönsson, L. J., & Martín, C. (2016). Pretreatment of lignocellulose: Formation of inhibitory by-products and strategies for minimizing their effects. *Bioresource Technology*, 199, 103–112.
114. Freitas, J. V., Nogueira, F. G., & Farinas, C. S. (2019). Coconut shell activated carbon as an alternative adsorbent of inhibitors from lignocellulosic biomass pretreatment. *Industrial Crops and Products*, 137, 16–23.
115. Lee, S. C. (2017). Removal and recovery of acetic acid and two furans during sugar purification of simulated phenols-free biomass hydrolysates. *Bioresource Technology*, 245, 116–122.
116. Schwartz, T. J., & Lawoko, M. (2010). Removal of acid-soluble lignin from biomass extracts using Amberlite XAD-4 resin. *BioResources*, 5(4), 2337–2347.
117. Kucera, D., Benesova, P., Ladicky, P., Pekar, M., Sedlacek, P., & Obruca, S. (2017). Production of polyhydroxyalkanoates using hydrolyzates of spruce sawdust: Comparison of hydrolyzates detoxification by application of overliming, active carbon, and lignite. *Bioengineering*, 4(2), 53.
118. Chen, K., Lyu, H., Hao, S., Luo, G., Zhang, S., & Chen, J. (2015). Separation of phenolic compounds with modified adsorption resin from aqueous phase products of hydrothermal liquefaction of rice straw. *Bioresource Technology*, 182, 160–168.
119. Priddy, S. A., & Hanley, T. R. (2003). Effect of agitation on removal of acetic acid from pretreated hydrolysate by activated carbon. In *Biotechnology for Fuels and Chemicals: The Twenty-Fourth Symposium* (pp. 353–364). Humana Press.
120. Jeřábek, K., Hankova, L., & Prokop, Z. (1994). Post-crosslinked polymer adsorbents and their properties for separation of furfural from aqueous solutions. *Reactive Polymers*, *23*(2–3), 107–112.
121. Carter, B., Squillace, P., Gilcrease, P. C., & Menkhaus, T. J. (2011). Detoxification of a lignocellulosic biomass slurry by soluble polyelectrolyte adsorption for improved fermentation efficiency. *Biotechnology and Bioengineering*, 108(9), 2053–2060.
122. Travália, B. M., Santos, N. T. D. G., Vieira, M. G. A., & Forte, M. B. S. (2019). Adsorption of fermentation inhibitors by layered double hydroxides in synthetic hemicellulose hydrolysate: A batch multicomponent analysis. *Industrial & Engineering Chemistry Research*, 58(40), 18822–18828.
123. Li, Y., Shao, J., Wang, X., Yang, H., Chen, Y., Deng, Y., & Chen, H. (2013). Upgrading of bio-oil: Removal of the fermentation inhibitor (furfural) from the model compounds of bio-oil using pyrolytic char. *Energy & Fuels*, 27(10), 5975–5981.
124. Huang, Q., Zhang, H., Xiong, L., Huang, C., Guo, H., Chen, X., & Chen, X. (2018). Controllable synthesis of monoacrylate-modified adsorption resins and enhancing adsorption toward fermentation inhibitors from rice straw hydrolysate. *Journal of Chemical Technology & Biotechnology*, 93(9), 2652–2658.
125. Yoshioka, K., Daidai, M., Matsumoto, Y., Mizuno, R., Katsura, Y., Hakogi, T., & Watanabe, T. (2018). Self-sufficient bioethanol production system using a lignin-derived adsorbent of fermentation inhibitors. *ACS Sustainable Chemistry & Engineering*, 6(3), 3070–3078.

126. Nwaneshiudu, I. C., & Schwartz, D. T. (2015). Rational design of polymer-based absorbents: Application to the fermentation inhibitor furfural. *Biotechnology for Biofuels*, 8, 1–8.
127. Hatano, K. I., Aoyagi, N., Miyakawa, T., Tanokura, M., & Kubota, K. (2013). Evaluation of nonionic adsorbent resins for removal of inhibitory compounds from corncob hydrolysate for ethanol fermentation. *Bioresource Technology*, 149, 541–545.
128. Chen, X. F., Zhang, L. Q., Huang, C., Xiong, L., Li, H. L., Wang, C., & Chen, X. D. (2019). Adsorption study of acid soluble lignin removal from sugarcane bagasse hydrolysate by a self-synthesized resin for lipid production. *Applied Biochemistry and Biotechnology*, 188, 585–601.
129. Shen, J., Kaur, I., Baktash, M. M., He, Z., & Ni, Y. (2013). A combined process of activated carbon adsorption, ion exchange resin treatment and membrane concentration for recovery of dissolved organics in pre-hydrolysis liquor of the kraft-based dissolving pulp production process. *Bioresource Technology*, 127, 59–65.
130. Soto, M. L., Moure, A., Domínguez, H., & Parajó, J. C. (2011). Recovery, concentration and purification of phenolic compounds by adsorption: A review. *Journal of Food Engineering*, 105(1), 1–27.
131. Hasan, A., & Fatehi, P. (2019). Cationic kraft lignin-acrylamide copolymer as a flocculant for clay suspensions:(2) Charge density effect. *Separation and Purification Technology*, 210, 963–972.
132. Hasan, A., & Fatehi, P. (2019). Flocculation of kaolin particles with cationic lignin polymers. *Scientific Reports*, 9(1), 2672.
133. Yasarla, L. R., & Ramarao, B. V. (2012). Dynamics of flocculation of lignocellulosic hydrolyzates by polymers. *Industrial & Engineering Chemistry Research*, 51(19), 6847–6861.
134. Feizi, Z. H., Kazzaz, A. E., Kong, F., & Fatehi, P. (2019). Evolving a flocculation process for isolating lignosulfonate from solution. *Separation and Purification Technology*, 222, 254–263.
135. Wang, S., Kong, F., Gao, W., & Fatehi, P. (2018). Novel process for generating cationic lignin-based flocculant. *Industrial & Engineering Chemistry Research*, 57(19), 6595–6608.
136. Chen, J., Eraghi Kazzaz, A., AlipoorMazandarani, N., Hosseinpour Feizi, Z., & Fatehi, P. (2018). Production of flocculants, adsorbents, and dispersants from lignin. *Molecules*, 23(4), 868.
137. Sun, Y., Liu, Z., & Fatehi, P. (2017). Flocculation of thermomechanical pulping spent liquor with polydiallyldimethylammonium chloride. *Journal of Environmental Management*, 200, 275–282.
138. Oveissi, F., Sitter, T., & Fatehi, P. (2016). PDADMAC as a flocculant for lignosulfonate of NSSC pulping process. *Biotechnology Progress*, 32(3), 686–691.
139. Sitter, T., Oveissi, F., & Fatehi, P. (2014). A process for producing lignocellulosic flocs from NSSC spent liquor. *Journal of Biotechnology*, 173, 19–23.
140. Saeed, A., Fatehi, P., & Ni, Y. (2012). An integrated process for removing the inhibitors of the prehydrolysis liquor of kraft-based dissolving pulp process via cationic polymer treatment. *Biotechnology Progress*, 28(4), 998–1004.
141. Yasarla, R. L., & Ramarao, B. V. (2012). Statistical analysis of the performance of polymeric flocculants for lignocellulosic hydrolyzates. *Journal of Bioprocess Engineering and Biorefinery*, 1(2), 237–241.
142. Shi, H., Fatehi, P., Xiao, H., & Ni, Y. (2012). Optimizing the poly ethylene oxide flocculation process for isolating lignin of prehydrolysis liquor of a kraft-based dissolving pulp production process. *Industrial & Engineering Chemistry Research*, 51(14), 5330–5335.
143. Zhuang, J., Xu, J., Wang, X., Li, Z., Han, W., & Wang, Z. (2017). Improved microfiltration of prehydrolysis liquor of wood from dissolving pulp mill by flocculation treatments for hemicellulose recovery. *Separation and Purification Technology*, 176, 159–163.
144. Liu, X., Fatehi, P., & Ni, Y. (2012). Removal of inhibitors from pre-hydrolysis liquor of kraft-based dissolving pulp production process using adsorption and flocculation processes. *Bioresource Technology*, 116, 492–496.
145. Yasarla, L. R., & Ramarao, B. V. (2013). Lignin removal from lignocellulosic hydrolyzates by flocculation with polyethylene oxide. *Journal of Biobased Materials and Bioenergy*, 7(6), 684–689.
146. Saeed, A., Fatehi, P., & Ni, Y. (2011). Chitosan as a flocculant for pre-hydrolysis liquor of kraft-based dissolving pulp production process. *Carbohydrate Polymers*, 86(4), 1630–1636.
147. Shi, H., Fatehi, P., Xiao, H., & Ni, Y. (2011). A combined acidification/PEO flocculation process to improve the lignin removal from the pre-hydrolysis liquor of kraft-based dissolving pulp production process. *Bioresource Technology*, 102(8), 5177–5182.
148. Ai, C., Meng, H., Lin, J., Zhang, T., & Guo, X. (2020). Combined membrane filtration and alcohol-precipitation of alkaline soluble polysaccharides from sugar beet pulp: Comparision of compositional, macromolecular, and emulsifying properties. *Food Hydrocolloids*, 109, 106049.

149. Yasarla, L. R. (2014). Separation of lignocellulosic hydrolyzates by polymer induced flocculation and tangential flow microfiltration. State University of New York College of Environmental Science and Forestry (Ph.D thesis)
150. Hasan, A., Yasarla, R., Ramarao, B. V., & Amidon, T. E. (2011). Separation of lignocellulosic hydrolyzate components using ceramic microfilters. *Journal of Wood Chemistry and Technology*, 31(4), 357–383.
151. Steinmetz, V., Villain-Gambier, M., Klem, A., Ziegler, I., Dumarcay, S., & Trebouet, D. (2020). In-situ extraction of depolymerization products by membrane filtration against lignin condensation. *Bioresource Technology*, 311, 123530.
152. Kumar, M., Isloor, A. M., Rao, T. S., Ismail, A. F., Farnood, R., & Nambissan, P. M. G. (2020). Removal of toxic arsenic from aqueous media using polyphenylsulfone/cellulose acetate hollow fiber membranes containing zirconium oxide. *Chemical Engineering Journal*, 393, 124367.
153. Schlackl, K., Bischof, R. H., & Samhaber, W. (2020). Negative retention by the nanofiltration of aqueous biomass hydrolysates derived from wood pulping. *Separation and Purification Technology*, 242, 116773.
154. Domingos, J. M., Teixeira, A. R., Dupoiron, S., Allais, F., & Lameloise, M. L. (2020). Simultaneous recovery of ferulic acid and sugars from wheat bran enzymatic hydrolysate by diananofiltration. *Separation and Purification Technology*, 242, 116755.
155. Wijaya, H., Sasaki, K., Kahar, P., Rahmani, N., Hermiati, E., Yopi, Y., & Kondo, A. (2020). High enzymatic recovery and purification of xylooligosaccharides from empty fruit bunch via nanofiltration. *Processes*, 8(5), 619.
156. Zdarta, J., Thygesen, A., Holm, M. S., Meyer, A. S., & Pinelo, M. (2020). Direct separation of acetate and furfural from xylose by nanofiltration of birch pretreated liquor: Effect of process conditions and separation mechanism. *Separation and Purification Technology*, 239, 116546.
157. Mahboubi, A., Elyasi, S., Doyen, W., De Wever, H., & Taherzadeh, M. J. (2020). Concentration-driven reverse membrane bioreactor for the fermentation of highly inhibitory lignocellulosic hydrolysate. *Process Biochemistry*, 92, 409–416.
158. Abejón, R., Rabadán, J., Garea, A., & Irabien, A. (2020). Comparison of supported ionic liquid membranes and polymeric ultrafiltration and nanofiltration membranes for separation of lignin and monosaccharides. *Membranes*, 10(2), 29.
159. Weerasuriya Arachchige, A. R. P. P., Mezule, L., & Juhna, T. (2020). Separation of reducing sugars from lignocellulosic hydrolysate: Membrane experiments & system dynamic modelling. *Agronomy Research*, *18*(Special Issue 1), 1099–1106.
160. Sjölin, M., Thuvander, J., Wallberg, O., & Lipnizki, F. (2019). Purification of sucrose in sugar beet molasses by utilizing ceramic nanofiltration and ultrafiltration membranes. *Membranes*, 10(1), 5.
161. Fayet, A., Teixeira, A. R., Allais, F., Bouix, M., & Lameloise, M. L. (2018). Detoxification of highly acidic hemicellulosic hydrolysate from wheat straw by diananofiltration with a focus on phenolic compounds. *Journal of Membrane Science*, 566, 112–121.
162. Wang, T., Meng, Y., Qin, Y., Feng, W., & Wang, C. (2018). Removal of furfural and HMF from monosaccharides by nanofiltration and reverse osmosis membranes. *Journal of the Energy Institute*, 91(3), 473–480.
163. Servaes, K., Varhimo, A., Dubreuil, M., Bulut, M., Vandezande, P., Siika-aho, M., & Bongers, B. (2017). Purification and concentration of lignin from the spent liquor of the alkaline oxidation of woody biomass through membrane separation technology. *Industrial Crops and Products*, 106, 86–96.
164. Oriez, V., Peydecastaing, J., & Pontalier, P. Y. (2020). Lignocellulosic biomass mild alkaline fractionation and resulting extract purification processes: Conditions, yields, and purities. *Clean Technologies*, 2(1), 91–115.
165. Gogoi, G., & Hazarika, S. (2017). Coupling of ionic liquid treatment and membrane filtration for recovery of lignin from lignocellulosic biomass. *Separation and Purification Technology*, 173, 113–120.
166. Roli, N. F. M., Yussof, H. W., Seman, M. N. A., Saufi, S. M., & Mohammad, A. W. (2016). Separating xylose from glucose using spiral wound nanofiltration membrane: Effect of cross-flow parameters on sugar rejection. *In IOP Conference Series: Materials Science and Engineering, 162*(1), 012035.
167. Chen, X., Yang, Q., Si, C. L., Wang, Z., Huo, D., Hong, Y., & Li, Z. (2016). Recovery of oligosaccharides from prehydrolysis liquors of poplar by microfiltration/ultrafiltration membranes and anion exchange resin. *ACS Sustainable Chemistry & Engineering*, 4(3), 937–943.
168. Luo, J., Zeuner, B., Morthensen, S. T., Meyer, A. S., & Pinelo, M. (2015). Separation of phenolic acids from monosaccharides by low-pressure nanofiltration integrated with laccase pre-treatments. *Journal of Membrane Science*, 482, 83–91.

169. Nguyen, N. D. T. N., Fargues, C., Guiga, W., & Lameloise, M. L. (2015). Assessing nanofiltration and reverse osmosis for the detoxification of lignocellulosic hydrolysates. *Journal of Membrane Science*, 487, 40–50.
170. Sainio, T., Kallioinen, M., Nakari, O., & Mänttäri, M. (2013). Production and recovery of monosaccharides from lignocellulose hot water extracts in a pulp mill biorefinery. *Bioresource Technology*, 135, 730–737.
171. Zhou, F., Wang, C., & Wei, J. (2013). Simultaneous acetic acid separation and monosaccharide concentration by reverse osmosis. *Bioresource Technology*, 131, 349–356.
172. Zhou, F., Wang, C., & Wei, J. (2013). Separation of acetic acid from monosaccharides by NF and RO membranes: Performance comparison. *Journal of Membrane Science*, 429, 243–251.
173. Koivula, E., Kallioinen, M., Sainio, T., Antón, E., Luque, S., & Mänttäri, M. (2013). Enhanced membrane filtration of wood hydrolysates for hemicelluloses recovery by pretreatment with polymeric adsorbents. *Bioresource Technology*, 143, 275–281.
174. Weng, Y. H., Wei, H. J., Tsai, T. Y., Chen, W. H., Wei, T. Y., Hwang, W. S., & Huang, C. P. (2009). Separation of acetic acid from xylose by nanofiltration. *Separation and Purification Technology*, 67(1), 95–102.
175. Colyar, K. R., Pellegrino, J., & Kadam, K. (2008). Fractionation of pre-hydrolysis products from lignocellulosic biomass by an ultrafiltration ceramic tubular membrane. *Separation Science and Technology*, 43(3), 447–476.
176. Sjöman, E., Mänttäri, M., Nyström, M., Koivikko, H., & Heikkilä, H. (2008). Xylose recovery by nanofiltration from different hemicellulose hydrolyzate feeds. *Journal of Membrane Science*, 310(1–2), 268–277.
177. Knutsen, J. S., & Davis, R. H. (2004). Cellulase retention and sugar removal by membrane ultrafiltration during lignocellulosic biomass hydrolysis. In *Proceedings of the Twenty-Fifth Symposium on Biotechnology for Fuels and Chemicals Held May 4–7, 2003, in Breckenridge, CO*, 585–599. Humana Press.
178. Maiti, S. K., Thuyavan, Y. L., Singh, S., Oberoi, H. S., & Agarwal, G. P. (2012). Modeling of the separation of inhibitory components from pretreated rice straw hydrolysate by nanofiltration membranes. *Bioresource Technology*, 114, 419–427.

8 Polyhydroxyalkanoates production from effluents – cheap renewable resources

Poorna Chandrika Sabapathy, Koushika Saravanan and Preethi Kathirvel

8.1 INTRODUCTION

8.1.1 THE NEED FOR BIOPOLYMERS

The contemporary utilization of restricted fossil resources for the production of polymers provokes prevailing worldwide problems such as the greenhouse effect and global warming. This is caused by the fact that these materials are utilized only during a relatively short time span. After that, they are often incinerated, elevating the atmospheric carbon dioxide concentration that contributes to the said heating effects. By incineration of plastic waste, the energy that is chemically stored therein is recovered as thermal energy. Braunegg et al. (2004) compared the heating value of plastic waste (approximately 42 MJ/kg) with the heating values of pit coal (approximately 28 MJ/kg), fuel oil (approximately 41 MJ/kg) and natural gas (45 MJ/kg). These heating values are rather high and, regarded simply from the energetic point of view, incineration of plastic waste is of interest. But it cannot be overlooked that the main problem arising from incineration is the same as for energy recovery from fuel oil, petrol, gasoline, natural gas and coal: carbon that was fixed over millions of years and that within this time was not part of the natural carbon cycle is converted to carbon dioxide that eventually accumulates in the atmosphere. When incineration is planned, strict emission standards have to be obeyed not only for carbon dioxide but also for highly toxic compounds such as dioxins and HCl deriving from poly (vinyl chloride) (Ojumu et al., 2004). Furthermore, the optimum energy recovery has to be evaluated. This includes the definition of the composition of the plastic waste (Braunegg et al., 2004). Additionally, a Swiss study showed that the capacities of the incinerators currently in use are insufficient to handle the tremendous amount of plastic waste (Hänggi, 1995). Besides, more and more waste of highly resistant plastics that are not incinerated is piled up every year. Recycling systems demand a certain degree of purity of the plastics to be reutilized, as well as a sorting accuracy; otherwise, they do not function sufficiently for a satisfactory solution of the problem. In addition, the collection costs are fairly high, and recycling has a negative impact on the mechanical properties of the materials, such as an increase in brittleness (Braunegg et al., 2004).

The environmental necessity to stop this negative development by switching to alternative strategies independent of fossil resources nowadays is generally undisputed. Already in 1992, the United Nations 'Rio Declaration on Environment and Development' explicitly specified the political intention and willingness of most countries to forcefully support the development of bio-based and biocompatible materials. Literally, Principle 4 of the 'Rio Declaration' states that: In order to achieve sustainable development, environmental protection shall constitute an integral

DOI: 10.1201/9781003500483-8
This chapter has been made available under a (CC-BY-NC-ND) 4.0 license

part of the development process and cannot be considered in isolation from it. With the tools of life cycle assessment (LCA) and cleaner production studies, much effort is contemporarily devoted to quantifying the environmental impact and feasibility of processes for production of polymeric materials (Sudesh and Iwata, 2008). In addition to the ecological considerations, the price of crude oil rocketed to a new all-time high of US $147 per barrel in 2008. Data for remaining amounts of fossil oil in Earth's interior are changing quickly owing to advanced methods for tracing and discharging of mineral oils. Nevertheless, one day, fossil feed stocks will finally be depleted. This causes an increasing awareness of the industrial branches involved for the exigency of fostering novel production techniques based on renewable resources and embedded into nature's closed cycles. With this 'white biotechnology', sustainable production of fine chemicals, bulk chemicals, polymers and fuels is achieved by the action of living organisms or parts thereof such as enzymes (Koller et al., 2010).

8.1.2 Polyhydroxyalkanoates

Production of polyhydroxyalkanoates (PHAs) has been investigated for more than 80 years, but recently a number of factors including increase in the price of crude oil and public awareness of the environmental issues have become a notable driving force for extended research on biopolymers. The versatility of PHAs has made them good candidates for the study of their potential in a variety of areas from biomedical/medical fields to food, packaging, textile and household material. While production costs are still a drawback to wider usage of these biopolymers, their application as low-volume high-cost items is becoming a reality. The future trend is to focus on the development of more efficient and economical processes for PHA production, isolation, purification and improvement of PHA material properties. (Keshavarz and Roy, 2010).

Mineral oil-based plastics (traditional plastics) have successfully replaced many other substances over the years and have been used extensively in domestic, medical and industrial applications. However, recent estimates on the earth's mineral resources, suggesting alarming rates of depletion of these valuable natural assets, have created renewed impetus to search for sustainable alternatives. The increasing cost and the awareness of consumers of the negative environmental impact of the fluid mineral fuels and related products have added to the drive to find novel raw materials for essential daily products with a 'green agenda'. Another serious point against continued large-extent use of the traditional plastics is their recalcitrance towards microbial degradation. In this context, attention has focused on research for the production of bioplastics (biodegradable polymers). For more than 70 years, petroleum-based plastics have been used in a variety of industrial and day-to-day applications owing to their versatility and durability (Ojumu et al., 2004; Zinn et al., 2001). However, they bear negative attributes including recalcitrance to biodegradation (Reddy et al., 2003), toxicity after incineration and massive waste accumulation into the landfills and the marine environment. In response to the problems associated with the synthetic polymers, the public tendency, the scientific interest and the governments' determination have worked in unison over the past two decades to support the development of a new class of plastics. The challenge for the new polymers is to retain the physico-chemical characteristics of the traditional plastics but benefit from biocompatibility and biodegradability (Lee, 1996).

While researchers were looking for a suitable alternative, they were unaware that the answer to their quest was already given in 1920s by the French microbiologist Maurice Lemoigne who discovered the polyester, poly (3-hydroxybutyrate), P(3HB) forming intracellular granules in Gram-positive bacterium *Bacillus megaterium* (Lemoigne, 1926) Polyhydroxybutyrate, P(3HB) is the first and most common biopolymer belonging to PHAs. Many years later, PHA containing 3HB and 3-hydroxyvalerate (3HV) was found in activated sludge (Wallen and Rohwedder, 1974). It took nearly a decade when (Findlay and White, 1983) reported PHAs with 11 varieties of linear and branched repeating units of four to eight carbon atoms. PHAs are the most versatile fully biodegradable polymers with properties similar to conventional plastics (Steinbüchel and Füchtenbusch, 1998). Other biodegradable polymers such as chemically synthesized plastics (e.g. polyglycollic acid and polylactic acid) and starch-based plastics (e.g. starch-polyethylene) have also appeared on the scene but they lack variability in structure and extensive material properties. Appreciable number of PHAs with more than 150 monomers (Steinbüchel and Lütke-Eversloh, 2003) have been identified with molecular masses ranging from 50,000 to 1,000,000 Da. As PHAs are biodegradable and immunologically inert, they have promising future applications, particularly in medical-related fields, despite their expensive production. The schematic representation of PHA production utilizing effluent is represented in Figure 8.1.

8.2 ECONOMIC FEASIBILITY – THE NEED FOR SUSTAINABLE AND RENEWABLE SUBSTRATES

The application of biotechnological processes for industrial production can be regarded as promising for sustainable development, although for a range of products biotechnological production strategies have not yet passed the test of economic viability. This is often caused by the cost of the raw materials. Here, a viable solution strategy can be identified in the utilization of a broad range of waste and surplus materials that can be upgraded to the role of feed stocks for the bio-smediated production of desired end products. Such materials are mainly produced in agriculture and industrial branches that are closely related to agriculture (Braunegg et al., 1998; Solaiman et al., 2006; Khardenavis et al., 2007; Khanna and Srivastava, 2005a). Especially, the economics of PHA production is determined to a great extent (up to 50% of the entire production costs) by the cost of the raw materials. This is caused by the fact that PHA accumulation occurs under aerobic conditions, resulting in high losses of the carbon substrate by intracellular respiration. Hence, only a maximum amount of less than 50% of the carbon source is directed towards biomass and PHA formation. The utilization of waste materials upgraded to the role of starting materials for PHA biosynthesis constitutes a viable strategy for cost-efficient biopolymer production and helps industry to overcome disposal problems. For many regions in the world, the industrial-scale realization of value-added conversion of low-cost agricultural feed stocks can provide a certain degree of geopolitical independence. The selection of the appropriate waste stream as a feedstock for biotechnological purposes mainly depends on the global region where a production plant will be constructed. To save transportation costs, facilities for the production of biopolymers, biofuels and biochemicals should be integrated into existing production lines, where the feed stocks directly accrue as waste streams. The availability of a convertible substrate all year round has to be ensured.

8.3 PHAS FROM EFFLUENTS – THE CHEAP SUBSTRATES AROUND THE GLOBE

To produce PHAs economically is a challenging task as it relies on the productivity, biomass of the organisms and the yield of PHA from it, the raw material used as carbon source and finally the recovery process (Choi and Lee, 1999). From all these, the cost of substrate contributes much to the overall production of PHA. As carbon source is the key factor for any fermentation process, it increases the cost up to 50% in the commercial production of PHA (Koller et al., 2008). Hence, economically viable production of PHA can be done by utilizing cheaper substrates which paves an eminent way for the industrial production of PHA, so that it can possibly replace the conventional plastics in all possible ways.

8.4 WASTE WATER SUBSTRATES FROM THE AGRO-INDUSTRY

8.4.1 EFFLUENT FROM H_2 REACTORS

Acid-rich effluent from a biohydrogen-producing reactor (HBR) was used as a primary substrate for the production of PHV using aerobic consortia as inoculum (biocatalysts) with anoxic

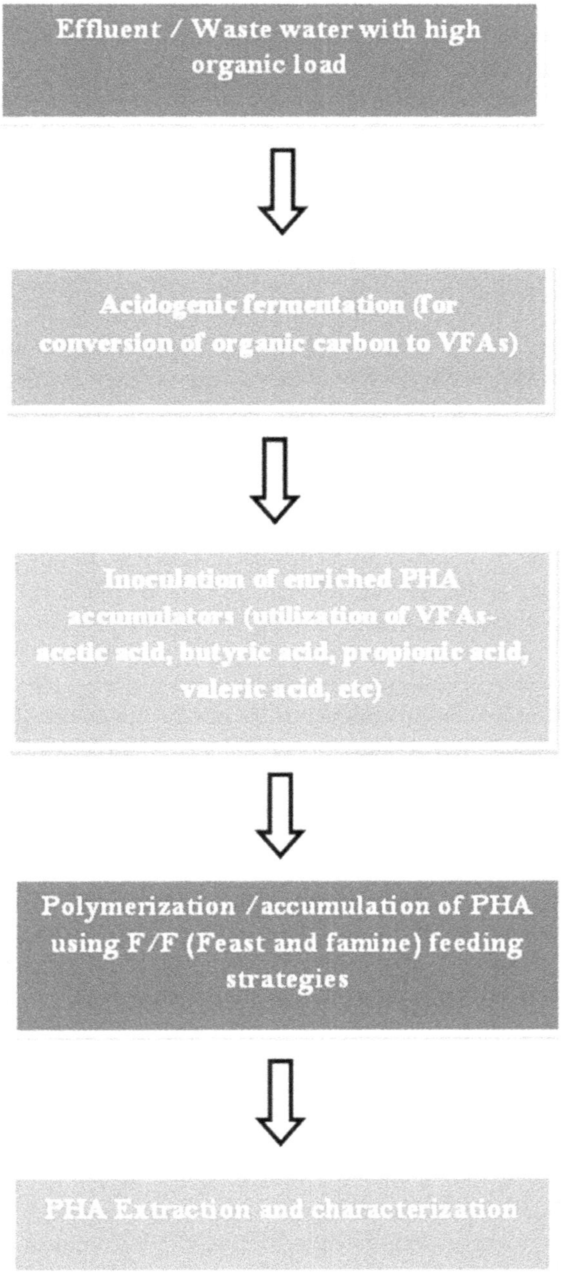

FIGURE 8.1 Schematic representation of commonly used methodology for the synthesis of PHA from effluent/waste water.

microenvironment. The VFA composition butyrate 33%, acetate 32%, propionate 11% other acids 26% was observed. In total, 25% PHV productivity was produced from the acidogenic effluent from water facilitate both product recovery and treatment of COD in the effluent. Neutral Redox condition showed a feasible microenvironment for PHB accumulation. VFA utilization relies mainly on the usage of substrates. At lower OLR (2.91 kg COD/m^3 day (44.75%) and 3.54 kg COD/m^3 day

(33.73%), higher reduction in VFA was observed, and production at higher OLR (4.58 & 7.53 kg COD/m^3 day), the amount of VFA fluctuated as there was both synthesis and utilization of VFA occurred (Venkata Mohan et al., 2012).

Using *Bacillus tequilensis* as biocatalyst for PHA from the spent wash coupled with biohydrogen production. The spent wash was initially used as substrate for the generation of biohydrogen, and the resultant acidogenic effluent was utilized for PHA production in a cost-effective manner. Maximum H_2 yield was 39.8 L, and PHA up to 40% DCW was obtained. A co-polymer of P (3HB- Co-3HV) was accumulated with high HB content than HV. The two-stage process was a promising approach for both substrate reduction and reduction in acidification through the recovery of value-added products (Amulya et al., 2014). Combined biohydrogen and biopolymer production from OMW using two stage system – VFAs produced by anaerobic fermentation (CSTR) followed by aerobic fermentation for polymer synthesis. Diluted OMW (1:4 V/V with tap water), with varied HRTs, was fed in the anaerobic reactors as the HRT defines the type of VFAs produced. Along with acetate, butyrate and propionate, valerate, isovalerate and isobutyrate in much lesser values were detected. The VFA-rich feed from the hydrogen fermentor was fermented aerobically with the enriched PHA-producing inoculum of bacteria (*Pseudomonas*.sp) and operated with subsequent feast and famine phases with limitation of nitrogen supply. The highest yield observed was 8.94% (w/w) dry weight of the biomass. Butyrate was the preferred substrate during the accumulation stage which states the fact that the PHA produced was polyhydroxybutyrate. Lower HRT values had positive effect on H_2 yield. Both H2 production and butyrate and acetate production were good at HRT 14.5, 27–33 h were good for total acidification of waste water and the production of propionate (Ntaikou et al., 2009).

Utilization of waste water shall serve as an interesting alternative for the cost-effective production of PHA. Biohydrogen reactor effluent serves as one of the potential substrate for the PHAs. Due to the high VFA content in the acidogenic effluent of biohydrogen reactors, these VFAs can be converted to PHA by exploiting suitable microorganisms. A novel strain *Pseudomonas otitidis* isolated from the mixed culture of PHA producing bioreactor was capable of producing PHA in both the synthetic acids and the acidogenic effluent from the reactor. In synthetic acids, the composition of the media was mimicked with that of the effluent from the reactor. The SA contained different organic loading rates (OLR) having acetate, propionate and butyrate, which were used for PHA production. The time taken for the maximum PHA production tended to increase with OLR. In SA OLR2 with 5 g/L of acetate, 0.5 g/L of propionate and 0.5 g/L of butyrate with 1.32 kg COD/m^3-day showed the highest PHA production as the strain belongs to the *Pseudomonas*. sp. Nitrogen limitation becomes an important factor; low nitrogen concentration (100 mg/L) was added in the reactor at the stage of PHA accumulation as it reduces the rate of protein synthesis and thus diverts the metabolic pathway towards the accumulation of PHA. As COD serves as the prime key in treating effluent, PHA production helps in reducing the COD of the effluent. With lesser OLR, higher removal efficiency was observed. The VFA composition of SA at 24 h for OLR 2 contained 90 ± 4% acetic acid, 4 ± 0.5% butyric acid, 5 ± 0.5% propionic acid, whereas AE had about 79 ± 3% acetic acid, 8 ± 1% butyric acid, 6 ± 0.5% propionic acid As in AE along with VFAs a lesser amount of carbohydrates was also present leading to the utilization of VFA removal than SE were only VFAs were present They utilized the acidogenic and synthetic effluents for P3(HB-co-HV) with high PHB content than PHV, concluding that these acidogenic effluent shall perform as better substrate for PHA production (Venkateswar Reddy et al., 2012).

8.4.2 Effluents from Sugarcane Industry

The effluent discharged from the sugar industry spoils the agricultural practices and aquatic organisms, thereby affecting the ecosystem greatly. The liquid waste effluent of sugar mills with high carbon and COD value was utilized for the synthesis of PHA using *Staphylococcus epidermidis* BU/SU1. The yield was contrasted with the synthetic mineral media for analysis. The effluent had about

50416 ppm COD, 28951 ppm BOD and 9720 ppm of total carbon content. After the fermentation process, the values reduced to 12600, 6119, and 4779 ppm. The fermentation process was carried out only for 48 h, leading to the production of 13 g/L of cell mass with commercially viable amount of P(3- HB) from the spent flow of sugar mill industry (Sarkar et al., 2014).

Bacillus megaterium and *Alcaligenes eutrophus* were grown in sugarcane effluent supplemented with different industrial waste medium yielding a cell mass of 0.250 in N_2-deficient medium and 0.358 in industrial waste medium for *B. megatherium* and 0.262 and 0.375 for *Alcaligenes eutrophus*. The yield of PHV was found to be more in *A. eutrophus* when compared with *B. megatherium*. The yield was 1.266 g/L (*A. eutrophus*) and 0.916 for *B. megatherium* (Kumaravel et al., 2010).

A three-step fermentation process for the PHA production using sugarcane molasses was carried out with two strategies: initially using acetate for culture selection and using fermented molasses for accumulation of PHA or utilizing the fermented molasses for both steps. The molasses was fermented acidogenically in a continuous stirred tank reactor (CSTR) under anaerobic conditions, an aerobic sequencing batch reactor (SBR) was used for PHA-accumulating culture selection and a batch reactor for PHA accumulation. Acetate and propionate were consumed at higher rates from the fermented molasses rather than other organic acids, after which butyrate and valerate rates increased. Fermented molasses with a pH of 5 gave high yield ranging from 0.22 g PHA/g molasses (0.26 PHA/g COD) to a volumetric production of 0.43 g PHA/h. An extensive study on the effect of pH, residual NH4+ and molasses matrix was done. With varied organic acid concentrations, the polymer composition differed. PHA accumulation was performed for selected cultures with fermented and clarified molasses as substrate (Albuquerque et al., 2007).

B. subtilus NG220 isolated from soil samples from sugarcane field area. The effluent had a high COD (1395± 317 mg/L) and BOD (1300 ± 238 mg/L). Maximum growth was observed in undiluted effluent after 72 h of incubation at 30°C. The organism produces about 4.928 g/L of PHB at 72 h under unoptimized conditions. In various dilutions, 20% −0.48, 40% −0.66, 60% −0.82, 80% −4.42, 100% −10.211 were the biomass (g/L) and 0.012, 4.928 PHB (g/L) for 80 and 100% was recorded (Singh et al., 2013).

P. aeruginosa NCIM 2948 produced 6.63 ± 0.05 g/L PHB concentration with the highest cell biomass and 4.14 ± 0.12 g/L of PHB concentration with 62.44% after 60 h of cultivation using cane molasses optimized with the composition as follows: cane molasses 40 g/L, urea 0.8 g/L, temperature-36°C and pH 7 and 175 rpm agitation speed (Tripathi et al., 2012).

8.4.3 Other agro-industrial waste water

With agro-industrial waste water like deproteinized jowar grain-based distillery spent wash, filtered rice grain-based distillery spent wash, PHA production shall be done effectively with low cost. Carbonaceous agro-industrial waste water could be explored as renewable substrates for the synthesis of PHA along with activated sludge. In this work, an addition of di-ammonium hydrogen phosphate (DAHP) resulted in the increase of PHB production (67%) in raw rice grain-based spent wash being used. Waste water from food processing and starch-rich grain-based industries with high COD values showing C:N ratio 50:1 (g/g) which was very optimal for maximum PHB accumulation in 96 h. The food processing waste water had a COD of 3.60 (g/L), VFA-6.40 (g/L), 2.75 (g/L) total sugars and the jowar grain-based distillery spent wash had a COD of 10.80 (g/L), VFA-0.65 (g/L), total sugars-0.225 (g/L). The rice grain-based distillery spent wash had a COD of 35 (g/L), VFA-1.46 (g/L), total sugars-5.40 (g/L) (Khardenavis et al., 2007).

In raw rice grain-based distillery spent wash had about 2.7 g/L (67% W/W) PHB with a highest biomass concentration of 6.6 g/L, corresponding to the productivity of 0.28 g/L/h and a yield of 0.212 (PHB g/COD consumed). Filtered food processing waste water gave 0.013 g/L/h and 0.021 g/L/h for deproteinized jowar grain- based distillery spent wash. Cassava waste water (CW) along with cooking oil and waste frying oil were investigated as cost- effective substrates for both rhamnolipid and PHA production from *P. aeruginosa* L2-1.

Industrial waste water from milk, wood and paper mill processing was acidogenically fermented for PHA production. Whey and paper mill effluent had nearly 100% readily available SCOD (soluble COD) for the process of fermentation. For whey, at retention time 95 h, the maximum of 0.93 g COD of VFA/influent SCOD and for paper mill effluent 0.75 g COD/g COD at RT 24 h were observed with high degree of acidification. Acetate, propionate and butyrate were the major products of fermentation. These experiments gave valuable data about the influence of RT and pH on regulating the monomeric composition of PHA and accompanying properties (Bengtsson et al., 2008).

8.4.4 Palm oil mill effluent (POME)

Palm oil mill effluent (POME) causes huge oxygen depletion in aquatic system because of the high organic and nutrient content. It constitutes different sugars like arabinose, xylose, glucose, galactose and mannose, COD-50000 mg/L, BOD of 25000 mg/L (Nakanishi & Hashimoto,1997). A mixed microbial consortium for PHA synthesis from high concentration of POME was used in a two-step process of acidogenesis and acid polymerization. In total, 5–8 g/L of VFA concentration was noted with a reduction of 80% of COD from 65 g/L at 40% of DCW maximum content of PHA was observed. In the anaerobic reactor, the palm oil fibres were used as support matrix. In total, 80% of COD removal was achieved at SRT of six days fermentation. The substrate volume decides the amount of biomass produced, and the amount of VFA corresponds to the amount of polymer produced. From the analysis of Do and oxygen uptake rate (OUR), it was significant that PHAs were stored during feast period and their degradation studied in the famine period as PHAs serves as internal source of carbon and energy (Salmiati et al., 2007).

Ralstonia eutropha JMP 134 produced PHA utilizing the VFAs from POME fermented anaerobically by using the same system of strategies of two-step fermentation. VFA from the first day of anaerobic fermentation at a pH of 4.43 was noted to be the best. The content of VFA from fresh fermented and distilled fermented POME (DFP) was taken. The DFP had the highest VFA concentration of 2.97 g/L acetic acid, 1.18 g/L of propionic acid and 3.04 g/L butyric acid. 0.048 g/L/h of PHA productivity in fed batch mode with 12% mol increase in 3HV with the addition of DFP (Setiadi et al., 2015).

A Bio-PoRec® system with aerobic feeding condition for high yield of PHA using POME showed maximum PHA production at a specific rate of 0.434 C- mol/C- mol/h with a yield of 0.80 C- mol/C- mol acetic acid at a microaerophilic condition. Acetic acid was found abundantly and is the most used fatty acid by the organism. A cyclic anoxic and aerobic condition was maintained for the production of needed electron acceptors (O_2 and N_2) in the reactor. They also studied the effect of C: N:P ratio and the feeding regime on the PHA production- 400 and 200 were the ratio of COD/N and COD/P for maximum optimal storage of PHA content. They reported that limitation of P caused higher accumulation of PHA when compared with the limitation of N (Din et al., 2012).

Acetic acid recovered from POME was used as sole carbon source for the generation of PHA in *Alcaligenes eutrophus*. The inhibition of acetic acid absorption to the anion exchange resin was solved by removing the sludge particles from POME, thus effectively separating the acetic acid to about 45% PHA content in dry cells corresponding to the yield of 0.32 g from it. The overall production was estimated to be 0.09 g PHA/L/h (Hassan et al., 1997).

Each ton of fresh fruit brunch for palm oil processing yields 1 ton liquid waste called POME with BOD of 37.5 kg, COD 75 kg, suspended solids 27 kg. Through partial anaerobic fermentation of POME, low molecular weight organic acids like acetic acid, propionic acid and butyric acid were produced using a pilot-scale filtration and evaporation system. The high solid fraction in POME was removed mechanically and clarified as it has more than 90% of water (Mumtaz et al., 2008).

Photosynthetic bacterium *Rhodobacter sphaeroides* (IFO 12203) produced PHA utilizing anaerobically treated POME devoid of sludge particles. More than 1.0 g of PHA/L from 5.5 g/L of organic acids corresponding to more than 30% of the DCW was obtained at the dilution rate of 0.072/d, with 0.024/d dilution 2 g of PHA/L from 15 g/L of organic acids (CDW more than 60%)

from POME. The activity of the cell for the accumulation of PHA was maintained by addition of ammonium and phosphate as anaerobically treated POME lacks these. With higher C/N ratio the PHA accumulation becomes directly proportional to that (Hassan et al., 1997).

8.4.5 Effluents of Dairy Industry

Along with the effluents of dairy industry (Whey), another inexpensive substrate, namely, starch was used for the production of PHB through fed batch culturing by *Azotobacter chroococcum* and recombinant *E. coli*. With oxygen limitation, *A. chroococuum* showed a cell concentration of 54 g/L with 64% PHB, without oxygen limitation, the values varied to be 71 g/L of cell concentration with 20% PHB content. Even in recombinant *E. coli* the oxygen limitation has notable changes, where it was controlled by the agitation speed of a stirred tank fermentor. 80% PHB content was recorded due to the oxygen limitation attained by agitation speed of 500 ppm (Kim, 2000).

8.4.6 Starchy Waste Water

Starchy waste water derived from textile, paper, fermentation, beverage and food processing with COD of 1100–10000 mg COD/L was successfully used for the synthesis of PHA through microbial acidogenesis and acid polymerization with total VFA reaching 4000 mg/L (utilizing 43% of organic carbon) at a COD loading rate of 2–35 g/L/d from the digestion of starchy waste water in a thermophilic upflow anaerobic sludge blanket (USAB) reactor using *A. eutrophus* to produce PHA. Utilizing 100 g TOC, 50 g PHA was produced (yield 28%) which was in range with the production from pure butyric and propionic acid (55 g PHA/100 g TOC). Butyric and propionic acid (48 and 53%) contributed to PHB production. The propionate composition controls the composition of PHA; the specific PHA formation rate increased from 10 to 35 mg PHA/g of biomass/h with an increase in the butyric acid concentration (Yu, 2001).

The cassava industry produces starch rich waste water with 30% of raw material input. The waste water treated in SBR with activated sludge which produced PHA content of 0.03–0.10 g PHA/g MLSS, but the removal of COD was not efficient, and the combined aerobic and anaerobic fermentation had no significant impact on the COD removal and PHA generation (Setyawaty et al., 2011).

Alcaligenes eutropus (WSH3) produced PHA from the organic waste water by a composite anaerobic acidification fermentation system. In total, 10 g/L of PHA from approximately 68.9% of cell mass (15.8 g/L DCW) was obtained. By the acidogenic fermentation, acids were produced which in turn were fermented to synthesize PHA. The amount of acid produced was found to increase with temperature (100% at 40°C). Rather than batch fermentation, fed batch fermentation exhibited good results with high yield of PHA in both acidified and concentrated waste water (Jin et al., 1999).

Cassava is among the major agricultural products estimated to be produced about 160 million tons/year worldwide. Production of cassava flour generates large amount of effluent rich in carbohydrate residue. (Contiero, 2009). CW with waste frying oil showed good yield of both the products (PHA-39% of DCW and rhamnolipid-660 mg/L) 17.6± 1.3% PHA accumulation, 3.3 ± 0.1 CDW (g/L) and 300.3 ± 18.1(mg/L) of Rhamnolipid was produced using CW alone (Costa et al., 2009).

Cassava starch waste water from SBR treatment system was used to produce PHA by *Bacillus tequilensis* MSU112. Anoxic and aerobic fermentation was employed on 4/18 h basis with total reaction period of 24 h. With different COD concentration of waste water (3000, 4000 and 5000 mg/L), the yield was about 79.2% (dry sludge weight) with 3346 mg/L of PHA concentration (COD-4000 mg/L), whereas COD concentration of 5000 mg/L had the highest COD removal efficiency (94.8%). The anoxic phase yielded high PHA than the aerobic condition (Chaleomrum et al., 2014).

Sago effluents along with waste substrates were studied for the generation of PHA using *A. eutrophus* MTCC 1285. In the molasses-based effluent highest PHB yield was recorded at a pH of 8.0 (Senthilkumar & Prabakaran, 2006).

By using a novel process, PHA from *Alcaligenes eutropus* was produced through two distinctive stages: cell growth with fructose and from acidified water PHA was synthesized from the VFAs. The work states that a good growth of cells was observed in fructose than in VFA as VFA was used as substrate for polymerization, giving a yield of 9.6 g/L PHA with a DCW of 15.9 g/L. Butyric acid was the most suitable VFA for *A. eutrophus* for the synthesis of PHA than others and also the next important consideration for PHA production was the total number of cells present in the fermentation medium (Ruan et al., 2003).

Forest industry waste water has large amount of fermentable organic water. Explained by several researchers, the three-stage process was the effective strategy for the production of PHA from waste water. Paper mill effluent waste water was acidogenically fermented, where the organic waste in the effluent gets converted into VFAs followed by an activated sludge system where the PHA producers were enriched by the feast and famine Phase of feeding, and finally the PHA was accumulated. About 74% of soluble COD was converted as VFA after the fermentation of the waste water. The maximum PHA content was the 48% with a yield of 0.11 kg/kg of influent COD. The accumulated PHA had 31–47 mol % hydroxybutyrate and 53–69 mol % hydroxyvalerate. The diluted waste water had the concentration of soluble COD -8750 mg COD/L, acetate -870 mg COD/L, propionate -170 mg COD/L, butyrate 50 mg COD/L, valerate 120 mg COD/L. During acidogenic fermentation, about 75% of soluble COD was converted to VFA. 18% converted to biomass and 7% was lost in the conversion. During the enrichment of PHA produce, 95% soluble COD was removed. From 1 kg soluble COD, 0.16 kg COD was utilized for biomass production etc. Yielding 75% VFA from the acidogenic fermentation the 0.85 kg COD was splitted for biomass enrichment (0.43 kg COD) and (0.41 kg COD) for PHA accumulated (0.13 kg TSS) yielding 0.11 kg PHA (Bengtsson et al., 2008).

Activated sludge treatment of municipal waste water for the production of PHA was investigated with three major factors taken into consideration, namely, acetate concentration influent, pH and SRT (sludge retention time) 31% of PHA was accumulated in the municipal waste water supplemented with acetate, whereas the sludge acclamations only with municipal waste water achieved 21% of sludge dry weight. The typical municipal waste water with COD 60–130 mg O/L, TOC of 30–130 mg C/L, acetate-0.2 mg/L and 1.7–5.6 mg P/L phosphate. Optimization of activated sludge process for better PHA production yielded 30% of PHA. With a short SRT of three days better PHA content (10%) was exhibited than a longer SRT of ten days (Chua et al., 2003).

Two-phase olive mill waste water (TPOMW-alpeorujo) where diluted at different concentrations and used as substrates for PHA production by three strains of *Azotobacter* sp. The yield of PHA increased when TPOMW was fermented anaerobically beforehand. The organism produced homopolymers having β- hydroxybutyrate. After 72 h of fermentation, 72% of COD reduction was observed. Alpeorujo had a COD of 175 g/L, N (15%), total phenolic content of 2.5% and total reducing sugars of 9.1% (Cerrone et al., 2010).

Mixed microbial consortia (MMC) of PHA producers yielded 1.50 g/L/d utilizing olive Mill waste water in a sequential process, thereby helping in the removal of phenols and recovery of PHA. With different OLR ranging from 2.40 to 8.40 g COD/L/d was investigated with dephenolized and fermented OMW. 4.70 g/COD/L/d was the optimal OLR with high storage rate and yield (339±48 mg COD g/g COD h and 0.56± 0.05 COD/COD). Direct biological treatment of OMW being impossible because of their high content of polyphenols, hindering the growth of bacteria. Hence, different physiochemical and chemical methods for treatment of OMW were manipulated. A single treatment can never satisfactorily make the waste water to be eco-friendly, a combined multi-step method for the valorization of OMW for PHA production and the recovery of polyphenol was done. Two different types of pretreated OMW were used. PHA accumulating microorganisms shall be selected based on the selective pressure into the SBR and during famine phase along with VFA other soluble COD was also consumed. During the initial stage the phenols removal was higher to about 80% concentration of reduction of COD (25%), and after acidogenic fermentation it was reduced further due to the production of methane. By considering dephenolized and the fermented OMW the PHA generated from the COD was about 14 and 22%, respectively. The influent COD to polymer conservation accounted to10% with a PHA production of 3.30 g COD/d with an abatement of 85% initial COD content of OMW (Campanari et al., 2014).

A two-stage pilot scale system for the synthesis of PHA from olive Mill waste was made using Municipal waste water treatment plant-derived mixed culture of anaerobic and aerobic cultures, which were initially used to treat OMW for acidification in a continuous mode. From the anaerobic reactor, the acidogenic effluent was treated aerobically with nutrition limitation to which an enriched culture of pseudomonas SP was added as limited inoculum. A comparison between clarified and unclarified acidogenic effluent was reported. The produced PHA consisted (3HB) 3-hydroxybutyrate and 3-hydroxyoctanoate (HO) units explaining that it shells either be a blend of these two homopolymer or 3HB-Co-3HO co-polymer which seems to be a rare occurrence naturally, exhibiting advanced properties. The final microbial consortia formed were found to be highly diverse which was evident with the average molecular mass of the obtained PHA (490 KDa) with a wide molecular weight distribution (PDI-5.15) (Ntaikou et al., 2014).

By batch and two-stage batch culture industrial effluent like corn stalk water, corn corb petroleum refinery effluent yielded a maximum yield of PHV 3.1 mg/L. *Bacillus megatherium* MTCC 8075 was exploited to produce PHB which was improved by two stage fermentation studies with a comparison on various nutrients limitation condition (N&P). The optimization studies revealed that glucose (6%) and peptone were the preferred C&N sources (Aswathy et al., 2015).

Cardboard industrial waste water was typically rich in carbohydrates with fixed nitrogen, these conditions favour the PHA production from bacteria. They have a high BOD (680–1250 mg/L) and COD (3400–5780 mg/L) and COD/BOD ratio b/w 3.95 bacillus SP NAIO isolated from soil accumulated up to 66.6% of DCW with 0.072 g/L/h (Bhuwal et al., 2014).

With a high COD content (100–200 COD/L), OMEs were of serious environment concern in the olive oil-producing countries. The high COD value of OMEs indeed is advantageous for PHA production as through acidogenic fermentation they produce more amounts of VFAs (Cerrone et al., 2010). OMEs were successfully exploited for the production of PHA using three sequential fermentation strategies proposed by Dionasi et al (2004). Utilizing various pretreatment steps the effluent was processed and used for the fermentation later. The pretreatment had specific effects on the COD removal and on the rate and yield of VFAs produced. Pretreatment along with centrifugation caused relatively 30–40% increased yield of VFA than that produced from untreated OME. PHA production was tested with centrifuged and fermented OME and centrifuged unfermented OME. Centrifuged and fermented OME with a fermentation yield from 25 to 36% at a primary concentration of 36.7 g COD per L and 9 to 13 g COD per L of VFA concentration was found favourable for PHA storage when compared with untreated OME. The initial specific rate of 417 mg COD per g COD per h with maximum HV (11%) content within the copolymer was observed. Even though the acids like acetic acid and butyric acid were predominant in VFA, the more amounts of propionic and valeric acids were also produced. These acids help in the increase of HV content in the copolymer P(HB-HV) there by increasing the thermal and mechanical properties (Dionisi et al., 2005).

Packed bed biofilm reactor (PBBR) was used for the anaerobic fermentation OMEs and SBR for the aerobic stage for production of PHA using microbial consortia. From 18%, the percentage of VFA was increased to about 32% of the overall COD by the anaerobic fermentation process. The SBR feed with OME from PBBR with an organic load rate (OLR) of 8.5 g COD L^{-1} d^{-1}, a maximum substrate utilization rate of 146 mg COD g^{-1} COD h^{-1}, and a storage yield of 0.36 g COD g^{-1} COD. From the experiment, it was known that not alone VFAs contribute to the PHA accumulation, half of the stored PHAs were produced from other substrates especially alcohol constituting about 22% of the total COD (Beccari et al., 2009).

Enterobacter aerogenes 12Bi isolated from the cooling towers of a petrochemical industry plant was grown on domestic waste water (DWW) for the first time. COD -100–300 mg/L, COD -100–500 mg/L, phosphorous 6–20 mg/L where the major contributes of typically DWW. As the DWW plays a key role in polluting different water bodies. Accompany with disposal of waste products in it. Various methods of treatment were investigated with one being the synthesis of PHA in it. With different concentration of DWW along with yeast nitrogen both medium being supplemented, expect for 100% in all other concentration the strain showed good growth. The organism had the highest growth at 24 h, the yield of PHB on the media with DWW was 96.25% which was observed after 18 h of growth with 100%. DWW and a highest biomass of 5.8 g/L was obtained at 80% DWW medium (Ceyhan and Ozdemir, 2011).

Waste water from the processing of milk and ice cream was exploded for the synthesis of PHAs in reactor system interesting an acidogenic reactor (AAR) for VFA Production, a conventional activated sludge production reactor (ASPR) for the production of both activated sludge, which was mixed together in PHA synthesis reactor (PHAR) for the accumulation of PHA.AAR(optimal pH approximately 6.0 ± 0.3; ORP (oxidation reduction potential) 85 ± 10 mV with VFA analysis of biomass) 5400 mg/L, F/M -0.8± HRT -17.3 h, MLSS concentration -1800 mg/L (average). The F/M ratio represents the optimal COD to MLSS ratio. In ASPR, the value of K_s, μ_m, Y_{obs} and k_d was derived as 37.16 mg/L COD, 0.51 mg MLSS/mg COD. In the PHAR kinetic study, the maximum yield coefficient (Y_{sp}max) was derived as 0.25 kg PHA/kg of COD being degraded. The PHAR growth kinetics was studies using a revised metabolic model (Chakravarthy et al., 2010). Mixed consortia of microorganisms to treat waste water shall reduce the operational cost as it does not require the maintenance of sterile condition & the reactor system. Mixed consortia is more advantageous than pure culture in both economical and waste management effectively. Using the designed synthetic waste water (DSW) as substrates an anoxic microenvironment was maintained for PHA production using mixed consortia. From the optimization studies, it was known that higher the organic load (carbon concentration) higher the accumulation of PHA can be observed which also corresponds to the time taken for accumulation also being increased (OLR 3 at 60th h (40.3%). From 12th to 60th h, PHA accumulation increased and there after decreased (72nd h, 26.3%). Lowering the concentration of N2 exhibited higher PHB accumulation. From the optimization studies performed N1 showed 45.1% at 60 h, N2–41.5%, N3–38%; like less N phosphorous concentration lessening showed higher PHA accumulation. Hence OLR 3, N1 and P1 were considered the optimal conditions for PHA production. In this work, the first report of the organism *Pseudomonas otitidis* on PHA accumulation was reported (Venkateswar Reddy et al., 2012).

8.5 CONCLUSION

It would be wise to use renewable and sustainable substrates for any value-added product production. As for PHA production to hit the common market, utilization of these industrial wastes shall be the only way, which shall pave the way for a new generation of truly biodegradable plastics.

ACKNOWLEDGEMENT

The authors thank the Department of Science and Technology (DST) for supporting the Department of Microbial Biotechnology, Bharathiar University, Tamil Nadu under DST-FIST scheme to have necessary facilities for the successful execution of this work.

REFERENCES

Albuquerque, M. G. E., Eiroa, M., Torres, C., Nunes, B. R., & Reis, M. A. M. (2007). Strategies for the development of a side stream process for polyhydroxyalkanoate (PHA) production from sugar cane molasses. *Journal of Biotechnology*, *130*(4), 411–421.

Amulya, K., Reddy, M. V., & Mohan, S. V. (2014). Acidogenic spent wash valorization through polyhydroxyalkanoate (PHA) synthesis coupled with fermentative biohydrogen production. *Bioresource Technology, 158*, 336–342.

Aswathy, M. (2015). Production of bio-plastics (polyhydroxybutyrate) from industrial effluent using batch and two stage batch culture studies. *Indian Journal of Science and Technology, 8*(32), 1–6.

Beccari, M., Bertin, L., Dionisi, D., Fava, F., Lampis, S., Majone, M., Valentino, F., Vallini, G., & Villano, M. (2009). Exploiting olive oil mill effluents as a renewable resource for production of biodegradable polymers through a combined anaerobic–aerobic process. *Journal of Chemical Technology and Biotechnology, 84*(6), 901–908.

Bengtsson, S., Werker, A., Christensson, M., & Welander, T. (2008). Production of polyhydroxyalkanoates by activated sludge treating a paper mill wastewater. *Bioresource Technology, 99*(3), 509–516.

Bhuwal, A. K., Singh, G., Aggarwal, N. K., Goyal, V., & Yadav, A. (2014). Poly-β-hydroxybutyrate production and management of cardboard industry effluent by new *Bacillus* sp. NA10. *Bioresources and Bioprocessing, 1*(9), 1–11.

Braunegg, G., Bona, R., & Koller, M. (2004). Sustainable polymer production. *Polymer-Plastics Technology and Engineering, 43*(6), 1779–1793.

Campanari, S., Silva, F. A., Bertin, L., Villano, M., & Majone, M. (2014). Effect of the organic loading rate on the production of polyhydroxyalkanoates in a multi-stage process aimed at the valorization of olive oil mill wastewater. *International Journal of Biological Macromolecules, 71*, 34–41. https://doi.org/10.1016/j.ijbiomac.2014.06.021

Cerrone, F., Sánchez-Peinado, M. M., Juárez-Jiménez, B., González-López, J., & Pozo, C. (2010).Biological treatment of two-phase olive mill wastewater (TPOMW, alpeorujo): Polyhydroxyalkanoates (PHAs) production by *Azotobacter* strains. *Journal of Microbiology and Biotechnology, 20*(3), 594–601.

Ceyhan, N., & Ozdemir, G. (2011). Poly-β-hydroxybutyrate (PHB) production from domestic wastewater using Enterobacter aerogenes 12Bi strain. *African Journal of Microbiology Research, 5*(6), 690–702.

Chakravarty, P., Mhaisalkar, V., & Chakrabarti, T. (2010). Study on poly-hydroxyalkanoate (PHA) production in pilot scale continuous mode wastewater treatment system. *Bioresource Technology, 101*(8), 2896–2899.

Chaleomrum, N., Chookietwattana, K., & Dararat, S. (2014). Production of PHA from cassava starch wastewater in sequencing batch reactor treatment system. *APCBEE Procedia, 8*, 167–172. https://doi.org/10.1016/j.apcbee.2014.03.023

Choi, J., & Lee, S. Y. (1999). Factors affecting the economics of polyhydroxyalkanoate production by bacterial fermentation. *Applied Microbiology and Biotechnology, 51*(1), 13–21.

Chua, A. S., Takabatake, H., Satoh, H., & Mino, T. (2003). Production of polyhydroxyalkanoates (PHA) by activated sludge treating municipal wastewater: effect of pH, sludge retention time (SRT), and acetate concentration in influent. *Water Research, 37*(15), 3602–3611.

Contiero, J. (2009). Cassava wastewater as a substrate for the simultaneous production of rhamnolipids and polyhydroxyalkanoates by *Pseudomonas aeruginosa*. *Journal of Industrial Microbiology & Biotechnology, 36*(8), 1063–1072.

Costa, S. G., Lépine, F., Milot, S., Déziel, E., Nitschke, M., & Contiero, J. (2009). Cassava wastewater as a substrate for the simultaneous production of rhamnolipids and polyhydroxyalkanoates by Pseudomonas aeruginosa. *Journal of Industrial Microbiology and Biotechnology, 36*(8), 1063–1072.

Din, M. F. M., Mohanadoss, P., Ujang, Z., van Loosdrecht, M., Yunus, S. M., Chelliapan, S., ... & Olsson, G. (2012). Development of Bio-PORec® system for polyhydroxyalkanoates (PHA) production and its storage in mixed cultures of palm oil mill effluent (POME). *Bioresource Technology, 124*, 208–216.

Dionisi, D., Carucci, G., Papini, M. P., Riccardi, C., Majone, M., & Carrasco, F. (2005). Olive oil mill effluents as a feedstock for production of biodegradable polymers. *Water Research, 39*(10), 2076–2084.

Findlay, R. H., & White, D. C. (1983). Polymeric beta-hydroxyalkanoates from environmental samples and *Bacillus megaterium*. *Applied and Environmental Microbiology, 45*(1), 71–78.

Hänggi, U. J. (1995). Requirements on bacterial polyesters as future substitute for conventional plastics for consumer goods. *FEMS Microbiology Reviews, 16*(2–3), 213–220.

Hassan, M. A., Shirai, Y., Kusubayashi, N., Karim, M. I. A., Nakanishi, K., & Hasimoto, K. (1997). The production of polyhydroxyalkanoate from anaerobically treated palm oil mill effluent by Rhodobacter sphaeroides. *Journal of Fermentation and Bioengineering, 83*(5), 485–488.

Hassan, M. A., Shirai, Y., Umeki, H., Yamazumi, H., Jin, S., Yamamoto, S., Abdul Karim, M. I., Nakanishi, K., & Hashimoto, K. (1997). Acetic acid separation from anaerobically treated palm oil mill effluent by ion exchange resins for the production of polyhydroxyalkanoate by *Alcaligenes eutrophus*. *Bioscience, Biotechnology, and Biochemistry, 61*(9), 1465–1468.

Jin, D., Chen, J., & Lun, S. (1999). Production of poly(hydroxyalkanoate) by a composite anaerobic acidification–fermentation system. *Process Biochemistry, 34*(9), 829–833.

Keshavarz, T., & Roy, I. (2010). Polyhydroxyalkanoates: Bioplastics with a green agenda. *Current Opinion in Microbiology, 13*(3), 321–326. https://doi.org/10.1016/j.mib.2010.02.006

Khanna, S., & Srivastava, A. K. (2005). Recent advances in microbial polyhydroxyalkanoates. *Process Biochemistry, 40*(2), 607–619.

Khardenavis, A. A., Kumar, M. S., Mudliar, S. N., & Chakrabarti, T. (2007). Biotechnological conversion of agro-industrial wastewaters into biodegradable plastic, poly β-hydroxybutyrate. *Bioresource Technology, 98*(17), 3579–3584.

Kim, B. S. (2000). Production of poly(3-hydroxybutyrate) from inexpensive substrates. *Enzyme and Microbial Technology, 27*(10), 774–777.

Koller, M., Atlić, A., Dias, M., Reiterer, A., & Braunegg, G. (2010). Microbial PHA production from waste raw materials. In G. Steinbüchel (Ed.), *Plastics from bacteria* (pp. 85–119). Springer. https://doi.org/10.1007/978-3-642-03287-5_6

Koller, M., Bona, R., Chiellini, E., Fernandes, E. G., Horvat, P., Kutscher, C., Hesse, P., & Braunegg, G. (2008). Polyhydroxyalkanoate production from whey by *Pseudomonas hydrogenovora*. *Bioresource Technology, 99*(11), 4854–4863.

Kumaravel, S., Hema, R., & Lakshmi, R. (2010). Production of polyhydroxybutyrate (bioplastic) and its biodegradation by *Pseudomonas lemoignei* and *Aspergillus niger*. *E-Journal of Chemistry, 7*(S1), S536–S542.

Lee, S. Y. (1996). Bacterial polyhydroxyalkanoates. *Biotechnology and Bioengineering, 49*(1), 1–14.

Lemoigne, M. (1926). Produits de déshydration et de polymérisation de l'acide β-hydroxybutyrique. *Bulletin de la Société Chimique de Biologie, 8*, 770–782.

Mumtaz, T., Abd-Aziz, S., Rahman, N. A. A., Yee, P. L., Shirai, Y., & Hassan, M. A. (2008). Pilot-scale recovery of low molecular weight organic acids from anaerobically treated palm oil mill effluent (POME) with energy integrated system. *African Journal of Biotechnology*, *7*(21), 3900–3905.

Nakanishi, K., & Hashimoto, K. (1997). The production of polyhydroxyalkanoate from anaerobically treated palm oil mill effluent by *Rhodobacter sphaeroides*. *Journal of Fermentation and Bioengineering, 83*(5), 485–488.

Ntaikou, I., Kourmentza, C., Koutrouli, E. C., Stamatelatou, K., Zampraka, A., Kornaros, M., & Lyberatos, G. (2009). Exploitation of olive oil mill wastewater for combined biohydrogen and biopolymers production. *Bioresource Technology, 100*(15), 3724–3730. https://doi.org/10.1016/j.biortech.2008.12.013

Ntaikou, I., Valencia Peroni, C., Kourmentza, C., Ilieva, V. I., Morelli, A., Chiellini, E., & Lyberatos, G. (2014). Microbial bio-based plastics from olive-mill wastewater: Generation and properties of polyhydroxyalkanoates from mixed cultures in a two-stage pilot scale system. *Journal of Biotechnology, 188*, 138–147. https://doi.org/10.1016/j.jbiotec.2014.08.030

Ojumu, T. V., Yu, J., & Solomon, B. O. (2004). Production of polyhydroxyalkanoates, a bacterial biodegradable polymers. *African Journal of Biotechnology, 3*(1), 18–24. https://doi.org/10.5897/AJB2004.000-2005

Reddy, C. S. K., Ghai, R., & Kalia, V. (2003). Polyhydroxyalkanoates: An overview. *Bioresource Technology, 87*(2), 137–146. https://doi.org/10.1016/S0960-8524(02)00212-2

Ruan, W., Chen, J., & Lun, S. (2003). Production of biodegradable polymer by *Alcaligenes eutrophus* using volatile fatty acids from acidified wastewater. *Process Biochemistry, 39*(3), 295–299.

Sarkar, K., Ray, B., Banerjee, R., Saha, S., Roy, S., & Chatterjee, S. (2014). Poly-β-hydroxybutyrate (bioplastic) production utilizing waste effluent of a sugar industry. *IOSR Journal of Environmental Science, Toxicology and Food Technology, 8*(4), 26–31.

Setiadi, T., Aznury, M., Trianto, A., & Pancoro, A. (2015). Production of polyhydroxyalkanoate (PHA) by *Ralstonia eutropha* JMP 134 with volatile fatty acids from palm oil mill effluent as precursors. *Water Science and Technology, 72*(11), 1889–1895. https://doi.org/10.2166/wst.2015.428

Setyawaty, R., Setiadi, T., Katayama-Hirayama, K., Kaneko, H., Hirayama, K., Indonesia, J., & No, G. (2011). Polyhydroxyalkanoate (PHA) production from tapioca industrial wastewater treatment: Operating conditions and influence on PHA content. *Environmental Research, 22*, 123–127.

Singh, G., Kumari, A., Mittal, A., Yadav, A., & Kumar, N. (2013). Poly-β-hydroxybutyrate production by *Bacillus subtilis* NG220 using sugar industry wastewater. *BioMed Research International, 2013*, Article ID 952641. https://doi.org/10.1155/2013/952641

Solaiman, D. K., Ashby, R. D., Foglia, T. A., & Marmer, W. N. (2006). Conversion of agricultural feedstock and coproducts into poly (hydroxyalkanoates). *Applied Microbiology and Biotechnology*, *71*(6), 783–789.

Steinbüchel, A., & Füchtenbusch, B. (1998). Bacterial and other biological systems for polyester production. *Trends in Biotechnology, 16*(10), 419–427.

Steinbüchel, A., & Lütke-Eversloh, T. (2003). Metabolic engineering and pathway construction for biotechnological production of relevant polyhydroxyalkanoates in microorganisms. *Biochemical Engineering Journal, 16*(2), 81–96.

Sudesh, K., & Iwata, T. (2008). Sustainability of biobased and biodegradable plastics. *CLEAN – Soil, Air, Water, 36*(5–6), 433–442.

Tripathi, A. D., Yadav, A., Jha, A., & Srivastava, S. K. (2012). Utilizing of sugar refinery waste (cane molasses) for production of bio-plastic under submerged fermentation process. *Journal of Polymers and the Environment, 20*(2), 446–453.

Venkateswar Reddy, M., & Venkata Mohan, S. (2012). Effect of substrate load and nutrients concentration on the polyhydroxyalkanoates (PHA) production using mixed consortia through wastewater treatment. *Bioresource Technology, 114*, 573–582. https://doi.org/10.1016/j.biortech.2012.03.019

Wallen, L. L., & Rohwedder, W. K. (1974). Poly-β-hydroxyalkanoate from activated sludge. *Environmental Science & Technology, 8*(6), 576–579. https://doi.org/10.1021/es60091a009

Yu, J. (2001). Production of PHA from starchy wastewater via organic acids. *Journal of Biotechnology, 86*(2), 105–112.

Zinn, M., Witholt, B., & Egli, T. (2001). Occurrence, synthesis and medical application of bacterial polyhydroxyalkanoate. *Advanced Drug Delivery Reviews, 53*(1), 5–21.

9 Production of biofuels from biomolecules obtained from microbial consortium

A review

Sindhu S and Krishna Prasad R

9.1 INTRODUCTION

Fossil fuel emissions contribute significantly to the climate change effect. Therefore, it is crucial to find a green, renewable, and environmentally friendly energy source for future needs. To achieve sustainable development, there is a need for a continuous energy supply at affordable prices. Converting wastes into useful forms of energy is the best way to achieve this, and biofuels such as biodiesel, biohydrogen, biogas, and bioethanol are the most sustainable options as they release fewer carbon dioxide emissions (Aziz et al., 2021).

One eco-friendly approach to generating hydrogen is by using waste residues from agriculture, inorganic wastes, industrial wastes, and lignocellulosic biomass. The biological conversion process includes biophotolysis, fermentation, and microbial electrolysis, which can be performed at ambient conditions. Macroalgae, also known as seaweed, are a sustainable raw material for biohydrogen generation. They are rich in carbohydrates and lack hemicellulose and lignin, which prevents biodegradation. Macroalgae also have the potential for CO_2 bioremediation and have a high biomass yield (Rezania et al., 2017).

Bioethanol can be produced from various sources such as switchgrass, cotton, paddy straw, coconut fibers, maize, bagasse and seaweed, diatoms and algae from seawater (Aparna et al., 2025). Bioethanol contains oxygen, which reduces vehicle emissions. However, bioethanol has a low volumetric energy density compared to crude-based gasoline, so a larger quantity of bioethanol is required. The presence of lignin in biomass affects the fermentation process as it hinders enzymes and microorganisms from breaking down cellulose compounds. The use of thermophilic bacteria has improved the fermentation process of lignocellulosic biomass (Akanksha Shukla et al., 2023).

Biogas is a sustainable form of energy produced through the anaerobic decomposition of organic residues. The interaction between microbial species and substrate biomass is essential for improving biogas yield. The substrates used for biogas production come from various sources such as food waste, industrial wastes, agricultural waste residue, and sewage effluent. Brewery effluents are rich in nutrients and can be a good source for biogas generation. Biological pretreatment of substrates using enzymes and microorganisms including amylase, protease, pectinase, and cellulase is commonly done. Fungal species like *Trametes villosa* and *Coriolopsis gallica*, as well as bacterial species like *Bacillus subtilis and Pseudomonas aeruginosa,* are often used.

Biodiesel is an efficient and sustainable fuel for future demand. The transesterification process is widely used worldwide for biodiesel production (Sindhu et al., 2025). It involves converting triglycerides from different substrates into fatty acid esters or biodiesel using alcohol (Arun Shankar et al., 2017, Shobana et al., 2020). Biodiesel can be blended with diesel and used in existing infrastructural

DOI: 10.1201/9781003500483-9
This chapter has been made available under a (CC-BY-NC-ND) 4.0 license

facilities. It emits lower greenhouse gases and is an environmentally friendly fuel. Biodiesel emissions are lower than those of Petro diesel, reducing sulfur dioxide emissions. Biodiesel also emits 50% less carbon monoxide than diesel. In 2018, the United States produced 7 billion liters of biodiesel (Murat Efgan Kibar et al., 2023).

Biofuels are a valuable source for maintaining economic, social, and environmental sustainability in a region. They offer advantages such as improving the rural economy and reducing carbon dioxide emissions. Biofuels from algae are considered to be a viable alternative as they are non-consumable and can grow rapidly in wastewater and saline environments, generating huge amounts of biomass (Aniruddha et al., 2022). The production of biofuels meets sustainable goals as it generates energy and valuable byproducts. The residues obtained in jatropha production can be used as fertilizers or pesticides and the glycerol produced as a byproduct in the transesterification process can be used for making soaps and lubricants. Biodiesel can be used as an alternative to coal or firewood to improve the rural economy, and cassava industries can sell starch products (Jeswani et al., 2020).

This review focuses on the role of microbial species in the digestion of biomass substrates from sources such as crop residues, lignocellulosic biomass, industrial wastes, and agricultural residues for the generation of biofuels such as bio-based hydrogen, bio-based methane gas, bio-based ethanol, bio-based butanol, and biodiesel. The role of microbial consortium in co-cultivation technology is also explored.

9.2 PRODUCTION OF BIODIESEL FROM MICROALGAE

Fossil fuels are scarce resources that are rapidly depleting from the Earth. Microalgae are unicellular plants that thrive in both saline and fresh habitats. They are efficient photosynthetic organisms that require less area for cultivation and use less water than conventional crops. Biofuels from microalgae involve a two-step mechanism of upstream and downstream processes. Advances in the upstream process involve selecting highly productive cultures for biodiesel generation. The downstream step targets high biodiesel yields by increasing lipid content in cells to improve biodiesel conversion.

Two-stage culture procedures can produce maximum biomass and high biofuel generation as they solve the complexity between cell development and biomass accumulation. The low fuel productivity of microalgae means that, although they have great potential as an alternative energy source, their practical usage is limited by their expensive production costs. To address the cost issue, it is necessary to employ a range of approaches aimed at enhancing the yield of microalgae production. The biodiesel production process can be optimized using photobioreactors, as well as through the application of genetic modification techniques such as electroporation.

Photobioreactors are highly durable systems used for cultivating microalgae, effectively regulating many critical parameters including light intensity, nutrient availability, pH levels, and carbon dioxide concentration. Numerous designs of photobioreactors have been devised to enhance the growing conditions for microalgae. Open reservoir reactors used for algal cultivation are considered cost-efficient systems. However, these approaches are associated with certain constraints such as water evaporation, challenges in maintaining optimal temperature conditions, and susceptibility to contamination. Photobioreactors have the potential to address these limitations by effectively regulating the physiological demands of agriculture depending on the desired scale of operation. Photobioreactors situated in outdoor environments enhance operational efficiency. Indoor microscale bioreactors have the capability to run continuously throughout the day using a light-emitting diode (LED) as a light source. This setup allows for meticulous examination of reciprocal interactions under diverse circumstances. Optimal photobioreactors, when appropriately designed to regulate flow and light transmission through channel configurations, have the potential to enhance biofuel yield while minimizing energy consumption. The classification of microalgae based on lipid content is provided in Table 9.1.

TABLE 9.1
Classification of microalgae based on lipid content

Microalgae	Content of lipid %
Chlorella sorokiniana species	23
Parietochloris incise species	63
Chlorella Minutissima species	58
Chlorella emersonii species	64

The utilization of algal-based technologies has proven to be a viable strategy in addressing the growing demand for energy and achieving sustainable development objectives. Sequestration technology for carbon based on microalgal systems is widely recognized as a prominent strategy for carbon sequestration. The simultaneous processes of carbon dioxide sequestration, effluent treatment, and biomass generation through microalgae provide added value. The utilization of algal species for sequestration and biofuel generation has been a focal point of scientific investigation over the past ten years. According to a recent study using the logistic model, it has been theoretically determined that the production of microalgae in an area spanning 100,000 km^2 has the potential to store around 2.35 gigatons of CO_2. This sequestration could result in a drop of approximately 5–8% in global CO_2 emissions for 2020. Microalgae have the potential to sequester around 65 million tonnes of carbon, which would translate to a price per gallon of $8.52. The cultivation of algae in open reservoirs has the capacity to utilize around 513 tonnes of CO_2 and produce approximately 280 tonnes of dry biomass per hectare annually. The carbon fixation efficiency exhibited by microalgal cells holds promising potential for mitigating the industrial flue emissions containing high concentrations of carbon dioxide. The effectiveness of microalgae in CO_2 sequestration is contingent upon a range of aspects, including the physiological characteristics of the algae, temperature of the pond, and the origin of the CO_2 (Harun Chowdhry and Bavin Loganathan, 2019; Kisoo Kim et al., 2022).

9.2.1 Recent designs of photobioreactors for microalgal cultivation

Microalgae cultivation is done in open reservoirs and photobioreactors. The growth of microalgae requires nutrients, including carbon dioxide and water, as well as a sufficient light source and optimal temperature. Microalgae tend to exhibit optimal development at 25°C with a light intensity of 140–200 $mE/m^2/s$. Various bioreactor designs such as the helical tube model, flat plate reactor, and vertical tube model have certain constraints that impede the growth of microalgae. These limitations include the deposition of cell debris, elevated shear stress, and the need for separate gas exchange mechanisms. The torus-shaped photobioreactor technology has the capability to prevent the formation of areas with high concentrations of cell debris, known as dead zones, and effectively captures light. A fermenter equipped with internal lighting can regulate temperature and gas exchange. The curved chamber photobioreactor is designed to improve photosynthesis reaction. The A-shaped reactor is designed to capture sunlight through multi-directional tubes. The high density of cells within the reactor can cause bubbles to form. Traditional methods of cultivating microalgae, like open ponds, are cost-effective in terms of construction expenses. Table 9.2 provides the limitations and advantages of different bioreactor designs.

Growing macro-scale microalgae in outdoor photobioreactors is advantageous because they utilize sunlight as a source of energy. The interior regions are less affected by temperature changes or bad weather, which can impact efficiency. Experiments with outdoor tubular photobioreactors showed more productivity than the inhouse system in the southern European region during the spring. It's important to note that high temperatures in the summer can negatively affect microalgae productivity, as the ideal temperature for cultivation is around 25°C. Spraying water and using

TABLE 9.2
Types of bioreactor design with their advantages and limitations

Bioreactor design	Advantages	Limitations
Torus shaped	Efficient mixing process with no dead zones	Issues during scaling up the reactor
Fermenter model	Temperature, light intensity can be adjusted	Efficiency of conversion of light is low
Curved chamber model	Surface to volume is large, good photosynthetic efficiency	Biofouling issues
Alpha-shaped reactor	Surface to volume is large	Formation of foam
Open pond type	Inexpensive and easy to construct	Poor biofuel productivity

a tarpaulin has been found to be an effective method for regulating temperature. However, using a sunshade can hinder microalgae growth by blocking light. The effectiveness of the shade in regulating light levels depends on the changing angles of sunlight over time. Spraying water in a 40 L tubular bioreactor significantly reduced temperature by 4–7°C during noon hours. Phase change materials (PCMs) like Glauber's salt and decanoic acid can be utilized to control the temperature of the system. PCMs can collect thermal energy during the day and release it at night, maintaining a consistent temperature. PCMs can regulate temperature within a range of 10°C and are considered a cost-effective method.

An optimal photobioreactor is one that minimizes hydrodynamic shear stress on cells while providing enough carbon dioxide, nutrients, and light. Using laboratory-scale photobioreactors is advantageous for cultivating microalgae compared to macro-scale reactors, because they offer conditions that closely resemble optimal conditions. Additionally, different designs can be used for this process. In macro-scale photobioreactors, solar radiation is the main source of light. In laboratory-scale bioreactors, the light flux can be manipulated to increase biomass concentrations. For example, *C. ellipsoidea* cultivated under blue LED lighting had higher lipid contents. Different chamber technologies such as bubble column photobioreactors, tanks with stirrers, and flat plate reactors have been utilized in the development of laboratory-scale photobioreactors. Bubble column photobioreactors are designed to maintain a consistent gas supply regardless of their placement. However, these systems can cause shear stress on algal cells, which can suppress cellular functionality and lead to cell death. Photobioreactors are utilized to achieve efficient mixing of microalgae, ensuring uniform distribution of nutrients and regulation of heat and light conditions. Flat plate photobioreactors have an extended surface area for effective light delivery. The use of laboratory-scale photobioreactors is limited in terms of mass production applications due to their smaller size compared to macro-scale reactors. To address this limitation, a high-throughput screening approach was presented, which improved the efficiency of light delivery by optimizing aspects such as light intensity, density factor, and cycle lengths. In this technology, LED lights were used to program and deliver specific light conditions to the microplate. The high-throughput screening technique was employed to analyze the photosynthetic efficiency (PE) of *Chlorella* species. The results showed that substantial PE conditions were observed at low Imax and with minimal cycles of 3 s.

Researchers have also developed a novel algal cultivation system that utilizes machine learning techniques. This method aims to overcome two main challenges faced by previous algal cultivation systems: the growth hindrance caused by mutual shading and high harvesting expenses. The researchers utilized a machine learning model called growth rate prediction to simulate the growth of microalgae. Additionally, the method enhances productivity by promoting cell aggregation and sedimentation, which is attributed to the hydrophobicity of the algal cell surface.

Lipids, the primary constituents of biofuel, can be obtained from microalgae through various methods including cell disruption techniques like electroporation. Different approaches such as milling beads, microwave application, and mechanical pressing are used to induce cell death, which results in the release of significant amounts of intracellular molecules. Electroporation allows for the collection of lipids from cells multiple times without causing cell death, though the yield of lipid extraction is lower. Electroporation is a technique that creates transient pores in the cell membrane, enabling the transportation of intracellular substances like lipids. The production expenses for microalgal biofuel exceed those of petroleum diesel. Approximately 60% of the total expenditure is attributed to harvesting and operation, while oil extraction constitutes 20% of the cost. Esterification processes account for 15% of the total cost, and cleaning activities contribute 5% (Licheng Peng et al., 2020; Angela Paul Peter et al., 2022).

9.2.2 Technology Advancement in Algal Cultivation for Biodiesel

Algal cells have multiple uses in biosequestration of CO_2 to generate biofuel and the removal of pesticides and pharmaceuticals from wastewater. Among various microalgae species, *Chlorella* shows significant potential as a strain for effectively sequestering carbon dioxide from hazardous emissions. The cultivation of *Chlorella sp.* has been employed as a bioremediation technique to mitigate the presence of CO_2 in emissions resulting from power plant combustion. At a concentration of approximately 40% (v/v) CO_2, the CO_2 fixation rate of *Chlorella species* is 2.3 g/L per day. *Chlorella vulgaris* has shown a CO_2 collection efficiency ranging from 70% to 99%. When exposed to an airflow with a CO_2 concentration of CO_2 above 1850 parts per million (ppm). *Chlorella vulgaris* demonstrated the ability to sequester nearly 74% of the CO_2 (Jalilian et al., 2020; Keffer and Kleinheinez, 2002).

Scenedesmus sp. grew under typical conditions with ambient CO_2 (0.036%), but after 30 days, it was able to withstand 100% CO_2 and achieved a biomass content almost three times higher. Nannochloropsis, a marine microalgae, is used for both carbon dioxide sequestration and biofuel production. Compared to freshwater species, marine microalgae are superior in biomass production even when carbon dioxide is limited. The marine environment provides a habitat that enables these species to undergo evolutionary changes, enhancing the efficiency and resilience of their photoconversion machinery. This adaptation facilitates the rapid conversion of carbon into biomass or bioenergy.

Chaetoceros muelleri with a CO_2 concentration of 10–20% showed a significant lipid output of 50 mg/L/d. *Isochrysis sp.* and *Chlorella salina*, the two marine strains, have been studied for their ability to adapt to different CO_2 levels. The capacity of these strains to sequester CO_2 and generate bioenergy depends on the physiology of the algal species. Algal physiology plays a crucial role in determining their bioenergy content and varies significantly among different species. The suitability of microalgal species for the biofuel or bioproduct industry is evaluated based on the prevalence of specific ingredients. Various microalgal strains exhibit variations in their morphological characteristics and biochemical composition including the proportions of lipids, carbohydrates, proteins, vitamins, and other constituents. Microalgal cells adapt their metabolism in response to various abiotic stress conditions, such as nutrient deprivation, exposure to heavy metals, changes in osmotic pressure, temperature fluctuations, pH imbalances, and variations in light intensity. This metabolic flexibility allows microalgae to efficiently allocate carbon resources toward the accumulation of carbohydrates and lipids. Table 9.3 provides biodiesel conversion rates for different microalgal strains.

A multitude of microalgal strains exhibit a wide range of biochemical compositions, including protein contents ranging from 17% to 70%, carbohydrate contents ranging from 10% to 50%, and lipid contents ranging from 10% to 50%. Microalgae can produce a significant amount of biomass per unit area of cultivation, making them highly suitable as feedstock for bioenergy applications. Compared to other options, microalgae are a sustainable source of oil which yield up to 100,000 L of bio-oil annually. Projections indicate that the global algal biofuel market will experience substantial growth, increasing from 5 billion US dollars in 2020 to 9 billion US dollars in 2027 (Adeniyi et al., 2018; Sivaramakrishnan et al., 2018; Hoofar Shokravi et al., 2022).

TABLE 9.3
Conversion of biodiesel using different microalgal strains (Khan et al., 2023)

Microalgae	Reaction conditions	Technique	% Conversion of biodiesel
Chlorella pyrenoidosa	77% content water in biomass, Ratio of methanol to biomass is 8:1, Sulfuric acid, 90°C, 30 min	Assisted with microwave	86
Aurantiochytrium sp.	40% water content in biomass, solvent ethanol, Potassium carbonate catalyst, 60°C, 1 h	Assisted with ultrasound	80
Spirulina platensis	40% water content in biomass, methanol, 300°C, 30 min, 67 bar pressure	Supercritical methanol	99
Nannochloropsis sp.	Water content is 80% in biomass, Solvent is mixture of ionic liquids and methyl alcohol, 65°C, 15 min	Microwave treatment	37
Nannochloropsis sp.	80% water content in biomass, ethanol solvent, sulfuric acid catalyst, 150°C, 2 h, 15 MPa	Supercritical carbon dioxide	25

TABLE 9.4
Studies on improving lipid synthesis for different algal species

Species	Approach	Improvement
Scenedesmus quadricauda	The expression of Acetyl-CoA carboxylase is regulated	Fatty acid content is increased 1.6 times
Haematococcus pluvialis	Fatty acid generation pathway is modified	Fatty acids content increased 24%
Chlamydomonas reinhardtii	Biosynthesis pathway for triacylglycerol is improved	58% increase in lipid contents
Chlorella pyrenoidosa	Increasing the nicotinamide adenine dinucleotide phosphate supply	3.2 times lipid content increased
Nannochloropsis oceanica	Improving photosynthesis reaction efficiency	41% increase in lipid content
Chlamydomonas reinhardtii	Competing pathways are blocked	75% increase in lipid content

9.2.3 Fourth generation microalgal biodiesel generation

Marine algae can be genetically modified in various ways. Electroporation, a method used for over 30 years to transfer genes in cells and bacteria, requires only a small amount of DNA and produces excellent results compared to other methods. Kilian and colleagues reported that microalgae have been engineered to knock out nitrogen metabolism genes for biofuel production (Kilian et al., 2011). Studies have also focused on enhancing lipid accumulation by manipulating microalgal lipid biosynthesis pathway such as regulating ACCase expression, modifying the fatty acid synthesis pathway, and modifying the triacylglycerol synthesis pathway. Blocking competing pathways through genetic modification has the potential to increase the TAG content of certain strains by up to 45-fold. The oil and biomass content of algae-based biofuels are important cost factors in bioeconomic analysis (Hoofar Shokravi et al., 2022). Table 9.4 provides information on studies conducted to improve lipid synthesis for different algal species.

9.3 SYNTHESIS OF BIODIESEL FROM FUNGI

Single-cell oils (SCOs) are derived from microorganisms. SCO production is not affected by change in seasons, geographical locations, or transport concerns. SCOs consist of triacylglycerols, free fatty acids, and polar lipids. Oleaginous microorganisms have a high lipid content inside the cells. These microbes thrive in nicotinamide adenine di-nucleotide phosphate for fatty acid accumulation. Proper identification of SCO-producing microorganisms is economically useful for biodiesel production. *Mucor circinelloides* is the fungi used in the synthesis of fatty acids. *M. circinelloides* produce 98% of lipids that can undergo saponification reaction to produce biodiesel.

The availability of low-cost substrates such as lignocellulosic biomass and industrial wastewater for SCO production, along with targeting high-value products from these substrates, can significantly reduce the cost of operation. Oleaginous filamentous fungi have high growth rate, do not require light energy, and produce high lipid content using various carbon sources for biodiesel production. Oleaginous microorganisms can produce lipid yield of more than 30% using low-cost carbon substrates. The amount of triacylglycerol synthesis depends on carbon source. A deficiency of nitrogen results in lipogenesis; the oil begins to accumulate on the cell wall, which prevents fungal growth.

Mortierella alpina grows on a glucose source and produces a 50% lipid production rate. *Aspergillus sp.* grows on potato dextrose and produces a 53% lipid yield at pH 5 and 30°C. Fungus *Mortierella alpina* grown on glucose with potassium nitrate as a nitrogen source synthesized 32% lipid content. *Aspergillus niger* species grown on wastewater from distilleries produced a lipid content of 3 g/L (Alok Patel et al., 2020; Sizwe et al., 2021; Subramaniam et al., 2010). The lipid generation using various oleaginous filamentous fungi for varied carbon substrates is given in Table 9.5.

The several advantages of oleaginous filamentous fungi in biorefineries are as follows:

- The lipid content of 90% and above is obtained along with high-value products useful in nutraceuticals.
- Profiles of lipids are rich in saponifiable fatty acids, allowing for the production of high-quality biodiesel.
- It forms pellets easily, reducing viscosity during the fermentation process.
- The carbon sources utilized include tomato waste, corn stover, brewery wastewater, and glycerol.

9.3.1 FACTORS AFFECTING ACTIVITY OF FUNGAL LIPASE

Carbon source: Carbon sources stimulate genes in microbes, improving fermentation and increasing cell metabolism activity, thus enhancing the activity of fungal lipase. The use of mustard

TABLE 9.5
Yield of lipid from oleaginous fungal species in varied carbon substrates

Fungi	Biomass g/L	Yield of lipid g/L	Substrate
Alternaria sp	14	7.6	Glucose
A. oryzae	4.35	39	Cellulose
Aspergillus tubingensis	16	31	Palm fibers
Umbelopsis isabelline	45	78	Corn stover
Mortierella ramanniana	7.5	3	Glycerol
Cunninghamella echinulate	12	4	Molasses

oil as a carbon source in *Aspergillus terreus* culture medium improved lipase yield. In media consisting of *Aspergillus sydowii,* the use of sucrose and mannitol as carbon source increased lipase yield. In media consisting of *Aspergillus niger,* the addition of fructose as a carbon source improved lipase yield.

Nitrogen source: Nitrogen is vital for lipase enzyme synthesis and stimulates lipase production in microbes. *Rhizopus sp.* showed high lipolytic activity with the addition of urea. In media consisting of *Aspergillus sp.* culture, the use of peptone as a nitrogen source improved lipase yield. *Trichoderma harzianum* provided maximum lipase yield when glucose and peptone were added in the culture medium. In *Aspergillus sydowii*, yeast extract and $NaNO_3$ were used as nitrogen sources to improve the yield of lipase.

Temperature: Higher lipase production was observed at 37°C. The production of lipase enzymes in *Aspergillus niger* culture medium was studied from 25 to 55°C and optimal results were achieved at 30°C. In *Botrytis cinerea* strain, optimal lipase yield was achieved at 38°C. *Rhizopus oryzae* showed the highest lipase yield at 50°C. Thermophilic fungi produce more saturated fatty acids than mesophilic fungi.

pH of the culture medium: Fungus lipase production was stimulated by conditions ranging from neutral pH to alkaline pH, *Rhodotorula glutinis* exhibited high lipase activity when the pH of the culture medium was maintained at neutral levels. In a medium containing *Aspergillus terreus*, the optimum pH for maximum lipase activity was pH 8. When maintained at pH 6, *M. circinielloides* showed high lipid yields.

Surfactants: They are organic molecules with long carbon chains that have hydrophobic and hydrophilic parts. They improve cell permeability and aid in the secretion of proteins. *Nomuraea rileyi* showed improved lipid activity when surfactant Tween 80 was available. The selection of the correct surfactant is crucial for enhancing lipase activity.

Metal ions: Metal ions are essential in the functioning of lipase-producing enzymes. Lipase production from *Aspergillus japonicas* was enhanced in the presence of Ca^{2+} ions while lipase activity was inhibited in the presence of Mn^{2+} ions. *Candida rugosa* strain also exhibited improved lipase activity in the presence of Ca^{2+} ions. The addition of metal ions such as Ca^{2+} and Mn^{2+} ions had no effect on lipase production in *Cladosporium tenuissimum.*

Molecular techniques in lipase generation: Gene lip3 in *Candida rugosa* was codon optimized, resulting in a 70-fold improvement in lipase production. Recombinant lipase is produced through metabolic engineering. Fermentation conditions are optimized to enhance lipase production using *Candida rugosa* strains in combination with recombinant *Pichia pastoris.* The growth rate of cells in the fermenter can be controlled by adjusting the proteolytic sensitivity of lipase (Kumar et al., 2023; Bharathi and Rajalakshmi, 2019; Saranya and Ramachandra, 2020). The fungal strains and their specific activities are provided in Table 9.6.

TABLE 9.6
Fungal strains and process conditions with specific activity

Fungal strain	Fermenter	Optimum conditions
Aspergillus niger	Solid-state fermenter	121 U/g. des, 30°C, pH 7
Penicillium verrucosum	Submerged fermentation	3.2 U/mL, 28°C, pH 7
Antrodia cinnamomea	Batch fermentation	26 U/mL, 45°C, pH 8
Penicillium chrysogenum	Solid-state fermenter	650 U/gds, 40°C, pH 9
Penicillium aurantiogriseum	Tributyrin agar plate	17 U/mL min, 30°C, pH 6.8
Aspergillus aculeatus	Potato dextrose agar	9.5 U/mL, 40°C, pH 9

9.3.2 Oleaginous Filamentous Fungi for Lipid Enhancement in Biodiesel Production

The two major phyla of oleaginous filamentous fungi are *Mucoromycota* and *Ascomycota*. *Mucor circinelloides* was the first oleaginous fungal strain used in gamma linolenic acid synthesis. SCO produced from fungal species is similar in properties to oils produced from vegetable sources. The biodiesel generated from SCO can be combined with conventional petrol in different ratios. The selection of fungal strains that yield high levels of triacylglycerol is essential for better biodiesel yield. The degree of unsaturation and chain length are important aspects to consider in SCO for biodiesel generation. The oil produced should be rich in monounsaturated and saturated fatty acids for the synthesis of biodiesel. SCO containing polyunsaturated fatty acids is useful in pharma applications. The desired acids for biodiesel generation are monounsaturated acids of fats like palmitoleic and oleic acid and unsaturated acids of fats such as palmitic and stearic acids. The fatty acid composition profile affects the various desired properties of biodiesel such as stability under oxidation conditions and melting point. Fungal strains are capable of metabolizing low-cost substrates. Gas chromatography-mass spectrometry is utilized to analyze the fatty acid profile. The selection of the correct fungal strain with high lipid content is essential for reducing costs during biodiesel production. The use of efficient screening methods for oleaginous filamentous fungi for SCO generation is required for downstream processing methods for biodiesel production. Lipid biosynthesis involves multiple enzymes such as malic enzymes, acetyl-CoA carboxylase, and ATP-citrate lyase. Nutrient imbalances such as excess carbon source or deficiency in nitrogen cause metabolic changes in lipid biosynthesis (Alok Patel et al., 2020; Sizwe et al., 2021).

Lignocellulosic polymers are hydrolyzed using cellulase enzymes to simple sugars. These sugars are utilized by oleaginous microorganisms. The limitations in such processes are due to the high cost of enzymes and microorganisms' productivity. *U. isabelline* yields 5 g/L lipids using acid-pretreated corn stover. *Colletotrichum sp.* provides 68 mg/g dry substrate using paddy straw substrate. *A. tubingensis* converts palm fiber into maximum lipid content of 37 mg/g dry substrate. The fungal bioconversions reduce the time of reaction and energy costs associated with the process. Direct transesterification is a process in which biomass reacts with methyl alcohol in the presence of catalyst. This reaction converts the biomass into fatty acid acyl esters. Methyl alcohol serves as an extraction and esterifying agent in this process. Sometimes a co-solvent like hexane is used to improve oil recovery from microbial cells. When wet biomass obtained from the *Mucor circinelloides* fungus was used, a 98% yield of fatty acid methyl ester was achieved using a heterogeneous catalyst and ethanol solvent. The fatty acids produced by oleaginous fungi are used to generate biodiesel, which provides energy. The synthesis of SCO is not affected by variation in seasons or cultivation location. The fatty acid profile has high saponification values for biodiesel generation (Sravan Kumar et al., 2018). Table 9.7 provides the lipid yield for different oleaginous fungal strains operated under different process conditions.

TABLE 9.7
Total lipid yield for different oleaginous fungal strains

Strain	Experimental conditions	Yield of total lipid (g/L)
Mucor ctenidius	150–200 rpm	22
Mortierella alpina	pH 3–8	18
Cunninghamella echinulate	Carbon to nitrogen ratio 55–100	3.2
Rhizopus arrhizus	Nitrogen source KNO_3	32
Mortierella ramanniana	Nitrogen source KNO_3, Metal ions of Cu, Zn, and Mg	29
Mortierella alpina	Temperature 25°C, 6 days	1.7
M. isabelline	100 g/L substrate glucose	18

The main advantages of biodiesel are as follows:

- Biodiesel has a much higher energy density.
- Biodiesel produces more energy than is consumed during its production.
- Biodiesel reduces greenhouse emissions by about 40% compared to fossil fuels.
- Biodiesel can be mixed with conventional diesel and used directly in existing combustion engines.
- Biodiesel has a good flash point and is biodegradable

9.3.3 Recent advancements in microbial lipids recovery

Cell disruption is a critical step in lipid extraction because it directly affects the transesterification process. In order to recover intracellular lipid products, cell disruption is necessary. Mechanical techniques for cell disruption involve breaking the cell wall through shear stress and abrasion. Bead milling, for example, utilizes steel beads to apply shear stress and disrupt the cell. This method has been proven effective for processing various species, such as *Chlorella vulgaris* algae, *Rhodotorula gracilis* yeast, *Bacillus cereus* bacteria, and *Penicillium citrinum* fungus.

Ultrasonication is another technique that involves the growth and collapse of bubbles during the rarefaction and compression phases. In the case of the *Trichosporon oleaginous* fungal strain, a lipid recovery of 43% was obtained using hexane as a solvent, 10% with water, 75% using methanol as a solvent, and 100% lipid recovery was achieved with a chloroform and methanol mixture as a solvent, at a frequency of 50 Hz.

The microwave process of lipid extraction utilizes electromagnetic waves with a frequency of up to 300 GHz. These waves disperse the water molecules inside the cell and subject them to uneven heating, resulting in the release of lipids through the cell disruption. However, in large industrial applications, microwaves may damage polyunsaturated acids due to the formation of hydroxyl radicals, which can affect the composition of the final product.

In electroporation techniques, a medium is passed between two electrodes at 50 kV with electrical power pulsing at 50 kHz. This pulsing causes the cell wall to fracture and release the lipids. Studies on *Chlorella vulgaris* using pulsed electric field in a stainless-steel electrode chamber with an inter-electrode gap of 15 mm resulted in a 50% lipid yield. For the target sample of *Auxenochlorella protothecoides*, a lipid extraction rate of 22% was obtained when a 35 kV/cm electric field was applied.

Biocompatible organic solvents can extract lipids from cells without destroying oleaginous microbes in algae. The solvent creates openings in the cell wall through which lipids are extracted. The large partition coefficient of solvents is desired because it prevents irreversible damage to the cell membrane.

Surfactants are non-toxic and biodegradable chemicals used to disrupt the cell wall and extract lipids. The cell membrane is negatively charged, so hydrophobic surfactants are used for this purpose. For example, Myristyltrimethylammonium is used in wet slurry biomass of *Scenedesmus sp.* and achieves a 100% yield of lipid. Another surfactant N-lauryl sarcosine is capable of extracting lipids from oleaginous yeast with a 98% yield.

Supercritical carbon dioxide behaves as both a liquid and a gas in its critical conditions of temperature and pressure. Its dissolving power increases significantly under these critical conditions, making it useful for extracting lipids from microbial cells. Supercritical carbon dioxide has low viscosity and high diffusivity. It solubilizes the oil, which is then depressurized, allowing the CO_2 to escape and leaving behind the oil.

In the first stage of lipid extraction, physical treatment, chemical treatment, or enzyme-based cell disruption processes are performed; in the second step, chemical solvents are used to recover the oil. Non-polar organic solvents are used to extract neutral lipids, which exist in the cytoplasm as globules. Polar solvents are used to extract attached polar lipids. In order to recover both forms of lipids,

TABLE 9.8
Lipid recovery using several cell disruption methods

Microbes	Cell disruption technique	% recovery of lipids
Scenedesmus sp	Enzyme-based technique	75
Chlamydomonas reinhardtii	Osmosis-based technique	84
Nannochloropsis sp	Surfactants based technique	79
Trichosporon oleaginous	Ultrasonication technique	100
Rhodotorula glutinis	Supercritical CO_2	99
Rhodosporidium diobovatum	Ionic liquid-based technique	97
Mortierella isabelina	Soxhlet extraction technique	100

a co-solvent containing both polar and non-polar solvents is used. The choice of solvent in the lipid extraction process depends on the microorganisms used, the reaction time, the initial lipid content in the microbial cells, and the interaction mechanism of the cell with the solvent (Sravan Kumar et al., 2018; Lee et al., 2010; Hidalgo et al., 2013). Table 9.8 provides information on the recovery of lipids from various microbes using different cell disruption technologies.

9.4 SYNTHESIS OF BIODIESEL FROM YEAST AND BACTERIA

9.4.1 Synthesis of Yeast Oils from Lignocellulosic Biomass Using Oleaginous Yeasts

Several non-conventional yeast species are considered oleaginous, but only a few species of yeast have been well characterized such as *Cutaneotrichosporon Oleaginosus, Cutaneum*, *Rhodotorula Toruloides, Gilutinis, L. starkeyi,* and *Yarrowia lipolytica.* Non-oleaginous yeasts like *S. cerevisiae* and *Candida utilis* can only store about 15% lipid relative to their body mass. An oleaginous microbe enters the lipid accumulation phase of its growth when it has depleted a particular nitrogen but still has an excess of carbon that is absorbed by the cells and converted into triacylglycerols.

Various oleaginous yeasts from the genera Cryptococcus, *Lipomyces, Rhodotorula, Saitoella*, and *Trichosporon* are involved in lipid production using hydrolysates of lignocellulosic biomass as a substrate. *Yarrowia lipolytica,* Vishniacozyma Psychrotolerans, *T.cutaneum ATCC 20271, Torulaspora delbrueckii, Trichosporonoides spathulata, Trigonopsis variabilis, R.fluvialis DMKU-SP314, R.toruloides strain such as* Y4, DSMZ 4444, and CCT 7815, *R.graminis* DBVPG 4620, *R.paludigenum* KM281510 and *Rhodotorula* species KM281508, *R.Glutinis*, *Pseudozyma aphidis, Meyerozyma Guilliermondii, Metschnikowia pulcherrima, Metschnikowia gruessii, L.starkeyi* ATCC 56304, *Lipomyces lipofer, Lipomyces tetrasporus, Lipomyces doorenjongii, Lipomyces kockii, Leucosporidiella creatinivora, Kodamaea ohmeri, Kurtzmaniella cleridarum, Geotrichum histeridarum, Galactomyces candidus, C.curvatus* ATCC 20509, *Candida diddensiae, Candida aff. Tenuis, Cutaneotrichosporon Dermatis, Cyberlindnera jadinii, C.humicola, C. vishniaccii* MTCC232, *Candida freyschussii* use corn cob, corn stover, hemicellulosic hydrolysate from Birch, Jerusalem artichoke extracts and hydrolysate, sugarcane top and bagasse hydrolysate, wheat straw, rice bran, sorghum stalk, groundnut shell, cassava bagasse, and switchgrass hydrolysate as a nutrient medium.

C. curvatus strains such as DSM 101032,MUcL 29819, ATCC 20509, and DSM 70022, *Y. lipolytica* strains such as CICC 31596, CCMA 0357, ACA DC 50109, polg modified and ATCC2046 modified, *L. starkeyi* strains such as NBRC10381, DSM 70295, and ATCC 58680, *L. lipofer* NRRL Y-1155, *R. toruloides* strains such as AS 2.1389 and ATCC 10788 and *R. babjevae* DVBPG 8058 used different carbon sources such as glucose, glucose and xylose, crude glycerol, food waste, distillery waste and mix of VFA (Mota et al., 2022).

9.4.2 Factors affecting the lipid production

The primary factors influencing lipid characteristics and synthesis are the type of substrate, carbon-to-nitrogen ratio, temperature, pH, dissolved oxygen concentration, and source of nitrogen. Ideal conditions for lipid production occur in a medium that is low in nitrogen and high in carbon. Only a small number of researchers have attempted to increase the lipid content and decrease the dry biomass content of *C. oleaginous, C. curvatus, R. toruloides, Y. lipolytica, R. glutinis, R. mucilaginosa,* and *R. kratochvilovae* by adjusting the carbon to nitrogen ratio. Genetic modifications to oleaginous yeast such as *Y. lipolytica* and *R.toruloides* have been used to boost lipid accumulation and, consequently, lipid yield (Sundaramahalingam et al., 2022).

The nutrient medium pH affects lipid accumulation in the yeast. On the other hand, few researchers have suggested that an alkaline pH of 8–11 is more suitable for the growth of *Y. lipolytica, R. toruloides,* and *C. curvatus*. Temperature and pH are factors that influence lipid production. The majority of oleaginous yeasts are mesophilic. So the culture temperature is around 30°C. While some yeasts, such as *Blastobotrys adeninivorans*, can thrive in temperatures as high as 45°C, others, such as *Rhodotorula glacialis*, *Leucosporidium sp.*, and *Mrakia sp.* (all of which are obligate psychrophilic), require temperatures as low as 4°C to grow and produce a high lipid yield. However, for facultative and mesophilic yeasts, culturing at 4°C affects the growth rate not the biomass accumulation (Thomas et al., 2019).

In addition to pH and temperature, macronutrients also affect lipid yield. Mathematical modeling was also used to examine the effects of limiting nutrients like nitrogen, phosphorus, and sulfur on the growth of *R. toruloides* in glucose-rich medium. The concentration of lipids changed most noticeably with the availability of nitrogen. Lipid synthesis is also affected by physical parameters such as fermentation time, agitation speed, optical density, aeration flow rate, and size (Liu et al., 2020; Zhang et al., 2022). The effect of inoculation medium on lipid production with *L. starkeyi* was studied. The production of lipids from lignocellulosic substrate using oleaginous yeast is provided in Table 9.9.

Genetic Engineering in Yeast for Efficient Bioconversion: Yeast strains have been genetically engineered to produce more lipids by increasing resistance to inhibitors and utilizing a wider range of carbon sources. Previously, a yeast strain of *S. cerevisiae* was used to produce bioethanol, but now it is being modified to prioritize the lipid storage. *S. cerevisiae* is a popular model organism in biofuel research due to its excellent genome database and ease of regulation. However, attempts to modify yeast strains for fatty acid synthesis and block ethanol production have been unsuccessful due to growth defects in *S. cerevisiae* (Lacerda et al., 2020).

To extract lipid from the yeast, cell-membrane-disruptive methods are used. The fatty acids are then converted into methyl esters through a transesterification process using a suitable nanocatalyst.

TABLE 9.9
Production of lipids from lignocellulose substrate using oleaginous yeast

Oleaginous yeast	Substrate	Lipid production g/L
Cryptococcus Curvatus	Sweet sorghum and bagasse, enzyme hydrolysate	11
Lipomyces starkeyi	Corncob, bagasse, acid hydrolysate	8
Rhodosporidium Toruloides	Starch from cassava, enzyme hydrolysate	14
Trichosporon Cutaneum	Corncob enzyme hydrolysate	10
Cryptococcus Vishniaccii	Sludge from paper mill	8

TABLE 9.10
Improvements in genetic engineering approach in lignocellulosic biomass by yeast strain

Yeast strain	Target gene	Traits	Enhancements
S. cerevisiae	AN25	Xylose transport enhancement	Xylose uptake increased 43 times
S. cerevisiae	△PHO13	Xylose catabolism enhanced	Xylose uptake increased 4-fold
S. cerevisiae	cbbM, sPRK	Carbon loss is reduced	Ethanol yield improved 1.1 times
Y. lipolytica	ssXYL1, ssXYL2	Xylose catabolism enhanced	30% yield of lipids
Y. lipolytica	ylXDH, ylXR	Heterologous xylose pathway	1.6 times lipid yield increased

Candida zeylanoides ATCC 20367 is grown using this glycerol as a nutrient source. Batch cultivation using either pure glycerol or glucose as the primary nutrient substrates yields similar results in terms of cell viability and biomass production (Singh et al., 2020; Mota et al., 2022). Table 9.10 provides an overview of the improvements in genetic engineering approach in lignocellulosic biomass using yeast strain.

Biodiesel has been produced using both traditional and cutting-edge fermentation methods, as well as a wide variety of oleaginous yeast strains. The efficiency and quality of biodiesel depend on optimizing fermentation conditions and transesterification techniques. Parameters such as carbon sources, C/N ratio, dissolved oxygen, pH, and temperature play an important role in lipid accumulation during submerged fermentation. In solid-state fermentation, microbes grow directly on the biomass and residues from agricultural biomass under optimal growth conditions. In the two-stage fermentation process, biomass generation and lipogenesis are controlled individually to simplify the optimization process (Ahuja et al., 2023).

9.4.3 Oleaginous bacteria as source of biodiesel

Like yeast and fungi, many strains of bacteria including *Streptomyces* and *Rhodococcus* have high lipid content under certain environmental conditions. *Rhodococcus opacus,* for example, contain more than 70% lipid on a dry basis. Pilot-scale fermentation and optimization have been extensively conducted on the *R. opacus* strain. Gram-negative bacterial strains, on the other hand, tend to accumulate fewer lipids. Bacterial species cultivated on olive oil or n-alkanes show increased lipid accumulation. *Aeromonas*, for instance, consists of fatty acids up to 12% of cellular dry weight with 30% being polyunsaturated fatty acid. Researchers have attempted to use high-carbon-content wastes as a substrate to reduce production cost by 45%. In addition to mitigating CO_2 emissions, the abundant extracellular lipids produced by certain chemolithotrophic bacteria can be used to make biodiesel. Clostridium, for example, synthesizes and stores medium-chain n-alkanes. The halotolerant Vibrio furnissii bacterium synthesizes and produces intracellular and extracellular hydrocarbons with properties resembling those of light oil and kerosene, ranging from C15 to C24 (Marri et al., 2020; Kumar et al., 2020). Table 9.11 provides information on lipid production from cellulosic biomass using oleaginous bacteria.

9.5 MANUFACTURE OF BIOETHANOL AND BIOBUTANOL FROM MICROBIAL CONSORTIUM

Bioethanol is produced from energy crops such as switch grass, cotton, giant miscanthus, residues from consumable crops like paddy straw, coconut fibers, maize, bagasse, and sources from seawater like seaweed, diatoms, and algae. The biofuels are classified based on substrates involved in the process into four generations as shown in Table 9.12.

TABLE 9.11
Lipid production from cellulosic biomass using oleaginous bacteria

Oleaginous microbes	Substrate	Lipid production %
Gordonia sp.	Orange peel	71
Rhodococcus opacus	Orange peel	83
Rhodococcus opacus	Hardwood	46
Rhodococcus opacus	Kraft lignin treated with oxygen	14
Rhodococcus opacus	Effluent from cellulose pretreatment	27

TABLE 9.12
Classification of biofuels based on substrates involved in the process

Biofuel Class	Substrates involved in process
Biofuel—First generation	Various consumable crops like maize, barley, corn, sugarcane.
Biofuel—Second generation	Various non-consumable crops like jatropha, cotton, grass
Biofuel—Third generation	Algal biomass, sea weeds, diatoms
Biofuel—Fourth generation	Genetically modified algae and microorganisms

Bioethanol has a 35% oxygen content, which reduces vehicle emissions. It is blended with gasoline and used as biofuel, reducing the demand for motor gasoline. However, bioethanol has a low volumetric energy density, so a larger quantity of bioethanol is required compared to crude-based gasoline. As a result, bioethanol is blended with conventional gasoline in different ratios. The United States accounts for 56% of global biobased ethanol production, mostly from edible and non-edible feedstocks.

The steps for bioethanol generation include pretreatment of feedstocks, enzyme hydrolytic process, and fermentation of glucose. The objective of pretreatment is to structurally modify the substrate to facilitate the action of enzymes, which then produce sugar monomers. The enzyme hydrolyzes the hemicellulose, cellulose polymers, and starch. The resulting hexoses and pentoses monomers are digested by microorganisms during the fermentation stage, which convert them into ethanol (Akanksha Shukla et al., 2023; Azra Maliha et al., 2023).

9.5.1 Pretreatment Methods of Feedstocks for Bioethanol Production

Physical pretreatment process: This treatment process relies on the supply of energy to break the lignin bonds in substrates and release sugar molecules. The temperature and pressure are adjusted simultaneously to achieve size reduction.

Mechanical process: This process involves breaking down the structural configuration of the feedstock through size reduction. Different milling techniques, such as ball milling, roll milling, and grinding are used. These techniques convert cellulose into a complete amorphous form, making it easier for hydrolytic enzymes to act on it. Ball milling techniques reduce the size and crystallinity of biomass, which loosens the hydrogen bonding of lignocellulosic biomass. However, ball milling has the disadvantages of consuming more energy and operating at lower efficiency.

Extrusion process: The extrusion technique combines mechanical process, chemical treatment, and thermal techniques to induce structural changes in biomass through high-power rotation. A shear force is created between the biomass, screw conveyor, and barrel, which increases the temperature and pressure in the barrel and enhances sugar recovery from biomass. The twin gear extruder is used in the pretreatment of rice straw, which removes the amorphous region and increases the crystallinity index by 50%.

Irradiation: Microwave irradiation breaks down complex cellulosic and hemicellulosic structures and increases the activity of enzymes for bioethanol production. Electron beam irradiation improves the digestion process of lignocellulosic biomass by enzymes. The glucose yield of treated rice straw is 52% higher than that of untreated rice straw after a hydrolysis time of 152 h. The yield of the irradiation process increases as the biomass size decreases.

Sonification: Ultrasonic pretreatment is an eco-friendly process that alters the physical structure and chemical nature of biomass. Ultrasonic vibration disrupts cellulose and hemicellulose materials by increasing the porosity of biomass resulting in the break down into simpler sugars. The frequency of the sonication process is 24 kHz and it requires 400 W of power. Ultrasonication-assisted pretreatment with alkalis results in 85% lignin removal.

9.5.1.1 Chemical pretreatment processes

Alkaline pretreatment: This process selectively removes lignin, which selectively improves the surface area and porosity of the biomass. Sodium hydroxide, ammonium hydroxide, and calcium hydroxide are commonly used chemicals in the process. The treatment involves dissolving the biomass in high temperatures and for a long period of time, which breaks the cellulosic hydrogen bonds. Sodium hydroxide specifically dissolves the lignin carbohydrate bond and the lignin's alkyl-aryl bond, enhancing enzyme activity. For example, alkaline hydrogen peroxide pretreatment has been found to be effective with 74% hemicellulose solubilization for wheat straw biomass. The dilute acids used in chemical pretreatment improve the digestion of cellulosic polymers. The effective concentration of dilute acids used in pretreatment is typically 4%.

Ionic liquids pretreatment: It disintegrates cellulose at ambient conditions releasing sugar molecules. They are considered "green solvents" due to their large thermal and chemical stability. Additionally, ionic liquids can be recycled for reuse and are non-volatile. Various types of ionic liquids such as imidazolium-based compounds $[(C_3N_2)\ Xn]^+$, ammonium compounds $[NX_4]^{+,}$ and phosphonium compounds $[PX_4]^+$ are used in pretreatment. Acidic ionic liquids have been found to be more efficient in pretreating lignocellulosic substrates. They disrupt the hydrogen bond network of cellulose improving enzyme digestibility. In fact, a concentration of 10% ionic liquid in biomass can disrupt cellulase enzymes. A combination of polyethylene glycol and the ionic liquid 3-methylimidazolium chloride has been found to be effective for enzyme conversion and bioethanol yield. For example, a pretreatment using 5% polyethylene glycol resulted in the production of 176 g/L of glucose after three days with an ethanol yield of 105 g/L.

9.5.1.2 Physicochemical pretreatment processes

Steam explosion: The process of steam explosion involves using saturated steam to treat lignocellulosic biomass, which leads to an increase in pressure that detaches fibers and dissolves lignin substances. However, this process has some disadvantages. For one, it only partially removes lignin. Additionally, it releases toxic chemicals like furfural. Steam explosion is typically conducted at pressure of 2.5–7 MPa and a temperature range of 180–280°C. It also results in a 60% recovery of glucose. To improve the digestion of cellulose fibers, an acid or alkali treatment is done as pretreatment.

Hot water pretreatment: In this method, cellulosic biomass is degraded using hot water at temperatures ranging from 160 to 250°C. The heating rate is set at 20°C/min for a duration of 20 min. When combined with sodium carbonate and supplied with 0.8 MPa oxygen, liquid hot water treatment is effective in removing hemicellulose polymer and lignin bonds, achieving a removal rate of up to 72% with an ethanol yield of 66 g/L. Another option is to combine hot water treatment with sodium hydroxide and oxygen at 0.8 MPa, which results in a glucose yield of 52% within an hour.

Ammonium fiber explosion process: The use of aqueous ammonia as a low-cost solvent can break the bonds formed by esters between cellulosic polymers. By combining hydrogen peroxide and ammonia, it is possible to achieve a 37% removal of lignin.

Carbon dioxide explosion: This method involves feeding carbon dioxide at high pressure 200°C through biomass. During the process, carbonic acid is produced and diffuses through the biomass, hydrolyzing hemicellulose. Then, the pressure is increased to improve the digestion of cellulose. When ammonium fiber explosion is combined with carbon dioxide assistance, a glucose yield of 94% is achieved. This process also increases the porosity between cellulose and hemicellulose, which enhances enzyme digestion activity.

Wet air oxidation: The biomass is oxidized at temperature ranging from 170 to with a pressure of 10–20 MPa, for a duration of 15 min. This combination results in an 89% removal of lignin. The pretreatment with oxygen leads to the formation of hydroxyl radicals and organic acids. For rice husks, the optimal parameters for wet air oxidation are a temperature of 185°C, a pressure of 0.5 MPa, and a reaction time of 15 min. This combination results in an 89% removal of lignin (Akanksha Shukla et al., 2023; Azra Maliha et al., 2023).

Biological pretreatment processes: The biological pretreatment using different microbial strains from fungi and bacteria and their lignin removal efficiency are provided in Table 9.13.

9.5.2 Synthesis of bioethanol from various biomass using microorganisms

First-generation biomass feedstocks such as cane sugar and beet sugar are sugar-based crops. Corn, barley, and wheat are starch-based crops, while sunflower and rapeseed are oil-based crops. Second-generation biomass consists of cellulosic biomass like wood and agricultural wastes. The presence of lignin affects the fermentation step as it hinders enzymes and microorganisms from dissolving cellulose compounds. The use of thermophilic bacteria has improved the lignocellulosic biomass fermentation process.

Barley straw is a useful biomass for the generation of bioethanol. The pretreatment of the feedstock is done using a decompression technique at 125–175°C and 3 MPa pressure. The hydrolysis step is

TABLE 9.13
Biological treatment using different fungal and bacterial strains and their efficiency of lignin removal (Dai et al., 2017; Naresh Kumar et al., 2017; Xie et al., 2017)

Fungi and bacterial species	Enzyme produced	Results of pretreatment
Fungal pretreatment		
Pleurotus florida	Cellulase	20% delignification, 83% recovery of cellulose
Pleurotus eryngii	Xylanase, laccase	43% removal of lignin, 86% recovery of cellulose
Trichoderma reesei	Cellulase	46% removal of lignin, 59% glucan digestion
Bacterial pretreatment		
***Galactomyces* sp.**	Cellulase, β-glucosidase	13% removal of lignin, 50% recovery of cellulose
Streptomyces griseorubens	Cellulase and xylanase	3% removal of lignin, 66% recovery of cellulose
Ochrobactrum oryzae	Xylanase	10% removal of lignin, 52% recovery of cellulose

carried out at 50°C for 72 h using cellulase enzymes. The fermentation step is done at 22°C for seven days using *Saccharomyces cerevisiae.* The bioethanol yield obtained from barley straw is 0.4–0.9 g/g. *Prosopis juliflora* is a good source of bioethanol. The pretreatment is done with mild nitric acid at 121°C, 0.01 MPa, and a biomass to liquid ratio of 1:10. Simultaneous saccharification and fermentation steps are carried out using cellulase enzymes at pH 4.9, and 41°C for 72 h. The bioethanol yield using mesquite stem is 0.67 g/g. Palm kernel cake is a useful source of bioethanol. The pretreatment of the kernel cake is done by steam explosion at 0.45 MPa pressure for 15 min. The hydrolysis step uses mannanase and cellulase at 50°C. The fermentation step is carried out using *Geobacillus thermoglucosidasius* at 60°C for 48 h with agitation at 250 rpm. The bioethanol yield using palm kernel cake is 0.47 g/g. Rice straw is used as a source for producing bioethanol. The pretreatment is done using microwave assisted sodium hydroxide process at 100–140°C for 2 min. The hydrolysis step is done using cellulolytic enzymes synthesized from *Trichoderma reesei* at pH 4.8, and 55°C for 72 h. The fermentation step is done with *Saccharomyces cerevisiae* at a temperature of 30°C, a time of 72 h, and a pH of 4.5. The bioethanol yield using rice straw biomass is 0.44 g/g. Sorghum stalks are an improved biomass for bioethanol production. The pretreatment step is done with mild sulfuric acid treatment. The fermentation step is performed using the enzyme *Thermoanaerobacterium aotearoense* with a total sugar concentration of 15 g/L and operating conditions of a temperature of 55°C. The bioethanol yield using sorghum stalks is 0.36 g/g.

Soybean straw is subjected to pretreatment using mild sulfuric acid of concentration 0.1 M at 121°C with agitation for 30 min. The fermentation is done using the enzyme *Thermoanaerobacterium aotearoense* with a total sugar concentration of 15 g/L at a temperature of 55°C with an agitation speed of 150 rpm. The bioethanol yield using soybean straw biomass is 0.34 g/g.

Starch-based food waste is used as feedstock in bioethanol production. The pretreatment is done by mild sulfuric acid treatment. Simultaneous saccharification and fermentation step is carried out using enzyme *Saccharomyces cerevisiae.* The ratio of inoculum to feedstock is 1:10, with a pH of 6, a temperature of 30°C and a duration of 94 h with agitation at 80 rpm.

The bioethanol production using corn starch uses the dry grind and wet mill process. Yeasts such as *Saccharomyces cerevisiae* and *Schizosaccaharomyces pombe* are capable of metabolizing starch. In the dry milling process, the corn is milled and mixed with water, then cooked at 80–90°C for 15–20 min. α amylase is added to assist the liquefaction process. Saccharification and fermentation occur simultaneously at a pH of 4.8–5 and a temperature of 30°C for 48 h. The yield of ethanol per kg of corn in the dry process is 0.323 and in the wet process is 0.291.

The steps in bioethanol generation from cellulosic biomass are as follows:

- Pretreatment of cellulose and hemicellulose to make them suitable for further processing.
- Enzyme hydrolysis of cellulose into simple sugars.
- Fermentation of hexoses and pentoses by microorganisms into bioethanol.
- Separation of bioethanol to concentrate the product.

Sugar cane bagasse is pretreated with dilute sulfuric acid and recombinant *Saccharomyces cerevisiae* in a solid-phase fermentation technique. The yield of bioethanol is 52 g/L (Prasad et al., 2020; Qu et al., 2021).

9.5.3 Bioethanol production from algae

Algae are excellent photosynthetic plants that grow in non-consumable water resources. Single and multicellular species of freshwater and marine algae are abundant in nature. Microalgae and macroalgae are classified based on size, and both are useful sources for bioethanol generation. The classification of algae based on pigments present in them is as follows: chloro-phyceae or green algal species, rhodophyceae or red algal species, phaeophyceae or brown algal species and cyanophyceae or blue-green algae species. Cyanophyceae is the most commonly used algal species due to its photosynthetic activity for the synthesis of bioethanol. The synthesis of bioethanol from the green algal species *Chlamydomonas reinhardtii* is widely studied. The microalgae *Chlorococum littorale* was used to generate bioethanol under dark fermentation conditions with a yield of 450 mol/g dry weight of algae at a temperature of 30°C. The process of intracellular fermentation is used with *Chlamydomonas reinhardtii* for the production of ethanol. Fermentation studies with the microalgae species *Nannochloropsis oculata* in soy sauce waste treatment for ethanol production were attempted. Algae substrate treated with mild sulfuric acid to separate glucose, which is then converted by fermentation to ethanol using *Chlamydomonas reihardtii*. Pretreatment with sodium hydroxide was used to convert *Chlorococcum infusionum* biomass to ethanol. An ethanol yield of 0.28-g ethanol/gram biomass was obtained for 0.75% sodium hydroxide, 120°C treatment for 30 min. Green algae *Spirogyra* is fermented by a combination of bacterial and yeast (*Saccharomyces cerevisiae*) species to produce ethanol. The ethanol generation using *Chlorococcum species* is improved by the hydrolysis step of microalgal biomass with enzymes. Ethanol is produced from the green algae *Chlamydomonas reinhardtii* by a highly efficient saccharification technique using *Trichoderma harzianum* enzymes. The biomass of *Chlorella sorokiniana* synthesizes ethanol by enzymatic saccharification of carbohydrates.

Brown algae *Laminaria* and *Sargassum* are commonly used for the synthesis of bioethanol. *Sargassum sagamianum* biomass was used as a source of bioethanol with various *Pichia stipitis* species. Brown algae *Saccharina japonica* was pretreated with mild acid and subjected to combined saccharification with fermentation to generate ethanol. Ethanol and protein production were done with brown algae biomass from *Laminaria digitata*. The biomass of *Saccharina latissima* was enzymatically hydrolyzed to produce ethanol. Ethanol is produced from the brown algae biomass of *Colpomenia sinuosa* by fermentation using a strain of yeast *Meyerozyma guilliermondii*. The red algae *Gracilaria verrucosa* were acid hydrolyzed to produce ethanol. Additionally, the enzyme treatment of freshwater red algae *Porphyridium cruentum* resulted in increased ethanol production through solid-state fermentation. *Eucheuma spinosum* biomass is also capable of generating ethanol from algae.

Blue-green algae or cyanobacteria are a valuable species for bioethanol production. *Microcystis aeruginosa* is capable of producing ethanol using various media compositions. Ethanol can also be generated from blue-green algae biomass from *Spirulina platensis* through saccharification with four different acids. The use of Spirulina also enhances ethanol production through increased carbohydrate productivity. *Leptolynbgya sps* found in agro-industrial wastewater treatment produces ethanol (Thummala Chandrasekhar et al., 2023; Shoyeb Khan et al., 2023). The bioethanol yield from different microalgae strains is provided in Table 9.14.

TABLE 9.14
Bioethanol yield from different microalgal strains and their process conditions

Microalgae biomass	Parameters for pretreatment processes	Process conditions for fermentation	Biobased ethanol yield g/g on dry basis
Scenedesmus di morphis	Enzymatic hydrolysis, 24 h, 750 rpm	*S. cerevisiae*, 34°C, agitation 150 rpm	0.266
Chlorella vulgaris	Mild sulfuric acid at 120°C for 20 min	*S. cerevisiae*, 30°C, agitation 200 rpm	0.25
Tetraselmis species	Chemical and enzyme hydrolysis, pH 5, 60°C	*S. cerevisiae*, 30°C, agitation 150 rpm, 48 h	0.314
Leptolyngbia valderiana	Mild sulfuric acid at 121°C for 20 min	*S. cerevisiae*, 30°C, agitation 200 rpm, 80 h	0.16
Chlorococum sp.	Supercritical carbon dioxide	*S. bayanus*, 30°C, agitation 200 rpm, 60 h	0.35
Scenedesmus acuminatus	2N sulfuric acid, pH 5.5	*S. cerevisiae*, 30°C, agitation 200 rpm, 80 h	0.12

9.5.4 Biobutanol production from different substrates using microorganisms

The butanol fermentation process involves fermenting starch-based crops or lignocellulosic crops using butanol-producing strains, which also generate byproducts of acetone and ethyl alcohol. This method is commonly referred to as the acetone-butyl alcohol-ethyl alcohol (ABE) technique.

One strain that produces butyl alcohol is *Clostridium acetobutylicum,* which ferments glucose to produce butyl alcohol, acetone, and ethyl alcohol with a yield of 10.4 g/L. Another bacterial species *Clostridium beijerinckii* digests glucose to produce butyl alcohol and isopropyl alcohol with a butanol yield of 15.2 g/L. *Clostridium saccharoperbutylacetonicum* ferments glucose to produce butyl alcohol, acetone, and ethyl alcohol with a yield of 16.2 g/L. *Clostridium saccharoperbutylicum* converts glucose to butyl alcohol, acetone, and ethyl alcohol with a butanol yield of 9.7 g/L. Lastly, *Clostridium pasteurianum* converts glucose to butanol and 1,3-propylene glycol with yield of 6.5 g/L.

Starch-based raw materials: Cassava starch is fermented using *Clostridium saccharoper butyl acetonicum* with butanol yield of 16.9 g/L. *C. acetobutylicum* can also be used on cassava substrate producing butyl alcohol yield of 13 g/L. A mutant strain of *C. acetobutylicum* ART18, obtained through room temperature plasma mutagenesis, can use gelatinized cassava flour for fermentation to produce butanol with yield of 16.3 g/L.

Lignocellulosic biomass as raw materials: Wheat bran is pre-treated with dilute acid and fermented using bacterial strain *C. beijerinckii* to yield butanol titer value of 8.8 g/L. Corn stover feedstock can be fermented using the strain *C. aceto butylicum* resulting in 6.6 g/L of butyl alcohol. The steam explosion technique is used for pre-treating corn stover, followed by a continuous fermentation process. Sugarcane bagasse can be used as a substrate in saccharification yielding 0.21 g/L/h of butanol. Corn straw can be pre-treated with a solvent resulting in 99% cellulose removal and a yield of 13.65 g/L of butanol. Molasses as raw material: Molasses is a secondary substance produced from the alcohol industry, containing various sugars and amino acids. *Clostridium acetobutylicum* can be used to ferment molasses to produce 18 g/L of butyl alcohol. Fermentatingmolasses with the strain *Clostridium beijerinckii* yields 11.33 g/L of butanol. *C. saccharoperbutylacetonicum* can also use molasses as a substrate in a four-stage continuous fermentation process, resulting in a yield of 13.75 g/L of butanol. Batch fermentation: This process involves fewer risks of microbial contamination during the fermentation stage. The butanol yield from a batch fermentation process generally does not exceed 21 g/L. The presence of butyric acid inhibits cell growth during batch fermentation. Increasing the carbon to nitrogen source ratio from 4.3 to 21.4 resulted in an increase in the total titer value from 1.58 to 19 g/L, respectively.

Continuous fermentation: The fresh culture is supplied to the fermenter, and the broth generated is separated from the fermenter at the same rate. Techniques like cell immobilization and cell recycling improve fermentation productivity by enhancing cell density. Cell immobilization is achieved through the adsorption and covalent binding of cells. Cell recycling is accomplished using ultrafiltration membranes made from cellulose triacetate and polysulfone (Lin et al., 2023; Shams Forruque Ahmed et al., 2023). The various feedstocks and microorganisms used during the fermentation process to produce butanol are provided in Table 9.15.

9.6 MANUFACTURE OF BIOHYDROGEN FROM MICROBIAL CONSORTIUM

Hydrogen is a clean source of fuel that only produces water vapor as a byproduct (Cabrol et al., 2017). Hydrogen can be obtained from various sources including biomass waste, making it an environmentally friendly, cost-efficient and renewable source of energy (Weber and Lipman, 2018). Hydrogen can be stored in compressed gas form, as a liquid, or in solid states. It is widely used in transportation vehicles, power generation plants, and various industrial processes (Zhang et al., 2021).

TABLE 9.15
Feedstocks and microorganisms used during fermentation process to produce butanol

Substrate	Fermentation operating conditions	Microorganisms	ABE (g/L)	Butanol yield (g/L)
Decayed potato	Fermentation for 96 h	*Clostridium beijerinckii*	12	7.9
Green coconut husk	Fermentation for 96 h	*Clostridium beijerinckii*	5.3	3.4
Switchgrass	Fermentation for 72 h	*C. beijerinckii*	20.24	11.21
Microalgal biomass	Fermentation for 48 h, 37°C	*Clostridium acetobutylicum*	15.47	12.67
Rice bran	Fermentation for 128 h	*C. saccharoperbutyl-acetonicum*	10.5	7.1
Corn stover	Fermentation for 72 h	*C. saccharobutylicum*	9	7.12
Barley straw	Fermentation with gas stripping	*C. beijerinckii*	47.2	30.86

TABLE 9.16
Biohydrogen production using various microalgae Yun et al. (2014); Maswanna et al. (2020)

Microalgae	Fermentation Parameters	Biohydrogen Yield
Chlorella vulgaris	3N KOH, 35°C, pH 7.4	43 mL/g
Tetraspora species	36°C, 18 h, 29 μmol of photons per ms	512 mL/L
Chlorella species	37°C, pH 7	1276 mL/L
Chlamydomonas species	25°C, pH 9	8.73 L/kg

Grey H_2 is produced through methane gas reformation using steam, which releases a significant amount of carbon dioxide (Katebah et al., 2022). Fossil fuels produce blue hydrogen in which some carbon dioxide is captured (Massarweh et al., 2023). Turquoise hydrogen is produced through methane pyrolysis, capturing most of the carbon dioxide (Hermesmann and Müller, 2022). Pink hydrogen is generated through the electrolysis process using nuclear power, while black hydrogen is produced through coal gasification (Ajanovic et al, 2022).

Recently, biohydrogen production has been explored as a cost-efficient source of energy from renewable biomass sources. Lignocellulosic materials, industrial residues, and municipal wastes are sources of biomass (Nikolaidis and Poullikkas, 2017). Biomass can be converted into biohydrogen through pyrolysis, gasification, biophotolysis, and fermentation processes. The biological process has the advantage of being able to operate at ambient conditions (Rezania et al., 2017).

Algae are a common marine biomass that is classified into microalgae and macroalgae based on size. Macroalgae or seaweed are raw materials used for biohydrogen generation. It is a rich source of carbohydrates and does not contain hemicellulose and lignin, which prevents biodegradation. Macroalgae have great potential for CO_2 bioremediation and have a high biomass yield (Sudhakar et al., 2018; Del Río et al., 2019). Macroalgae are further classified based on pigment color, including brown macroalgae like Saccharina and Sargassum, green macroalgae like Ulva and Codium, and red macroalgae like Gelidium and Gracilaria. Macroalgae contains 55% carbohydrates in its dry biomass including laminarin and mannitol (Lee et al., 2010). Table 9.16 provides information on the types of microalgae, fermentation process parameters, and corresponding biohydrogen yield.

Cyanobacteria are involved in the biophotolysis of water molecules to produce biohydrogen. Biohydrogen is produced by cyanobacteria in the presence of nitrogen-fixing strains that contain nitrogenase enzymes (Sharma and Arya, 2017). The biophotolysis technique allows each mole of glucose to produce 12 mol of hydrogen as follows.

$$C_6H_{12}O_6 + 6H_2O \rightarrow 6CO_2 + 12H_2$$

9.6.1 Biohydrogen Production by Biophotolysis Process

Biophotolysis is a process that involves the splitting of water into H_2 and O_2 gas by microalgae or cyanobacteria using a light source. This photochemical reaction generates electrons that are then transmitted through electron carriers in the Calvin cycle, producing adenosine triphosphate (ATP) molecules. Biophotolysis can be done directly or indirectly, with or without sunlight.

In direct photolysis, sunlight is used to split the water molecules. The role of hydrogenase is to generate hydrogen without producing harmful greenhouse gases, while also releasing oxygen into the atmosphere.

$$2H_2O + \text{light-energy} \rightarrow 2H_2 + O_2$$

The photons produced by sunlight are utilized to charge the electron transport, and the generated electrons are used in the photosynthesis process in photosystem to create ATP molecules. *Chlamydomonas reinhardtii* and *Chlorella vulgaris* are commonly used as microalgae in direct biophotolysis. This process is catalyzed by photocatalysts such as titanium dioxide or metal oxides. The light energy is absorbed by the photocatalysts causing water to split into hydrogen gas molecules and oxygen molecules. Titanium dioxide acts as a semiconductor component where high-energy photons strike the surface of the semiconductor exciting electrons into electron-hole pairs. The protons released from the semiconductor surface create hydrogen gas molecules (Jiménez-Llanos et al., 2020).

The inherent advantages of direct biophotolysis include the ability to produce biohydrogen and oxygen simultaneously from water. The process utilizes water as a simple substrate and employs simple cultivation techniques. However, a disadvantage is that the buildup of oxygen during the process inhibits biohydrogen formation. Additionally, there are challenges in separating hydrogen and oxygen as high-purity compounds. The Fe-hydrogenase enzyme used in direct biophotolysis is sensitive to the oxygen generated during the process.

The first step of the indirect photolysis process or photosystem I is the reduction of carbon dioxide to carbohydrates through photosynthesis. The second stage of photosystem II involves the conversion to hydrogen. In the photo fermentation process, carbohydrates are broken down into H_2, CH_3COOH, and CO_2. Cyanobacteria produce nitrogenase enzymes for nitrogen fixation and hydrogen evolution reactions, and they require minimal nutrients for survival. The carbon dioxide molecule acts as a carrier for electrons between the first step of photosynthesis and the second step involved in hydrogen generation. The reactions involved in this process are provided below, which take place in the presence of a photochemical agent:

$$6\ CO_2 + 12\ H_2O \rightarrow C_6H_{12}O_6 + 6\ O_2$$

$$C_6H_{12}O_6 + 12\ H_2O \rightarrow 6\ CO_2 + 12\ H_2$$

During the aerobic phase, cyanobacteria or microalgae use light energy to fix carbon dioxide into carbohydrates. The lack of oxygen results in the electron transport stops functioning, highlighting the need for the activation of hydrogenase, an oxygen-sensitive enzyme that produces biohydrogen (Kumar et al., 2019). Generally, four steps are involved in indirect photolysis:

- Photosynthesis reaction to produce glucose
- Concentration of biomass
- Performance of the photo fermentation process in an aerobic scenario
- Hydrogen evolution.

9.6.2 Biohydrogen Generation by Photo Fermentation of Biomass

Fermentation converts biomass into biohydrogen using microorganisms such as yeasts and bacteria. The process breaks down sugar complexes into simple molecules using enzymes supplied by microorganisms. Photo fermentation produces biohydrogen using strains like *Rhodobium, Rhodobacter, Rhodospirillum,* and *Rhodopseudomonas.* These purple non-sulfur bacterial species can convert hydrogen ions or protons into hydrogen gas molecules. Oxygen is not produced during the fermentation step. The bacteria can use various substrates like alcohol, amino acid, carbohydrates, and pyruvate. The reactions involved in photo fermentation are as follows:

Using carbohydrate: $C_6H_{12}O_6 + 6H_2O \rightarrow 6CO_2 + 12H_2$
Using acetate: $2CH_3COOH + 2H_2O \rightarrow 4H_2 + 2CO_2$

The nitrogenase enzyme acts as a catalyst in hydrogen evolution during photochemical fermentation. The presence of micro and macronutrients is crucial for the growth and activity of algae and bacterial species (Saravanan et al., 2022). Table 9.17 provides the biohydrogen yield of various bacterial species.

The advantages of photo fermentation process:

- Photosynthetic bacterial species are active across a wide range of wavelengths.
- Photosynthetic bacteria can process a wide range of substrate biomass.
- It can process effluent generated by the dark fermentation step.

The limitations of the photo fermentation process are as follows:

- The conversion efficiency of light is low.
- The yield of biohydrogen production is low.

9.6.3 Biohydrogen Generation by Dark Fermentation of Biomass

In the dark fermentation process, biomass is converted to biohydrogen using bacterial species involved in fermentation. These bacterial species produce hydrogenase enzymes that assist in the production of hydrogen. The hydrogen protons neutralize the electrons generated during the oxidation of biomass, resulting in hydrogen production under anaerobic conditions. The dark fermentation process can be carried out using mixed flow reactors, packed bed reactors, or fluidized bed reactors. Specifically, the dark fermentation of rice straw is performed at a temperature of 55°C. The pH is maintained between 5.5 and 6.5 for optimal biohydrogen production (Sillero et al., 2022).

TABLE 9.17
Photo fermentation bacterial species and their maximum hydrogen yield Lu et al. (2021)

Microorganisms	Yield of hydrogen	Efficiency
Rhodo pseudomona and Rhodo bacter	Maximum 160 mL/gCS	16% energy conversion
Rhodospirillum and Rhodobium	140 mL (g TS)$^{-1}$	10% energy conversion

Fermentation is an energy-intensive process that can produce biohydrogen under optimal conditions. The process is environmentally friendly with lower greenhouse gas emissions. However, the fermentation process is sensitive to change in pH and temperature, which can affect its operational efficiency (Mishra et al., 2019). Table 9.18 provides information on the types of biomass, process conditions, and corresponding biohydrogen yield.

The advantages of the dark fermentation process are as follows:

- The rate of dark fermentation is larger than that of photo fermentation.
- Dark fermentation processes can utilize various substrates obtained from different sources.
- Dark fermentation does not require a direct light source, allowing for operation 24 h a day.
- The reactor configuration required for this process is simple and economical.

The reaction for dark fermentation of glucose to produce acetic acid with hydrogen production is as follows:

$$C_6H_{12}O_6 + 2H_2O \text{ —-> } 2CH_3COOH + 2CO_2 + 4H_2$$

The reaction for dark fermentation of glucose to produce acetic acid with hydrogen production is as follows:

$$C_6H_{12}O_6 \text{ —-> } CH_3CH_2CH_2\,COOH + 2CO_2 + 2H_2.$$

The optimum hydrogen yield obtained from various anaerobic bacterial species is provided in Table 9.19.

TABLE 9.18
Type of biomass, Inoculum, Process conditions and biohydrogen yield (Zhang L et al., 2019; Yin Y et al., 2019)

Biomass type	Inoculum	Process conditions	Biohydrogen Production Rate
Seaweed, Ulva reticulate	Digested sludge	pH 6, 37°C, 68 h	87.5 mL/g
Laminaria japonica	Digested sludge	pH 7, 55°C, 18 h	16 mL/g
Municipal waste	*Clostridium lentocellum*	pH 7.5, 55°C, 3 h	5.7 mL/g
Corn cob waste	Mixed activated sludge	pH 7, 37°C, 116 h	114 mL/L

TABLE 9.19
Optimum hydrogen yield obtained from anaerobic bacterial species (Cao et al., 2022)

Generic name of bacteria	Species name of bacteria	Biohydrogen yield (moles/ moles glucose)
Citro bacter	*C. amalonaticus*	1.3
Klebsiellae	*Enterobacter aerogenes*	2.16
Entero bacter	*Entero bacter cloacae*	4
Escherichia	*Escherichia coli*	2.1
Clostridium	*C. acetobutylicum*	2.0

9.6.4 Biohydrogen Production by Microbial Electrolysis of Biomass

The microbial electrolysis cell is a module used to generate biohydrogen through a biological and electrochemical system. The process involves two steps: the breakdown of organic substances into carbon dioxide, electrons, and protons by microbes in the anode surface and the generation of hydrogen by the protons released on the cathode. A biofilm of microbes forms on the electrode surface to oxidize the substrate. Microbial fuel cells can convert organic mass to hydrogen without the use of oxygen at low current supply. The voltage supplied affects the charged species of electrons and protons, which combine on the cathode surface to generate hydrogen molecules. Organic waste materials are a good source of biohydrogen production (Rahul Gautam et al., 2023). Microbial electrolysis cells can utilize various substrate wastes such as food wastes, industrial wastes, domestic wastes, and vegetable wastes. Food industry wastes are rich in carbohydrates like starch and glucose, while dairy wastes are rich in protein like casein and carbohydrates. The performance of microbial electrolysis cells is influenced by factors such as inoculum, current efficiency, type of electrodes, and hydrogen production rate. Commonly used bacterial species as electrochemical active bacteria in microbial electrolysis cells include *Geobacter, Shewanella, Rhodoferax spp.*, and *Rhodopseudomonas spp.* Algal species are also used in microbial electrolysis cells. The reactions involved at the cathode and anode are classified below requiring a circuit voltage greater than 0.11 V:

Reaction at anode surface:

$$C_2H_4O_2 + 2H_2O \rightarrow 2CO_2 + 8H^+ + 8e^-$$

Reaction at cathode surface:

$$8e^- + 8H^+ \rightarrow 4H_2$$

Glucose and cellulose substrates are fermented into end products that are difficult to convert to hydrogen in subsequent steps. The microorganisms are unable to extract energy from these products. In order for reaction to be spontaneous and irreversible, the change in Gibbs free energy must be less than zero. However, the hydrogen generation from various organic compounds has a positive Gibbs free energy (Ariadna Segundo-Aguilar et al., 2021). For the degradation of acetate at 1 bar, 25°C and pH 7, the Gibbs free energy is 104.6 KJ/mol. The reaction for acetate degradation is as follows:

$$CH_3COO- + 4H_2O \rightarrow 2\ HCO_3- + H+ + 4\ H2\ (\Delta GrO= +104.6\ \text{kJ/mol})$$

To degrade the substrate, additional energy must be supplied through applied voltage. Table 9.20 provides several physico-biological parameters that affect microbial electrolysis cells. Table 9.21 presents the biohydrogen yield for different substrates under different operating parameters.

$E_{eq} = -\ \Delta Gr^O/nF$
E_{eq} = Equilibrium voltage
ΔGr^O = Gibbs Free energy change
n = Electrons involved in the reaction
F = Faraday's constant

9.7 MANUFACTURE OF BIOGAS FROM MICROBIAL CONSORTIUM

Biogas is a form of non-conventional energy generated through the anaerobic decomposition of organic waste. The produced biogas consists of methane (ranging from 50 to 75% volume), carbon dioxide (ranging from 25 to 50% by volume) and small amounts of nitrogen gas, hydrogen sulfide, and hydrogen. However, if carbon dioxide and hydrogen sulfide are absent, the calorific value of

TABLE 9.20
Physico-biological parameters affecting microbial electrolysis cell Hou et al. (2017); Yange et al. (2015)

Substrate	Anode	Cathode	Electrode Distance	Microorganisms
Dyes	Brush of graphite	Nickel foam coated with TiO_2	2.5 cm	Mixed microbial consortium culture
Sodium acetate	Stainless steel frame with carbon fiber	Mesh made of stainless steel	1.5 cm	Mixed microbial consortium culture
Activated sludge wastes	Carbon fiber	Mesh made of stainless steel	2 cm	Mixed microbial consortium culture
Stalk of corn	Brush of graphite mesh	Platinum coated with carbon cloth	1.5 cm	Mixed microbial consortium culture
Sugar industry effluents	Graphite	Ni foam, SS mesh 304	1.5 cm	Mixed Culture
Glycerol	Graphite brush	Carbon fabric platinum mesh	3 cm	Mixed Culture

TABLE 9.21
Biohydrogen yield for various substrates at different operating parameters by microbial electrolysis (Hou et al., 2017; Yange et al., 2015)

Substrate	Applied Voltage (V)	pH, Temperature	Biohydrogen yield
Dyes	0.8	7/25°C	113 mL
Sodium acetate	0.5	7.2/25°C	1.46 mL/h
Wasted activated sludge	0.8–1.2	6.8/30°C	25.6 mL/d
Corn stalk	0.8	6.8/30°C	387 mL H_2/g corn stalk
Glycerol	0.9	7/30°C	2 m^3/d

the biogas increases to 42 MJ/kg. The production of biogas involves metabolic processes controlled by microbial species. The interactions between these microbes and the substrate are crucial for enhancing biogas yield. The substrate for biogas production can be obtained from sources such as industrial effluent, food waste, agricultural waste, and sewage. Industrial effluent from the brewing industry is commonly used due to its rich organic nutrients.

There are several reasons why biogas is considered a self-sustainable non-conventional energy source.

- The process generates energy to sustain itself and produce additional biogas.
- It does not rely on non-renewable fossil fuels.
- It is a renewable energy source not contributing to carbon emissions.
- It helps to reduce greenhouse gas emissions.

The purpose of pre-treating the substrate before the main biogas production process is as follows.

- To enhance the ability of microorganisms to degrade the substrate by improving its surface properties.
- To remove any toxic substance that could inhibit biogas generation.

TABLE 9.22
Different Pretreatment methods for various substrates (Li et al., 2021; Sinbuathong et al., 2021; Avila et al., 2021)

Pretreatment types	Dried substrates	Pretreatment conditions
By chemical pretreatment	Dried *Pontederia crassipes*	5% H_2SO_4 for 1 h
By chemical pretreatment	Dried sun hemp	1% sodium hydroxide treatment
By physical pretreatment	Waste from paddy straw	Microwave irradiation treatment at 190°C for 4 min
By physical pretreatment	Waste from plant residues	Ball mill treatment for 4 h, 150°C
By biological pretreatment	Algae species	Hydrolytic enzymes treatment
By biological pretreatment	Wastes from fruits and vegetables	Viscozyme enzyme treatment

- To increase the rate of hydrolysis, which is an important step in the biogas production process.
- To improve the nutrient intake of microorganisms ultimately increasing the yield of biogas.

Physical pretreatment techniques are performed using mechanical disintegration and ultrasonic irradiation methods. The objective of mechanical disintegration is to increase the surface area of biomass by breaking it into smaller sizes. Ultrasonic waves are used in irradiation techniques to disintegrate biomass substrates. Ultrasonication generates highly reactive free radicals that chemically react with organic substances. Microwave treatment breaks the hydrogen bonds in cell walls and degrades the substrates.

Chemical pretreatment involves the use of acids, alkalis, solvents, or oxidation processes. Acid pretreatment breaks the hydrogen bonds in polymeric substrates and disintegrates them into simpler compounds. Alkaline treatment involves the saponification of fats and oils found in organic substrates. Calcium hydroxide and sodium hydroxide are used to disintegrate lignin and hemicellulose during the pretreatment stage.

Biological pretreatment involves the use of enzymes and microorganisms to biodegrade the substrates. The enzymes used in pretreatment of organic wastes include pectinase, cellulase, protease, and amylase. Fungal strains such as *Trametes villosa* and *Coriolopsis gallica* as well as bacterial species like *Bacillus subtilis and Pseudomonas aeruginosa* are used in this process. A comprehensive list of the different pretreatment methods for various substrates can be found in Table 9.22.

9.7.1 Biochemical mechanism of biogas production

Anaerobic digestion consists of four steps: hydrolysis, acidogenesis, acetogenesis, and methanogenesis (Figure 9.1).

During hydrolysis, microbes produce several enzymes that break down complex substances into simpler ones. Bacterial species involved in this step include *Clostridia sp.,* Bacteroides *sp., Fusobacterium sp.*, and *Streptococcus sp.*

In the acidogenesis/fermentation step, hydrolytic products are fermented into short-chain saturated fatty acids, ethanol, H_2, and CO_2. The simple compounds formed in this step such as formic acid, carbon dioxide, hydrogen gas, and acetic acid can be used directly in the methanogenesis step. Microorganisms involved include *Thermotoga maritima, Caldicellulosiruptor saccharolyticus*, and *Escherichia coli.*

Acetogenesis involves the reduction of carbon dioxide to acetic acid and the fermentation of organic acids into acetate. *Clostridium aceticum* is a homoacetogen that reduces carbon dioxide to acetic acid.

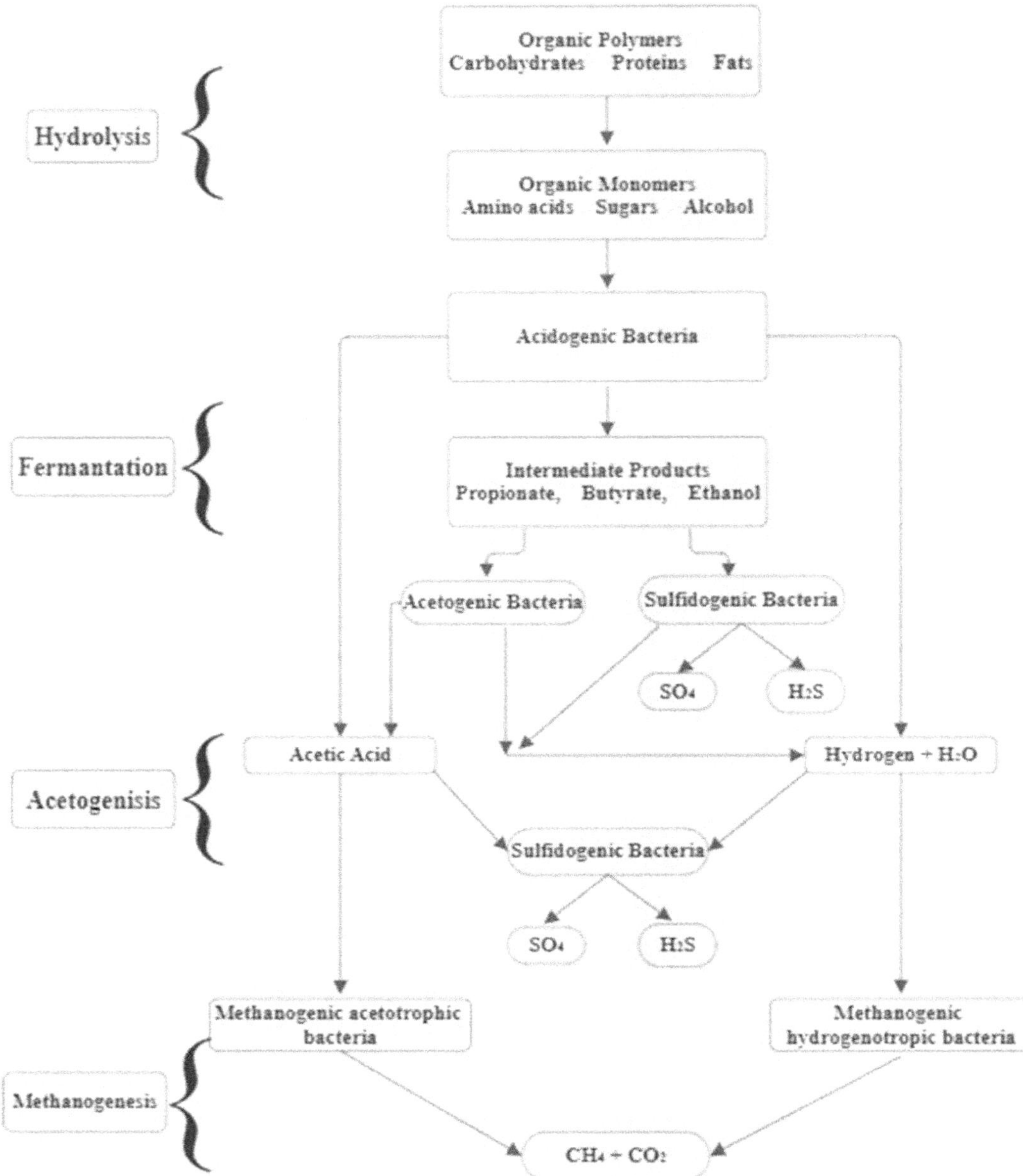

FIGURE 9.1 Steps involved in biochemical mechanism of biogas production by anaerobic digestion.

$$2CO_2 + 4H_2 \leftrightarrow CH_3COOH + 2H_2O$$

Syntrophobacter wolinii, breaks down propionic acid to acetate acetogen.

$$CH_3CH_2CH_2OH + 2H_2O \leftrightarrow CH_3COOH + 3H_2 + CO_2$$

Syntrophomonas wolfei, ferments butyric acid into acetate acetogen.

$$CH_3CH_2CH_2CH_2OH+2H_2O \leftrightarrow CH_3COOH+2H_2$$

Acetobacterium woodii ferments glucose to acetic acid.

$$C_6H_{12}O_6 +2H_2O \leftrightarrow 2CH_3COOH+2CO_2 +4H_2$$

In the methanogenesis step, organic matter is fermented into methane gas, carbon dioxide, and hydrogen. Substrates utilized in methanogenesis include methylamine, CO_2, HCOOH, CH_3OH, and CH_3COOH. Commonly used methanogens in this step include *Methanosaeta, Methanococcoides, Methanosalsus, Halomethanococcus, Methanogenium*, and *Methanoculleus* (Neeraj Raja Ram and Nikhil, 2022; Ramansu Goswami et al., 2016; Venkateswar et al., 2020). There are three pathways involved:

- Methylotrophic methanogenesis: Methyl amines and methyl alcohol are decarboxylated to methane.
- Hydrogenotrophic methanogenesis: Reduction of hydrogen and carbon dioxide to methane.
- Acetotrophic methanogenesis: Acetate decarboxylation to methane.

9.7.2 Factors Influencing Microbial-Substrate Interaction During Biogas Production

pH and alkalinity: Volatile fatty acids are generated during the acidogenesis step, which results in a reduction of pH that affects microbial growth. The optimal pH for methanogens in the methanogenesis step is between 6.5 and 7.4 as it is conducive to breaking down acetic acid into methane. Maintaining the pH level is considered essential for the formation of biofilm on substrates. If the pH falls below 7 or rises above 8, the biofilm detaches from the substrate during the hydrolysis step. Volatile fatty acids diffuse into the cytoplasm of the cell where they generate protons and corresponding volatile fatty acid anions. Total alkalinity is required to prevent the system from becoming acidic. Carbonates, hydroxide, phosphate, volatile fatty acids, and ammonium all have an influence on the total alkalinity of the system. The optimum range of total alkalinity for the anaerobic digestion process is 3000–5000 $CaCO_3$/L.

Temperature: The growth levels of microorganisms are affected by the temperature at which the reaction occurs. The optimal temperature ranges are mesophilic (25–45°C) and thermophilic (45–60°C). Bacterial enzymes such as amylase, cellulase, and lipase are active during thermophilic conditions. Solubilization of substrates occurs at a high rate in thermophilic conditions during the hydrolysis step. This leads to more generation of volatile fatty acids in the acidogenesis step, resulting in a drop in pH. If the temperature is below 25°C, the solubility of gaseous substances increases in the digester. The dissolution of methane, carbon dioxide, and hydrogen increases resulting in a decrease in pH affecting the methanogenesis stage.

Ratio of parts of carbon source to parts of nitrogen source (C/N): The requirement of nitrogen gas for the synthesis of protein and nucleic acid is determined by the carbon content supplied to microorganisms. Lower C/N ratios affect methanogens as it inhibits ammonia generation, and a high C/N ratio results in higher generation of volatile fatty acids, which affect the bacterial species involved in the hydrolytic step and acidogenic stage. The optimum value of the C/N ratio is between 20 and 30. Protein-rich substrates have a low C/N ratio, whereas substrates rich in carbohydrates have a high C/N ratio. The carbon to nitrogen ratio using algae as biomass is reported as 5.3–10.2. A carbon-to-nitrogen ratio above 35 results in low yield of biogas.

Retention time: The time required for the substrate inside an anaerobic digester is known as the hydraulic retention time, while the total time that bacterial species reside in the digester is calculated as the solid retention time. A longer hydraulic retention time enhances substrate removal and has a proactive effect on the acidogenesis and methanogenesis stages. The hydraulic retention time varies based on parameters such as the temperature of the digester, substrate concentrations, and

TABLE 9.23
Optimal parameter range for microbial biogas production

Parameter	Optimum range
Alkalinity (VFA/TA)	0.3–0.4
Temperature	Mesophilic 30–40°C, Thermophilic 40–55°C
Hydraulic Retention Time	15–30 days
Carbon to Nitrogen ratio	20–35
pH	7–7.5
Trace elements	< 100 μM

microbial population count. In tropical countries like India, digester hydraulic retention times range from 40 to 60 days, while colder countries like China have hydraulic retention times of 100 days.

Trace element requirements: Cu^{2+} is essential in the hydrolytic and methanogenesis steps. The optimal range for copper is less than 100 mg/L for maximum biogas synthesis. Nickel is needed in the methanogenesis step where methyl coenzyme M reductase enzymatically reduces methyl coenzyme to methane gas. The optimal nickel concentration for biogas production is 0.8–50 mg/L. Fe is essential for the activity of proteolytic enzymes and cellulase. During the acidogenesis step, the presence of Fe inhibits the generation of sulfides. The Fe concentration needed for biogas generation is less than 4000 mg/L at the optimum level. High concentrations of Zn^{2+} affect methanogens, and the optimal range for Zn^{2+} is 0.5 mg/L for biogas production. Trace elements such as selenium and tungsten are required for the activity of enzyme dehydrogenase during the acetogenesis stage, while molybdenum is required for the activity of dehydrogenase during the methanogenesis stage. The optimal range for sodium ions is less than 350 mg/L to maintain the osmotic pressure of methanogens (Neeraj Raja Ram and Nikhil, 2022; Ramansu Goswami et al., 2016). Table 9.23 provides the optimal ranges for various parameters during microbial biogas generation.

9.7.3 Biogas production from different feedstocks

The various organic wastes used in anaerobic digestion to produce biogas include lignocellulosic wastes, food waste, leather waste, waste-activated sludge, and animal manure.

Lignocellulosic wastes are derived from waste generated in gardens, crops, and wood, which contain cellulose polymers, hemicellulose polymers, and lignin cross-linked polymers. The lignin and hemicellulose are cross-linked bonded polymers that need to be removed through pretreatment. The global rice straw production is 730 million tons/year.

Food wastes consist of carbohydrates, proteins, and lipids. Sources of food waste include cooked waste, fruit waste, vegetable waste, and meat waste. If the fat, oil, and grease percentage exceed 6%, it can affect microbial reactions.

Leather waste contains chromium, which is toxic to microorganisms and should therefore be removed through pretreatment methods. The biogas production from different organic wastes is provided in Table 9.24, while the biogas yield from various microalgae feedstock is tabulated in Table 9.25.

9.7.4 Development in bioreactor technology for biogas production

Bioconversion occurs at three temperature regimes: psychrophilic (10–25°C), mesophilic (25–40°C), and thermophilic regimes (40–55°C).

The Upflow Anaerobic Sludge Blanket Reactor (UASB) consists of an internal settler and a biogas separator. Waste water is pumped through a sludge bed using a peristaltic pump. The organic substrates are degraded to produce biogas, which helps mix the sludge and water in the bed. The use of mechanical agitators is avoided, reducing installation costs. Biogas is separated and collected

TABLE 9.24
Biogas Yield from organic wastes by anaerobic digestion (Moreno et al., 2021; Undiandeye et al., 2022)

Wastes from residues	Microbial species	Parameters	Biogas yield
Urban solid waste	*Saccharomyces cerevisiae*	Ratio of substrate to inoculum is 0.5:0.5, 35°C	51 g/L
Leaves from sugar beet	*Neurospora intermedia* and *Aspergillus niger*	25°C, 0.9:1 ratio of inoculum to substrate	516 mL/g VS
Food waste	Microbes present in anaerobically digested sludge waste	2% substrate to inoculum ratio, 37°C	883 mL/g VS
Wood waste	*Methanothermobacter crinale*	50°C, 30 d	224 L/kg of cedar
Municipal solid waste	*Methanoculleus bourgensis*	37°C, 135 d	21%

TABLE 9.25
Biogas yield from various microalgae strains (Xiao et al., 2019; Damtie et al., 2021)

Microalgae	Parameters	Biogas yield (mL/g VS)
Chlorella pyrenoidosa	Retention time 30 min, feed rate 40 L/h	348
Chlorella vulgaris	35°C, 40 d	239
Chlamydomonas reinhardtii	38°C, 20 days hydraulic retention time, loading rate of organic substrates 4 g VS/d	464
Chlorella species	35°C, 46 d	252

in a three-phase separator operating at low pressure, increasing the surface area for gas to liquid diffusion. The sludge water reaches the settler section, where biomass settles.

UASB reactors commonly use organic loadings of up to 15 kg chemical oxygen demand per cubic meter for different substrates. The removal efficiency of UASB is 60–70% for chemical oxygen demand and 75–85% for biological oxygen demand at 25–35°C. When municipal wastewater is used, UASB produces one cubic meter of biogas for every three kilograms of chemical oxygen demand. The solid residence time for this system is one year, and the hydraulic retention time is 12 h. The design criteria for municipal effluents typically maintain a maximum up flow velocity of 0.5–1 m/h to prevent solid particle washing. Increasing the solid retention time improves bacterial growth on the surface, leading to increased digestion of organic matter. The reactor volume depends on the hydraulic retention time (Cayetano R.D. A et al., 2022).

In the Anaerobic Fixed Bed (AFB) system, methanogenic bacteria are immobilized on granular activated carbon, plastics, quartz, or foam polymers. This surface forms a biofilm where microorganisms break down the substrate and release biogas.

Anaerobic fluidized bed reactor: The immobilization of microbial cells on the surface of quartz particles, pumice stone, sandstone, or alumina with a particle size less than 5 mm fluidizes in the bed. The substrate passes through the reactor at a sufficient velocity. The active microbial cells degrade the substrate and release biogas. The reactor operates at low temperatures and is capable of handling both high and low chemical oxygen demand waste effluent. The volume of the medium expands as microbes grow over its surface.

Anaerobic dynamic membrane bioreactor: The anaerobic digestion step with membrane filtration technique is known as an anaerobic dynamic membrane bioreactor. The membrane support materials include woven metallic mesh, nylon polymer screen, or silk fabric. The biofilm grows over the surface of the supporting material and acts as a pseudo-membrane layer that degrades the substrates. Self-forming dynamic membrane occurs naturally over support during filtration, whereas pre-coated dynamic membrane is formed when substrate is passed at pre-set conditions.

Two-phase methane fermentation process: In the case of high chemical oxygen demand of the substrate, the acidogenic bacteria grow ten times faster than methanogenic bacteria. The volatile fatty acids generated and hydrogen buildup reduce methane formation. The two-phase process involving acidogenic and methanogenic fermentation steps has been developed. The acidogenic reactor operated with a chemical oxygen demand load of 20–60 kg/m^3/day produces 3–13 kg/m^2 day of biogas.

Integrated microbial electrolysis cell: The process combines the anaerobic digestion principle with a microbial electrolysis cell to achieve electro-methanogenesis. The bacterial biofilm is developed on the cathodic surface, and electroactive bacteria grow on the anode of the electrochemical cell. The substrate biofilm of electrotrophic methanogens present on the cathode surface reduces carbon dioxide to methane. The direct electron transfer between the anodic surface containing electroactive bacteria and the cathodic surface containing electrotrophic methanogens also results in methane formation (Neeraj Raja Ram et al., 2022; Ramansu Goswami et al., 2016).

9.8 ENVIRONMENT SUSTAINABILITY OF BIOFUELS

Greenhouse gas emissions emitted by the transport sector are rising at a faster rate than in other areas. Fossil fuels account for 88% of the fuel used in the transport sector. In an effort to reduce dependence on crude oil, there has been extensive exploration of alternatives such as biofuels. In 2018, global bioethanol production reached 110.4 billion liters, while biodiesel production reached 41 billion liters. Currently, biofuels make up 3.5% of the total transportation fuels used worldwide. The majority of biofuel production is concentrated in Brazil and the United States, which together account for 69% of global biofuel production. Europe contributes 9% to global biofuel production. Biodiesel in America is produced from corn, while in Brazil, it is produced from sugarcane. Other sources for biofuel include corn, sugar beet, wheat, and palm oil.

Biofuels offer environmental, economic, and social sustainability benefits to communities. The advantages of biofuels include rural development, a renewable energy source, and a reduction in carbon dioxide emissions. However, there are limitations to their application, such as pollution of land and water, deforestation, and rising food prices. These limitations can be mitigated by using biofuels derived from algae, as they are non-consumable and can grow rapidly in wastewater and saline water.

There are various factors that contribute to greenhouse gas emissions in the production of biofuels. These include the use of non-renewable fuels for growing feedstocks, the fossil fuel requirements for pesticide and fertilizer manufacturing, and for the installation of biofuel plants. The use of nitrogen fertilizer also leads to emission of nitrous oxides, which have a greenhouse effect 300 times stronger than carbon dioxide. However, byproducts from biofuels such as proteins can have a positive impact on the greenhouse effect. Additionally, the conversion of forest land or grass lands to grow feedstocks for biofuels releases stored carbon into the atmosphere, which offsets the benefits of using biofuels.

Biofuels production requires a large quantity of water for washing plants and seeds as well as for irrigating water-intensive crops like sugar cane, oil palm, and maize. This extensive water usage for crop cultivation has a significant impact on water quality in the area. Additionally, the production of biodiesel and bioethanol results in wastewater that pollutes water sources. Water pollution is also a concern due to the use of fertilizers and pesticides in biofuels production. Furthermore, improper cultivation practices contribute to soil erosion by removing the top layer of soil. However, environmental quality related to biofuels feedstock production can be improved through conservation tillage and crop rotation techniques.

The production of biofuels contributes to sustainable goals by utilizing byproducts and exploring alternative feedstocks. For example, residues from jatropha production can be used as fertilizers or pesticides. Glycerol, a byproduct of the transesterification process, can be used to make soaps and lubricants. Biodiesel can be used as an alternative to coal or firewood, for grinding wheat, thereby improving the rural economy. Additionally, cassava industries can sell starch products (Jeswani et al., 2020).

9.8.1 Environmental effects of biofuels

The global warming potential of bioethanol from consumable crops ranges from 4 to 160 gCO_2 eq. MJ^{-1}. Ethanol made from sugarcane meets the renewable energy directive by reducing global warming potential compared to petrol by 60%. This is achieved through the use of fewer agro-chemicals, high sugarcane yields, and the production of electricity in cogeneration plants. The global warming potential of first- generation biodiesel also varies, ranging from 4 to 110 gCO_2 eq. MJ^{-1}. Biodiesel made from palm oil meets the renewable energy directive by reducing emissions by 60%, while sunflower oil biodiesel only reaches a 35% reduction target.

A life cycle impact assessment study of corn-based ethanol produced in China shows that it has a global warming potential 40% greater than petrol due to the fossil energy consumed during production. Sugar beet-based bioethanol, on the other hand, has a low global warming potential of 20% due to constraints in water resources that affect crop yield. Soybean biodiesel produced in Brazil and the United States has 60% less emissions compared to fossil fuels due to its higher yield and lower input costs. The use of bagasse as fuel in molasses-based ethanol production reduces greenhouse gas emissions from 110 to 50 gCO_2 eq. MJ^{-1}.

Land use change, such as deforestation of tropical rainforests in Brazil for sugarcane cultivation, an increase in soybean cultivation in Middle America, and deforestation of peat land in Southeast Asia for palm cultivation, also contributes to global warming potential. Palm biodiesel grown in peat lands has emissions 40 times higher than diesel. Rapeseed and sunflower biodiesel have global warming potentials 40% higher than conventional diesel emissions.

Lignose cellulosic-based ethanol derived from forest and agriculture residues generates lower emissions compared to energy crops due to the emissions of N_2O from energy crops. The residual lignin co-generates heat, power, and electricity. Feedstocks such as forest residue, corn waste, and grass straw generate energy and other valuable products, offsetting emissions from biofuels production. This results in a negative global warming potential, avoiding greenhouse gas emissions. Jatropha biodiesel has a greenhouse gas emission of 20 gCO_2 eq. MJ^{-1}.

The global warming potential for third-generation algae biodiesel ranges from −2400 to 2900 gCO_2 eq. MJ^{-1}. This suggests that microalgae biodiesel can either increase or decrease global warming potential depending on the assumptions made. The high emissions are a result of low algae yield and the extensive use of energy for cultivation, harvesting, and drying. Studies have shown that higher emission savings can be achieved by using feedstocks such as CO_2 from cement plants, wastewater, and nutrients from anaerobic digestion units.

In terms of energy use, biofuels consume fossil-based energy ranging from 0.05 to 0.90 MJ MJ^{-1} for first generation substrates and −0.59 to 0.88 MJ MJ^{-1} for second generation substrates. The negative values are due to the production of value-based products and the co-generation of electricity. The results vary depending on the type of feedstocks, agricultural practices, and conversion technologies. The fossil fuel demand for algae growth ranges from 0.16 to 40 MJ MJ^{-1} with algae grown in open ponds requiring less energy than those grown in photo bioreactors.

Water usage is another important factor to consider. The water requirements for first-generation crops are much larger and compete with the water needs for growing food crops. The consumption of blue water or surface water for biofuels varies depending on the crops and country. For example, bioethanol produced from sugar beets requires less water due to limited irrigation in countries where these crops are cultivated. In Portugal, corn cultivation for bioethanol production consumes

86 m^3 GJ^{-1} of water. In European countries, water consumption levels for bioethanol and biodiesel production are 3.4 m^3 GJ^{-1} and 2 m^3 GJ^{-1}, respectively.

Biodiversity is also impacted by the cultivation methods and the use of chemicals and fertilizers for growing feedstocks. Second-generation biofuels have positive effects on biodiversity as lignocellulose requires fewer fertilizers, pesticides, has a longer growth cycle, and requires less manual labor. The growth of monocultures like Eucalyptus and switchgrass may negatively affect biodiversity in the region due to habitat loss. Third-generation biofuel feedstocks, such as large-scale algae cultivation, can pose significant risks to coastal biodiversity due to the invasion of algae species (Jeswani et al., 2020).

9.8.2 Advancement in Enzyme treatment of biomass toward sustainability

Enzymatic Advancement: In second-generation biofuel production, the conversion of lignocellulosic substances into pentose and hexose sugar is complex. The process of hydrolysis using sulfuric acid breaks the hydrogen bonds between cellulose fibers. The difficulty of extracting sugar and the requirement of high energy are areas of concern. The use of enzymes is an environmentally friendly and energy-efficient alternative process.

Hydrolytic enzymes: Glycosyl hydrolase: This enzyme has identical stereochemistry to its substrates. The important component of glycosyl hydrolase is cellulase, which hydrolyzes cellulose to produce hexose. The enzymes found in cellulase are endoglucanases, exoglucanases, and β-glucosidases. Hemicellulases such as L-arabinofuranosidase are involved in xylan hydrolysis. Mannanases degrade hemicellulose into mannose.

Carbohydrate esterases: Carbohydrate esterases remove esters from carbohydrates. Microorganisms secrete different glycosyl hydrolases for cellulose and hemicellulose breakdown. Microorganisms also develop carbohydrate esterases to remove esters from polysaccharides. Carbohydrate esterases are classified into 16 classes broadly categorized as hemicellulose deacetylating (class 1 to class 7 and class 16) and pectin deacetylating classes (class 8 and class 12).

Auxiliary activity proteins: These proteins break glycosidic bonds through an oxidation process. They include carbohydrate-active enzymes that act on lignocellulose and laccases, which can directly target lignin removal. The enzyme manganese peroxidase can oxidize lignin compounds and phenolic compounds. Cellobiose dehydrogenase enzymes efficiently oxidize dextrins of cellulose, maltose, and lactose. Lytic polysaccharide monooxygenases are effective in the hydrolysis of cellulosic biomass.

The steps involved in the enzymatic hydrolysis of biomass are as follows:

- Diffusion of enzyme molecules to the surface of substrate particles
- Diffusion through the pores of particles to the adsorption site
- Enzymatic hydrolysis takes place on the cellulose surface

In the enzymatic pathway from marine algae, microalgal cellulose is converted to cellobiose, which is then converted to glucose using biomass *Chlorococcum sp.* This conversion is achieved through the use of cellulase enzymes at a pH of 5 and a temperature of 50°C. *Hindakia tetrachotoma*, algal biomass is enzymatically hydrolyzed using β-glucosidase and α-amylase resulting in a glucose yield of 95% (Saurabh Singh et al., 2024). The various enzymes generated from algal biomass are listed in Table 9.26.

9.8.3 Microalgae biofuels for greener future

Algae are green-pigmented microorganisms that can be found in all major river bodies. Algae are tolerant to saline content, pH, temperature, and light intensities. Microalgae are a rich carbon source

TABLE 9.26
Enzymes generated from algal biomass

Algal biomass	Pretreatment	Enzyme	Yield
Hindakia tetrachotoma	Acidic	β - glucosidase from E. coli	92% glucose
Chlorella sp.	Hydrothermal	Glucoamylases	12 g/L of ethanol
Microalgae	Acidic	Cellulase synthesized from Trichoderma reesei	60% ethanol
K. alvarezii	Fungal	Amyloglucosidase	38% ethanol

that can be used for renewable energy, health supplements like omega-3 fatty acids, cosmetics, and pharmaceutical molecules. They are also involved in wastewater treatment and greenhouse gas mitigation. Various bioproducts obtained from microalgae include antimicrobial drugs, anticancer drugs, vitamins, and antioxidants. Algal biofuels have an oxygen level of 10–40% and release low levels of sulfur emissions compared to petroleum products, which have no oxygen and release sulfur emissions.

Microalgae have immense growth potential under the sun and can convert 10% of received solar energy into a biomass yield of 280 tons per hectare per year. Additionally, they are not edible, so they do not affect the human food chain, and they can be grown regardless of seasonal conditions. Microalgae require a simple pretreatment process due to the absence of lignocellulosic matter. They also have a lipid content above 50%, which meets the requirement for biodiesel production. The microalgal species *B. braunii* contains 80% oil in its biomass.

Bioethanol is a clean biofuel with inherent advantages:

- Bioethanol has high octane number that prevents knocking.
- Additionally, bioethanol emits less CO_2 due to the presence of oxygen.
- Another advantage is that ethanol can be used in present-day engines without any modifications.
- In fact, a mixture of bioethanol and petrol at different ratios can be used in combustion engines without any modifications.

Microalgae contain carbohydrates such as glycogen and starch, which can be fermented to convert them into sugar and then into bioethanol. These carbohydrates can be extracted from algal cells using enzymes, acids, or solvents. The extracted sugar is then converted to ethanol through microbial fermentation. It is important to carry out the fermentation step in aseptic conditions to prevent that could reduce the yield of bioethanol.

The process of algae processing involves several steps.

- Algae bio-culture is generated to produce biomass rich in carbohydrates
- Water is removed, and algae is harvested
- The biomass is subjected to various pretreatment
- The sugars are fermented to ethanol

Large-scale cultivation of microalgae is a sustainable way to harness biomass for ethanol production. Ocean-scale cultivation of algae is emerging as a solution for large-scale production, as it takes advantage of ocean waves to mix the cultures and utilizes the availability of dissolved nutrients.

To produce ethanol, microorganisms require fermentable sugars as substrates. The yield of bioethanol depends on various parameters such as the pH, temperature of reaction, oxygen levels, substrate concentration, and the type of microorganism used. For example, *Scenedesmus dimorphus* produces sugar through sulfuric acid treatment, while *Chlorella vulgaris* results in

TABLE 9.27
Biodiesel extraction from microalgae at different transesterification conditions

Microalgae	Reaction conditions	Biodiesel (%, w/w)
Botryococcus braunni	Catalyst used CH_3ONa, 55°C, 150 min	84
Chlorella minutıssima	Sulfuric acid transesterification, 120°C, 90 min	82
Chlorella protothecoides	Immobilized lipase obtained from Candidia sp.	98
Spirulina sp	KOH transesterification, 55°C, 120 min	96

11.8 g/L of bioethanol (Imran Khan et al., 2018; Indrajeet Singh et al., 2023). Table 9.27 provides information on the yield of biodiesel obtained from microalgae through different transesterification processes.

9.8.4 Sustainable biofuels production using co-cultivation systems

Diverse microbial species from the same community or different communities are developed to complete complex tasks. The artificial microbial consortium interacts through different modes such as commensalism, mutualism, competition, and parasitism. Co-cultivation improves the scope of using a wide variety of substrates. Lignocellulose is a common source of substrate employed in target product generation. The target product module is incorporated into cellulolytic microbes to generate targeted products and introduce cellulase systems into microbes. The consolidated bioprocessing system involves production of enzymes, hydrolysis of substrates, and microbial fermentation, all steps done in a single reactor. Co-cultivation systems consisting of *Clostridium species* and *Thermoanaerobacter species* can generate ethanol from cellulose. *Clostridum thermocellum–T. saccharolyticum* co-cultivation consortium is used to generate ethanol from cellulose with a yield value of 38 g/L.

The sequential utilization of sugars by microbes in which hexose is utilized, and pentose is leftover results in decreased operational efficiency. This utilization is called carbon catabolic repression. Microbial consortia avoid such a situation by shifting the interaction mode to commensalism instead of competition. An *Escherichia coli* binary culture was developed to produce ethanol from lignocellulose. The *Escherichia coli* strain is genetically engineered to hydrolyze hemicellulose to xylo oligosaccharides, and other strains develop an enzyme to convert it to ethanol. *C. thermocellum,* a cellulolytic microbial strain, is co-cultured with *Thermoanaerobacter* strains to achieve final ethanol production of 7.6 g/L. In this process, *C. thermocellum* strains are responsible for cellulose degradation, and *Thermoanaerobacter* strains are responsible for ethanol generation. A microbial consortium consisting of *Clostridium phytofermentans* and *S. cerevisiae* was used to generate 22 g/L of ethanol. *Clostridium phytofermentans* play the role of degrading of cellodextrin, and *S. cerevisiae* converts it into ethanol.

Biobutanol production is achieved using a co-cultivation of a microbial consortium consisting of *C.thermocellum* and *C. beijerinckii* species. In this process, *C. thermocellum* produces reducing sugar from cellulose, and *C. beijerinckii* converts the reducing sugars to biobutanol. The yield of biobutanol was 11 g/L. Biodiesel production from a co-cultured microbial consortium consisting of phototrophic algae and heterotrophic fungi species. Co-culturing of *Aspergillus awamori* and *Chlorella minutissima* to synthesize biodiesel from glycerol (Yujla Jiang et al., 2019; Argyros et al., 2011). The biofuels and chemicals produced by co-cultivation technology are given in Table 9.28.

TABLE 9.28
Biofuels and chemicals from co-cultivation process using microbial consortium

Microbial strains	Substrates	Product	Titer value
Clostridium thermocellum–Thermoanaerobacterium saccharolyticum	Microcrystalline cellulose	Bioethanol	39 g/L
Clostridium thermocellum–Kluyveromyces marxianus	Glucan	Bioethanol	9.8 g/L
Clostridium phytofermentans–Saccharomyces cerevisiae	Cellulose	Bioethanol	22.5 g/L
Clostridium thermocellum–Clostridium beijerinckii	Corn cobs	Biobutanol	11 g/L
Thermoanaerobacterium reesei–Lactobacillus pentosus	Microcrystalline cellulose	Lactate	35 g/L
Escherichia coli strains	Glycerine	Muconic acid	2 g/L

The reserves of fossil fuels are depleting rapidly, and various environmental concerns associated with their emissions demand that they be replaced with renewable sources of energy. Microalgae have a rapid growth rate and possess a notable capacity for biomass production per unit area of cultivation, making them highly suitable as feedstock for bioenergy applications. Algal biomass has a significant growth rate and high potential in carbon sequestration as well as the ability to generate various biofuels. The pretreatment of lignocellulosic biomass to remove lignin is an essential step in bioethanol production. Several factors such as feedstock varieties, pretreatment techniques, fermentation techniques, product purification, and other downstream steps are considered in the commercialization of biofuels production. Lignocellulose cultivation does not compete with arable lands, solving the issues of food security. The selection of pretreatment process and processing criteria for fermentation and saccharification steps determines the economic cost involved in the bioconversion process.

Various useful co-products are generated in biofuels manufacture such as glycerol during biodiesel synthesis and carboxylic acids during biomass fermentation. Biorefineries should focus on environmental considerations, so the development of technology for biofuel production should prioritize the generation of valuable byproducts and proper waste management practices. The use of solid-state fermenters for fermentation and saccharification is cost effective as it utilizes a single reactor instead of two for this process. This chapter discusses in detail the various species of algae used for biodiesel, bioethanol, and biobutanol manufacture. Modifying the gene structure in algal or fungal cells improves the yield of bioethanol. The utilization of laboratory-scale photobioreactors presents a very advantageous approach for cultivating microalgae compared to macro-scale reactors, as it offers a system that closely approximates optimal conditions. Cyanobacteria is involved in the biophotolysis of water molecules to produce biohydrogen. Biohydrogen is produced by cyanobacteria in the presence of nitrogen-fixing strains containing nitrogenase enzymes.

ACKNOWLEDGMENT

The authors would like to thank Center of Excellence in Advanced Materials and Green Technologies (COE-AMGT) and Department of Chemical Engineering and Materials Science, Amrita School of Engineering, Coimbatore, Amrita Vishwa Vidyapeetham, India for their help in publishing this chapter.

REFERENCES

Adeniyi, O. M., Azimov, U., and Burluka, A. (2018). Algae biofuel: Current status and future applications. *Renewable Sustainable Energy Reviews,* 90, 316–335. https://doi.org/10.1016/j.rser.2018.03.067.

Ahuja, V., Arora, A., Chauhan S., Thakur, S., Jeyaseelan, C., and Paul, D. (2023). Yeast-mediated biomass valorization for biofuel production: B A Literature Review. *Fermentation*, 9(9), 784. https://doi.org/10.3390/fermentation9090784.

Ajanovic, A., Sayer, M., and Haas, R. (2022). The economics and the environmental benignity of different colors of hydrogen. *International Journal of Hydrogen Energy,* 47(57), 24136–24154. https://doi.org/10.1016/j.ijhydene.2022.02.094.

Akanksha, S., Deepak, K., Madhuri, G., Anil, K., Abhineet, G., Tabarak, M., and Anand, M. (2023). Strategies of pretreatment of feedstocks for optimized bioethanol production: Distinct and integrated approaches. *Biotechnology for Biofuels and Bioproducts*, 16, 44. https://doi.org/10.1186/s13068-023-02295-2.

Alok, P., Dimitra, K., Emma, R., Petros, K., Ulrika, R., Paul, C., and Leonidas, M. (2020). An Overview of Potential Oleaginous Microorganisms and Their Role in Biodiesel and Omega-3 Fatty Acid-Based Industries. *Microorganism,* 8(3), 434. https://doi.org/10.3390/microorganisms8030434.

Angela Paul, P., Apurav Krishna, K., Kit Wayne, C., Shih-Hsin, H., Wei-Hsin, C., Jo-Shu, C., Rambabu, K., Fawzi B., and Pau Loke, S. (2022). Continuous cultivation of microalgae in photobioreactors as a source of renewable energy: Current status and future challenges. *Renewable and Sustainable Energy Reviews,* 154, 111852. https://doi.org/10.1016/j.rser.2021.111852.

Aniruddha, R., Rajendran, A., and Subramanian, S. (2022). A study on biofuel generation from microalgae species. *Materials Today Proceedings*, 57(4), 1660–1665. https://doi.org/10.1016/j.matpr.2021.12.269.

Aparna, P., Krishna Prasad, R., and Marali, B. (2025). Recent advancements and challenges in the lignocellulosic and algal biomass-based bioethanol production: A review. *Biofuels*, 16(5), 499–518. https://doi.org/10.1080/17597269.2024.2432148.

Argyros, D. A., Tripathi, S. A., Barrett, T. F., Rogers, S. R., Feinberg, L. F., Olson, D. G., Foden, J. M., Miller, B. B., Lynd, L. R., and Hogsett, D. A. (2011). High ethanol titers from cellulose by using metabolically engineered thermophilic, anaerobic microbes. *Applied Environmental Microbiology*, 77(23), 8288–8294. https://doi.org/10.1128/AEM.00646-11

Ariadna, S.-A., Gonzalez-Gutierrez, Linda V., Paya, V. C., Feliu, J., Buitron, G., and Cercado, B. (2021). Energy and economic advantages of simultaneous hydrogen and biogas production in microbial electrolysis cells as a function of the applied voltage and biomass content. *Royal Society of Chemistry*, 5, 2003–2017. https://doi.org/10.1039/D0SE01797C.

Arun Shankar, A., P. R. Pentapati., and Krishna Prasad, R. (2017). Biodiesel synthesis from cottonseed oil using homogeneous alkali catalyst and using heterogeneous multi walled carbon nanotubes: Characterization and blending studies. *Egyptian Journal of Petroleum*, 26(1), 125–133. https://doi.org/10.1016/j.ejpe.2016.04.001.

Avila, R., Carrero, E., Vicent, T., and Bl´anquez, P., (2021). Integration of enzymatic pretreatment and sludge co-digestion in biogas production from microalgae. *Waste Management*, 124, 254–263. https://doi.org/10.1016/j.wasman.2021.01.042.

Aziz, M, Darmawan, A, and Juangsa, F. (2021). Hydrogen production from biomasses and wastes: A technological review. *International Journal of Hydrogen Energy,* 46(68), 33756–33781. https://doi.org/10.1016/j.ijhydene.2021.07.189.

Azra, M., and Bassam, A.-H. (2023). A review on the current status and post-pandemic prospects of third-generation biofuels. *Energy Systems,* 14, 1185–1216. https://doi.org/10.1007/s12667-022-00514-7.

Bharathi, D., and Rajalakshmi, G. (2019). Microbial lipases: An overview of screening, production and purification. *Biocatalysis and Agricultural Biotechnology,* 22, 101368. https://doi.org/10.1016/j.bcab.2019.101368.

Cabrol, L., Marone, A., Tapia-venegas, E., Steyer, J., Ruiz-filippi, G., and Trably, E. (2017). Microbial ecology of fermentative hydrogen producing bioprocesses: Useful insights for driving the ecosystem function. *FEMS Microbiology Reviews,* 41(2),158–181. https://doi.org/10.1093/femsre/fuw043.

Cao, Y., Liu, H., Liu, W., Guo, J., and Xian, M. (2022). Debottlenecking the biological hydrogen production pathway of dark fermentation: Insight into the impact of strain improvement. *Microbial Cell Factories,* 21, 166. https://doi.org/10.1186/s12934-022-01893-3.

Cayetano, R. D. A., Kim, G. B., Park, J., Yang, Y. H., Jeon, B. H., Jang, M., and Kim, S. H. (2022). Biofilm formation as a method of improved treatment during anaerobic digestion of organic matter for biogas recovery. *Bioresource Technology,* 344,126309. 126309.

Chandrasekhar, T., Varaprasad, D., Gneneswari, P., Swapna, B., Riazunnisa, K., Anu Prasanna, V., Korivi, M., Wee, Y. J., and Lebaka, V. R. (2023). Algae: The reservoir of bioethanol. *Fermentation,* 9(8), 712. https://doi.org/10.3390/fermentation9080712.

Dai, Y., Zhang, H.S., Huan, B., and He, Y. (2017). Enhancing the enzymatic saccharification of bamboo shoot shell by sequential biological pretreatment with Galactomyces sp. CCZU11–1 and deep eutectic solvent extraction. *Bioprocess and Biosystems Engineering,* 40, 1427–36. https://doi.org/10.1007/s00449-017-1800-4.

Damtie, M. M., Shin, J., Jang, H. M., Cho, H. U., Wang, J., and Kim, Y. M. (2021). Effects of biological pretreatments of microalgae on hydrolysis, biomethane potential and microbial community. *Bioresource Technology,* 329, 124905. https://doi.org/10.1016/j.biortech.2021.124905.

Del Río, P. G., Gomes-Dias, J. S., Rocha, C. M., Romaní, A., Garrote, G., and Domingues, L. (2019). Recent trends on seaweed fractionation for liquid biofuels production. *Bioresource Technology*, 299, 122613. https://doi.org/10.1016/j.biortech.2019.122613.

Harun, C., and Bavin, L. (2019). Third-generation biofuels from microalgae: A review. *Current Opinion in Green and Sustainable Chemistry*, 20, 39–44. https://doi.org/10.1016/j.cogsc.2019.09.003.

Hermesmann, M., and Müller, T. E. (2022). Green, turquoise, blue, or grey? Environmentally friendly hydrogen production in transforming energy systems. *Progress in Energy and Combustion Science,* 90, 100996. https://doi.org/10.1016/j.pecs.2022.100996.

Hidalgo, P., Toro, C., Ciudad, G., and Navia, R. (2013). Advances in direct transesterification of microalgal biomass for biodiesel production. *Reviews in Environmental Science and Biotechnology,* 12,179–199. https://doi.org/10.1007/s11157-013-9308-0.

Shokravi, H., Heidarrezaei, M., Shokravi, Z., Ong, H. C., Lau, W. J., Din, M. F. Md and Ismail, A. F.. (2022). Fourth generation biofuel from genetically modified algal biomass for bioeconomic development. *Journal of Biotechnology*, 360, 23–36. https://doi.org/10.1016/j.jbiotec.2022.10.010.

Hou, Y., Zhang, R., Yu, A., Huang, L., Liu, Y., and Zhou, Z. (2017). Accelerated azo dye degradation and concurrent hydrogen production in the single-chamber photocatalytic microbial electrolysis cell, *Bioresource Technology,* 224, 63–68. https://doi.org/10.1016/j.biortech.2016.10.069.

Jeswani, H. K., Chilvers, A., and Azapagic, A. (2020). Environmental sustainability of biofuels: A review. *Proceedings Royal Society A,* 476, 20200351. https://doi.org/10.1098/rspa.2020.0351.

Jiménez-Llanos, J., Ramírez-Carmona, M., Rendón-Castrillón, L., and Ocampo-López, C. (2020). Sustainable biohydrogen production by Chlorella Sp. microalgae: A review. *International Journal of Hydrogen Energy,* 45(15), 8310–8328. https://doi.org/10.1016/j.ijhydene.2020.01.059.

Katebah, M., Al-Rawashdeh, M., and Linke, P. (2022). Analysis of hydrogen production costs in Steam-Methane Reforming considering integration with electrolysis and CO_2 capture. *Cleaner Engineering and Technology,* 10, 100552. https://doi.org/10.1016/j.clet.2022.100552.

Keffer, J. E., and Kleinheinz, G. T. (2002). Use of chlorella vulgaris for CO_2 mitigation in a photobioreactor. *Journal of Industrial Microbiology and Biotechnology*, 29, 275–280. https://doi.org/10.1038/sj.jim.7000313.

Khan, S., Das, P., Abdul Quadir, M., Thaher, M. I., Mahata,C., Sayadi, S., and Al-Jabri, H. (2023). Microalgal feedstock for biofuel production: Recent advances, challenges, and future perspective, *Fermentation,* 9(3), 281. https://doi.org/10.3390/fermentation9030281.

Kilian, O., Benemann, C. S. E., Niyogi, K. K., and Vick, B. (2011). High-efficiency homologous recombination in the oil-producing alga *Nannochloropsis* sp. *Proceedings of the National Academy of Sciences,* 108(52), 21265–21269. https://doi.org/10.1073/pnas.1105861108.

Kisoo, K., Junsang, Y., and Won Gu, L. (2022). Recent advances in photobioreactor systems for sustainable and enhanced microalgal biofuel production. *Sustainable Energy & Fuels,* 6, 5459. https://doi.org/10.1039/D2SE01345B.

Kumar, A., Verma, V., Dubey, V. K., Srivastava, A., Garg, S. K., Singh, V. P., and Arora, P. K. (2023). Industrial applications of fungal lipases: A review. *Frontiers in Microbiology* 14, 1142536. https://doi.org/10.3389/fmicb.2023.1142536.

Kumar, M., Rathour, R., and Gupta, J. (2020). Bacterial production of fatty acid and biodiesel: Opportunity and challenges. *Refining Biomass Residue for Sustainable Energy and Bioproducts,* 21–49. https://doi.org/10.1016/B978-0-12-818996-2.00002-8.

Kumar, M., Oyedun, A. O., and Kumar, A. (2019). A Comparative analysis of hydrogen production from the thermochemical conversion of algal biomass. *International Journal of Hydrogen Energy,* 44(21), 10384–10397. https://doi.org/10.1016/j.ijhydene.2019.02.220.

Lacerda, M. P., Oh, E. J, and Eckert, C. (2020). The model system Saccharomyces cerevisiae versus emerging non-model yeasts for the production of biofuels. *Life,* 10(11), 299, https://doi.org/10.3390/life10110299.

Lee, J. Y., Yoo, C., Jun, S. Y., Ahn, C. Y., and Oh, H. M. (2010). Comparison of several methods for effective lipid extraction from microalgae. *Bioresource Technology,* 101(1), S75–S77. https://doi.org/10.1016/j.biortech.2009.03.058

Lee, J. -H., Lee, D. -G., Park, J. -I., and Kim, J. -Y. (2010). Bio-hydrogen production from marine brown algae and its bacterial diversity. *Korean Journal of Chemical Engineering,* 27, 187–192. https://doi.org/10.1007/s11814-009-0300-x.

Li, F., He, X., Srishti, A., Song, S., Tan, H. T. W., Sweeney, D. J., Ghosh, S., and Wang, C. H. (2021). Water hyacinth for energy and environmental applications: A review. *Bioresource Technology*, 327, 124809. https://doi.org/10.1016/j.biortech.2021.

Licheng, P., Dongdong, F., Huaqiang, C., Zezheng, W., and Huaiyuan, Q. (2020). Biofuel production from microalgae: A review. *Environmental Chemistry Letters,* 18, 285–297. https://doi.org/10.1007/s10311-019-00939-0.

Lin, Z., Cong, W., and Zhang, J. (2023). Biobutanol production from acetone–butanol–ethanol fermentation: Developments and prospects. *Fermentation,* 9(9), 847. https://doi.org/10.3390/fermentation9090847.

Liu, W., Mao, W., Zhang, C., Lu, X., Xiao, X., and Zhao, Z. (2020). Co-fermentation of a sugar mixture for microbial lipid production in a two-stage fermentation mode under non-sterile conditions. *Sustainable Energy and Fuels*, 4, 2380–2385. https://doi.org/10.1039/D0SE00003E.

Lu, C., Li, W., Zhang, Q., Liu, L., Zhang, N., Qu, B., et al. (2021). Enhancing photo- fermentation biohydrogen production by strengthening the beneficial metabolic products with catalysts. *Journal of Cleaner Production,* 317, 128437. https://doi.org/10.1016/j.jclepro.2021.128437.

Marri, V. B., Kotha, M. M., and Gaddale, A. P. R. (2020). Production process optimisation of *Sterculia foetida* methyl esters (biodiesel) using response surface methodology. *International Journal of Ambient Energy*, 43(1), 1837–1846. https://doi.org/10.1080/01430750.2020.1723692.

Massarweh, O., Al-khuzaei, M., Al-Shafi, M., Bicer, Y., and Abushaikha, A. S. (2023). Blue hydrogen production from natural gas reservoirs: A review of application and feasibility. *Journal of CO_2 Utilization,* 70, 102438. https://doi.org/10.1016/j.jcou.2023.102438.

Maswanna, T., Lindblad, P., and Maneeruttanarungroj, C. (2020). Improved biohydrogen production by immobilized cells of the green algae Tetraspora sp. CU2551 incubated under aerobic condition. *Journal of Applied Phycology,* 32, 2937–2945. https://doi.org/10.1007/s10811-020-02184-3.

Mishra, P., Krishnan, S., Rana, S., Singh, L., Sakinah, M., and Ab Wahid, Z. (2019). Outlook of fermentative hydrogen production techniques: An overview of dark, photo and integrated dark-photo fermentative approach to biomass. *Energy Strategy Reviews,* 24, 27–37. https://doi.org/10.1016/j.esr.2019.01.001.

Moreno, A., Magdalena, D., Oliva, J. A., Greses, J. M., Lozano, C. C., Latorre-S´anchez, M., Negro, M. J., Susmozas, A., Iglesias, R., Llamas, M., Tom´as-Pejó, E., and Gonz´alez- Fern´andez, C. (2021). Sequential bioethanol and methane production from municipal solid waste: An integrated biorefinery strategy towards cost-effectiveness. *Process Safety and Environmental Protection,* 146, 424–431. https://doi.org/10.1016/j.psep.2020.09.022.

Mota, M. N., Múgica, P., and Sá-Correia, I. (2022). Exploring Yeast Diversity to Produce Lipid-Based Biofuels from Agro-Forestry and Industrial Organic Residues. *Journal of Fungi,* 8(7), 687; https://doi.org/10.3390/jof8070687.

Muhammad Imran, K., Jin Hyuk, S., and Jong Deog, K. (2018). The promising future of microalgae: Current status, challenges, and optimization of a sustainable and renewable industry for biofuels, feed, and other products. *Microbial Cell Factories,* 17, 36. https://doi.org/10.1186/s12934-018-0879-x.

Murat Efgan, K., Lina, H., Begum Tuna, Ç., Buse, B., and Brahim Ben, A. (2023). Assessment of homogeneous and heterogeneous catalysts in transesterification reaction: A mini review. *Chemical and Biochemical Engineering Reviews*, 10(4), 412–422. https://doi.org/10.1002/cben.202200021.

Naresh Kumar, M., Ravikumar, R., Thenmozhi, S., and Kirupa Sankar, M. (2017). Development of natural cellulase inhibitor mediated intensified biological pretreatment technology using Pleurotus florida for maximum recovery of cellulose from paddy straw under solid state condition. *Bioresource Technology,* 244, 353–361. https://doi.org/10.1016/j.biortech.2017.07.105.

Neda, J., Ghasem, D., and Najafpour, M. K. (2020). Macro and micro algae in pollution control and biofuel production – A review. *ChemBioEng Reviews,* 7, 1–17. https://doi.org/10.1002/cben.201900014.

Neeraj Raja, R., and Nikhil, G. N. (2022). A critical review on sustainable biogas production with focus on microbial-substrate interactions: Bottlenecks and breakthroughs. *Bioresource Technology,* 19, 101170. https://doi.org/10.1016/j.biteb.2022.101170.

Nikolaidis, P., and Poullikkas, A. (2017). A comparative overview of hydrogen production processes. *Renewable and Sustainable Energy Reviews* 67, 597–611. https://doi.org/10.1016/j.rser.2016.09.044.

Prasad, S., Kumar, S., Yadav, K. K., Choudhry, J., Kamyab, H., Bach, Q. V., Sheetal, K. R., Kannojiya, S., and Gupta, N. (2020). Screening and evaluation of cellulolytic fungal strains for saccharification and bioethanol production from rice residue. *Energy,* 190, 116422. https://doi.org/10.1016/j.energy.2019.116422.

Qadeer, S., Khalid, A., and Mahmood, S. (2017). Utilization oleaginous bacteria and fungi for cleaner energy production. *Journal of Cleaner Production,* 168,917–928. https://doi.org/10.1016/j.jclepro.2017.09.093.

Qu, C., Dai, K., Fu, H., and Wang, J. (2021). Enhanced ethanol production from lignocellulosic hydrolysates by Thermoanaerobacterium aotearoense SCUT27/DargR1864 with improved lignocellulose-derived inhibitors tolerance. *Renewable Energy*, 173, 652–661. https://doi.org/10.1016/j.renene.2021.04.018.

Rahul, G., Nayak, J. K., Ress, N. V., Wilckens, R. S. and Ghosh, U. K. (2023). Bio-hydrogen production through microbial electrolysis cell: Structural components and influencing factors. *Chemical Engineering Journal* 455, 140535. https://doi.org/10.1016/j.cej.2022.140535.

Ramansu, G., Chattopadhyay, P., Shome, A. Banerjee, S. N., Chakaborty, A. K., Mathew, A. K., and Chaudhury, S. (2016). An overview of physico-chemical mechanisms of biogas production by microbial communities: A step towards sustainable waste management. *3 Biotech,* 6(1), 72. https://doi.org/10.1007/s13205-016-0395-9.

Rezania, S., Din, M. F. M., Taib, S. M., Sohaili, J., Chelliapan, S., Kamyab, H., and Saha, B. B. (2017). Review on fermentative biohydrogen production from water hyacinth, wheat straw and rice straw with focus on recent perspectives. *International Journal of Hydrogen Energy*, 42(33), 20955–20969. https://doi.org/10.1016/j.ijhydene.2017.07.007.

Saranya, G., and Ramachandra, T. V. (2020). Novel biocatalyst for optimal biodiesel production from diatoms. *Renewable Energy,* 153, 919–934. https://doi.org/10.1016/j.renene.2020.02.053.

Saravanan, A., Kumar, P. S., Aron, N. S., Jeevanantham, S., Karishma, S., Yaashikaa P., Chew, K. W., Show, P. L. (2022). A review on bioconversion processes for hydrogen production from agroindustrial residues. *International Journal of Hydrogen Energy,* 47(88), 37302–37320. https://doi.org/10.1016/j.ijhydene.2021.08.055.

Saurabh, S., Morya, R., Jaiswal, D. K., Keerthana, S., Kim, S.-H., Manimekalai, R., encio de Araujo Pereira, A. P., Verma, J. P. (2024). Innovations and advances in enzymatic deconstruction of biomass and their sustainability analysis: A review. *Renewable Sustainable Energy Reviews,* 189, 113958. https://doi.org/10.1016/j.rser.2023.113958.

Shams Forruque, A., Kabir, M., Mehjabin, A., Oishi, F. T. Z., Ahmed, S., Mannan, S., Mofijur, M., Almomani, F., Badruddin, I. A., and Kamangar, S. (2023). Waste biorefinery to produce renewable energy: Bioconversion process and circular bioeconomy. *Energy Reports,* 10, 3073. https://doi.org/10.1016/j.egyr.2023.09.137.

Sharma, A., and Arya, S. K. (2017). Hydrogen from algal biomass: A review of production process. *Biotechnology Reports,* 15, 63–69. https://doi.org/10.1016/j.btre.2017.06.001.

Shobana, M., Krishna Prasad, R., Udaya Bhaskar, R. R., and Kumaresan, D. (2020). Kinetics and characterization of transesterification of cottonseed oil to biodiesel using calcined clam shells as catalyst. *Biofuels*,11(5), 597–605.https://doi.org/10.1080/17597269.2017.1378994.

Sillero, L., Solera, R., and Pérez, M. (2022). Effect of the hydraulic retention time on the acidogenic fermentation of sewage sludge, wine vinasse and poultry manure for biohydrogen production. *Biomass and Bioenergy,* 167, 106643. https://doi.org/10.1016/j.biombioe.2022.106643.

Sinbuathong, N., and Sillapacharoenkul, B. (2021). Enhancement of biogas production from sun hemp using alkaline pretreatment. *International Journal of Hydrogen Energy,* 46(6), 4870–4878. https://doi.org/10.1016/j.ijhydene.2020.04.058.

Sindhu, S., Vijay Kirushnan, V. M., Amritha, A., Sanjay Kumaar, V. S., Shobika, N. V., Dhamothar, P., and Swetha, S. (2025). Chapter 13. A review of extraction of biodiesel from non-edible oils and microalgae using nanocatalysts. Nature -based Technologies for waste water treatment and Bioenergy production, IWA publisher. https://doi.org/10.2166/9781789064100_0233

Singh, G., Sinha S., Kumar, K. K., Gaur, N. A., Bandyopadhyay, K. K., and Paul, D. (2020). High density cultivation of oleaginous yeast isolates in 'mandi' waste for enhanced lipid production using sugarcane molasses as feed. *Fuel,* 276, 118073. https://doi.org/10.1016/j.fuel.2020.118073.

Singh, I., Pandey, A., Shangdiar, S., Rai, P. K., Kumar, A., Amesho, K. T. T., and Bux, F. (2023). Towards sustainable energy: Harnessing microalgae biofuels for a greener future. *Sustainability,* 15(18), 14029, https://doi.org/10.3390/su151814029.

Sivaramakrishnan, R., and Incharoensakdi, A. (2018). Microalgae as feedstock for biodiesel production under ultrasound treatment – A review. *Bioresource Technology,* 250, 877–887. https://doi.org/10.1016/j.biortech.2017.11.095.

Sizwe, I. M., Obinna, T. E., Roopnarain, A., Ndaba, B., Sekoai, P. T., Habimana, O., and Pohl, C. H. (2021). The potential of single-cell oils derived from filamentous fungi as alternative feedstock sources for biodiesel production. *Frontiers in Microbiology,* 12, 637381. https://doi.org/10.3389/fmicb.2021.637381.

Sravan Kumar, Y., Bhartia, Lalit, R. K., Kumara, R., Tiwaria, B. Zhangb, X. and Tyagia, R. D. (2018). Recent developments of downstream processing for microbial lipids and conversion to biodiesel. *Bioresource Technology,* 256, 515–528. https://doi.org/10.1016/j.biortech.2018.01.129.

Subramaniam, R., Dufreche, S., Zappi, M., and Bajpai, R. (2010). Microbial lipids from renewable resources: Production and characterization. *Journal of Industrial Microbiology and Biotechnology,* 37(12), 1271–1287. https://doi.org/10.1007/s10295-010-0884-5.

Sudhakar, K., Mamat, R., Samykano, M., Azmi, W., Ishak, W., and Yusaf, T. (2018). An overview of marine macroalgae as a bioresource. *Renewable and Sustainable Energy Reviews,* 91, 165–179. https://doi.org/10.1016/j.rser.2018.03.100.

Sundaramahalingam, M. A., Sivashanmugam, P., Rajeshbanu, J., and Ashokkumar, M. (2022). A review on contemporary approaches in enhancing the innate lipid content of yeast cell. *Chemosphere,* 293, 133616. https://doi.org/10.1016/j.chemosphere.2022.133616.

Thomas, S., Sanya, D. R. A., Fouchard, F., Nguyen, H. V., Kunze, G., and Neuv´eglise, C. (2019). *Blastobotrys adeninivorans* and *B. raffinosifermentans*, two sibling yeast species which accumulate lipids at elevated temperatures and from diverse sugars. *Biotechnology for Biofuels,* 12, 1–15. https://doi.org/10.1186/s13068-019-1492-x.

Undiandeye, J., Gallegos, D., Lenz, J., Nelles, M., and Stinner, W. (2022). Effect of novel Aspergillus and Neurospora species-based additive on ensiling parameters and biomethane potential of sugar beet leaves. *Applied Science,* 12(5), 2684. https://doi.org/10.3390/app12052684.

Venkateswar Reddy, M., Kumar, G., Mohanakrishna, G., Shobana, S., and Al-Raoush, R. I. (2020). Review on the production of medium and small chain fatty acids through waste valorization and CO_2 fixation. *Bioresource Technology*, 309, 123400. https://doi.org/10.1016/j.biortech.2020.123400.

Weber, A. Z., and Lipman, T. E. (2018). Fuel Cells and Hydrogen Production: Introduction. Meyers, R. A., Ed. Springer. pp. 1–8.

Xiao, C., Liao, Q., Fu, Q., Huang, Y, Chen, H., Zhang, H., Xia, A., Zhu, X., Reungsang, A., and Liu, Z. (2019). A solar-driven continuous hydrothermal pretreatment system for biomethane production from microalgae biomass. *Applied Energy*, 236, 1011–1018. https://doi.org/10.1016/j.apenergy.2018.12.014.

Xie, C., Gong, W., Yang, Q., Zhu, Z., Yan, L., Hu, Z., and Peng, Y. (2017). White-rot fungi pretreatment combined with alkaline/oxidative pretreatment to improve enzymatic saccharification of industrial hemp. *Bioresource Technology,* 243,188–195. https://doi.org/10.1016/j.biortech.2017.06.077

Yang, N., Hafez, H., and Nakhla, G. (2015). Impact of volatile fatty acids on microbial electrolysis cell performance. *Bioresource Technology,* 193, 449–455. https://doi.org/10.1016/j.biortech.2015.06.124.

Yin Y., Hu J., and Wang J. (2019). Fermentative hydrogen production from macroalgae Laminaria japonica pretreated by microwave irradiation. *International Journal of Hydrogen Energy,* 44(21),10398–10406. https://doi.org/10.1016/j.ijhydene.2019.03.034.

Yujia, J., R. Wu., J. Zhou., A. He., J. Xu., F. Xin., W. Zhang., J. Ma., M. Jiang., and W. Dong. (2019). Recent advances of biofuels and biochemicals production from sustainable resources using co-cultivation systems. *Biotechnology for Biofuels,* 12, 155. https://doi.org/10.1186/s13068-019-1495-7.

Yun, Y. -M., Kim, D. -H., Oh, Y. -K., Shin, H.-S., and Jung, K. -W. (2014). Application of a novel enzymatic pretreatment using crude hydrolytic extracellular enzyme solution to microalgal biomass for dark fermentative hydrogen production. *Bioresource Technology*, 159, 365–372. https://doi.org/10.1016/j.biortech.2014.02.129.

Zhang, L., Li, Y., Liu, X., Ren, N., and Ding, J. (2019). Lignocellulosic hydrogen production using dark fermentation by Clostridium lentocellum strain Cel10 newly isolated from Ailuropoda melanoleuca excrement. *RSC Advances,* 9(20), 11179–11185. https://doi.org/10.1039/C9RA01158G.

Zhang, L., Lee, J. T. E., Ok, Y. S., Dai, Y., and Tong, Y. W. (2022). Enhancing microbial lipids yield for biodiesel production by oleaginous yeast *Lipomyces starkeyi* fermentation: A review. *Bioresource Technology*, 344, 126294. https://doi.org/10.1016/j.biortech.2021.126294.

Zhang, L., Zheng, H., Wan, T., Shi, D., Lyu, L., and Cai, G. (2021). An integrated control algorithm of power distribution for islanded microgrid based on improved virtual synchronous generator. *IET Renewable Power Generation*, 15, 2674–2685. https://doi.org/10.1049/rpg2.12191.

10 Plastics and microplastics
The state-of-the-art in advanced treatment technologies

Sheikh Mohammed, Karmuhil Mathimozhiyazh Vetriselvan, Sekaran Ganesan, and Ramani Kandasamy

10.1 INTRODUCTION

Plastics are synthetic compounds made up of carbon chain monomers linked by the atoms of hydrogen, nitrogen, and sulfur. These plastics are categorized into thermoplastics and thermosets. Thermoplastics are the plastics where the used polymers can be heated to soften them to produce different products, whereas the thermosets are the single-time application plastics, unlike the thermoplastics, these polymers are denser and have hard cross-linked molecular chains due to which they don't lose their fragility when heated. In the past 50 years, the production of this plastics is raised 20 times globally, estimating around 6,900 million tons are dumped in landfills (Brooks et al., 2018). Despite this, plastic used in the food and beverage industries and for packaging is being utilized once, contributing 61% of global beach litter. The studies show that around 19–23 million tons of wastes dispersed into the aquatic system in 2016 are expected to reach 53 million tons by 2030 (Borrelle et al., 2020). The dispersed nature of these polymers results in significant negative effects on both land and water creatures (Galloway & Lewis, 2016). These plastics degrade into MPs owing to factors such as UV light, chemicals, and bacteria (Ter Halle et al., 2016). These MPs measure about less than 5 millimeters. MPs are categorized into primary and secondary MPs. Primary MPs are manufactured in industries in different forms and shapes which is been utilized in personal care products, whereas the secondary MPs are the plastics which are fragmented from their original composition through environmental factors. MPs are a global problem due to their impact on human health through skin penetration, ingestion, and inhalation. And also, at the level of toxicity, it affects in the mode of cellular level in human health. Being as a vector, it has the ability to amplify the pollutants in the environment such as antibioticsn and plasticizer (Sun & Wang, 2023).

Plastic waste has accumulated significantly in the soils of several tropical and subtropical nations, where agricultural and municipal plastic wastes are often buried or disposed of in wide-open spaces or landfills. Landfilling plastic waste doesn't completely eradicate it due to its detrimental environmental impact retention; instead, it extends the challenge for eternity. Toxic substances can seep out of waste landfills if not handled properly, leading to damage of the nearby ecosystem (Narevski et al., 2021). Landfills get a large number of MPs from several sources. Water that drains through landfills forms leachate, which discharges MPs into the aquatic environment (Kazour et al., 2019). Two major sources of MPs in the landfill leachate are due to the solid waste and the wastewater treatment plant residue (Golwala et al., 2021). The MPs present in the landfill interact with the inorganic and organic contaminants. Owing to this, it acts as a vector for these contaminants to enter the ecosystem (Bank & Hansson, 2019). Moreover, the labors working in the site of the landfill experience harmful effects like skin disease, respiratory disease, etc. In addition, the MPs enter into the aquatic system through the wastewater treatment plants to the oceans, sea bead, and the coastal areas. Around 95% of the MPs do not undergo any treatment in the wastewater treatment plant,

DOI: 10.1201/9781003500483-10

This chapter has been made available under a (CC-BY-NC-ND) 4.0 license

and it led to the discharge into the aquatic environment. And around 90% of the MPs are from the landfill/terrestrial environment, where it undergoes partial decomposition by the physico-chemical and biological factors and are released into the landfill leachate (Akhbarizadeh et al., 2018). The MPs bearing leachate percolate into the groundwater system and other aquatic environments and cause adverse effects.

Three primary pathways for MPs to enter the human body include: inhaling, ingesting, and contacting the skin (Rahman et al., 2021). MPs may serve as endocrine disruptors through modifying hormonal signaling pathways vital for the healthy functioning of the reproductive system. They can also harm reproductive tissues, such as ovaries and testes, due to their abrasive properties. Moreover, marine species may ingest MPs, leading to obstructions in their digestive systems, starvation, and eventual death (Ghosh et al., 2023). Hence, there is an urgent need to develop efficient tactics to avoid and minimize the discharge of MPs into the environment. To date, no report on the effective removal of MPs in wastewater treatment plants and landfills. Standardizing methodologies for collecting, detecting, and characterizing MPs is crucial, as previously detailed in reviews (Araújo et al., 2018). However, very few research studies have focused on the removal of MPs in anaerobic digestion (Zhang et al., 2020), wastewater treatment, etc. Nevertheless, these evaluations have not thoroughly covered many techniques or technologies that may be used, nor have they addressed the issues of integrating these technologies into current wastewater treatment processes for MPs removal, degradation, or upcycling. Landfills, which are another source of pollution on land and a significant area of microplastic (MP) contamination, have not been adequately considered in these evaluations. The process of fragmentation and degradation of MPs in landfills, the accumulation of MPs in leachates, and the effectiveness of landfills and leachate treatment facilities in eliminating MPs are areas that require more research. Moreover, the literature has not thoroughly explored the relationship between MPs, different pollutants, and biofilms in wastewater streams, which might reduce the effectiveness of MPs removal. This chapter focuses on recent advancements in enhancing removal effectiveness, scalability, and specificity. It critically examines important technical flaws along with areas that need more research and improvement. The main emphasis is on evaluating the benefits, existing constraints, and future actions for converting effective laboratory approaches into practical solutions for widespread plastic and MP contamination. And also, this chapter discusses the latest treatment options for MPs and plastic waste, as well as offering guidance on innovative potential in the field of environmental engineering.

10.2 CURRENT CHALLENGES IN PLASTIC WASTE MANAGEMENT

Waste is accumulating in urban areas due to population migration. As wealth, urbanization, and population levels rise, waste generation also tends to grow. Several countries lack organized landfills for disposing of municipal solid waste. Cities opt to dispose of solid trash at dump yards where it is either buried or left untreated. Dumping is prevalent in India due to a lack of knowledge and the necessity for land to dispose of the large quantities of trash produced by families and neighboring regions. Plastic manufacturing in India is a profitable industry, but the absence of an effective waste management system to handle the staggering 15,342 tons of plastic waste generated daily is a significant concern. Data from the Central Pollution Control Board (CPCB) reveals that plastic constitutes 8% of the total solid waste, with Delhi being the largest contributor, followed by Kolkata and Ahmedabad . Despite the seeming simplicity of recycling plastic, the reality is far more complex. Even if plastic waste is successfully recovered before being released into the environment and subsequently processed for recycling, the recycled plastic obtained after use contains over 10,000 additives that are crucial for transforming it into everyday items, posing significant challenges to the recycling process (Abel et al., 2021). The vast variety of plastic types presents a significant hurdle in recycling due to the uncertainty surrounding the composition when manufacturing products from recycled plastic waste. Furthermore, over 2,400 of these additives are deemed potentially hazardous, compounding the challenges associated with the recycling process (Wiesinger et al., 2021).

These additives present in post-consumer recycled plastics cause them to differ significantly from raw resins, rendering them unsuitable for numerous applications. Mechanical recycling processes do not remove additives and involve shredding plastics before remelting, which shortens the polymer chains. Unlike metals that can be recycled indefinitely, the shredding process in plastic recycling leads to a decrease in quality with each cycle. Over time, the plastic loses its recyclability and must be either disposed of or utilized for its calorific value. In underdeveloped nations, the issue is exacerbated by inadequate or non-existent infrastructure for collecting and sorting plastic wastes (Browning et al., 2021). Thermoset polymers, including polyesters, polyurethanes, silicones, and epoxy, possess a crosslinked structure that prevents them from being melted and reshaped once they have been produced. Consequently, post-consumer thermoset plastics are generally considered non-recyclable. Despite the technological challenges, the economic hurdles confronting conventional recycling are equally formidable. At present, only pure waste plastic streams, such as polyethylene terephthalate and high-density polyethylene bottles, are commercially recycled, while potentially recyclable plastics like polystyrene, polypropylene, polyethylene films, and mixed polyolefins are typically discarded (Larraín et al., 2021). Low oil prices adversely impact the recycling industry by reducing the cost of virgin resin, making it less economically viable. Implementing regulations that mandate minimum recycled content targets is crucial for boosting the demand for recycled products and ensuring the economic sustainability of recycling operations.

10.3 TREATMENT TECHNOLOGIES FOR PLASTIC WASTE

10.3.1 Conventional treatment technologies for plastic waste

Waste plastics and MPs have caused significant pollution in the natural environment. Existing treatment systems for waste plastics often require harsh reaction conditions or prolonged reaction times, resulting in high energy consumption and capital costs. Recent review articles focused on advanced plastic treatment methods primarily emphasize specific techniques like pyrolysis or photodegradation, or specific types of polymeric wastes, despite the availability of numerous research papers on the subject. There are two basic strategies for disposing of plastic waste: recycling and degradation. Recycling methods can be further classified into primary (reprocessing into similar products), secondary (reprocessing into lower-performance products), tertiary (recovery of chemical intermediates), and quaternary (energy recovery through incineration) (Okan et al., 2018). Primary and secondary recycling involve mechanical reprocessing, while tertiary is resource recovery, and quaternary is energy recovery. Degradation methods aim to convert plastic waste into carbon dioxide and water through microbial degradation or oxo-biodegradation (pretreatment combined with biodegradation). Pretreatment technologies for oxo-biodegradation include photodegradation, thermodegradation, mechanochemical degradation, and others. The illustrative schematic representation delineating the current cutting-edge methodologies for plastic waste stream management and mitigation is depicted in Figure 10.1.

The predominant approach for valorizing post-consumer polymeric waste streams involves secondary recycling via mechanical reprocessing, wherein the plastic waste undergoes size reduction and melt processing to yield recycled polymeric feedstocks suitable for manufacturing recycled polymer products and components (Mazhandu et al., 2020). Conversely, the viability and efficiency of recycling operations are contingent upon the inherent chemical and physical characteristics of the plastic waste feedstock, which are determined by factors such as the source, compositional makeup, and physical state of the waste material (Damayanti & Wu, 2021). Tertiary recycling, also referred to as chemical recycling, involves the depolymerization and cleavage of the polymer backbone, facilitating the recovery of the constituent monomers or oligomers with reduced molecular weights. This approach enables the production of recycled thermoplastic resins from the depolymerized feedstocks (Quienne et al., 2022). The following delineates some of the prevalent technologies that can be employed for tertiary/chemical recycling of plastic waste (Table 10.1).

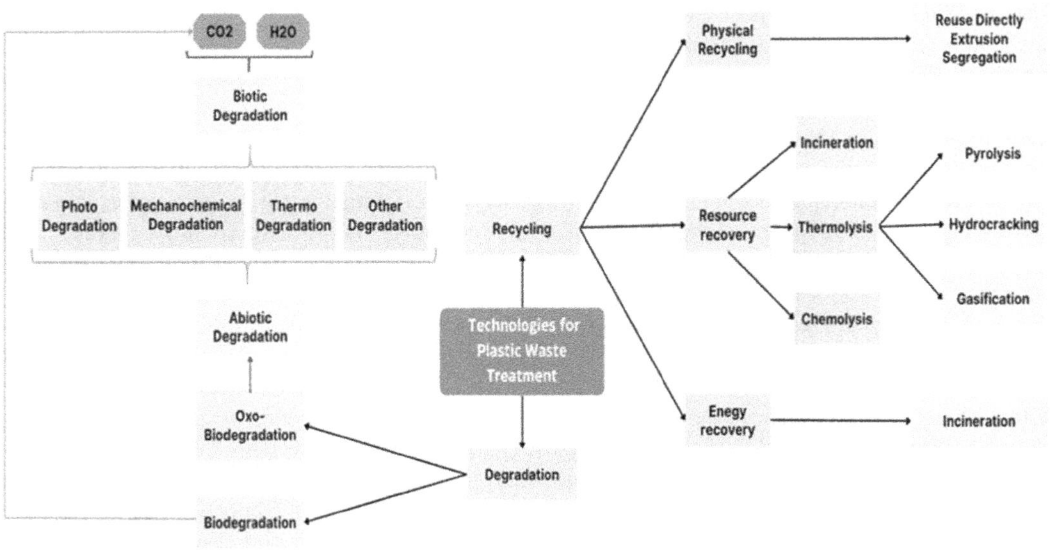

FIGURE 10.1 Technologies for plastic waste treatment.

TABLE 10.1
Chemical recycling route of plastic waste

Chemical recycling	Plastic waste
Glycolysis	PET, Polyamide (PA), Polyurethane (PU)s, Polylactic acid (PLA), Polycarbonate (PC)
Hydrolysis	PET, PA, PUs, PLA, PC
Ammonolysis	PET, PUs
Phosphorolysis	PUs
Dehydrochlorination	Polyvinyl chloride (PVC)
Pyrolysis	PET, PS, PVC, HDPE
Gasification	PS, HDPE, PUs
Hydroliquefication	HDPE

Quaternary recycling entails the recovery of the embodied energy content within polymeric waste streams via combustion processes (Siddiqui, 2009). The plastic waste undergoes controlled incineration, whereby the calorific value is harnessed and converted into usable forms such as thermal energy and electricity. These recycling strategies represent a hierarchical continuum of options, progressing from primary to quaternary methods, with the aim of optimizing resource utilization and minimizing the processing costs incurred by recyclers and converters.

10.3.2 Advanced treatment technologies for plastic waste

10.3.2.1 Elesctrocatalytic oxidation

The electrocatalytic conversion of polymeric materials can be facilitated via two distinct pathways: direct anodic oxidation and indirect mediated oxidation. Direct oxidation involves the electrophilic attack on the polymer substrate by hydroxyl radicals (OH) generated from water discharge at the anode surface. Conversely, indirect oxidation predominates when highly oxidizing intermediates play a dominant role in the polymer degradation process. Under the application of an external potential of 0.55 V in a phosphoric acid (H_3PO_4) electrolyte at 200°C, polyvinyl alcohol (PVA) underwent successful conversion, yielding hydrogen gas at a rate of 9.5 mol/min (Chow et al., 2017). The reductive dechlorination of the polymeric substrate occurs via an electron transfer process from the cathodic TiO_2/C catalyst at elevated temperatures. Concomitantly, the polymer undergoes anodic oxidation facilitated by hydroxyl radicals (·OH), inducing the formation of carbonyl and hydroxyl functionalities along the polymer backbone. This is followed by subsequent chain scission, yielding low molecular weight oxygenated organics such as alcohols, carboxylic acids, and esters. Ultimately, these degradation products undergo partial mineralization, yielding carbon dioxide and water as the final oxidation products. The electrocatalytic degradation of polymeric waste streams has the potential to yield a singular product stream that can be directly converted into fuel precursors. However, electrolysis alone may not generate as diverse an array of fuel components as a coupled pyrolysis-electrolysis approach. Solar thermally assisted electrolytic conversion has been demonstrated for the depolymerization of polypropylene (PP), yielding hydrogen gas and C1-C5 hydrocarbon fuel fractions. Furthermore, increasing the reaction temperature from 350 to 390°C and applying higher electrolysis currents up to 400 mA facilitated enhanced depolymerization and conversion of the PP (Jiang et al., 2020).

10.3.2.2 Photocatalytic oxidation

Photocatalysis is a technology that imitates the natural process of photosynthesis. Usually, it consists of three specific stages: (1) the stimulation of charge carriers within the photocatalyst by absorbing light, (2) the following separation and movement of the electron-hole pairs formed by the light, and (3) the happening of redox reactions on the surface of the catalyst. Photocatalytic oxidation involves the breakdown of polymeric substrates into smaller molecules using ultraviolet (UV) radiation and a photocatalyst. The photocatalyst is the main factor responsible for driving the conversion process. In order to commence photocatalytic activity, the energy of the incident photons must be equal to or greater than the band gap energy of the photocatalyst material. Furthermore, the reduction potential of the electrons that are excited by light in the conduction band must be higher than that of the substance to be reduced, whereas the oxidation potential of the holes created in the valence band must be greater than that of the substance to be oxidized. Photocatalytic valorization of plastic waste often involves using the holes in the valence band of the photocatalyst to help break down the polymer through oxidation, resulting in organic products or complete conversion to carbon dioxide. The electrons in the conduction band can be used to reduce protons and generate hydrogen, convert carbon dioxide into carbon-based fuels, or activate molecular oxygen for further involvement in polymer oxidation processes (Rafey et al., 2023). Conventional photocatalyst materials have a restricted ability to catalyze the process of reducing carbon dioxide by light, leading to a poor level of specificity and production of the necessary C^{2+} hydrocarbon fuel products. In order to efficiently convert plastic waste into longer-chain carbon compounds at normal temperature and pressure, it is crucial to develop rational design strategies to improve the performance of photocatalysts and optimize the mechanisms that control the breaking and joining of carbon-carbon bonds. By using solar irradiation as the main energy source to convert plastic feedstocks into fuel products through photocatalysis, the process becomes a thermal and more efficient compared to pyrolytic methods. Implementing these photocatalytic treatment methods could potentially lower operational costs and offer an effective solution for plastic waste remediation.

10.3.3.3 Fenton oxidation

The Fenton process represents an advanced oxidative treatment technology that is frequently employed for the degradation of recalcitrant chemical compounds that are resistant to conventional remediation methods. Fenton oxidation facilitates the conversion of polymeric substrates into lower molecular weight species through the generation of highly reactive hydroxyl radicals (·OH) via the iron-catalyzed decomposition of hydrogen peroxide (H_2O_2). The Fenton-mediated oxidative degradation of plastics is typically conducted under relatively mild reaction conditions. Owing to the rapid kinetics of H_2O_2 decomposition, the conversion process exhibits high efficiency, rendering it advantageous for large-scale applications. However, the substantial consumption of H_2O_2 during the process contributes to increased operational costs. Through chemical oxidation pathways, the Fenton reaction can regulate the depolymerization of plastic waste, yielding high-value fine chemical products. When the Fenton reagent is introduced to plastic, it causes the cleavage of the C-C bond, resulting in the production of hydroxyl radicals (·OH). Consequently, the polymer undergoes decomposition, resulting in the formation of various dicarboxylic acids. The chemical reaction between hydrogen peroxide (H_2O_2) and ferrous ions (Fe^{2+}) results in the formation of ferric ions (Fe^{3+}) and hydroxyl radicals (·OH). In addition, the compound H_2O_2 is catalyzed by the ion Fe^{3+} to produce $\cdot HO_2$, which can further react with H_2O_2 to generate additional OH. Furthermore, the formation of R· occurs as a result of the reaction between ·OH and RH. The polymer undergoes C-C bond cleavage, resulting in the formation of carbon dioxide (CO_2) and water (H_2O). A novel chemical technique utilizing sulfonation and the Fenton reaction was devised to convert LDPE and HDPE into organic acids. The conversion of LDPE and HDPE into carboxylic acids resulted in yields of around 87.5% and 88.8%, respectively (Chow et al., 2016). At a temperature of 65°C, the sulfonated PVC also underwent Fenton oxidation and decomposed into carboxylic acids, achieving a yield of around 75.5% (Chow et al., 2017). Clearly, polyethylene (PE) has a higher efficiency and speed in the production of carboxylic acids compared to PVC. Sulfonated polyethylene (PE), polypropylene (PP), and PVC have been reported to undergo photo-Fenton oxidation. This process results in the creation of carbon dioxide (CO_2) as the principal product. Through photo-reduction, the CO_2 can be further converted into acetic acid. Catalytic pyrolysis at low temperatures is an effective method for converting plastic waste into valuable products, which helps to address the increasing difficulties in managing these waste streams. Nevertheless, the retrieval and reuse of catalysts, which are highly sought after for promoting polymer conversion processes, present a notable obstacle due to catalytic deactivation caused by the creation of coke. Furthermore, the wide range of plastic waste varieties requires the creation of catalysts that may be widely used and have strong effectiveness in breaking down different types of polymers. Hence, it is imperative to develop and create catalytic systems that are extremely efficient, versatile, and can be reused in order to facilitate effective plastic waste conversion procedures. Due to progress in research and development, advanced oxidation technologies have emerged as promising options for converting plastic waste into desirable fuel products at normal temperature and pressure. These technologies offer significant energy savings compared to traditional thermal treatment processes. These methods strive to create goods of exceptional purity by carefully regulating the pathways of conversion. One major drawback of advanced oxidation processes (AOPs) is that the liquid product streams obtained have a very low calorific value. Additionally, highly effective catalysts are needed to assist the desired reactions. However, improved oxidation technologies have great potential for converting plastic trash in the near future.

10.4 ADVANCED TREATMENT TECHNOLOGIES FOR MICROPLASTICS

To address the emerging concern of MPs pollution, numerous review articles have been published on MP removal techniques. However, despite the promising potential of AOPs for MPs treatment, comprehensive reviews focusing specifically on AOPs for MP removal are scarce. Consequently, there is a pressing need to consolidate recent research findings on the application of various AOPs, such as UV photolysis, UV/H_2O_2, ozonation, UV/catalyst systems, heat-activated persulfate, heat-activated peroxy-mono-sulphate, and plasma-based processes, for the remediation of MPs in the environment.

10.4.1 Homogeneous AOPs

Photolysis is a light-induced degradation process in which chemical species undergo transformation upon exposure to electromagnetic radiation, particularly in the ultraviolet (UV) region of the spectrum. The absorption of photons initiates the generation of reactive intermediates and radical species, such as hydroxyl radicals (•OH), triplet excited states of organic matter (3OM•), singlet oxygen ($1O_2$), hydrated electrons (e−aq), superoxide radical anions (O_2•−), carbonate radicals (CO_3•−), and organoperoxy radicals (ROO•). These highly reactive species possess the potential to attack and decompose recalcitrant contaminants through various oxidation and reduction pathways. Photolytic processes have been predominantly explored for the degradation of plastics present in the natural environment, as these processes harness solar radiation as the primary energy source. Consequently, there is a relative paucity of research investigations focused on the application of photolysis for the removal of MPs within engineered environmental remediation systems or treatment facilities. The studies have shown that ultraviolet (UV) radiation can cause physical and chemical changes in different types of plastic, such as polyethylene (PE), polystyrene, polyethylene terephthalate (PET), and PVC. These changes can lead to the breakdown of the plastics, although the degradation process is complex. The process of UV photolysis has been found to cause the production of cracks on the surface of plastic samples. This leads to an increase in surface roughness and eventually results in the plastic breaking into smaller particles, ranging in size from nanometers to micrometers. Furthermore, studies have found that plastics degrade when exposed to several UV wavelength ranges, including UV-C (200–280 nm), UV-B (280–315 nm), and UV-A (315–400 nm). This provides additional evidence supporting the effectiveness of photolytic processes in breaking down plastics (Suhrhoff & Scholz-Böttcher, 2016). Nevertheless, due to the fact that photolytic processes primarily impact the outer layer of plastic materials, it is not possible to fully break them down in a short period of time. Therefore, prolonged exposure is required for significant deterioration to take place. Moreover, the degree of fragmentation and the subsequent distribution of particle sizes depend on the original dimensions of the plastic or MP particles. Prolonged photolysis can potentially result in the creation of plastic particles in the nano-size range as time passes. The effectiveness of the UV/H_2O_2 method in causing physicochemical alterations in polystyrene has been proven (Liu et al., 2021). Significant changes in the external structure, increased brittleness, carbonyl index (CI), degree of crystallization, glass transition temperatures, water repellence, and average molecular weight were observed during the treatment process. As expected, the chemical oxidation, aided by hydroxyl radicals (•OH), led to an augmentation in surface roughness, crystallinity, and embrittlement. The presence of surface oxidation was further confirmed by noticeable alterations in the color of the treated samples. The confidence interval (CI) of the polystyrene samples showed an approximately two-fold increase in comparison to the original polystyrene. Nevertheless, the mean molecular weight and hydrophobicity declined due to chain scission processes and the creation of polar functional groups (such as carbonyl groups) on the surface of the treated polystyrene, respectively. In addition, the study assessed the deterioration of polystyrene by the utilization of UV/H_2O and UV/Cl_2 methods. Not unexpectedly, both treatments produced comparable outcomes to the UV/H_2O_2 procedure, as the UV/H_2O and UV/Cl_2 processes efficiently generated hydroxyl radicals and chlorine radicals (Cl• and Cl_2•−), respectively. However, the study highlighted that the full breakdown of MPs may take a long time, and the oxidation mainly occurred on the surface of the MPs. This happened even though there were rapid changes in the MPs' physical and chemical properties, such as polarity, crystallinity, molecular weight, and brittleness, which were facilitated by oxidation caused by radicals.

10.4.2 Heterogeneous AOPs

10.4.2.1 UV-induced photocatalysis

UV radiation is widely used as a light source in many water treatment methods, such as UV disinfection, UV photolysis, and UV-induced photocatalysis, for treating both drinking water and wastewater. UV radiation is commonly used to activate various photocatalysts in order to degrade stubborn pollutants. This activation helps generate reactive oxygen species (ROS), including hydroxyl radicals (•OH) and superoxide radical anions ($O_2^{\bullet-}$), during photocatalytic reactions. The study examined the use of TiO_2 photocatalysts to eliminate MPs (Fadli et al., 2021). In addition, the TiO_2 was modified with silver (Ag) or a mixture of Ag and reduced graphene oxide (RGO) to improve the separation of charges and reduce the recombination of electrons and holes. This enhancement leads to an overall improvement in the catalytic performance of TiO_2 for the treatment of MPs. The study employed PE particles with sizes ranging from 100 to 150 μm as the model substrate. The samples were evaluated for changes in weight. Under UV irradiation, the presence of TiO_2 and modified TiO_2 photocatalysts significantly enhanced the oxidation process, leading to the efficient decomposition of PE particles. Significantly, the catalyst composed of 3% Ag/TiO_2 and 1% RGO attained a breakdown rate of 76% for PE after a treatment duration of 4 h. On the other hand, pure TiO_2 was only able to break down 56% of PE throughout the same period of treatment when exposed to UV light. The increased removal efficiency reported with the Ag/TiO_2-RGO catalyst can be attributed to the notable enhancement in charge transfer and separation of electrons and holes aided by the inclusion of Ag and RGO during the photocatalytic process under the explored experimental conditions. In contrast, G. Liu et al. (2012) investigated the application of a different photocatalyst, boron-doped cryptomelane (B-OMS-2), to break down PE. The study observed the degradation of PE at specific time intervals (0, 32, 64, 96, 128, and 288 h) when exposed to UV radiation with a wavelength of 254 nm. Using the specific parameters of the experiment, the maximum degradation of PE reached 19.9% after 288 h of UV irradiation with the presence of B-OMS-2. Nevertheless, without boron doping, the weight reduction of PE was restricted to a mere 9.5%, underscoring the advantageous impact of boron doping in augmenting the photocatalytic efficacy of cryptomelane for PE decomposition.

10.4.2.2 Solar-induced photocatalysis

Due to the fact that the solar spectrum consists of just a tiny portion (about 5%) of ultraviolet (UV) radiation, considerable research has been focused on expanding the photoresponse range of photocatalysts to include visible light in order to degrade different pollutants. Visible light-induced photocatalysis is a technology that uses solar energy to address environmental issues. It is considered environmentally friendly and has attracted significant attention for its potential in environmental remediation applications. Titanium dioxide (TiO_2) and zinc oxide (ZnO) have been widely studied as potential candidates for visible light-active photocatalysts, with the goal of improving the efficiency of degradation processes when exposed to visible light. Tofa et al. (2019) created zinc oxide (ZnO) nanorods with platinum (Pt) deposits and tested their ability to oxidize low-density polyethylene (LDPE) films, which were 50 μm thick, using visible light. The addition of Pt onto ZnO nanorods led to a significant increase in the absorption of visible light, reaching up to 78%. Surface oxidation of LDPE was seen throughout the photocatalytic treatment, as indicated by a progressive increase in the CI and vinyl index. This suggests the production of oxidized functional groups on the surface of the polymer. Additional photocatalysts, such as $NiAl_2O_4$ (Venkataramana et al., 2021) and hydroxy-rich BiOCl (Jiang et al., 2021), have been formulated to facilitate the decomposition of LDPE, HDPE, and PP when exposed to visible light. Surface oxidation caused by photocatalysis results in a weight loss of either 12.5% or 5.4%, depending on the type of photocatalyst used. This is because the bandgap energy is influenced by the properties of the catalysts.

10.4.2.3 Biodegradation

There has been little research attention on using organismal bioaccumulation as a bioremediation method to reduce the spread of MPs in aquatic ecosystems (Arossa et al., 2019). The researchers suggested that the attachment and clustering of MP particles onto the outer skeletons of small aquatic organisms hindered their feeding processes, thus acting as a crucial limitation on the ideal growth patterns of marine animal communities (Van Franeker et al., 2011). Bioremediation is the process of using various biological agents, including bacteria, fungus, or higher eukaryotic organisms (Zhou et al., 2022). Bacterial species have received greater study attention than fungi and higher eukaryotes in relation to the removal of MPs (Tang & Kristanti, 2022). Nevertheless, several fungal taxa, such as *Penicillium, Aspergillus*, and *Fusarium*, have also demonstrated the ability to degrade MPs. Nevertheless, these organisms have a restriction when it comes to excreting MPs, and their ability to respond to these contaminants can vary. Considerable attention has been focused on the isolation, alteration, and application of enzymes derived from these microbes to aid in the degradation of MPs. Hydroxylases, laccases, peroxidases, and reductases derived from actinomycetes and bacteria have been found to break down polyethylene (PE) (Amobonye et al., 2021), while cutinases, laccases, lipases, and ureases of bacterial and fungal origin have shown the potential to degrade PU. However, the functioning of these enzymes is limited by the physicochemical properties of the reaction environment, including pH, temperature, and ionic strength. The inherent forms of these enzymes frequently exhibit deficiencies in terms of stability, activity, and recyclability (Jabloune et al., 2020). Various techniques, such as immobilizing enzymes or their associated microbes on organic or inorganic substrates, have been suggested to improve their stability, capacity to be reused, and rates of breaking down MPs (Hou et al., 2014). However, the feasibility of bioaugmentation using MP-degrading microorganisms may be reduced due to several constraints. These drawbacks include the lengthy duration required, partial biodegradation, variable effectiveness of biodegradation, and ambiguity over their capacity to colonize the system. Biocatalysts and genetic engineering have the potential to overcome certain constraints, while there are still technical obstacles that need to be resolved.

10.5 ENVIRONMENTAL AND ECONOMIC ASSESSMENT

Conducting a thorough life cycle assessment (LCA) of polymeric products is extremely important in the context of the circular economy and sustainable practices. In accordance with the guidelines set by the European Environment Agency, the practical tactics aimed at implementing a circular economic model involve extending the lifespan of products. Multiple research papers have contended that the circular economy encourages the reduction of material and energy flows and the minimization of waste (Stahel, 2016). Based on the empirical evidence provided by research (Labuschagne & Brent, 2005), the new technological improvements based on life cycle evaluations require a specific focus on the manufacturing stage. During the production phase, it is crucial to recognize that plastic waste can be treated through disposal, incineration, or recycling methods. Based on the findings from LCA studies (Lahtela et al., 2019) and the guidelines provided by the European Food Safety Authority (EFSA), recycling plastic trash is generally considered to be the more environmentally favorable choice. The quality of the recycled polymer product depends mostly on the physicochemical qualities of the polymer, the processing conditions, and the purity of the input waste stream. Several research studies have attempted to tackle economic and ecological concerns by restricting the extensive use of chemical recycling methods. In order to achieve sustainable production methods, it is essential to carry out a thorough life cycle analysis throughout the manufacturing stage (Vuarnoz et al., 2018) developed an energy management technique that effectively reduced emissions during the first life cycle stage. However, there is a lack of research that investigates a life cycle model using an iterative looping technique for the injection molding process, together with a comparative assessment of different plastic products. LCA methodologies can aid in the comparative evaluation of various options for particular materials and products, thereby enabling a comprehensive rating system. The cradle-to-gate LCA paradigm refers to the process of evaluating the environmental impact of material production from its initial stages to the point of leaving the factory (Marcelino-Sádaba et al., 2017). The results of this LCA can be used as inputs for future iterations of the assessment.

10.6 FUTURE DIRECTIONS AND RESEARCH NEEDS

The discovery of new DNA sequences, enzymes, metabolic pathways, and metabolically active compounds with unique or improved metabolic functions plays a crucial role in advancing biotechnological applications for breaking down polymers (De Fátima Alves et al., 2018). Metagenomics is a genetic analytical method that allows the study of microbial communities without the need for culturing. It has enabled researchers to conduct extensive investigations into complex microbiomes and uncover specific metabolic processes involved in the breakdown of polymers. Due to the widespread presence of plastic goods in everyday life, the ways in which contaminants enter aquatic habitats are complex and varied. Future research endeavors concerning MPs should give priority to the following areas. Developing policy frameworks and regulatory actions to address the sources of MP contamination, together with attempts to increase public awareness and knowledge about MP-related issues. Implementing rigorous surveillance and oversight of wastewater containing MPs released by relevant industrial companies, together with improving or creating equipment to effectively remove MPs from drinking water sources. Strengthening ecological strategies to combat MP pollution in environmentally vulnerable and representative regions. Enhanced exploitation of biodegradable resources, such as starch, cellulose, and lignin, in the manufacturing of plastic goods. Assessing the possible hazards linked to the intake of MPs through polluted sources of drinking water, using epidemiological techniques. To tackle these complex challenges, it is important to take a multidisciplinary approach that combines knowledge from various fields such as sociology, engineering, epidemiology, and technology. This approach will help us gain a comprehensive understanding and fill the gaps in our knowledge, especially when it comes to the environmental factors and human activities that contribute to MP pollution.

10.7 CONCLUSION

This chapter offers a thorough study of the latest treatment technologies used to address and reduce plastic and MP contamination. The explanation covers a wide range of creative methods, such as enhanced oxidation processes, membrane-based filtration techniques, bioremediation tactics, electrochemical decomposition pathways, and novel hybrid approaches. The chapter highlights recent advancements in improving the effectiveness of removing plastic impurities, increasing the ability to scale up the process, and enhancing the selectivity for stubborn plastic pollutants. Also, it examines the existing technology gaps and suggests key areas that require additional research and development efforts. The focus is mostly on evaluating the advantages, current constraints, and potential paths for converting innovative laboratory-scale methods into practical solutions for addressing widespread plastic and MP contamination. Additionally, it emphasizes the necessity of performing thorough LCAs of polymeric products, in line with the principles of circular economy and sustainable practices promoted by the European Environment Agency. Moreover, the importance of metagenomics and the discovery of new biocatalysts, enzymes, and metabolic pathways in developing biotechnological treatments for polymer breakdown, while also providing guidance for future research directions has also been emphasized. Furthermore, it accentuates the need for a multidisciplinary approach encompassing sociological, engineering, epidemiological, and technological domains to bridge the knowledge gaps, particularly concerning environmental factors and anthropogenic activities contributing to MP proliferation.

ACKNOWLEDGMENT

The authors are highly thankful to the Department of Science and Technology, Ministry of Science and Technology, New Delhi, for funding the project under the "Scheme for Young Scientist and Technologists (SYST-SEED)" Project No: SP/YO/2019/1360(G).

REFERENCES

Abel, B. A., Snyder, R. L., & Coates, G. W. (2021). Chemically recyclable thermoplastics from reversible-deactivation polymerization of cyclic acetals. *Science*, 373(6556), 783–789. https://doi.org/10.1126/science.abh0626

Akhbarizadeh, R., Moore, F., & Keshavarzi, B. (2018). Investigating a probable relationship between microplastics and potentially toxic elements in fish muscles from northeast of Persian Gulf. *Environmental Pollution*, 232, 154–163. https://doi.org/10.1016/j.envpol.2017.09.028

Amobonye, A., Bhagwat, P., Singh, S., & Pillai, S. (2021). Plastic biodegradation: Frontline microbes and their enzymes. *Science of the Total Environment*, 759, 143536. https://doi.org/10.1016/j.scitotenv.2020.143536

Araújo, C. F., Nolasco, M. M., Ribeiro, A. M., & Ribeiro-Claro, P. J. A. (2018). Identification of microplastics using Raman spectroscopy: Latest developments and future prospects. Water *Research (Oxford)*, 142, 426–440. https://doi.org/10.1016/j.watres.2018.05.060

Arossa, S., Martin, C., Rossbach, S., & Duarte, C. M. (2019). Microplastic removal by Red Sea giant clam (Tridacna maxima). *Environmental Pollution* (1987), 252, 1257–1266. https://doi.org/10.1016/j.envpol.2019.05.149

Bank, M. S., & Hansson, S. V. (2019). The Plastic Cycle: A novel and holistic paradigm for the Anthropocene. *Environmental Science & Technology*, 53(13), 7177–7179. https://doi.org/10.1021/acs.est.9b02942

Borrelle, S. B., Ringma, J., Law, K. L., Monnahan, C. C., Lebreton, L., McGivern, A., Murphy, E. L., Jambeck, J., Leonard, G. H., Hilleary, M. A., Eriksen, M., Possingham, H. P., De Frond, H., Gerber, L. R., Polidoro, B., Tahir, A., Bernard, M., Mallos, N. J., Barnes, M., & Rochman, C. M. (2020). Predicted growth in plastic waste exceeds efforts to mitigate plastic pollution. *Science*, 369(6510), 1515–1518. https://doi.org/10.1126/science.aba3656

Brooks, A., Wang, S., & Jambeck, J. (2018). The Chinese import ban and its impact on global plastic waste trade. *Science Advances*, 4(6). https://doi.org/10.1126/sciadv.aat0131

Browning, S., Beymer-Farris, B. A., & Seay, J. (2021). Addressing the challenges associated with plastic waste disposal and management in developing countries. *Current Opinion in Chemical Engineering*, 32, 100682. https://doi.org/10.1016/j.coche.2021.100682

Chow, C. F. S., Wong, W., Chan, C. S., Li, Y., Tang, Q., & Gong, C. (2017). Breakdown of plastic waste into economically valuable carbon resources: Rapid and effective chemical treatment of polyvinylchloride with the Fenton catalyst. *Polymer Degradation and Stability*, 146, 34–41. https://doi.org/10.1016/j.polymdegradstab.2017.09.016

Chow, C. F. S., Wong, W., Ho, K. Y. F., Chan, C. S., & Gong, C. (2016). Combined chemical activation and fenton degradation to convert waste polyethylene into high-value fine chemicals. *Chemistry (Weinheim. Print)*, 22(28), 9513–9518. https://doi.org/10.1002/chem.201600856

Damayanti, D., & Wu, H. (2021). Strategic possibility routes of recycled PET. *Polymers (Basel)*, 13(9), 1475. https://doi.org/10.3390/polym13091475

De Fátima Alves, L., Westmann, C. A., Lovate, G. L., De Siqueira, G. M. V., Borelli, T. C., & Guazzaroni, M. (2018). Metagenomic Approaches for understanding new concepts in Microbial science. *International Journal of Genomics (Print)*, 2018, 1–15. https://doi.org/10.1155/2018/2312987

Fadli, M. H., Ibadurrohman, M., & Slamet, S. (2021). Microplastic pollutant degradation in water using modified TiO_2 photocatalyst under UV-Irradiation. *IOP Conference Series: Materials Science and Engineering*, 1011(1), 012055. https://doi.org/10.1088/1757-899x/1011/1/012055

Galloway, T. S., & Lewis, C. (2016). Marine microplastics spell big problems for future generations. *Proceedings of the National Academy of Sciences of the United States of America*, 113(9), 2331–2333. https://doi.org/10.1073/pnas.1600715113

Ghosh, S., Sinha, J. K., Ghosh, S. K., Vashisth, K., Han, S., & Bhaskar, R. (2023). Microplastics as an emerging threat to the global environment and human health. *Sustainability (Basel)*, 15(14), 10821. https://doi.org/10.3390/su151410821

Golwala, H., Zhang, X., Iskander, S. M., & Smith, A. L. (2021). Solid waste: An overlooked source of microplastics to the environment. *Science of the Total Environment*, 769, 144581. https://doi.org/10.1016/j.scitotenv.2020.144581

Hou, J., Guo, D., Ye, Y., & Chen, V. (2014). Enzymatic degradation of bisphenol-A with immobilized laccase on TiO_2 sol–gel coated PVDF membrane. *Journal of Membrane Science*, 469, 19–30. https://doi.org/10.1016/j.memsci.2014.06.027

Jabloune, R., Khalil, M., Moussa, I., Simao-Beaunoir, A., Lerat, S., Brzeziński, R., & Beaulieu, C. (2020). Enzymatic degradation of *p*-Nitrophenyl esters, polyethylene terephthalate, cutin, and suberin by Sub1, a suberinase encoded by the plant Pathogen. *Streptomyces scabies Microbes and Environments*, 35(1), n/a. https://doi.org/10.1264/jsme2.me19086

Jiang, R., Lu, G., Yan, Z., Liu, J., Wu, D., & Wang, Y. (2021). Microplastic degradation by hydroxy-rich bismuth oxychloride. *Journal of Hazardous Materials (Print)*, 405, 124247. https://doi.org/10.1016/j.jhazmat.2020.124247

Jiang, T., Zhao, X., Gu, D., Yan, C., Jiang, H., Wu, H., Wang, B., & Wang, X. (2020). STEP polymer degradation: Solar thermo-coupled electrochemical depolymerization of plastics to generate useful fuel plus abundant hydrogen. *Solar Energy Materials and Solar Cells*, 204, 110208. https://doi.org/10.1016/j.solmat.2019.110208

Kazour, M., Terki, S., Rabhi, K., Jemaa, S., Khalaf, G., & Amara, R. (2019). Sources of microplastics pollution in the marine environment: Importance of wastewater treatment plant and coastal landfill. *Marine Pollution Bulletin*, 146, 608–618. https://doi.org/10.1016/j.marpolbul.2019.06.066

Labuschagne, C., & Brent, A. C. (2005). Sustainable Project Life Cycle Management: The need to integrate life cycles in the manufacturing sector. *International Journal of Project Management*, 23(2), 159–168. https://doi.org/10.1016/j.ijproman.2004.06.003

Lahtela, V., Hyvärinen, M., & Kärki, T. (2019). Composition of plastic fractions in waste streams: Toward more efficient recycling and utilization. *Polymers (Basel)*, 11(1), 69. https://doi.org/10.3390/polym11010069

Larraín, M., Van Passel, S., Thomassen, G., Van Gorp, B., Nhu, T. T., Huysveld, S., Van Geem, K. M., De Meester, S., & Billen, P. (2021). Techno-economic assessment of mechanical recycling of challenging post-consumer plastic packaging waste. *Resources, Conservation and Recycling*, 170, 105607. https://doi.org/10.1016/j.resconrec.2021.105607

Liu, G., Liao, S., Zhu, D., Yue, H., & Zhou, W. (2012). Innovative photocatalytic degradation of polyethylene film with boron-doped cryptomelane under UV and visible light irradiation. *Chemical Engineering Journal*, 213, 286–294. https://doi.org/10.1016/j.cej.2012.09.105

Liu, X., Sun, P., Qu, G., Jing, J., Zhang, T., Shi, H., & Zhao, Y. (2021). Insight into the characteristics and sorption behaviors of aged polystyrene microplastics through three type of accelerated oxidation processes. *Journal of Hazardous Materials*, 407, 124836. https://doi.org/10.1016/j.jhazmat.2020.124836

Marcelino-Sádaba, S., Kinuthia, J., Oti, J., & Seco, A. (2017). Challenges in Life Cycle Assessment (LCA) of stabilised clay-based construction materials. *Applied Clay Science*, 144, 121–130. https://doi.org/10.1016/j.clay.2017.05.012

Mazhandu, Z. S., Muzenda, E., Mamvura, T. A., Belaid, M., & Nhubu, T. (2020). Integrated and consolidated review of plastic waste management and bio-based biodegradable plastics: Challenges and opportunities. *Sustainability*, 12(20), 8360. https://doi.org/10.3390/su12208360

Narevski, A. C., Novaković, M., Petrović, M., Mihajlović, I., Maoduš, N., & Vujić, G. (2021). Occurrence of bisphenol A and microplastics in landfill leachate: Lessons from South East Europe. *Environmental Science and Pollution Research*, 28(31), 42196–42203. https://doi.org/10.1007/s11356-021-13705-z

Okan, M., Aydın, H. M., & Barsbay, M. (2018). Current approaches to waste polymer utilization and minimization: A review. *Journal of Chemical Technology and Biotechnology*, 94(1), 8–21. https://doi.org/10.1002/jctb.5778

Quienne, B., Cuminet, F., Pinaud, J., Semsarilar, M., Cot, D., Ladmiral, V., & Caillol, S. (2022). Upcycling bio-based polyurethane foams into thermosets: Toward the closing of the loop. *ACS Sustainable Chemistry & Engineering*, 10(21), 7041–7049. https://doi.org/10.1021/acssuschemeng.2c00950

Rafey, A., Pal, K., Bohre, A., Modak, A., & Pant, K. K. (2023). A state-of-the-art review on the technological advancements for the sustainable management of plastic Waste in consort with the generation of energy and value-added chemicals. *Catalysts*, 13(2), 420. https://doi.org/10.3390/catal13020420

Rahman, A., Sarkar, A., Yadav, O. P., Achari, G., & Slobodní, K. J. (2021). Potential human health risks due to environmental exposure to nano- and microplastics and knowledge gaps: A scoping review. *Science of the Total Environment*, 757, 143872. https://doi.org/10.1016/j.scitotenv.2020.143872

Siddiqui, M. N. (2009). Conversion of hazardous plastic wastes into useful chemical products. *Journal of Hazardous Materials (Print)*, 167(1–3), 728–735. https://doi.org/10.1016/j.jhazmat.2009.01.042

Suhrhoff, T. J., & Scholz-Böttcher, B. M. (2016). Qualitative impact of salinity, UV radiation and turbulence on leaching of organic plastic additives from four common plastics-A lab experiment. *Marine Pollution Bulletin*, 102(1), 84–94. https://doi.org/10.1016/j.marpolbul.2015.11.054

Sun, A., & Wang, W. (2023). Human exposure to microplastics and its associated health risks. *Environment & Health (Washington, D.C.)*, 1(3), 139–149. https://doi.org/10.1021/envhealth.3c00053

Stahel, W. R. (2016). The circular economy. *Nature,* 531, 435–438.

Tang, K. H. D., & Kristanti, R. A. (2022). Bioremediation of perfluorochemicals: Current state and the way forward. *Bioprocess and Biosystems Engineering*, 45(7), 1093–1109. https://doi.org/10.1007/s00449-022-02694-z

Ter Halle, A., Ladirat, L., Gendre, X., Goudounèche, D., Pusineri, C., Routaboul, C., Tenailleau, C., Duployer, B., & Perez, É. (2016). Understanding the fragmentation pattern of marine plastic debris. *Environmental Science & Technology*, 50(11), 5668–5675. https://doi.org/10.1021/acs.est.6b00594

Tofa, T. S., Fei, Y., Laxman, K., & Dutta, J. (2019). Enhanced visible light photodegradation of microplastic fragments with plasmonic platinum/Zinc oxide nanorod photocatalysts. *Catalysts*, 9(10), 819. https://doi.org/10.3390/catal9100819

Van Franeker, J., Blaize, C., Danielsen, J., Fairclough, K., Gollan, J., Guse, N., Hansen, P., Heubeck, M., Jensen, J., Guillou, G. L., Olsen, B., Olsen, K., Pedersen, J., Stienen, E., & Turner, D. M. (2011). Monitoring plastic ingestion by the northern fulmar Fulmarus glacialis in the North Sea. *Environmental Pollution (1987)*, 159(10), 2609–2615. https://doi.org/10.1016/j.envpol.2011.06.008

Vega, G. C., Gross, A., & Birkved, M. (2021). The impacts of plastic products on air pollution - A simulation study for advanced life cycle inventories of plastics covering secondary microplastic production. *Sustainable Production and Consumption*, 28, 848–865. https://doi.org/10.1016/j.spc.2021.07.008

Venkataramana, C., Botsa, S. M., Shyamala, P., & Muralikrishna, R. (2021). Photocatalytic degradation of polyethylene plastics by NiAl2O4 spinels-synthesis and characterization. *Chemosphere*, 265, 129021. https://doi.org/10.1016/j.chemosphere.2020.129021

Vuarnoz, D., Cozza, S., Jusselme, T., Magnin, G., Schafer, T. M., Couty, P., & Niederhäuser, E. (2018). Integrating hourly life-cycle energy and carbon emissions of energy supply in buildings. *Sustainable Cities and Society*, 43, 305–316. https://doi.org/10.1016/j.scs.2018.08.026

Wiesinger, H., Wang, Z., & Hellweg, S. (2021). Deep Dive into Plastic Monomers, Additives, and Processing Aids. *Environmental Science & Technology*, 55(13), 9339–9351. https://doi.org/10.1021/acs.est.1c00976

Zhang, X., Chen, J., & Ji, L. (2020). The removal of microplastics in the wastewater treatment process and their potential impact on anaerobic digestion due to pollutants association. *Chemosphere*, 251, 126360. https://doi.org/10.1016/j.chemosphere.2020.126360

Zhou, Y., Kumar, M., Sarsaiya, S., Sirohi, R., Awasthi, S. K., Sindhu, R., Binod, P., Pandey, A., Bolan, N., Zhang, Z., Singh, L., Kumar, S., & Awasthi, M. K. (2022). Challenges and opportunities in bioremediation of micro-nano plastics: A review. *Science of the Total Environment*, 802, 149823. https://doi.org/10.1016/j.scitotenv.2021.149823

11 Biodegradation mechanisms and its applications in wastewater treatment

Sarojini Devi Nagesh, Renuka Devi Ravi, Rekha Pachaiappan, Padmavathi Rajangam, Geetha Arunachalam, and Kovendhan Manavalan

11.1 INTRODUCTION

In the modern life, plastic materials are playing a major role for various types of utilization due to its excellent properties. After their lifetime it was filled on the land and produces a problem to the environment causing soil, water, and air pollutions. Instead of regular incineration process, the biodegradation like microbial assemblages can degrade it more effectively. However, this area of research has not received as much attention as plastic degradation with single microbial strains. Within this context, the phenomenon of hydrocarbon and xenobiotic biodegradation with the aid of microbial consortia has received extensive research attention. Yu et al. (2019) found that when microorganisms work together, they can have higher biodegradation efficiencies than when they work alone. This can happen when they remove potentially hazardous degradation intermediates or play a direct part in biodegradation. Through metabolic cross-feeding or the production of metabolites that cause co-metabolic degradation, individual members of a microbial consortium can also indirectly enhance biodegradation (Hu et al., 2020). The term "plastic biodegradation" primarily describes the process by which anaerobic microbes that are capable of employing polymers as a carbon source for their own development convert polymeric materials into renewable energy and biomass while there is no air present (Ali & Sun, 2019). A wide range of polymers made from synthetic materials, such as PET, PU, PS, PVC, PE, PP, and PS, have been used extensively as fundamentals for human existence. However, garbage is a weak growth substrate due to their unique physical features and the very nature of the material, which inhibits biodegradability (Biffinger et al., 2014). Although a number of research initiatives on the subject of plastic biodegradation are centered on isolating single degradative microorganisms, it is clear that bacterial and fungal consortiums have enormous potential for the biodegradation and bioremediation of plastic waste. In the presence of microbial ensembles, polyester polyurethane (PSPU) and poly-acrylic polymers biodegraded more efficiently than when sole strains or specific members of the community were involved (Vargas-Suárez et al., 2019). Likewise, Gaytán et al. (2020) revealed the effectiveness of a bacterial consortium in breaking down a copolymer of PU and acrylate. On the other hand, it was also reported (Zafar et al., 2014) that fungal compost consortia degrade PSPU coupons. It is unclear, though, whether the fungal strains degrade the coupons alone or in a consortium. Furthermore, a variety of microbial consortia have been investigated for the degradation of plastics, including weathered polyethylene (WPE), polycaprolactone (PCL), PE, PP, and PS (Nakamura et al., 2006; Syranidou et al., 2017a, 2017b). The enzymatic fractionation of the polymeric chain into low molecular weight (MW) compounds, such as oligomers as dimers, and monomers for short, is the first step in the biodegradation of

DOI: 10.1201/9781003500483-11
This chapter has been made available under a (CC-BY-NC-ND) 4.0 license

plastic waste. This is accomplished by protein binding to the polymer and catalyzing its hydrolytic in nature cleavage. Eventually, the process leads to the mineralization of these low MW compounds into H_2O and CO_2. According to reports, bacteria, fungi, and algae are capable of breaking down polymers like PU and PE.

Biodegradation is a natural process by which organic substances are broken down into simpler compounds by the action of microorganisms such as bacteria, fungi, and other biological agents. This process is crucial for the recycling of organic matter in the environment and plays a significant role in maintaining ecological balance. Understanding the mechanisms of biodegradation is essential for addressing environmental concerns, waste management, and the development of sustainable practices.

11.2 BIODEGRADABLE TECHNOLOGY

Biodegradable technologies are those that have been developed to use various ways for product packaging, manufacturing, and medicine. The trade-off between biodegradability and performance is a key barrier to widespread adoption. Figure 11.1 represents effect of compost on microbe and soil physicochemical characteristics.

11.2.1 Types of biodegradation

Biodegradation is classified into many kinds based on the nature of the organic substance being degraded and the unique processes involved. Table 11.1 provides the ISO standards for degradable methods from the year 1995 to till date.

11.2.1.1 Aerobic biodegradation

This form of biodegradation happens when oxygen is present. Organic substances are broken down by aerobic microbes into carbon dioxide, water, and other simple byproducts. This is the most prevalent kind of biodegradation, and it is employed in wastewater treatment, composting, and natural decomposition.

11.2.1.2 Anaerobic biodegradation

This type of biodegradation occurs in the absence of oxygen. Anaerobic microbes degrade organic molecules, creating methane and carbon dioxide. This method is frequently used in anaerobic digestion to handle organic waste, such as in landfills and biogas generation.

11.2.1.3 Composting

Composting is a sort of aerobic biodegradation that is used to decompose organic waste materials such as food scraps, yard debris, and agricultural leftovers. Microorganisms such as bacteria and fungus decompose organic materials to produce nutrient-rich compost that may be used as a soil conditioner.

11.2.1.4 Petroleum hydrocarbon biodegradation

Certain bacteria are capable of breaking down hydrocarbons contained in petroleum products such as oil and gasoline. This biodegradation method has the potential to reduce the environmental effect of oil spills and polluted areas (Varjani et al., 2017).

11.2.1.5 Plastic biodegradation

Enzymatic activity in some microorganisms may break down some types of plastics, such as polyhydroxyalkanoates (PHA) and polyesters. While this is a work in progress, it has the potential to alleviate concerns of plastic pollution (Amobonye et al., 2021).

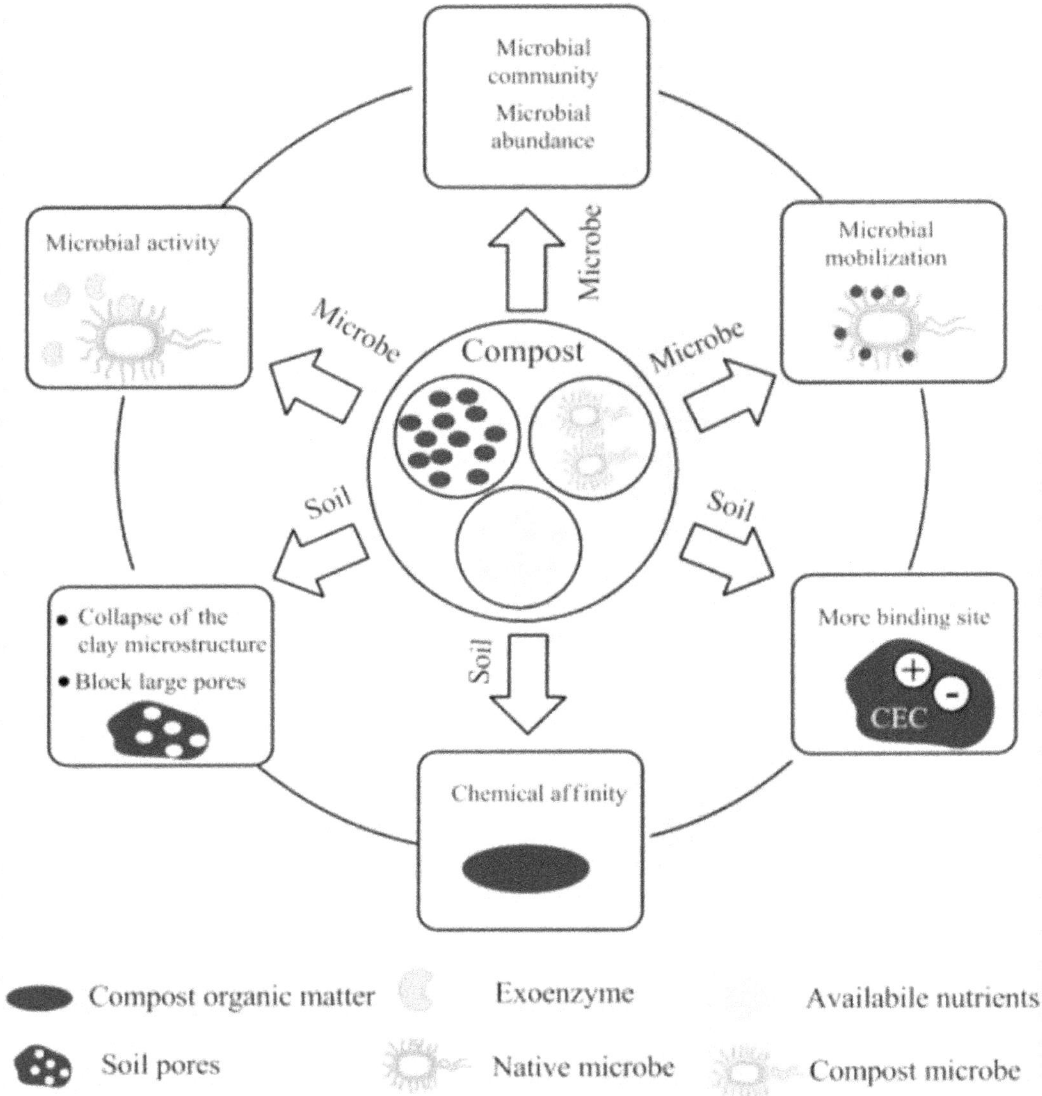

FIGURE 11.1 The above given diagram describes effect of compost on microbe and physicochemical characteristics.

Source: Adapted from Ren et al. (2018).

11.2.1.6 Pharmaceutical and personal care product biodegradation

Microorganisms in wastewater treatment systems may break down many medications and personal care goods. Some drugs, however, are persistent and may need sophisticated therapeutic approaches (Caracciolo et al., 2015).

11.2.2 Bio-deterioration

Biodegradation deterioration is the surface-level breakdown of a material that alters its mechanical, physical, and chemical properties. The abiotic factors that cause deterioration were previously

TABLE 11.1
Development of degradable methods

Year	Test Method	Standard
Before 1995	Photo-degradation test	ISO 4892
1995	Fungal erosion test	ISO 486
2001	Biodegradable test	ISO 14851
2005	Disintegration	ISO 169291
2014	Soil biodegradability test	ISO 17556
2017	Packaging compostability test	ISO 18606
2022	Degradation of plastics in water	ISO 22404

mentioned. The biological aspects of deterioration are the main topic of this section. Microorganisms growing on the surface or within a particular material are the primary cause of deterioration (Hueck, 2001). Microorganisms can function mechanically, chemically, or enzymatically. The composition and characteristics of polymer materials influence the development of microorganisms. Important factors to consider are the particular environmental circumstances, such as humidity, weather, and air pollution.

The lichenaceae, bacteria, protozoa, algae, and fungi are among the many different types of microorganisms that are involved in biodeterioration (Wallström et al., 2005). They have the ability to form associations with biofilms, an organized organization. When this microbial mat cooperates, it can cause significant harm to a variety of materials (Flemming, 1998). The emergence of distinct species of microbes, arranged in a particular sequence, intensifies microbial degradation and thus promotes the synthesis of simple molecules.

According to recent research, some microorganisms may be able to obtain nutrients from air pollutants (Zanardini et al., 2000; Nuhoglu et al., 2006). According to Mitchell and Gu (2000), a variety of polymer materials have been exposed to sulfur dioxide, aliphatic, and aromatic hydrocarbons found in urban air. These pollutants that have been adsorbed may also encourage other microbial species to colonize the material. These microorganisms may also find nourishment in organic dyes.

11.2.2.1 Physical way

A type of glue secreted by microorganisms allows them to stick to material surfaces (Capitelli et al., 2006). This material is a polymer-based complex matrix, such as proteins and polysaccharides. This slime matter seeps into porous structures, changing the distribution and size of pores as well as the degrees of moisture and heat transfers. The slime matrix's job is to shield microorganisms from adverse environments, such as desiccation and UV rays. Within the materials, filamentous microorganisms grow their mycelia framework. The mechanical penetration of apices causes pore enlargement and fractures in the materials. As a result, the material's resistance and durability are reduced.

11.2.2.2 Chemical way

Microorganisms can produce polymers outside of cells that function as surfactants to aid in the transitions between hydrophilic and hydrophobic phases. The spreading rate of organisms is favored by these interactions. Furthermore, slime promotes the accumulation of air pollutants, which in turn favors the growth of microorganisms and speeds up the breakdown (Zanardini et al., 2000). The chemical biodeterioration is caused by various types of microbial flora that grow into the building components over time. Inorganic substances such as ammonia, nitrites, hydrogen sulfide, thiosulfates, and simple sulfur are used by chemolithotrophic bacteria as sources of energy and electrons. They can release active chemicals as nitrous acid (e.g., Nitrosomonas spp.), nitric acid (e.g., Nitrobacter spp.), or sulphuric acid (e.g., Thiobacillus spp.). Organic substrates serve as sources of carbon, energy, and electrons for chemoautotrophic microorganisms. Oxalic, citric, gluconic, glutaric, glyoxalic, oxaloacetic, and fumaric acids are among the organic acids that are released. Abiotic and/or biotic hydration of various polymers (e.g., PBS, PBA, and PLA) releases succinic acid, adipic acid, lactic acid, and other acids along with butanediol (Lindström et al., 2004).

Water seeps into the polymer matrix, potentially causing swelling. Water leaking in causes the polymer to hydrolyze, resulting in the formation of monomers and oligomers. As pores form as a result of progressive degradation, the matrix's microstructure is altered, and oligomers and monomers are liberated. The breakdown products simultaneously alter the pH inside the pores, typically exhibiting some acid-base properties. These acids function in different ways. Some substances have the ability to react with other substances and accelerate surface erosion. In order to create stable complexes, other cations (such as Ca^{2+}, Al^{3+}, Si^{4+}, Fe^{2+}, Mn^{2+}, and Mg^{2+}) can be sequestered from the matrix. When it comes to fixing cations, organic acids perform better than mineral acids. They are thought to be one of the primary causes of biodeterioration. Furthermore, certain microorganisms such as filamentous bacteria and fungi have the ability to extend their mycelia framework by using these organic acids as carbon sources. Oxidation processes can also lead to chemical biodeterioration. Through oxidation processes, certain fungi and chemolithotrophic germs can absorb iron and/or manganese cations from the matrix. To recover iron atoms, they employ particular proteins found in cellular membranes that ensnare siderophores, or iron-chelating substances secreted by other microbes. In photosynthetic structures, siderophores can participate in redox reactions when oxygen is present. It is possible to couple the oxidation of cations and the catalytic hydrocarbon degradation by some extracellular enzymes, especially the peroxidases (Hofrichter, 2002; Otsuka et al., 2003).

11.2.2.3 Enzymatic way

Polyurethane, polyvinyl chloride, and polyamide are examples of materials that are thought to be recalcitrant polymers; however, they are susceptible to microbial biodeterioration (Howard, 2002; Shokrollahzadeh et al., 2008). The production of lipases, esterases, ureases, and proteases is thought to be the cause of these polymers' susceptibility to microbes (Flemming, 1998).

Cofactors, or cations found in the material matrix and coenzymes produced by microorganisms, are necessary for the breakdown of particular bonds by the enzymes involved in biodeterioration. Two distinct mechanisms—bulk and surface erosion—may be involved in the biodeterioration of thermoplastic polymers (von Burkersroda et al., 2002; Pepic et al., 2008). Bulk erosion occurs when a polymer's entire mass is broken up into fragments, and bond cleavage modifies the MW. Enzymes do not cause this lysis; instead, chemicals (such as H_2O, acids, bases, transition metals, and radicals) or radiations do. They are too big to fit inside the matrix structure. Surface erosion results in the loss of matter but does not alter the MW of the matrix's polymers. Bulk erosion of the polymer occurs when the rate of chemical diffusion through the material surpasses the rate of polymer bond cleavage. Bond cleavage mostly takes place at the matrix's surface if it happens more quickly than chemical diffusion (von Burkersroda et al., 2002; Pepic et al., 2008). Several authors have described the erosion mechanisms of polymers: bulk erosion for PLA and PLGA, surface erosion for aliphatic–aromatic copolyesters (Muller, 2005), PHB (Tsuji and Suzuyoshi, 2002), and polyanhydrides.

11.2.3 Environmental treatment

Biodegradation is a natural process in which microorganisms such as bacteria and fungus degrade organic molecules into simpler, non-toxic chemicals. Biodegradation is a key method in environmental rehabilitation for cleaning up polluted places and managing pollution. It is very helpful for removing organic pollutants such as petroleum hydrocarbons, solvents, and different organic compounds. Here are some essential considerations about biodegradation's significance in environmental remediation (Francesco Agostini et al., 2012):

- **Natural Attenuation:** In certain circumstances, polluted areas may rely on natural attenuation, in which existing microorganisms in the environment break down toxins over time. This procedure can be time-consuming and may not be successful for all pollutants.
- **Enhanced Bioremediation:** Environmental engineers and scientists frequently use techniques like enhanced bioremediation to speed up and improve the effectiveness of the biodegradation process. To stimulate the growth of pollutant-degrading bacteria, particular microorganisms (biostimulation) or nutrients (bioaugmentation) can be introduced into the polluted region.
- **Bioremediation procedures:** Biodegradation is used in numerous bioremediation procedures, including:
  a. In situ bioremediation: Treating toxins on-site rather than excavating or removing them.
  b. Ex-situ bioremediation: Extracted contaminated material is treated in a controlled setting, such as a bioreactor, before being returned to the site.
  c. Phytoremediation: The use of plants to facilitate pollutant breakdown, absorption, or sequestration.
- **Substrate Selection**
  Microorganisms require specific substrates in order to break down various pollutants. Environmental scientists choose acceptable substrates for biodegradation, such as oxygen, nitrogen, or other organic compounds.
- **Monitoring and Evaluation:**
  It is critical to conduct regular monitoring and evaluation of the remediation process to confirm that biodegradation is effectively lowering pollutant concentrations and that the site is becoming less hazardous.
- **Limitations:**
  While biodegradation is effective for some organic pollutants, it may not be effective for inorganic contaminants such as heavy metals. Furthermore, the effectiveness of bioremediation is dependent on factors such as pollutant type, site circumstances, microbial activity, and environmental parameters.
- **Sustainability:**
  Biodegradation is frequently seen as an ecologically beneficial and sustainable approach to repair since it depends on natural processes and might be less invasive than other remediation approaches.
- **Regulatory Considerations:**
  Regulatory bodies are frequently involved in the approval and oversight of bioremediation projects to ensure that they are carried out safely and effectively.

11.3 BIODEGRADATION KINETICS IN WASTEWATER TREATMENT

Biodegradation kinetics was important in wastewater treatment processes, especially in biological treatment methods including activated sludge systems, biofilters, and lagoons. Biodegradation is the process by which microorganisms degrade organic materials in wastewater into simpler, more stable molecules, lowering pollution load and improving water quality. Table 11.2 provides the biodegradation mechanisms utilized in the wastewater treatment. Understanding the dynamics of this process is critical for building and running efficient wastewater treatment systems. The following are some important characteristics of biodegradation kinetics in wastewater treatment (de Lucas et al., 2005).

TABLE 11.2
Biodegradation mechanisms employed in wastewater treatment

Biodegradation mechanism	Description	Application in wastewater treatment
Aerobic process	Organic matter is broken down by microorganisms in the presence of oxygen.	1. Activated Sludge Process: Aerobic bacteria are frequently used in municipal wastewater treatment to break down organic pollutants. 2. Aerated Lagoons: Aerobic microbial activity is encouraged in sizable basins that feature aeration systems.
Anaerobic process	In the absence of oxygen, microorganisms disintegrate organic matter to produce biogas.	1. Anaerobic Digestion: used for generating methane for energy by relating to sludge. 2. Up flow Anaerobic Sludge Blanket (UASB): Industrial wastewater treated by anaerobic digestion.
Facultative process	Microorganisms are able to adjust to both anaerobic and aerobic environments.	1. Stabilization Ponds: Man-made or natural ponds where wastewater is treated by facultative bacteria. 2. Lagoon Systems: For flexible treatment, mix anaerobic and aerobic zones.
BOD (biochemical oxygen demand) reduction	Measurement of oxygen required by microorganisms to decompose organic matter.	1. BOD Test: Used to evaluate wastewater's organic strength and treatment effectiveness. 2. Treatment plants with integrated BOD removal tanks lower BOD levels.
Nitrification	Aerobic bacteria that convert ammonia to nitrate.	1. Biological nitrogen removal is a two-step process that produces nitrogen gas by first turning ammonia into nitrate. 2. Nitrification should be used in activated sludge systems in order to remove nitrogen.
Denitrification	Nitrate is reduced by anaerobic bacteria to nitrogen gas.	First, denitrification Basins: Engineered to eliminate surplus nitrogen from wastewater. Second, Biological Nutrient Removal (BNR): Combined nitrification and denitrification processes carried out simultaneously.
Phosphorus removal	Using bacteria to sequester and accumulate phosphorus	1. Enhanced Biological Phosphorus Removal (EBPR): Phosphorus removal through activated sludge process. 2. Phosphorus removal procedures are included in biological nutrient removal (BNR)

Reaction Rate Kinetics:

Reaction rate kinetics describes the rate at which micro-organisms breakdown organic contaminants in wastewater. This rate is often stated mathematically using models such as the Monod equation, which connects the specific growth rate of microorganisms to the concentration of substrate. The Monod equation is often used to describe the link between biodegradation rate and substrate concentration (organic matter).

Equation of Monod,

$$\alpha \cdot = \cdot \alpha \cdot \max \cdot * \cdot (R / (Kr + \cdot R))$$

where

α—specific growth rate of microorganisms.
α max—maximum specific growth rate.
R—concentration of the substrate.
Kr—half-saturation constant

Maximum Specific Growth Rate (αmax):

This parameter represents the maximum rate at which microorganisms can consume the organic substrate. It is influenced by factors such as the type of microorganisms present, temperature, and pH.

Half-Saturation Constant (Kr):

Kr is the substrate concentration at which microorganisms operate at half their maximum growth rate. It indicates the affinity of microorganisms for the substrate. Lower Ks values indicate higher affinity.

Haldane Equation:

$$\alpha = \left(\alpha \max * S\right) / \left(Kr + R + \left(R^2 / Ki\right)\right)$$

where

Ki—inhibition constant.

Biomass Growth:

Microorganisms proliferate and develop during biodegradation. The Yoon-Nelson model, which explains how biomass concentration varies over time, may also be used to estimate the rate of biomass increase. The kinetics of biodegradation are critical for improving the design and operation of biological wastewater treatment systems. Engineers and operators may change operational parameters such as hydraulic retention time (HRT), aeration, and nutrient input to guarantee successful organic pollutant removal while maintaining a stable and healthy microbial population in the treatment system by understanding these dynamics. This, in turn, aids in obtaining the appropriate effluent quality and fulfilling regulatory wastewater discharge criteria.

11.3.1 Biodegradation pathways and intermediate products

Organic contaminants in wastewater biodegrade via numerous routes, resulting in the development of intermediate products before the pollutants are eventually mineralized into simpler, more stable molecules. The type of the contaminants, the microbial populations involved, and the ambient circumstances all influence the particular routes and intermediates. Figure 11.2 represents the typical diagram involved in the treatment of wastewater.

Aerobic biodegradation pathway

- **Hydrolysis:** Organic compounds may undergo hydrolysis, breaking down complex molecules into simpler ones.
- **Oxidation:** Microorganisms oxidize organic pollutants to produce intermediate compounds such as alcohols, ketones, and aldehydes.
- **Fermentation:** In some cases, complex organic compounds are fermented into organic acids, alcohols, and other simpler compounds.
- **Mineralization:** Finalize mineralization, the pinnacle of aerobic biodegradation, is the conversion of organic compounds into carbon dioxide (CO_2) and water (H_2O).

Examples of intermediate products: Water, ethanol, carbon dioxide, and aspartic acid.

Pathway of anaerobic biodegradation

- **Hydrolysis:** Complex organic compounds are hydrolyzed into simpler forms.
- **Acidogenesis:** Microorganisms convert hydrolyzed products into organic acids, alcohols, and other intermediates.
- **Methanogenesis:** Some anaerobic bacteria further convert these intermediates into methane (CH_4) and carbon dioxide.

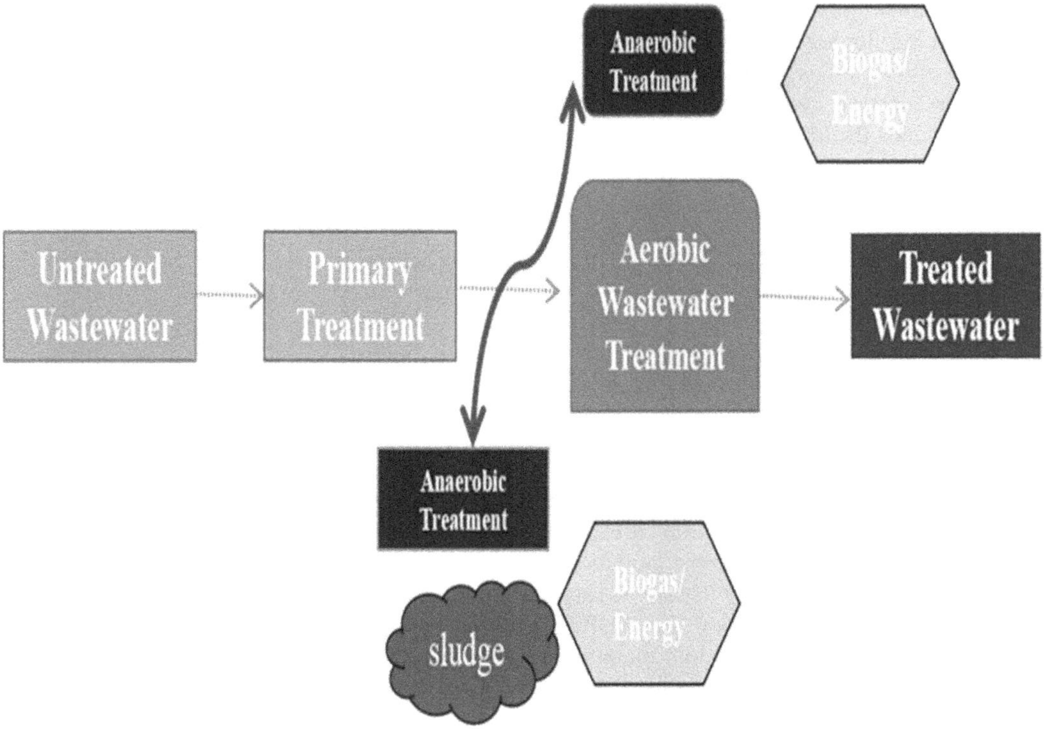

FIGURE 11.2 Schematic representation of wastewater treatment process.

Examples of intermediate products: Acetic acid, propionic acid, butyric acid, carbon dioxide, and methane.

11.3.2 Factors influencing biodegrading efficiency

Factors influencing biodegradation efficiency in wastewater treatment, biodegradation efficiency is influenced by a number of factors, both intrinsic to the wastewater and related to the biological treatment processes. Understanding and managing these factors is critical for optimizing the performance of biological treatment systems.

- **Nature of the wastewater:** The kind and quantity of organic and inorganic pollutants, pH, temperature, and the presence of hazardous compounds are all factors. Toxic substances in high quantities can hinder the development of microorganisms and limit their biodegradation efficiency.
- **Temperature:** Temperature is an important factor in biodegradation effectiveness. Microbial activity increases as temperature rises, although various microbial communities have ideal temperature ranges. The ideal temperature range for most typical wastewater treatment bacteria is 20 to 35°C. Temperature extremes can impede or prevent biodegradation.
- **pH:** The pH of wastewater influences microbial growth and activity. Because various microorganisms have different pH optimal, keeping the pH in the treatment system within the proper range for the given microbial population is critical for successful biodegradation.
- **Oxygen availability:** The availability of dissolved oxygen is critical for aerobic biodegradation processes. Microorganisms require oxygen to properly digest organic materials. Insufficient aeration or oxygen delivery might result in incomplete biodegradation.

- **The hydraulic retention time (HRT):** The HRT is the average amount of time that wastewater stays in the treatment system. Longer HRTs can promote more thorough biodegradation by giving microorganisms more time to digest organic substances. Excessively lengthy HRTs, on the other hand, may overburden the system and diminish efficiency.
- **Nutrient availability:** For development and metabolism, microorganisms require vital nutrients such as nitrogen and phosphorus. When these nutrients are insufficient, microbial activity and, as a result, biodegradation efficiency suffer. In rare circumstances, nutrient supplementation may be required.
- **Concentration of microbial biomass:** The concentration and health of the microbial biomass in the treatment system are crucial. Biodegradation efficiency may be hampered if the biomass content is too low. Excess biomass, on the other hand, might result in solids accumulation and impaired treatment efficiency. Proper mixing and aeration are required to ensure that microorganisms come into touch with the organic materials in the wastewater. A sufficient supply of oxygen and enough mixing facilitate effective biodegradation.
- **Retention time:** The amount of time that microorganisms spend in contact with organic materials in wastewater is critical. Longer retention duration can result in more thorough biodegradation, but this must be balanced with the total capacity and hydraulic loading of the treatment system.
- **Microbial community:** The composition and diversity of the microbial community in the treatment system can impact biodegradation efficiency. Different microbial species have varying abilities to degrade specific compounds, so the selection and maintenance of the right microbial community are crucial.
- **Toxic substances:** The presence of toxic compounds or chemicals in the wastewater can inhibit microbial activity and biodegradation. Effective pretreatment or removal of toxic substances may be necessary.
- **Sludge management:** Proper management of the sludge produced during the treatment process is essential. Inefficient sludge management can lead to the accumulation of solids, which can reduce the treatment system's efficiency. Biodegradation efficiency is a complex interplay of these factors, and successful wastewater treatment relies on the optimization of these parameters to achieve the desired treatment goals while considering the specific characteristics of the wastewater and treatment system in use. Table 11.3 gives the aspects for biomass growth and sludge management.

11.3.3 Petrochemical wastewater treatment plant

The maximum biodegradation yield of wastewater contaminants in terms of COD, total hydrocarbons, ethylene dichloride, and vinyl chloride was observed to be 89%, 80%, 99%, and 92%, respectively. According to a study of activated sludge wastewater treatment of APC, it was found that normal-alkanes, aromatic hydrocarbons, and polycyclic hydrocarbons were the most prevalent chemical compounds in the biological treatment influent. Activated sludge yielded 67 aerobic bacterial species, mostly belonging to the genera Pseudomonas, Comamonas, Acidovorax, Flavobacterium, Cytophaga, Sphingomonas, and Acinetobacter. In any bioremediation program, these isolates with their varied catabolic activity would be regarded as consortium members. In conclusion, the data demonstrate that even in cases where bioremediation processes measures, such as residual petroleum concentrations and phytotoxicity, signaled the end of the course of bioremediation, the original characteristics of the contaminated soils could not be restored after a year of bioremediation treatment, regardless of the initial sludge concentration in the systems. Additionally, the information showed that the pollutant had a long-term effect on the soil's bacterial solidarity. There may be a correlation between the hydrocarbon transformation process and the qualitative and quantitative changes in the culturable bacterial population in the soil. Further research is required to ascertain the frequency of these alterations on the soil ecosystem. When Davarnejad et al. (2014)

TABLE 11.3
This table discusses the aspects for biomass growth and sludge management

Aspect	Biomass growth	Sludge management
Micro-organisms involved	Protozoa, bacteria, and additional microbes.	Mainly composed of bacterial cells.
Nutrient requirements	Carbon, nitrogen, phosphorus, trace elements, etc.	Nutrient supplementation may be required.
Growth conditions	Controlled by adjusting aeration, pH, temperature, and nutrient levels.	Influenced by operational parameters such as sludge age.
Formation of biomass	Microorganisms grow and reproduce in the treatment system.	Excess biomass, called waste activated sludge (WAS), is produced.
Aeration	Oxygen is provided through aeration to support microbial growth and activity.	Used to mix and aerate the sludge, facilitating settling and removal of solids.
Sludge settling	Microorganisms in the activated sludge settle in secondary clarifiers.	Separation of biomass from treated wastewater in clarifiers.
Waste Activated Sludge (WAS)	Excess biomass, known as WAS, is periodically removed from the system to control sludge age.	Collected WAS is subjected to various treatment and disposal processes.
Sludge treatment	May include processes like anaerobic digestion, aerobic digestion, or dewatering.	Sludge is treated to reduce volume and stabilize it.
Disposal/Reuse options	Sludge can be incinerated, land-applied, used for energy generation (biogas), or landfill disposal.	Treated sludge may be reused as a soil conditioner or for other beneficial purposes.
Regulatory compliance	Must adhere to environmental regulations governing sludge quality and disposal.	Compliance with local, state, and federal regulations is essential to ensure safe management.

compared the use of iron and aluminum anodes for the removal of COD from petrochemical wastewater, they found that, under ideal circumstances, Fe anode had a higher capacity to remove COD (67.3%) than Al anode (53.9%). Comparably, dos Santos et al. (2014) looked into the removal of real petrochemical wastewater using platinized titanium (Ti/Pt) and BDD anodes; it was found that the BDD system performed better, lowering COD from 2.75×103 to 200 mg/L.

Additionally, the authors calculated the cost to be 56.2 kWh/m^3. For the advanced petrochemical wastewater treatment of particular pollutants, like dimethyl phthalate (DMP) and 1,2-dichlorobenzene (o-DCB), a general understanding of degradation pathways is helpful. In the presence of H_2O_2 solution, Ren et al. (2018) treated dimethyl phthalate using a graphite anode and CeO_2 catalyst; O_2 was first converted to •OOH, which was then translated into H_2O_2 to produce more. In order to remove o-DCB, Zazou et al. (2019) compared the anode materials Pt, BDD, and Ti/RuO_2-IrO_2 4 (DSA); under five ideal circumstances, approximately 90.0% COD removal was accomplished. Furthermore, in the BDD-based ECO system, the authors suggested a thorough degradation pathway 6 for o-DCB. By oxidative dehydration with •OH, the o-DCB first changed into 7 2-chlorophenol; subsequent de-chlorination changed it to catechol; and finally, the effect of •OH changed it into o-benzoquinone and o-benzoquinone. The degradation of phenols by aerobic and anaerobic degradation was discussed in Figure 11.3. By •OH oxidation, both compounds yielded oxalic acid, formic acid, maleic acid, and malonic acid.

11.3.4 Degradation of Plastic Wastes and Polyesters

Plastic wastes can break down via biodegradation (biotic) or physicochemical (abiotic) methods. In any degradation process, the breakdown of the polymeric material by mechanical forces

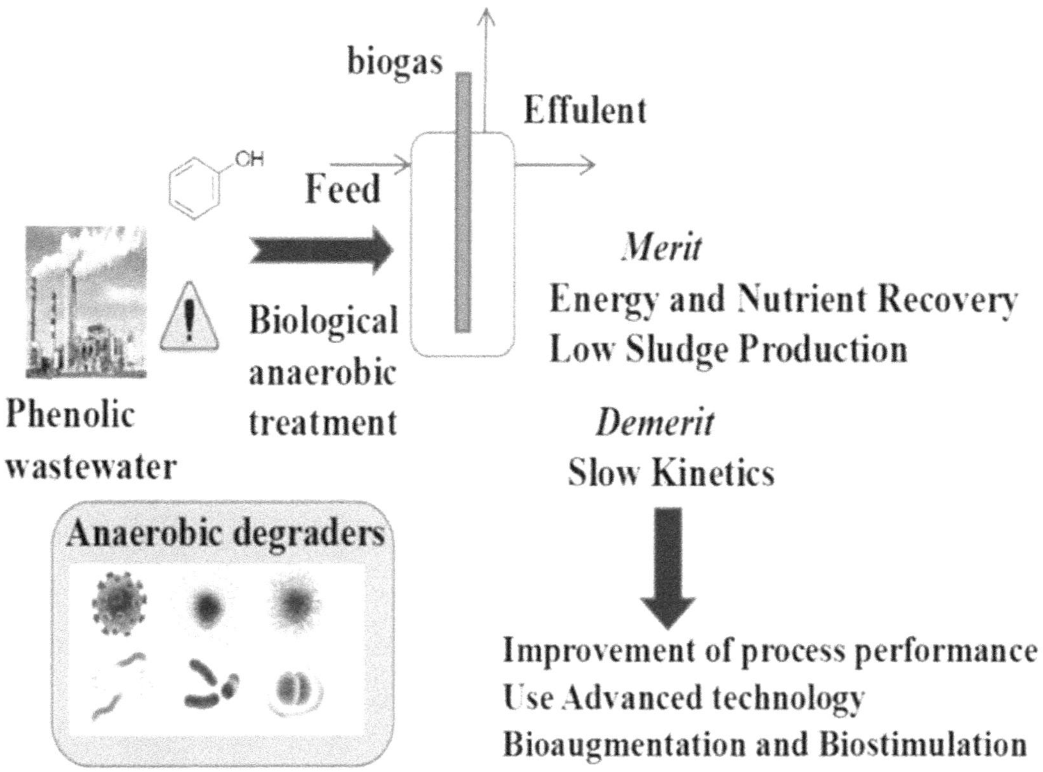

FIGURE 11.3 Diagram representing the mechanism of degradation of phenolic substance present in wastewater.

is typically regarded as the initial and most important step (Kyrikou & Briassoulis, 2007). The factors affecting degradation of plastics were shown in Figure 11.4. Plastics can degrade in the natural environment via one or more of the four primary processes: photodegradation, hydrolysis, thermo-oxidative degradation, and biodegradation. Common plastics like HDPE, LDPE, and PP degrade naturally in environments like marine environments. Photodegradation, which is mostly caused by UV-B radiation, starts the process, which is followed by thermo oxidation and, to a lesser extent, hydrolysis. Plastics fragment (become smaller pieces) and the polymer's MW decrease as a result of degradation processes. Microbes can then metabolize these low MW compounds.

Creating a transient mechanical and physical scaffold for the gradual regeneration of newly formed tissues is a crucial component of polymer applications in biomedicine. For the design of many medical devices, knowledge of a polymer's rate of degradation is essential. For example, PLA's slow rate of degradation makes it possible to produce orthopedic implants with a long lifespan, like screws and plates (Jansen et al., 1991; Kundungal et al., 2019; Kyrikou et al., 2007). However, because of their quick degradation, PGA-based biomaterials are mostly utilized in the production of sutures and drug delivery systems (Laist, 1997; Muhonja et al., 2018). Furthermore, it is necessary to maintain a balance in the rate of polymer degradation to ensure that the scaffold or implanted device can sustainably supply the necessary mechanical strength for the regeneration of newly formed tissue over time. In a particular instance, following arthroscopic surgery, a PLA-based implant did not regenerate the tissue and did not exhibit any signs of degradation. As a result, the patient experienced certain clinical complications (Muller et al., 2005). Numerous factors, including the polymer's nature, composition, MW, crystallinity, structure, thickness, surface properties, and conditions in the environment, influence the degradation process. Damage rate also

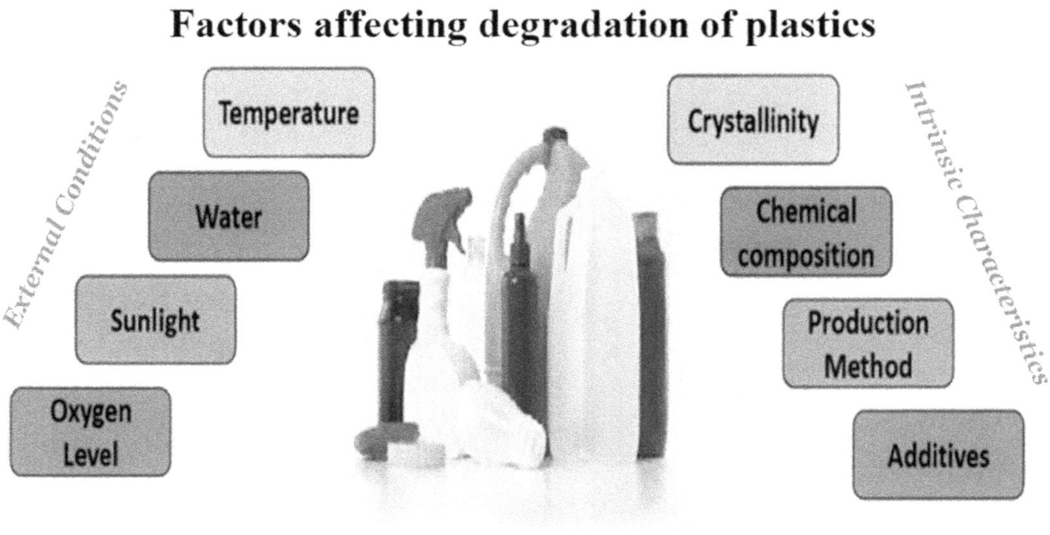

FIGURE 11.4 Factors affecting degradation of plastics.

affects a medical device's or implant's mechanical strength. For example, the rate of degradation is directly correlated with MW; longer polymer chains at higher MWs result in slower degradation (Nakamiya et al., 1997). The direct correlation between MW and degradation rate can, however, be proportionally impacted by the degree of crystallinity of certain polyesters, such as PLLA (Nomura et al., 1998). There is debate regarding the indirect impact of crystallinity on degradation rate because some studies indicate that polyesters with higher levels of crystallinity degrade more quickly because of their increased hydrophilicity (Oberbeckmann et al., 2016; Ojha et al., 2017). On the other hand, some groups show a slower rate as sample crystallinity increases.

The essential chemical characteristics of polymers, in addition to the implant's or device's physical characteristics and influence, determine the rate of degradation. The physical characteristics are crucial because the contact surface area of the implants with bodily fluids influences water diffusion and, in turn, the hydrolysis of the polymer structures. Consequently, there is a range of reported degradation rates for various polyesters. With the exception of PGA and its copolymer PLGA, the majority of polyesters remain stable in the body for at least a year. For use in medical applications, this polymer has been copolymerized from LA and GA to create a relatively quickly degradable polymer. Altering the molar ratios of LA to GA can also change the rate at which PLGA degrades. One way to double the rate of degradation from 100 to 50 days is to increase the weight ratio of GA to LA from 25:75 to 50:50. The two main processes by which polyesters degrade in bulk or on the surface of implants are hydrolytic and enzymatic. While enzymatic degradation heavily relies on the enzyme that is in charge of breaking down a particular molecule, hydrolytic degradation is autocatalytic and works by hydrolyzing the carboxylic groups of hydroxy acids. For example, PCL is enzymatically degraded lipase-type when Rhizopus delemer lipase, Rhizopus arrhizus lipase, and Pseudomonas lipase are present. Out of all these enzymes, Pseudomonas lipase is the most rapid, breaking down the highly crystalline PCL completely in four days, whereas hydrolytic degradation takes years. Bulk hydrolysis is the usual process used to break down polyesters. Certain polyesters may degrade more quickly if certain enzymes are present. A polymeric structure may experience an abrupt loss of structural stability due to bulk degradation. When designing biomedical devices, it is imperative to consider the biocompatibility and toxicity of any degradation products resulting from a polymer. When a polymer breaks down in large quantities, its byproducts are released into the surrounding environment, including the host tissue. For example, the breakdown of PLA or

TABLE 11.4
Polyesters and its mechanisms of degradation

Polyesters	Degradation byproducts pKa	Mechanism of degradation
PLA	Lactic acid (3.85)	Hydrolysis through the action of enzymes
PGA	Glycolic acid (3.83)	Both enzymatic and non-enzymatic hydrolysis
PPC	CO_2 and Water	Hydrolysis, or enzyme mediation
PHB	3-Hydroxybutyric acid (4.41)	Hydrolysis via nonspecific esterase enzymes
PBS	Succinic acid (4.21 and 5.64 for the first and second hydroxyl group)	Enzymatic hydrolytic degradation
PCL	Caproic acid (4.88)	Hydrolytic degradation
PPF	Fumaric acid (pKa2 = 4.44)	Hydrolysis

PLGA can release acidic byproducts that lower the pH of nearby tissues, causing inflammation and necrosis of nearby cells. Therefore, in order to systematically study the biological behavior of the host environment upon polymer degradation, it is essential to quantify the products of polymer biodegradation. The acidity of the final products after degradation of polyesters is measured using the average logarithmic acid dissociation constant, or pKa, of the intermediate degradation products. The main mechanisms of the degradation of various polyesters are listed in Table 11.4.

11.3.5 Microbes in wastewater treatment

Microbial populations are important in wastewater treatment techniques. The removal of impurities and pollutants from sewage and other sources of wastewater to make it safe for release into the environment or reuse is referred to as wastewater treatment. The major participants in these therapeutic processes are microorganisms, principally bacteria and some archaea. They decompose organic materials, eliminate nutrients, and lower the number of infections (Vasant Kumar et al., 2023).

- **Primary Treatment:** Physical methods such as sedimentation and flotation are utilized in the main treatment stage to remove big solid particles as well as some organic debris. While the primary aim of this stage is physical separation, it can nonetheless result in the production of microbial aggregation and biofilms.
- **Secondary Treatment:** Secondary treatment is a biological process in which microbial populations play an important role. There are two basic secondary treatment methods: activated sludge and trickling filters.

  Activated Sludge: Aeration tanks are employed in this process to deliver oxygen to a mixed population of microorganisms. These microorganisms, which include bacteria and protozoa, degrade organic materials in wastewater.

  Trickling Filters: Trickling filters employ a fixed-bed biofilm system in which wastewater is trickling over a material that favors microbial growth (such as rock or plastic). Organic material is broken down by microorganisms adhering to the media.
- **Tertiary Treatment:** Tertiary treatment is frequently used to polish the effluent further to remove leftover nutrients, suspended particles, and pathogens. Nitrification and denitrification are important microbial mechanisms for eliminating nitrogen molecules.

  Anaerobic Digestion: Microorganisms operate in the absence of oxygen to break down organic waste and create biogas (methane and carbon dioxide) in anaerobic digestion. This technology is commonly used for sludge treatment since it may drastically reduce sludge volume while creating sustainable energy.

11.3.5.1 Nutrient needs for microorganism

Biodegradation is the process by which microorganisms degrade organic molecules such as pollution or garbage into simpler and more ecologically friendly chemicals. To carry out these activities successfully, microorganisms engaged in biodegradation require certain food requirements.

- **Carbon (C):** Carbon is the major source of energy as well as the building blocks for microbiological organisms. Microorganisms consume carbon molecules in the organic substances they degrade in biodegradation.
- **Nitrogen (N):** Nitrogen is essential for the creation of enzymes and proteins required by microorganisms to perform biodegradation processes. It is frequently derived from the organic nitrogen contained inside the biodegradable substance itself.
- **Phosphorus (P):** Phosphorus is required for the production of nucleic acids (DNA and RNA), which are required for microbial growth and replication during biodegradation. Microorganisms require trace elements such as iron, manganese, and molybdenum as cofactors for numerous enzymes engaged in biodegradation processes. These elements are required for particular biodegradative enzymes to operate properly.
- **Other Electron Acceptors besides Oxygen (O_2):** Microorganisms in aerobic biodegradation require molecular oxygen (O_2) as an electron acceptor for respiration. Alternative electron acceptors such as nitrate, sulfate, or carbon molecules are employed in anaerobic biodegradation, depending on the unique metabolic pathways of the microorganisms involved.
- **Water (H_2O):** Water is required for all biological activities, including biodegradation.
- **Specific Substrates:** Organic pollutants or waste products are required as the principal substrate for microorganisms participating in biodegradation. Different bacteria have distinct preferences for the organic substances that they may breakdown. Some microorganisms, for example, specialize in hydrocarbon degradation (e.g., oil-degrading bacteria), whereas others specialize in organic acid or complex polymer degradation.

The availability and balance of these nutrients, as well as ambient factors such as temperature, pH, and oxygen levels, all have an impact on the rate and effectiveness of biodegradation processes. To guarantee the effective and efficient removal or transformation of organic pollutants, it is critical to optimize these conditions in diverse biodegradation applications such as bioremediation of polluted areas, composting, and wastewater treatment. The variety of microorganisms and substrates involved in biodegradation processes makes biodegradation difficult.

11.3.5.2 Fungal and bacterial roles in plastic degradation

A significant factor in the deterioration of polymeric materials is fungus. To break down as much of this substrate as possible, fungi mycelia can effectively pierce the surface of polymeric materials and move deeper into their mass. Additionally, the fungus's mycelia have the ability to secrete extracellular enzymes, such as depolymerases, which degrade the polymeric substrate into oligomers, dimers, and monomers—that is, low MW fragments. The fungi then absorb these monomers and use their intracellular enzymatic system to either mineralize or assimilate them. Compared to bacterial enzymes, fungi produce and secrete a much greater quantity of enzymes. According to this theory, it has been frequently reported that brown- and white-rot fungi are effective degraders of polymeric materials. Fungal enzymatic systems are thought to be responsible for the degradation of polymers because they release a variety of extracellular enzymes, such as laccase (Lac), manganese peroxidase (MnP), lignin peroxidase (LiP), and versatile peroxidase. These enzymes have the ability to break down and ultimately mineralize lignin (Ameen et al., 2015). In addition to having some physical traits in common with lignin, such as hydrophobicity, polymeric materials also have chemical structures similar to lignin (e.g., ether bonds, non-phenolic aromatic rings, carbon skeleton, etc.), which are oxidized during the degradation process of lignin. Due to their physical and chemical similarities, lignin-modifying enzymes (LMEs) like MnP and Lac can break down certain plastic polymers like PE and PP (Ali et al., 2021). In contaminated water or soil, bacterial strains have the ability to break down plastic polymeric materials. According to Yoshida et al. (2016), a number of studies have shown that the biodegradation of plastics by specific bacteria can be a promising bioremediation strategy for contaminated ecosystems. According to our review of the literature, bacterial strains including Pseudomonas, Bacillus, and Streptomyces have demonstrated high degradation efficiency when it comes to different plastic polymers (Matjašič et al., 2021). These findings also demonstrate the need for additional research on the bacterial role in plastic biodegradation in order to evaluate the efficacy of bacterial consortia and the potential of various bacterial species. In any event, fungi degrade plastics more quickly than bacterial strains do (Muhonja et al., 2018). However, compared to fungi, which need more stable conditions, bacteria can grow and break down polymeric materials more easily.

11.3.5.3 Algal role in synthetic plastic polymer degradation

Few studies have examined the potential of algal species to reduce white pollution as of yet. One noteworthy finding concerned the capacity of filamentous algae to colonize the surface of plastic waste materials because these materials provide the necessary environmental conditions for algal growth, namely sunlight, nutrients, and water (Moog et al., 2019; Ali et al., 2021). Microalgae are a viable candidate because they do not contain endotoxins and do not require organic carbon sources for growth, unlike bacterial and fungal systems, which may be regarded as biological pollutants due to their endotoxins Furthermore, a number of bacterial and fungal species, including Pestalotiopsis microspore and Ideonella sakaiensis, which are employed in the production of PETase, are ill-suited to the marine environments where the majority of plastic waste is deposited (Tanasupawat et al., 2016). It was discovered that a number of non-toxic and non-hazardous algal species from the families Bacillariophyceae, Chlorophyceae, and Cyanophyceae could grow on polythene surfaces and create algal biofilms in a variety of contaminated aquatic environments, including wastewaters, lakes, and ponds. According to Sarmah and Rout (2018), freshwater non-toxic cyanobacteria, namely, Phormidium lucidum and Oscillatoria subbrevis, are easily isolated and grow quickly. They can effectively colonize on PE surfaces and degrade LDPE without the need for pretreatment. Furthermore, Moog et al. (2019) produced an engineered PETase that exhibited activity against PET and the copolymer PETG (polyethylene terephthalate glycol) by effectively using the diatom Phaeodactylum tricornutum as a microbial factory. Furthermore, Kumar et al. (2017) discovered that following algal colonization on PE, surface deterioration was noticed. Additionally, they discovered that the degradation percentages of the blue-green alga Anabaena spiroides, the diatom Navicula pupula, and the green alga Scenedesmus dimorphus were 3.74, 8.18, and 4.44%, respectively. Furthermore, Spirulina sp. has been shown by Khoironi et al. (2019) to be able to decrease the tensile strength of PET and PP by 0.9939 and 0.1977 MPa/day, respectively. They discovered that the decreasing carbon in PP and PET was 36.7% and 48.61, respectively, based on EDX analysis. Furthermore, the evolution of CO_2 showed that PET degraded more quickly than PP. By producing ligninolytic enzymes and exopolysaccharides, algae can adhere to a plastic surface and initiate the degradation process (Sarmah & Rout, 2018). According to Chinaglia et al. (2018), the biodegradation process starts when the extracellular enzymes secreted in the liquid media interact with macromolecules on the plastic surface. It is possible to genetically modify microalgae to create a microbial cell factory that secretes and produces enzymes that break down polymers. For example, green microalgae Chlamydomonas reinhardtii was genetically engineered to produce PETase, and it was subsequently tested against PET. The development of holes and cavities on the plastic surface confirmed the surface degradation (Kim et al., 2020). These investigations have demonstrated the potential of synthetic biology as a means of creating a sustainable approach to the biological breakdown of PET by means of microalgae.

More research and analysis are needed to fully understand the mechanism and the effectiveness of algae as plastic degraders. One of the most promising technologies for the advanced treatment and nutrient recovery of wastewater is the microalgae-based wastewater treatment process, which has gained increasing attention in recent years (Lutzu et al., 2021).

Many researchers have demonstrated the viability of using microalgae as a supplement to tertiary wastewater treatment because of their high efficiencies in removing nutrients in the advanced treatment of wastewaters from agriculture, industry, and municipalities (Pizarro et al., 2002; Whitton et al., 2015; Kumar et al., 2017; Moog et al., 2019; Ali et al., 2021). Urban, agricultural, and industrial activities generate large amounts of wastewater with excessive nutrients, which would inevitably lead to eutrophication in the aquatic environment. It was also noted that the biomass production of microalgae in wastewater treatment could bring significant additional value by using algal biomass as feedstock in biorefinery applications (Chinnasamy et al., 2010; Zhou et al., 2011; Lutzu et al., 2021). This was in spite of the original idea of using microalgae for wastewater treatment to remove the excess nutrients of secondary effluent and eliminate the risk of eutrophication in natural water bodies (Oswald & Golueke, 1960). Because microalgae can remove nutrients from wastewater to a very low level, they can meet the increasingly strict discharge and reuse standards. As a result, microalgae cultivated on waste streams offer significant benefits over traditional cultivation and treatment processes (Whitton et al., 2015). Because microalgae absorb a lot of pollutants, wastewater treatment becomes less expensive (Lutzu et al., 2021). Using inorganic carbon sources from wastewater treatment plants, microalgae can be converted into carbon-neutral fuel (Raheem et al., 2015). Microalgae-based wastewater treatment has the potential to reduce wastewater because they can survive on the water and nutrients found in wastewater without or with limited supplemental water and nutrients. The cost of production and greenhouse gas emissions related to fertilizers derived from fossil fuels (Clarens et al., 2010). Furthermore, value-added products such as biogas, biofuels, fertilizers, and animal feed can be produced from the harvested microalgae (Raheem et al., 2015). Various insect species as efficient biodegraders of plastic numerous invertebrates, including the larger wax moth Galleria mellonella (Bombelli et al., 2017), the Indian meal moth Plodia interpunctella (Yang et al., 2014), and superworms Zophobas atratus (Yang et al., 2020), have demonstrated the biodegradation of plastic polymers. Certain social insects have demonstrated comparable skills, such as termites, which are characterized by cooperative brood care, group integration, labor division, and generational overlap within their colonies. Their intestinal microbial symbionts are typically responsible for this exceptional activity against the degradation of plastic polymers (Yang et al., 2014). Some species of invertebrates can consume wood or other polymeric materials. In fact, symbiotic yeasts have been found in the digestive tract of Lasioderma serricorne. Shen and Dowd, (1991) have shown that these yeasts can produce enzymes that can hydrolyze and degrade phenolic compounds and esters. Furthermore, according to Ali et al. (2019), termites' digestive tracts perform a variety of specific functions because of microbial consortia that coexist symbiotically in their guts and offer significant advantages to their hosts in exchange. Within this framework, Riudavets et al. (2007) documented the degradation activity of the rice weevil (Sitophilus oryzae), the cigarette beetle (L. serricorne), and the lesser grain borer (Rhyzopertha dominica). on food packaging and polyester, low-density polyethylene (LDPE), and biaxially oriented polypropylene (BOPP) multilayer films (Yang et al., 2014). The presence of Bacillus sp. and Enterobacter asburiae in the gut of waxworms (larvae of P. interpunctella) allows the worms to consume and digest PE films. According to Yang et al. (2015), who studied the Bacillus sp. YP1 genome, 182 genes are present and are in charge of the xenobiotics' catabolic activity. According to Brandon et al. (2018), assessment of mealworms' (T. molitor larvae) capacity for digesting PS and PE, 49% of PE was converted and mineralized into CO_2. Furthermore, in mealworms fed PS and PE, the MW of ingested polymers dropped by 13 and 40%, respectively. This capability was linked to Citrobacter and Kosakonia's metabolic activity. Additionally, T. molitor was shown to be able to consume PS foam quickly, with a 50% daily degradation rate (Yang et al., 2015). Yang et al. (2020), however, expanding on their findings, discovered that Z. atratus, the PS foam-fed superworm, digested 0.58 mg/day/superworm, four times more than T. molitor. Also, Bombelli et al. (2017) research on G. mellonella's capacity to break down PP and PE revealed that the worm could break down 92% of plastic materials at a rate estimated to be 1.84 mg per day. Zhang et al. (2020) have shown that Aspergillus flavus's ability to produce Lac and Lac-like multi-copper oxidases is the primary cause of G. mellonella's capacity to biodegrade plastic. However, Cassone et al. (2020) linked Acinetobacter sp.'s presence and activity to G. mellonella's potential. According to Lou et al. (2020), the activity of Bacillus and Serratia resulted in a loss of plastic mass in 150 G, mellonella larvae that were fed either PE or PS.

11.4 KEY CHALLENGES AND FUTURE PROSPECTS

Challenges

- **Pollutant Diversity:** Wastewater includes a wide spectrum of pollutants, such as organic materials, nutrients, heavy metals, and emerging contaminants. Biodegradation mechanisms must be adaptable enough to deal with this variety.
- **Emerging Pollutants:** Pharmaceuticals, personal care products, and microplastics are examples of new and emerging pollutants. Understanding these chemicals and properly biodegrading them are continuing issues.
- **Nutrient Imbalance:** It is critical to keep the appropriate balance of nutrients, notably nitrogen and phosphorus, in wastewater. Nutrient imbalances in receiving bodies of water can cause eutrophication and water quality concerns.
- **Harmful Compounds:** Some wastewater pollutants are harmful to microorganisms or hinder their function. Toxic chemicals can be difficult to manage and remove.
- **Microorganism Adaptation:** Microorganisms can adapt to changing environments, thereby decreasing their efficacy in biodegradation processes. Microbial community management and control can be difficult.

Future prospects

- **Pathways of Advanced Biodegradation**: Ongoing research is being conducted to find and optimize biodegradation routes for a broader spectrum of toxins, including new pollutants. Understanding the genetics and biochemistry of microorganisms involved in degradation is required.

Technologies for Bioremediation: Bioremediation methods like as biofilters, biopiles, and phytoremediation are being developed and applied more widely. These techniques can improve the biodegradation of certain contaminants. Advances in the creation and usage of biodegradable products, such as biodegradable plastics and textiles, can help lower the burden of non-biodegradable elements in wastewater and the environment.

- **Bioaugmentation and Biostimulation:** Bioaugmentation is the introduction of specialized bacteria or enzymes to improve biodegradation. The process of enhancing circumstances for native microorganisms is known as biostimulation. Both techniques are gaining popularity.
- **Genetic Engineering:** A emerging subject is the genetic engineering of microbes for targeted biodegradation of certain pollutants. Engineered microbes can be programmed to degrade certain contaminants more efficiently.
- Real-time monitoring, sensing technology, and automation can all help to enhance biodegradation processes. These technologies aid in maintaining optimal microbial activity conditions and adapting to changing influent characteristics.
- **Circular Economy and Resource Recovery:** Biodegradation may be integrated into a circular economy model in which valuable resources such as energy and nutrients are reclaimed from wastewater.

- **Green Infrastructure**: Including green infrastructure solutions in wastewater treatment, such as artificial wetlands and planted swales, can stimulate natural biodegradation processes and improve water quality.

11.4.1 Public Education and Awareness

Educating the public about the necessity of proper wastewater disposal and the effects of emerging contaminants can help limit the entry of pollutants into the wastewater stream. Developing and implementing legislation and policies to handle new pollutants and promote sustainable wastewater management. To summarize, the future of biodegradation processes in wastewater treatment will require a combination of technological advances, research into new pollutants, and an emphasis on sustainability.

11.5 CONCLUSION

With view to the topic biodegradation mechanism in wastewater treatment process conclusion can be elucidated as follows. Precisely, we can utter that to develop an efficient wastewater process, it is necessary to understand the presence of micro-pollutants. It is must to know about the various microorganisms and its role toward the biodegradation of pollutants. In order to enhance the degradation efficiency, the target pollutants and microbial communities need to be optimized. Furthermore, it is necessary to apply new genetic engineering expertise to select and amplify the most efficient microbes in order to breakdown contaminants. So that the wastewater treatment reactors can be manufactured with a lesser investment and can get the good results with in less time. This chapter provides in detail about the concepts underlying in biodegradation and its utilization in wastewater treatment.

ACKNOWLEDGMENT

The author RP thanks the Solar Energy Research Center (SERC-Chile) research fellowship (ANID/FONDAP/1523A0006).

REFERENCES

Agostini, F., Sundberg, C., & Navia, R. (2012). Is biodegradable waste a porous environment? A review. *Waste Management & Research: The Journal for a Sustainable Circular Economy*, 30(10). https://doi.org/10.1177/0734242X12452444

Ali, H. R., & Ropy, A. (2019). The differences in the digestive system and enzymes between soldiers and workers of the subterranean termite, Psammotermes hypostoma Desneux (Rhinotermitidae: Isoptera). *Egyptian Academic Journal of Biological Sciences. A, Entomology*, 12(3), 49–61. 1.

Ali, S. S., Elsamahy, T., Al-Tohamy, R., Zhu, D., Mahmoud, Y. A. G., Koutra, E., … & Sun, J. (2021). Plastic wastes biodegradation: Mechanisms, challenges and future prospects. *Science of the Total Environment*, 780, 146590. https://doi.org/10.1016/j.scitotenv.2021.146590

Ali, S. S., & Sun, J. (2019). Effective thermal pretreatment of water hyacinth (Eichhornia crassipes) for the enhancement of biomethanation: VIT® gene probe technology for microbial community analysis with special reference to methanogenic Archaea. *Journal of Environment Chemistry Engineering*, 7, 102853. https://doi.org/10.1016/j.jece.2018.102853

Ameen, F., Hadi, S., Moslem, M., Al-Sabri, A., & Yassin, M. A. (2015). Biodegradation of engine oil by fungi from mangrove habitat. *The Journal of General and Applied Microbiology*, 61(5), 185–192. https://doi.org/10.2323/jgam.61.185

Amobonye, A., Bhagwat, P., Singh, S., & Pillai, S. (2021). Plastic biodegradation: Frontline microbes and their enzymes. *Science of the Total Environment,* 759, 143536. https://doi.org/10.1016/j.scitotenv.2020.143536

Biffinger, J. C., Barlow, D. E., Pirlo, R. K., Babson, D. M., Fitzgerald, L. A., Zingarelli, S., Nadeau, L. J., Crookes-Goodson, W. J., & Russell Jr., J. N. (2014). A direct quantitative agar-plate based assay for analysis of Pseudomonas protegens Pf-5 degradation of polyurethane films. *International Biodeterioration & Biodegradation*, 95, 311–319. https://doi.org/10.1016/j.ibiod.2014.09.005

Bombelli, P., Howe, C. J., & Bertocchini, F. (2017). Polyethylene bio-degradation by caterpillars of the wax moth Galleria mellonella. *Current Biology*, 27(8), R292–R293. https://doi.org/10.1016/j.cub.2017.02.060

Brandon, A. M., Gao, S. H., Tian, R., Ning, D., Yang, S. S., Zhou, J., … & Criddle, C. S. (2018). Biodegradation of polyethylene and plastic mixtures in mealworms (larvae of Tenebrio molitor) and effects on the gut microbiome. *Environmental Science & Technology*, 52(11), 6526–6533. https://doi.org/10.1021/acs.est.8b02301

Capitelli, F., Principi, P., & Sorlini, C. (2006). Biodeterioration of modern materials in contemporary collections: Can biotechnology help? *Trends in Biotechnology*, 24(8), 350–354. https://doi.org/10.1016/j.tibtech.2006.06.001

Caracciolo, A. B., Topp, E., & Grenni, P. (2015). Pharmaceuticals in the environment: Biodegradation and effects on natural microbial communities. A review. *Journal of Pharmaceutical and Biomedical Analysis*, 106, 25–36. https://doi.org/10.1016/j.jpba.2014.11.040

Cassone, B. J., Grove, H. C., Elebute, O., Villanueva, S. M., & LeMoine, C. M. (2020). Role of the intestinal microbiome in low-density polyethylene degradation by caterpillar larvae of the greater wax moth, Galleria mellonella. *Proceedings of the Royal Society B*, 287, 20200112. https://doi.org/10.1098/rspb.2020.0112

Chinaglia, S., Tosin, M., & Degli-Innocenti, F. (2018). Biodegradation rate of biodegradable plastics at molecular level. *Polymer Degradation and Stability*, 147, 237–244. https://doi.org/10.1016/j.polymdegradstab.2017.12.011

Chinnasamy, S., Bhatnagar, A., Claxton, R., & Das, K. C. (2010). Biomass and bioenergy production potential of microalgae consortium in open and closed bioreactors using untreated carpet industry effluent as growth medium. *Bioresource Technology*, 101(17), 6751–6760. https://doi.org/10.1016/j.biortech.2010.03.094

Clarens, A. F., Resurreccion, E. P., White, M. A., & Colosi, L. M. (2010). Environmental life cycle comparison of algae to other bioenergy feedstocks. *Environmental Science & Technology*, 44(5), 1813–1819. https://doi.org/10.1021/es902838n

Davarnejad, R., Mohammadi, M., & Ismail, A. F. (2014). Petrochemical wastewater treatment by electro-Fenton process using aluminum and iron electrodes: Statistical comparison. *Journal of Water Process Engineering*, 3, 18–25. https://doi.org/10.1016/j.jwpe.2014.08.002

de Lucas, A., Rodríguez, L., Villaseñor, J., & Fernández, F. J. Biodegradation kinetics of stored wastewater substrates by a mixed microbial culture. *Biochemical Engineering Journal*, 26, 191–197. https://doi.org/10.1016/j.bej.2005.04.015

Dos Santos, E. V., Sena, S. F. M., da Silva, D. R., Ferro, S., De Battisti, A., & Martínez-Huitle, C. A. (2014). Scale-up of electrochemical oxidation system for treatment of produced water generated by Brazilian petrochemical industry. *Environmental Science and Pollution Research*, 21, 8466–8475. https://doi.org/10.1007/s11356-014-2779-x

Flemming, H.-C. (1998). Relevance of biofilms for the biodeterioration of surfaces of polymeric materials. *Polymer Degradation Stability,* 59, 309–315. https://doi.org/10.1016/S0141-3910(97)00189-4

Gaytán, I., Sánchez-Reyes, A., Burelo, M., Vargas-Suárez, M., Liachko, I., Press, M., Sullivan, S., Cruz-Gómez, M. J., & Loza-Tavera, H. (2020). Degradation of recalcitrant polyurethane and xenobiotic additives by a selected landfill microbial community and its biodegradative potential revealed by proximity ligation-based metagenomic analysis. *Frontiers in Microbiology*, 10, 2986. https://doi.org/10.3389/fmicb.2019.02986

Hofrichter, M. (2002). Review: Lignin conversion by manganese peroxidase (MnP). *Enzyme and Microbial Technology*, 30, 454–466.

Howard, G. T. (2002). Biodegradation of polyurethane: A review. *International Biodeterioration and Biodegradation*, 49, 245–252. https://doi.org/10.1016/S0964-8305(02)00051-3

Hu, B., Wang, M., Geng, S., Wen, L., Wu, M., Nie, Y., Tang, Y.-Q., & Wu, X.-L. (2020). Metabolic exchange with non-alkane-consuming Pseudomonas stutzeri SLG510A3–8 improves n-alkane biodegradation by the alkane degrader Dietzia sp. strain DQ12–45-1b. (A. J. M. Stams, Ed.). *Applied Environmental Microbiology*, 86(8), e02931–e02919. https://doi.org/10.1128/AEM.02931-19

Hueck, H. J. (2001). The biodeterioration of materials: An apraisal. *International Biodeterioration and Biodegradation*, 48, 5–11. https://doi.org/10.1016/S0964-8305(01)00061-0

Jansen, B., Schumacher-Perdreau, F., Peters, G., & Pulverer, G. (1991). Evidence for degradation of synthetic polyurethanes by Staphylococcus epidermidis. *Zentralblatt für Bakteriologie,* 276, 36–45. https://doi.org/10.1016/S0934-8840(11)80216-1

Khoironi, A., Anggoro, S., & Sudarno, S. (2019). Evaluation of the interaction among microalgae Spirulina sp, plastics polyethylene terephthalate and polypropylene in freshwater environment. *Journal of Ecological Engineering*, 20(6), 161–173. https://doi.org/10.12911/22998993/108637

Kim, H. R., Lee, H. M., Yu, H. C., Jeon, E., Lee, S., Li, J., & Kim, D. H. (2020). Biodegradation of polystyrene by Pseudomonas sp. isolated from the gut of superworms (larvae of Zophobas atratus). *Environmental Science & Technology*, 54(11), 6987–6996. https://doi.org/10.1021/acs.est.0c01495

Kumar, R. V., Kanna, G. R., & Elumalai, S. (2017). Biodegradation of polyethylene by green photosynthetic microalgae. *International Biodeterioration and Biodegradation*, 8(381), 2. https://doi.org/10.4172/2155-6199.1000381

Kundungal, H., Gangarapu, M., Sarangapani, S., Patchaiyappan, A., & Devipriya, S. P. (2019). Efficient biodegradation of polyethylene (HDPE) waste by the plastic-eating lesser waxworm (Achroia grisella). *Environmentai Science Pollution Result International,* 26, 18509–18519. https://doi.org/10.1007/s11356-019-05038-9

Kyrikou, I., & Briassoulis, D. (2007). Biodegradation of agricultural plastic films: A critical review. *Journal of Polymers and the Environment,* 15, 125–150. https://doi.org/10.1007/s10924-007-0053-8

Laist, D. W. (1997). Impacts of marine debris: Entanglement of marine life in marine debris including a comprehensive list of species with entanglement and ingestion records. In: Coe, J. M., & Rogers, D. B. (Eds.), *Marine Debris: Sources, Impacts, and Solutions*. New York: Springer, pp. 99–139. https://doi.org/10.1007/978-1-4613-8486-1_10

Lindström, A., Albertsson, A. C., & Hakkarainen, M. (2004). Quantitative determination of degradation products an effective means to study early stages of degradation in linear and branched poly(butylene adipate) and poly(butylene succinate). *Polymer Degradation and Stability*, 83(3), 487–493. https://doi.org/10.1016/j.polymdegradstab.2003.07.001

Lou, Y., Ekaterina, P., Yang, S. S., Lu, B., Liu, B., Ren, N., … & Xing, D. (2020). Biodegradation of polyethylene and polystyrene by greater wax moth larvae (Galleria mellonella L.) and the effect of co-diet supplementation on the core gut microbiome. *Environmental Science & Technology*, 54(5), 2821–2831. https://doi.org/10.1021/acs.est.9b07044

Lutzu, G. A., Marin, M. A., Concas, A., & Dunford, N. T. (2021). Nutrient enrichment of wastewater generated during hydraulic fracturing with animal wastewater to enhance microalgae growth. *Chemical Engineering Transactions*, 86, 115–120.

Matjašič, T., Simčič, T., Medveščcek, N., Bajt, O., Dreo, T., & Mori, N. (2021). Critical evaluation of biodegradation studies on synthetic plastics through a systematic literature review. *Science of the Total Environment*, 752, 141959. https://doi.org/10.1016/j.scitotenv.2020.141959

Mitchell, R., & Gu, J. D. (Eds.). (2010). *Environmental microbiology*. John Wiley & Sons. https://doi.org/10.1002/9780470495117

Moog, D., Schmitt, J., Senger, J., Zarzycki, J., Rexer, K. H., Linne, U., … & Maier, U. G. (2019). Using a marine microalga as a chassis for polyethylene terephthalate (PET) degradation. *Microbial Cell Factories*, 18, 1–15. https://doi.org/10.1186/s12934-019-1220-z

Muhonja, C. N., Makonde, H., Magoma, G., & Imbuga, M. (2018). Biodegradability of polyethylene by bacteria and fungi from Dandora dumpsite Nairobi-Kenya. *PLoS One,* 13(7), e0198446. https://doi.org/10.1371/journal.pone.0198446

Müller, R. J., Schrader, H., Profe, J., Dresler, K., & Deckwer, W. D. (2005). Enzymatic degradationbof poly (ethylene terephthalate): Rapid hydrolyse using a hydrolase from T. fusca. *Macromology Rapid Communication*, 26, 1400–1405. https://doi.org/10.1002/marc.200500410

Nakamiya, K., Ooi, T., & Kinoshita, S. (1997). Non-heme hydroquinone peroxidase from Azo tobacter beijerinckii HM121. *Journal of Fermentation and Bioengineering*, 84, 14–21. https://doi.org/10.1016/S0922-338X(97)82780-8

Nakamura, H., Nakamura, T., & Noguchi, Imagawa K. (2006). Photodegradation of PEEK sheets under tensile stress. *Polymer Degradation and Stability*, 9, 740–746. NF EN ISO 13432, 2000. https://doi.org/10.1016/j.polymdegradstab.2005.06.003

Nomura, N., Shigeno-Akutsu, Y., Nakajima-Kambe, T., & Nakahara, T. (1998). Cloning and sequence analysis of a polyurethane esterase of Comamonas acidovorans TB-35. *Journal of Fermentation and Bioengineering*, 86, 339–345. https://doi.org/10.1016/S0922-338X(99)89001-1

Nuhoglu, Y., Oguz, E., Uslu, H., Ozbek, A., Ipekoglu, B., Ocak, I., & Hasenekoglu, I. (2006). The accelerating effects of the microorganisms on biodeterioration of stone monuments under air pollution and continental-cold climatic conditions in Erzurum, Turkey. *Science Total Environment*, 364, 272–283. https://doi.org/10.1016/j.scitotenv.2005.06.034

Oberbeckmann, S., Osborn, A. M., & Duhaime, M. B. (2016). Microbes on a bottle: Substrate, reason and geography influence community composition of microbes colonizing marine plastic debris. *PLoS One*, 11(8), e0159289. https://doi.org/10.1371/journal.pone.0159289

Ojha, N., Pradhan, N., Singh, S., Barla, A., Shrivastava, A., Khatua, P., Rain, V., & Bose, S. (2017). Evaluation of HDPE and LDPE degradation by fungus, implemented by statistical optimization. *Scientific Reports*, 7, 39515. https://doi.org/10.1038/srep39515

Oswald, W. J., & Golueke, C. G. (1960). Biological transformation of solar energy. *Advances in Applied Microbiology*, 2, 223–262. https://doi.org/10.1016/S0065-2164(08)70127-8

Otsuka, Y., Sonoki, T., Ikeda, S., Kajita, S., Nakamura, M., & Katayama, Y. (2003) Detection and characterization of a novel extracellular fungal enzyme that catalyzes the specific and hydrolytic cleavage of lignin guaiacylglycerol β-aryl ether linkages. *European Journal of Biochemistry*, 270(11), 2353–2362. https://doi.org/10.1046/j.1432-1033.2003.03545.x

Pepic, D., Zagar, E., Zigon, M., Krzan, A., Kunaver, M., & Djonlagic, J. (2008). Synthesis and characterization of biodegradable aliphatic copolyesters with poly (ethylene oxide) soft segments. *European Polymer Journal*, 44, 904–917. https://doi.org/10.1016/j.eurpolymj.2007.11.035

Pizarro, C., Kebede-Westhead, E., & Mulbry, W. (2002). Nitrogen and phosphorus removal rates using small algal turfs grown with dairy manure. *Journal of Applied Phycology*, 14(6), 469–473. https://doi.org/10.1023/A:1022338722952

Raheem, A., Azlina, W. A. K. G. W., Yap, Y. H. T., Danquah, M. K., & Harun, R. (2015). Thermochemical conversion of microalgal biomass for biofuel production. *Renewable and Sustainable Energy Reviews*, 49, 990–999. https://doi.org/10.1016/j.rser.2015.04.186

Ren, X., Zeng, G., Tang, L., Wang, J., Wan, J., Wang, J., Deng, Y., da, Y., & Peng, B. (2018) The potential impact on the biodegradation of organic pollutants from composting technology for soil remediation. *Waste Management*, 72, 138–149. https://doi.org/10.1016/j.wasman.2017.11.032

Riudavets, J., Salas, I., & Pons, M. J. (2007). Damage characteristics produced by insect pests in packaging film. *Journal of Stored Products Research*, 43(4), 564–570. https://doi.org/10.1016/j.jspr.2007.03.006

Sarmah, P., & Rout, J. (2018). Biochemical profile of five species of cyanobacteria isolated from polythene surface in domestic sewage water of Silchar town, Assam (India). *Current Trends in Biotechnology and Pharmacy*, 12(1), 7–15.

Shen, S. K., & Dowd, P. F. (1991). Detoxification spectrum of the cigarette beetle symbiont Symbiotaphrina kochii in culture. *Entomologia Experimentalis et Applicata*, 60(1), 51–59. https://doi.org/10.1111/j.1570-7458.1991.tb01522.x

Shokrollahzadeh, S., Azizmohseni, F., Golmohammad, F., Shokouhi, H., & Khademhaghighat, F. (2008). Biodegradation potential and bacterial diversity of a petrochemical wastewater treatment plant in Iran. *Bioresource Technology*, 99(14), 6127–6133. https://doi.org/10.1016/j.biortech.2007.12.034

Syranidou, E., Karkanorachaki, K., Amorotti, F., Franchini, M., Repouskou, E., Kaliva, M., Vamvakaki, M., Kolvenbach, B., Fava, F., Corvini, & P., Kalogerakis, N. (2017a). Biodegradation ofweathered polystyrene films in seawater microcosms. *Science Replied,* 7(1), 17991. https://doi.org/10.1038/s41598-017-18366-y

Syranidou, E., Karkanorachaki, K., Amorotti, F., Repouskou, E., Kroll, K., Kolvenbach, B., Corvini, P., Fava, F., & Kalogerakis, N. (2017). Development of tailored indigenous marine consortia for the degradation of naturally weathered polyethylene films. *PLoS One,* 12(8), e0183984. https://doi.org/10.1371/journal.pone.0183984

Tanasupawat, S., Takehana, T., Yoshida, S., Hiraga, K., & Oda, K. (2016). Ideonella sakaiensis sp. nov., isolated from a microbial consortium that degrades poly (ethylene terephthalate). *International Journal System Evolotion Microbiology,* 66, 2813–2818. https://doi.org/10.1099/ijsem.0.001058

Tsuji, H., & Suzuyoshi, K. (2002). Environmental degradation of biodegradable polyesters 1. Poly(e-caprolactone), poly[(R)-3-hydroxybutyrate], and poly(L-lactide) films in controlled static seawater. *Polymer Degradratation Stability*, 75, 347–355. https://doi.org/10.1016/S0141-3910(01)00240-3

Vargas-Suárez, M., Fernández-Cruz, V., & Loza-Tavera, H. (2019). Biodegradation of polyacrylic and polyester polyurethane coatings by enriched microbial communities. *Applied of Microbiology Biotechnology,* 103(7), 3225–3236. https://doi.org/10.1007/s00253-019-09660-y

Varjani, S. J. (2017) Microbial degradation of petroleum hydrocarbons. *Bioresource Technology,* 223, 277–286. https://doi.org/10.1016/j.biortech.2016.10.037

Vasant Kumar, Rutika Sehgal, Reena Gupta, Chapter 13- Microbes and wastewater treatment, Editor(s): Maulin P. Shah, Susana Rodriguez-Couto, Ashok Kumar Nadda, Achlesh Daverey, Development in Wastewater Treatment Research and Processes, Elsevier, 2023, Pages 239–255.

Von Burkersroda, F., Schedl, L., & Göpferich, A. (2002). Why degradable polymers undergo surface erosion or bulk erosion. *Biomaterials,* 23, 4221–4231. https://doi.org/10.1016/S0142-9612(02)00170-9

Wallström, S., Strömberg, E., & Karlsson, S. (2005). Microbiological growth testing of polymeric materials: An evaluation of new methods. *Polymer Testing*, 24(5), 557–563. https://doi.org/10.1016/j.polymertesting.2005.02.005

Whitton, R., Ometto, F., Pidou, M., Jarvis, P., Villa, R., & Jefferson, B. (2015). Microalgae for municipal wastewater nutrient remediation: Mechanisms, reactors and outlook for tertiary treatment. *Environmental Technology Revised*, 4(1), 133–148. https://doi.org/10.1080/21622515.2015.1105308

Yang, J., Yang, Y., Wu, W.-M., Zhao, J., & Jiang, L. (2014). Evidence of polyethylenebiodegradation by bacterial strains from the guts of plastic-eating waxworms. *Environmental Science Technology,* 48(23), 13776–13784. https://doi.org/10.1021/es504038a

Yang, Y., Chen, J., Wu, W.-M., Zhao, J., & Yang, J. (2015). Complete genome sequence of Bacillus sp. YP1, a polyethylene-degrading bacterium from waxworm's gut. *Journal of Biotechnology,* 200, 77–78. https://doi.org/10.1016/j.jbiotec.2015.02.034

Yang, Y., Wang, J., & Xia, M. (2020). Biodegradation and mineralization of polystyrene by plastic-eating superworms Zophobas atratus. *Science Totally Environment,* 15(708), 135233. https://doi.org/10.1016/j.scitotenv.2019.135233

Yoshida, S., Hiraga, K., Takehana, T., Taniguchi, I., Yamaji, H., Maeda, Y., Toyohara, K., Miyamoto, K., Kimura, Y., & Oda, K. (2016). A bacterium that degrades and assimilates poly(ethyleneterephthalate). *Science*, 351, 1196–1199.

Yu, K., Yi, S., Li, B., Guo, F., Peng, X., Wang, Z., Wu, Y., Alvarez-Cohen, L., & Zhang, T. (2019). An integrated meta-omics approach reveals substrates involved in synergistic interactions in a bisphenol A (BPA)-degrading microbial community. *Microbiome,*7(1), 1–13. https://doi.org/10.1186/s40168-019-0634-5

Zafar, U., Nzeram, P., Langarica-Fuentes, A., Houlden, A., Heyworth, A., Saiani, A., & Robson, G. D. (2014). Biodegradation of polyester polyurethane during commercial composting and analysis of associated fungal communities. *Bioresource Technolnolgy,* 158, 374–377. https://doi.org/10.1016/j.biortech.2014.02.077

Zanardini, E., Abbruscato, P., Ghedini, N., Realini, M., & Sorlini, C. (2000). Influence of atmospheric pollutants on the biodeterioration of stone. *International Biodeterioration Biodegradation,* 45, 35–42. https://doi.org/10.1016/S0964-8305(00)00043-3

Zazou, H., Oturan, N., Çelebi, M. S., Hamdani, M., & Oturan, M. A. (2019). Cold incineration of 1, 2-dichlorobenzene in aqueous solution by electrochemical advanced oxidation using DSA/Carbon felt, Pt/Carbon felt and BDD/Carbon felt cells. *Separation and Purification Technology*, 208, 184–193. https://doi.org/10.1016/j.seppur.2018.03.030

Zhang, J., Gao, D., Li, Q., Zhao, Y., Li, L., Lin, H., Bie, Q., & Zhao, Y. (2020). Biodegradation of polyethylene microplastic particles by the fungus Aspergillus flavus from the guts of wax moth Galleria mellonella. *Science Totally Environment*, 704, 135931. https://doi.org/10.1016/j.scitotenv.2019.135931

Zhou, W. G., Li, Y. C., Min, M., Hu, B., Chen, P., & Ruan, R. (2011). Local bioprospecting for highlipid producing microalgal strains to be grown on concentrated municipal wastewater for biofuel production. *Bioresource Technology,* 102(13), 6909–6919. https://doi.org/10.1016/j.biortech.2011.04.038

12 Biopolymers types, characterization, and application
An overview

Padmavathi Rajangam, Sarojinidevi Nagesh, and Rekha Pachaiappan

12.1 INTRODUCTION

A number of factors, including population growth, industrialization, globalization, wearable technology, and a dangerous planet, have combined to increase demand for plastics and/or flexible materials. Due to the petroleum-based nature of the chemical industry, synthetic plastics that can be produced quickly and in huge quantities have satisfied the increasing demand for lightweight materials that may be used for a variety of single-use applications. The need for plastics made mostly of petroleum, which are not biodegradable, has resulted in unsustainable environmental effects. The most notable is how microplastics, which are found in many different ecosystems, affect both plant and wildlife, with the ocean being the largest and most diversified ecosystem. In addition to plastic pollution, other elements that contribute to the environment's degradation include deforestation, the greenhouse effect, industrial pollution, and a host of other things that release additional gases into the atmosphere, including carbon dioxide, methane, SO_2, nitrous oxide, and many others. Alternative materials or methods to the current petroleum-based plastic applications are desperately needed in order to alleviate some of these problems and advance the objective of green economies, which includes mitigating the effects of climate change. Among the main avenues being investigated are the concepts of green chemistry, sustainability, eco-friendly engineering, and bio alternatives. Because biopolymers can flow into current renewable carbon or nitrogen cycles, they have become a viable option (Ilyas et al., 2020; Mahmoud et al., 2020).

Generally, polymers from renewable resources can be classified into three groups:

1. Natural polymers, such as starch, protein, and cellulose.
2. Synthetic polymers from natural monomers, such as poly (lactic acid) (PLA).
3. Polymers from microbial fermentation, such as poly (hydroxybutyrate) (PHB).

Today, plastic-based materials are used in many different contexts, including everyday products as well as commercial and industrial areas. The inherent qualities of plastics, such as their light weight, affordability, durability, and resistance to chemicals, have led to a steady increase in their production worldwide. Furthermore, the increased demand for plastic products is said to be caused by a number of factors, including changes in lifestyle, ongoing urbanization, fast economic expansion, and population rise (Ilhan Chang et al., 2019; Vicki Flaris et al., 2016).

The primary disadvantage of using plastic extensively, however, is that it can be difficult to properly dispose of it at the end of its life cycle, which leads to its accumulating in the environment. Millions

DOI: 10.1201/9781003500483-12

This chapter has been made available under a (CC-BY-NC-ND) 4.0 license

of tons of plastic are expected to be discharged into the environment in the upcoming years. Tons of plastic debris, including microplastics (particles between 1 and 5000 μm in size), end up in the oceans each year, drastically changing the marine ecosystem and the lives of the creatures that dwell there. Moreover, millions of tons of CO_2 will be released into the atmosphere during the course of the product's life cycle, from both the final combustion and the production operations. Massive emissions of greenhouse gases, such CO_2, cause abrupt and permanent changes in the weather, which furthers the cause of global warming. The global temperature increased by C and the CO_2 content increased to about 390 ppm as a result of the industrial revolution. The latter increased by C in 2019, while the former increased to over 400 ppm. In the next 20 to 40 years, these levels could surpass 450 ppm and C based on present trends (Antonella Patti et al., 2022; Fan-Long Jin et al., 2018).

Biopolymers are synthetic polymers derived from natural sources that are either fully biosynthesized by live organisms or chemically synthesized from biological components. For many years, researchers have looked into the usage of biopolymers from various sources in pharmaceutical and therapeutic applications (Smith et al., 2016). The primary characteristic that sets biopolymers apart from polymers derived from fossil fuels is their sustainability, particularly when paired with biodegradability. It is now possible to create biodegradable biopolymers from renewable resources as an alternative to polymers derived from fossil fuels. They are frequently made from different combinations of starch, sugar, natural fibers, and other organic biodegradable ingredients. When bacteria in soil, compost, or marine debris come into contact with the biopolymers, they break down. Furthermore, compared to traditional incineration, the use of biodegradable biopolymers for waste disposal greatly lowers carbon dioxide emissions due to their ability to be broken down by ground-dwelling bacteria.

As a result, the application of biodegradable biopolymers is highlighted from the perspective of preventing global warming. The critical state of the environment has worsened recently as a result of global warming, which has expedited the development of systems with sustainable material usage from the perspective of efficiently using finite carbon resources and preserving finite energy resources. In addition, the price of petroleum feedstock has skyrocketed, and consumers are becoming more interested in products made from "green" (or renewable) resources (Antonio Soldo et al., 2020). For usage in biomedical applications, biopolymers can be shaped into a variety of shapes, including scaffolds, films, hydrogels, and nanocomposites. Biopolymers can be utilized separately or combined to create a variety of composites for usage in a range of applications. Biopolymers are employed in numerous different industrial applications besides the pharmaceutical and medical fields.

The synthesis of polymers from renewable resources has emerged as one of the materials industries with the quickest rate of growth in recent years. The possibility that these polymers could supplant polymers derived from fossil fuels is what is driving their development. The following is a summary of the primary motivators behind this drive: (1) insufficient supplies of fossil fuels; (2) volatile fossil fuel prices; (3) fossil fuels' role as a feedstock for climate change; (4) their sporadic use as political weapons; and (5) their connection to the issue of waste disposal brought on by polymers developed from fossil fuels.

12.2 CLASSIFICATION OF BIOPOLYMERS

Depending on the scale, biopolymers are categorized differently (Figure 12.1). Biopolymers can be broadly classified as biodegradable or non-biodegradable, or alternatively as bio-based or non-bio-based biopolymers, depending on how biodegradable they are. Based on the type of repeating unit they contain, biopolymers can be divided into three groups: (i) polysaccharides, which are made of sugars (like cellulose found in plants); (ii) proteins, which are made of amino acids (like myoglobin found in muscle tissues); and (iii) nucleic acids, which are made of nucleotides (DNA, an organism's genetic material). Biopolymers can be categorized as bioplastics, biosurfactants, biodetergents, bioadhesives, biofloculants, and so forth, depending on their intended use (Sneha Mohan et al., 2020).

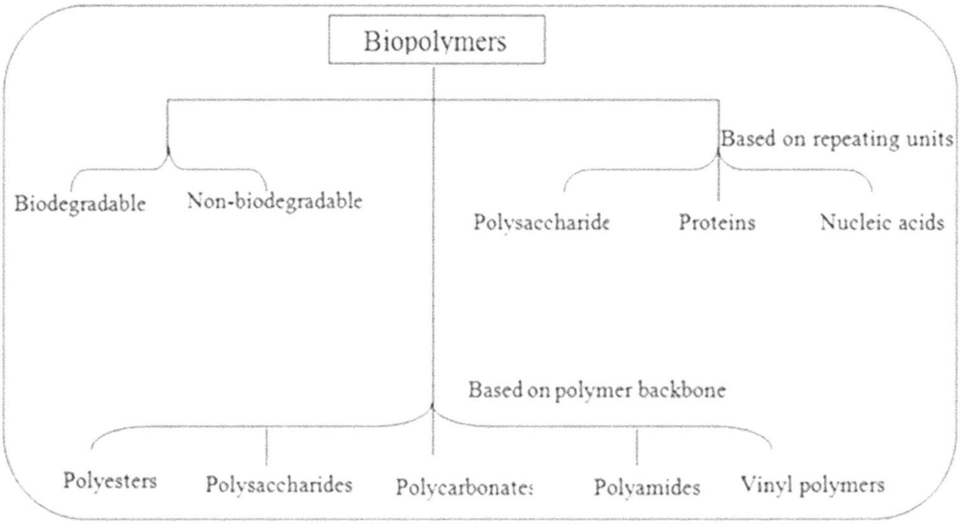

FIGURE 12.1 Different classes of biopolymers.

Source: Sneha Mohan et al. (2016).

12.2.1 Biopolymers production process

To enable their use in various applications, biopolymers can be produced in a variety of ways:

i. A large number of biopolymers can be found in nature and are separated from the plants and algae that thrive there. Agar and alginates are separated from different brown algae, commonly known as seaweeds, or from red algae in the genus Gelidium.
ii. Extracting biopolymers from incredibly natural sources is rare. Hyaluronic acid, which is taken out of newborns' umbilical cords, is one instance of an exception.
iii. Another method for producing biopolymers is by the in vitro synthesis of biopolymers using separated enzymes in cell-free environments. Using heat-stable DNA polymerases in the polymerase chain reaction (PCR) to create monodisperse specified DNA molecules is one example. Another illustration is dextran, which can be manufactured using isolated dextran sucrase on a technological level.
iv. Biopolymers produced during fermentation are employed in industry, such as polysaccharides. Biopolymers can be produced extracellularly or intracellularly by biotechnological means. This has a number of detrimental effects on the downstream process that obtains the biopolymers in a purified form as well as production restrictions.

12.2.2 Polysaccharides

They can be hetero-polysaccharides, which include two or more sugars, or homo-polysaccharides, which are made up of a single monosaccharide. While hetero comprises multiple copies of oligosaccharides, such as gellan and xanthan, homo-polysaccharides are composed of linear chains of polysaccharides, such as pullulan, levan, curdlan, or bacterial cellulose. It is possible to attach other components such as acyl groups, amino acids, and inorganic residue. A vast range of glycosidically connected structures based on 40 distinct monosaccharides is available through polysaccharides. Mostly produced by prokaryotes from hexoses and pentosessome sugars are also present. Polyglucoside acrylates have been reported to possess certain material qualities, including water absorption, biocompatibility, and reinforcing effects. These are a few significant structural polysaccharides that are crucial for the synthesis of biopolymers. The physical properties of polysaccharides including solubility, gelation, and surface characteristics are dictated by monomers sequence, chain shapes, and molecular weight. In the organism, polysaccharides play crucial role in membranes and intracellular communication and act as storage molecules (Lovegrove A. et al., 2015).

12.2.3 Pectin

Plant middle lamella contains a naturally occurring polysaccharide that is commercially produced from citrus peels and contains 10 to 15% pectin, and 20 to 30% pectin under some acidic circumstances. Pectin's molecular structure is made up of chains of D-galacturonic acid (GalA) units connected by (1–4) glycosidic bonds. Because of its gel-forming properties, fruit jelly is made with it. Gel formation is contingent upon the molecule size and esterification level. Pectin is a water-soluble biopolymer; however, there are certain variables that can alter its solubility, such as an increase in viscosity due to gel formation. Deesterification and depolymerization are two processes that might break down dissolved pectin. Pectin finds significant application in the pharmaceutical industry for a range of medications, ionotropic gelation, and gel coating.

12.2.4 Casein

The term "milk protein" also refers to its four primary parts (αS1, αS2, β, κ). Based on how these fractions interact with water, they are arranged within the casein micelle. It has a molecular weight of 1000–20,000 g.*mol*–1. Its pH is more than 6.5, and it exhibits heat-stable qualities. It is utilized in a wide range of industries, including biomedical applications, controlled releases, and adhesives. There is a film available in the market that is used to wrap food that resembles plastic wrap but is edible. Citrus pectin, salts, and milk casein are combined to make this film. The film's strength and moisture resistance make it 500 times more effective at preventing oxygen from reaching food than plastic film made of petroleum.

12.2.5 Agar gum

Agar gum is a polysaccharide derived from rhodophyceae that is made up of linked galactose molecules. Because of its rheological characteristics, agar gum can be used as an emulsifier, thickener, and stabilizer. Furthermore, after dissolving in boiling water, agar gum possesses a thermogelation feature that enables the creation of robust gels upon cooling back to room temperature. Without endangering the environment, agar gum efficiently increases the strength of sand, particularly cohesiveness. In a recent attempt to strengthen soils, researchers used 3% (to soil mass) thermally treated agar gum, which increased the unconfined compressive strength of soil up to 10 MPa in a dry state.

12.2.6 Gelatin

Animal products are used to make gelatin, a protein. It is created by partially hydrolyzing collagen that is extracted from animal tissues, skin, and bones. They are primarily made of type I collagen, which is cysteine-free. Based on the process and composition of their manufacture, there are primarily two types of gelatin. Because they lack amide groups, type A, which is produced by acid hydrolyzing collagen, has 18.5% nitrogen, while type B, which is produced by alkaline hydrolyzing collagen, has 18.5% nitrogen. It melts at high temperatures and exists as coils; as the temperature is lowered, it transforms from coils to helices. Gelatin (Figure 12.2) is vulnerable to proteases, although collagen is resistant to them. Since gelatin contains numerous functional

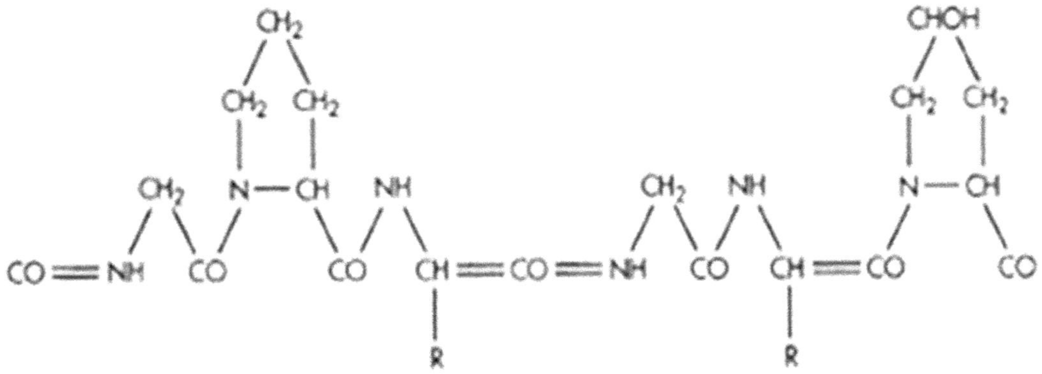

FIGURE 12.2 Structure of gelatin.

Source: Sneha Mohan et al. (2016).

groups, such as -NH, -SH, and -COOH, it can be altered using biomolecules and nanoparticles for a variety of uses.

In the biomedical fields of bone, tissue engineering, wound dressing, gene transfection, and medication delivery, gelatin finds extensive use. Gelatin is utilized to speed up the healing process following sports-related injuries and improve hair quality (Sneha Mohan et al., 2016).

12.2.7 Starch

While the structure of starch, a naturally occurring biopolymer, is similar to that of cellulose, the internal bonding is different. The components that make up starch are amylose and amylopectin, a semi-crystalline polymer. Starch (Figure 12.3) is the main type of carbohydrate that plants employ to store energy; in animals, it is referred to as glycogen.

Glycogen and starch are both polymers of glucose that have varying degrees of branching and distinct glycosidic bonds between glucose monomers. Whereas amylopectin is a very big molecule formed of (1–4)-linked a-D-glucopyranose chains with a-(1–6) branches, amylose is a linear polymer made up of a-D-glucopyranosyl units. One of the most prevalent natural polymers, starch is also inexpensive and biodegradable. Many commercial goods can be manufactured from starch that has been properly processed. Their weak mechanical qualities and susceptibility to moisture have limited their application to a number of niche markets. Research has indicated that the mechanical and barrier qualities of starch products can be enhanced with the addition of fibers. When the composite is being prepared, the tensile strength and flexibility will be enhanced by the dispersion of nano and micro-structured fibers in the polymer matrix. There is no denying the importance of starch to both humans and plants. Although plants use it as a source of energy storage, people require it for a variety of industrial products as well as a necessary component of their nutrition. Numerous uses for starch and its derivatives have already been investigated, including the production of paper, textiles, and adhesives. They are an environmentally beneficial substitute for synthetic additives found in many other items, such as plastics, detergents, pharmaceutical tablets, cosmetics, oil-drilling fluids, and pesticides, due to their renewable and biodegradable nature (Ravindra et al., 2017).

12.2.8 Cellulose

β-1, 4-linked glucan chains are the monomer unit of cellulose (Figure 12.4). Hydrogen bonds are generated between oxygen atoms and hydroxyl groups inside and between nearby chains. Cellulose

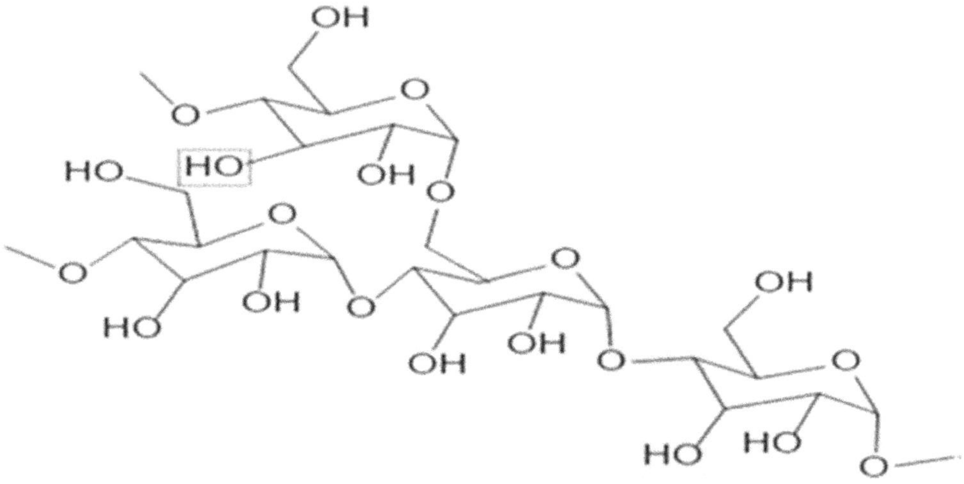

FIGURE 12.3 Structure of starch with α (1/4) and α (1/6) glycosidic linkages.

Source: Rahul Singh et al. (2021).

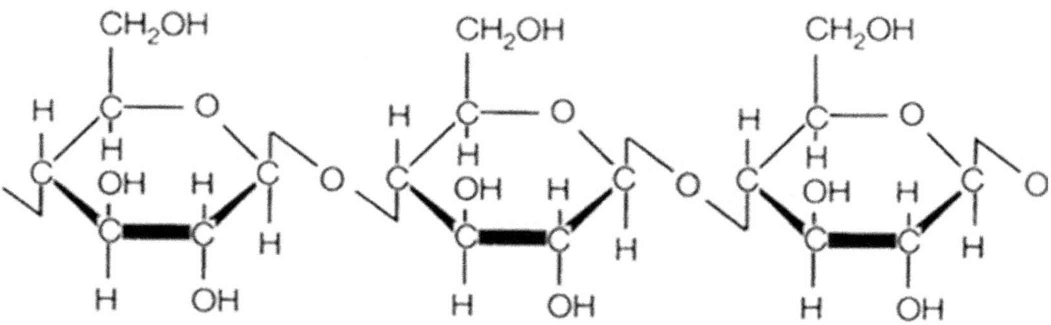

FIGURE 12.4 The structural representation of cellulose.

Source: Sneha Mohan et al. (2016).

microfibrils are formed when glucan chains are grouped side by side by van der Waals forces and hydrogen bonding. After then, crystalline cellulose is created by stacking these cellulose microfibrils together. The polar -OH groups in the cellulose chain bundle the chains together by forming many hydrogen bonds with the OH groups on neighboring chains. Because of the extremely regular chain stacking, hard, durable crystalline areas are formed, which increases the stability and strength of the bundled chains. In wood pulp, the length of the chain is only a few hundred sugar units, but in cotton, it reaches around 6,000 units. It is the most prevalent naturally occurring organic polymer and is regarded as a nearly limitless supply of raw materials for the growing market for environmentally and biologically acceptable products. Strong hydrogen bonds cause it to be insoluble in most solvents. It is consequently chemically changed to produce derivatives such as acetal, ester, and ether (Mehmet Isik et al., 2014).

The most prevalent biological material on Earth, cellulose, is made up of glucose monomers but is connected by beta glycosidic linkages, which give it a more streamlined structure that allows it to pack tightly and give wood its mechanical strength (Swarup Roy et al., 2020).

12.2.9 Chitin and Chitosan

Chitin is a nitrogen-containing polymer that is mostly found in the exoskeleton, or outer covering, of insects, crustaceans, and arachnids. It is chemically related to cellulose and creates a semitransparent horny substance. Chitin's structure is similar to that of cellulose, a polysaccharide made of β-(1–4) linked nacetyl glucosamine that forms crystalline nanofibrils or whiskers. The second most prevalent naturally occurring polysaccharide in the exoskeleton of insects and the outer shell of crustaceans is chitin.

Most chemical and inorganic solvents do not dissolve chitin. The de-acetylated derivative of chitin, chitosan (Figure 12.5), is a cationic polymer that is the second most abundant natural biopolymer after cellulose. It can form polyelectrolyte complexes with other polysaccharides. It is made up of N-acetyl-D-glucosamine and β-(1–4)-linked D-glucosamine. It is utilized as a material for wound dressings because of its facile application, water sorptivity, oxygen permeability, blood coagulating capabilities, and cytokine induction (interleukin-8), which stimulates fibroblast migration and proliferation.

Chitosan has been utilized extensively in the casting of independent films because of its strong film-forming properties. It can be used as a coating on a variety of surfaces to increase the surface's permeability against different gases and moisture. The chitosan coating improved the paper's permeability to water vapor. Chitosan coatings can be applied to polypropylene films that have been activated by CO or NH molecules, making the film surfaces hydrophilic and preventing the transfer of ethylene, carbon dioxide, and oxygen.

Using nanoclays added to chitosan can further improve its barrier qualities. Interesting qualities of chitosan include its inexpensive cost, chemical inertness, excellent mechanical strength, biodegradability, biocompatibility, and good film-forming abilities. Chitosan finds widespread usage in many products and applications, encompassing anything from cosmetics and pharmaceuticals to water treatment and plant protection. Different chitosan qualities are needed for each application, and these properties vary according on the molecular weight and degree of acetylation (Santosh Kumar et al., 2020; Mariana Adina Matica et al., 2019).

12.2.10 Polylactic acid (PLA)

Biodegradable thermoplastic aliphatic polyester polylactic acid, often known as polylactide (PLA, Poly), is made from renewable resources such as maize starch, tapioca roots, chips, starch, or sugarcane. The main process used to produce PLA is ionic polymerization of lactide, which is the ring closure of two lactic acid molecules. A ring-opening polymerization occurs at temperatures between 140 and 180°C, facilitated by catalytic tin compounds (such as tinoxide). By using different microorganisms to digest lactic acid from renewable resources like starch, lactide itself can be produced. Polycondensation is another direct method of producing PLA from lactic acid. Low molecular weight polymers are the result of this technique, though, and there are issues with solvent disposal during commercial production.

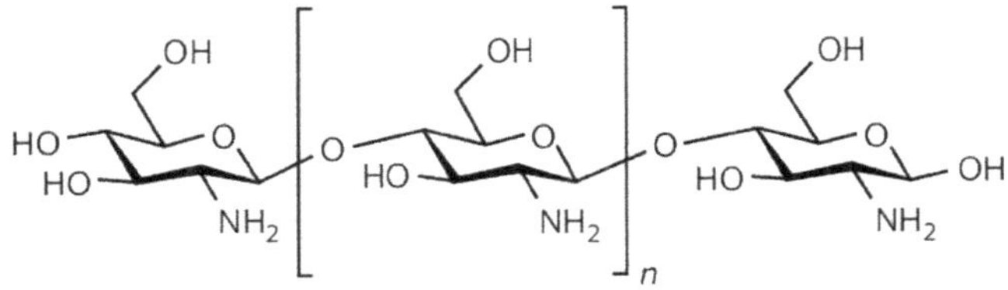

FIGURE 12.5 The structure of chitosan biopolymer.

Source: Sneha Mohan et al. (2016).

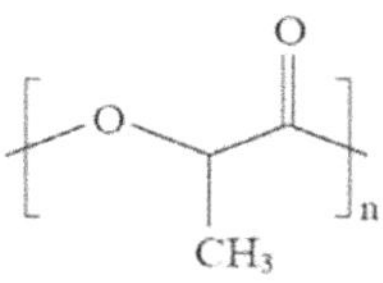

FIGURE 12.6 Structural formula of PLA.

Source: Sneha Mohan et al. (2016).

The main determinants of PLA's characteristics are its molecular mass, degree of crystallinity, and maybe its co-monomer content. Increases in T, tensile strength, elastic modulus, and strain following fracture are all correlated with increasing molecular mass. The material exhibits hydrophobic or water-repellent properties because of the CH side group. Numerous organic solvents, including dichloromethane and similar substances, are soluble in PLA (Figure 12.6). Compared to other biodegradable polymers, PLA is more transparent and has better workability and weather resilience (Rafael Balart et al., 2021).

12.2.11 Collagen

The most prevalent protein in humans is collagen. It creates a framework to give strength and structure in the bones, muscles, skin, and tendons. Collagen is a protein that the body naturally produces and performs a variety of vital roles in health. A lot of health issues are linked to the body's natural collagen breaking down and running out. The body receives exogenous collagen for medical and aesthetic uses, which includes aiding in tissue healing and repair.

Collagen makes up around 30% of the protein in the human body, with types I, II, and III accounting for 80–90% of total collagen. Among these, type I collagen fibrils are the material that keeps the entire body together since they are stronger than steel. In addition to helping to replace dead skin cells, collagen provides the skin with strength and structure. Medical products that contain collagen might come from human, bovine, porcine, or ovine origins. Wound sites attract new skin cells when collagen dressings are applied. Some factors that can be controlled to harm collagen formation are exposure to sunshine, smoking, and consuming large amounts of sugar (Antonella Patti et al., 2022).

12.3 SOURCES AND PREPARATION OF BIOPOLYMERS

Polymeric biomaterials are artificially produced or altered polymers intended for a range of uses. One way to synthesize novel biopolymers that are truly biorenewable is to engineer plants to produce them. These polymers are made in large quantities and then shaped for a particular end use, just like all other polymer industries.

In addition, a wide range of biopolymers, including viscous solutions and plastics, polyesters, polyamides, and polysaccharides, are produced by microorganisms (Table 12.1).

The molecular weight and composition of the polymer determine its physical properties (Hernandez et al., 2014). Through genetic modification of microorganisms, the characteristics of different biopolymers produced with their assistance can be modified to suit high-value medical applications like drug delivery and tissue engineering. Microorganisms assist in the production of biopolymers, which need particular nutrients and regulated environmental conditions. They can be made directly by fermentation or indirectly through the chemical polymerization of monomers that are made by fermentation. The majority of biopolymers don't negatively impact biological systems and are biocompatible. It is thought that the synthesis of biopolymers originating from bacteria occurs either as a defense mechanism or as a storage material (Sukan A et al., 2015). Enzymes, microbes, and natural processes can all break them down so that the environment can eventually

TABLE 12.1
Some biopolymers, their sources, and preparation

Polymer	Method/source	Example of bacteria used for synthesis
Hybrid plastics	Adding denatured algae biomass to petroleum-based plastics like polyurethane and polyethylene as fillers	Filsmentous green algae, cladophorales
Cellulose-based plastics	Biopolymer of glucose	30% of the biomass produced after extraction of algal oil is known to contain cellulose
Poly lactic acid (PLA)	Polymerization of lactic acid lactic acid	Bacterial fermentation of algal biomass
Bio polyethylene	Ethylene produced from ethanol, by a chemical reaction called cracking, ethanol derived from natural gas or petroleum	Bacterial fermentation of algal biomass
Poly esters	Biomass	Bacteria like Akaligeneseurrophus, *E. coli*, etc.

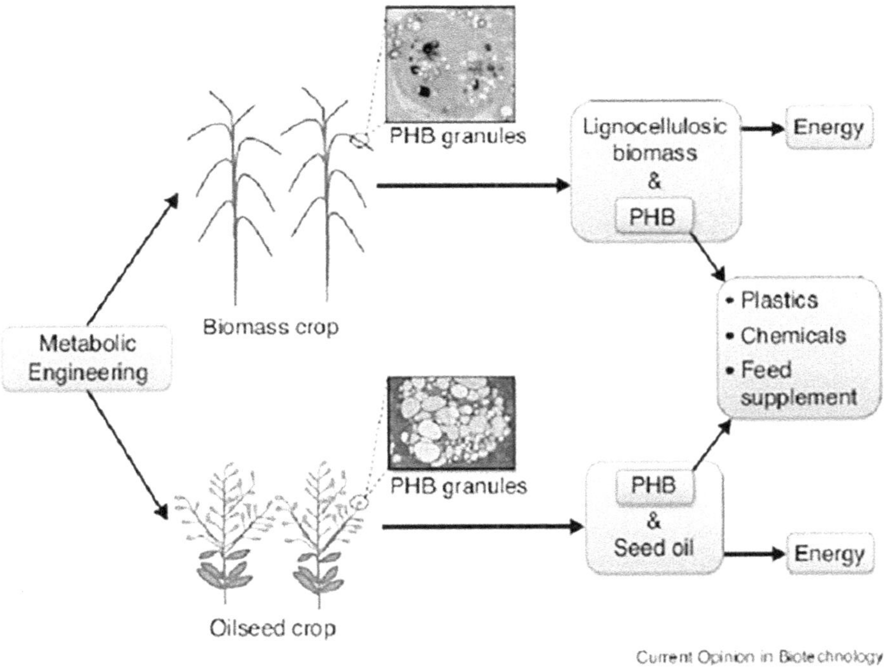

FIGURE 12.7 Schematic representation of the production of polyhydroxybutyrate (PHB) in both biomass and oilseed crops.

Source: Snell et al. (2015).

absorb them again. A type of plastic called biopolymers, also known as organic plastics, is made from biomass sources that are renewable, like vegetable oil, corn starch, pea starch, and so forth (Figure 12.7).

Sustainable development can be facilitated by concentrating more on biopolymers, which can also help to reduce CO_2 emissions and conserve fossil fuels (Koyama et al., 1995). Algae are one of the best microorganisms for plastic production feedstock because of their high yield and adaptability to a variety of environments. Utilizing carbon and offsetting greenhouse gas emissions from factories or power plants is made possible by the use of algae. In the history of bioplastics, algae-based plastics have emerged as a new trend in contrast to the more conventional uses of feedstocks like potatoes and corn to make plastics. Although algae-based plastics are still in their infancy, once they enter the market, they should find use in a variety of sectors. Microbial plastics are currently thought to be a significant source of polymeric materials with excellent commercialization potential. They can create emulsions, stabilize suspensions, flocculate particles, change the way fluids flow, and encapsulate materials (Tirrell et al., 1996).

12.4 VARIOUS METHODS OF CHARACTERIZATION

The majority of methods employed in polymer characterization can also be applied to biopolymer characterization. Biopolymer characterization serves two objectives:

- Creation of processing parameter
- Identifying the performance characteristics of the end-user.

The most significant characteristics that are of interest through characterization are molecular mass, size, polydispersity, degree of association, conformation, interaction, and so forth. The following is a list of characterization methods that are employed in the analysis of biopolymers.

12.4.1 Fourier transform infrared spectroscopy (FTIR)

The different functional groups and interactions found in biopolymers can be examined using FTIR. By examining the spectra, relations such as amide linkage and hydrogen bonding can be readily identified (Theophile et al., 2015). ATR-FTIR spectroscopy, or attenuated total reflection (ATR) sampling device-based Fourier transform infrared spectroscopy, is one of several possible methods. It is simple to use, allows for routine analysis in both laboratory and field settings, and calls for little upfront preparation of samples. VIS–NIR spectroscopy is a well-recognized substitute for determining the components of biological materials. The various vibrational modes of the molecules, which result from their interaction with electromagnetic radiation absorbed at particular wavelengths, have an impact on the near-infrared spectrum. This method can be applied to the authentication of various complex constituents found in biological materials, including proteins and carbohydrates. Chemometrics makes it possible to gain pertinent information from spectra in order to create calibration models that enable categorization and compositional prediction of organic samples. Using variable-temperature Fourier transform infrared (FT–IR) absorption spectroscopy, the thermotropic phase behavior of a series of recently developed self-forming synthetic biopolymers has been studied (Bista et al., 2011). The FTIR method has been widely used in numerous studies to investigate the mechanical and physical characteristics of biopolymers. Characterizing the ATR spectral intensity fluctuations of immature and mature cotton fibers was done using two-dimensional (2D) correlation analysis (Liu et al., 2012). Verification of the interactions between different biopolymers in its composites can also be done via FTIR analysis (Flores-Hernández et al., 2014), displays the FTIR spectra of keratin, chitosan-starch films, and composites made with 20%. Because starch is present in the chitosan-starch film, the band at 3400 per cm is attributed to hydrogen-bonded hydroxyl groups, as shown in Figure 12.8 (a).

The primary vibrations linked to the keratin structure were found in the vicinity of 3300 per cm, as depicted in Figure 12.8a. These vibrations correlate to a variety of amide bands. Moreover, the methyl group's asymmetric CH vibration is attributed to the peak at 2945 per cm. Figure 12.8b displays three characteristic peaks between 995 and 1150 per cm, which are attributed to C–O bond stretching. The main peaks related to chitosan-starch films are seen at 700–770 per cm, which correspond to the saccharide structure in Figure 12.8 (b).

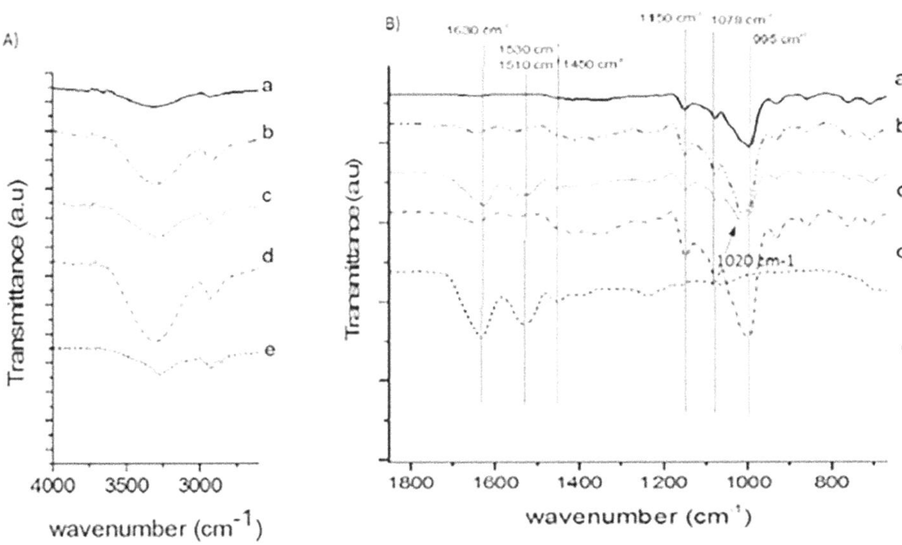

FIGURE 12.8 The composite films' infrared spectra range from 4000 to 2500 per cm (a) and 1800 to 700 per cm in (b). Chitosan-starch films (a), chitosan-starch-short biofiber (20%), chitosan-starch-long biofiber (20%), chitosan-starch-ground quill (20%), and keratin (Flores-Hernández CG et al., 2014) are the different forms of chitosan-starch.

The C = O group is identified by the band at 1630 per cm, the NH group's in-plane bending is indicated by the peaks at 1530 per cm and 1510 per cm, and the bending of the CH_3 group for keratin is linked to the signal at 1430 per cm. The morphological characteristics and thermomechanical properties of the composite are correlated with the FTIR results. According to the spectrum, composites with large and short fibers achieve a higher storage modulus than the composite with ground quill. Better dispersion is also achieved in these composites.

12.4.2 X-RAY DIFFRACTION ANALYSIS

It is possible to effectively investigate the crystallinity of the biopolymers using X-ray diffraction techniques. The X-ray diffraction data of native wheat starch, compressed starch foam, and compressed starch/fiber foam are shown in Figure 12.9 (Teixeira et al., 2014). The natural wheat starch exhibited an A-type crystal-like semi-crystalline structure with peaks. Diffractograms showing a broad amorphous peak and no discernible residual A-type crystallinity are the result of the gelatinization/compression processes that occur during the composite preparation, which reduce crystallinity. The spectrum makes it evident that the processes of gelatinization and high compression caused structural disruption to the starch granules. About 2-|12.0, 17.3, and 19.5, which are typical for the crystallographic parameters of VH-type crystals for destructured starch prepared from solution, small peaks were discovered. With regard to the starch/fiber sample, the resulting spectrum little peaks were discovered at approximately 2-| 12.0, 17.3, and 19.5, which correspond to the crystallographic parameters of VH-type crystals for deformed starch that has been prepared in solution. For the fiber/starch sample, the spectrum was acquired.

12.4.3 NMR SPECTROSCOPY

The NMR technique makes it simple to determine the molecular dynamics of water adsorbed on biopolymer surfaces and the functional groups of biopolymers (Blicharska et al., 2010). The

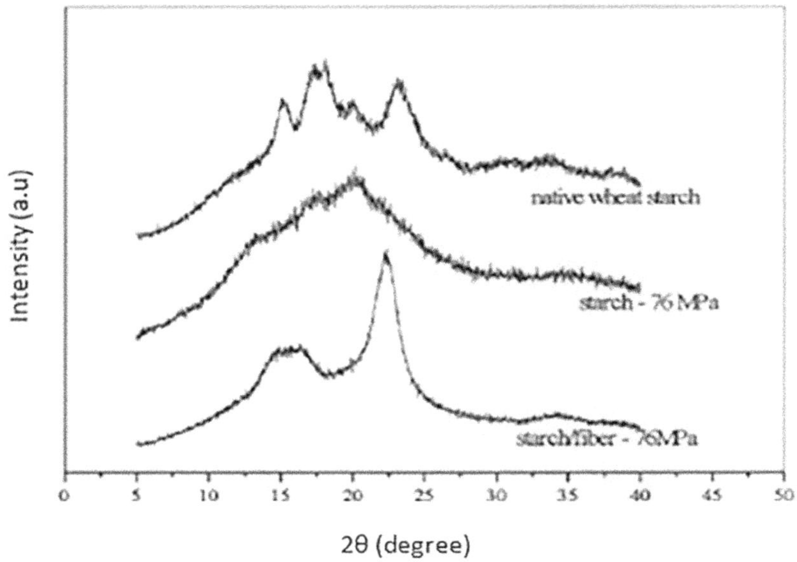

FIGURE 12.9 X-ray diffraction profile for native starch, starch (76 MPa) and starch/fiber (76 MPa).

Source: Flores-Hernández et al. (2014).

relaxation times obtained from NMR spectroscopy, along with their correlation with temperature and magnetic field, have shown to be a valuable resource for understanding the molecular structure, phase transition, conformational exchange, solubility, and diffusion of biopolymers. Numerous investigations into the spin-lattice relaxation times (T1), T2, and T1q in the rotating frame of various biopolymers have previously been published (Rachocki A et al., 2006). In cellulose and its derivatives, the molecular cause of nuclear spin relaxation has been investigated (Rachocki A et al., 2006). Considerable research has been done on the effect of temperature on nuclear-spin relaxation in biopolymers found in cell walls in order to better understand the behavior of the main functional groups (Tang et al., 2000). In order to look into structure–hydration relationships in the biopolymer, the temperature dependence of the starch chain's relaxation times has been studied (Calucci et al., 2004).

12.4.4 Scanning Kelvin Probe Microscopy (SKPM)

In material science, SKPM (Figure 12.10) has grown to be an extremely powerful tool (Kitamura et al., 1998), giving up a surface mapping of electrostatic potential (Koley et al., 2001). The rejection of charged species in membrane applications, like heavy metal removal and water softening, is significantly influenced by electrical properties. For the purposes of reverse osmosis (RO) and nanofiltration (NF), a higher membrane charge may enhance ion rejection. For the removal of ions, electrostatic interaction becomes significant if the membrane is electrically charged. To determine their electrical potential, SKPM was used to characterize the nanocomposites that showed the best flows.

12.5 NATURAL FIBERS AND THEIR KINDS

A composite material is typically a material structure that helps achieve superior performance by combining two macroscopically identifiable materials. The terms "continuous" and "discontinuous phases" are often used to describe these two material systems. The discontinuous phase is known

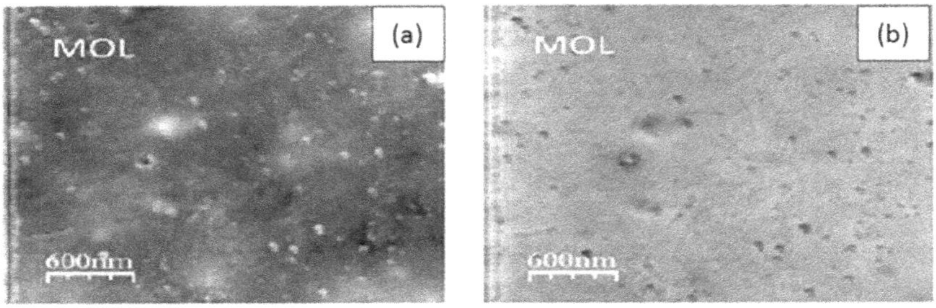

FIGURE 12.10 SKPM views of MOL (Lignin) nanofiltration composites and CTA (cellulose triacetate). The figure's left side displays topography, while the right-side displays surface potential mapping.

Source: Koley et al. (2001).

as the reinforcement phase, and the continuous phase is called the matrix phase. When compared to the matrix phase, the reinforcement phase is typically more robust and stiff. There are two primary forms of reinforcement available: particulate matter (which comes in various shapes and sizes) and fiber, which includes whiskers. As a result, these comprised fiber-reinforced composites (FRCs) and particle-reinforced composites, the two primary categories of composites. Typically, one of the following makes up. Polymer matrix composites, ceramic matrix composites, and metal matrix composites are the terms used to describe natural fibers and their types that use these matrices. Laminar composites, also referred to as laminates or laminated composites, are another type of composite. Usually, laminates are made up of two or more layers, each of which is made of a different or related substance. Laminated composite structures are frequently advised for use in lightweight structural applications because of their strong rigidity.

Since they include at least one component (such as a matrix or reinforcement) made from easily accessible renewable resources, natural fiber reinforced composites (NFRCs) are referred to as bio-composite materials (Satyanarayana et al., 1990). These days, they are used to construct structural components by many different industries, including the aerospace, military, marine, and building engineering sectors. A lot of engineering and structural sectors were interested in producing these materials because they could reduce weight and improve product efficiency (Pickering et al., 2006). Furthermore, as Figure 12.11 illustrates, using natural fibers as reinforcing material instead of artificial synthetic fibers (carbon and glass) has certain advantages from a technical, financial, and environmental standpoint. Based on these reviews, it appears that NFRCs are a great choice for creating structural materials.

Natural fibers lack the necessary mechanical strength, despite their advantages for the environment and their use in some construction, automotive, and household soundproofing applications. Because these fibers are less resistant to moisture absorption than synthetic or man-made fibers, their use is restricted in structurally based noise control applications. Because of their improved mechanical properties, hybrid composite materials are currently becoming more popular as structural materials. A material structure that combines multiple reinforcement and filler materials with an intricate matrix mixture is referred to as "hybrid". The main advantage of using multiple fibers in a hybrid composite material system is that even if one of the fibers doesn't have the desired qualities, it will still be offset by the other fiber. Due to appropriate material design considerations, hybridization also aids in improving the composite's efficiency and cost balance (Ahmad et al., 2022). The biological resources that are readily available to us include animals, plants, minerals, and vegetables. As illustrated in Figure 12.11, natural fibers can be extracted from these sources and are being used in place of synthetic fibers in a wide range of engineering products (Gurupranes et al., 2023). Alpaca fiber, bird feathers, wool, silk, sheep and rabbit wool, goat hair, Angora goat mohair, hog bristle, ox hair, Siberian weasel, camelhair, and horsehair are some examples of animal natural fibers (De et al., 2008).

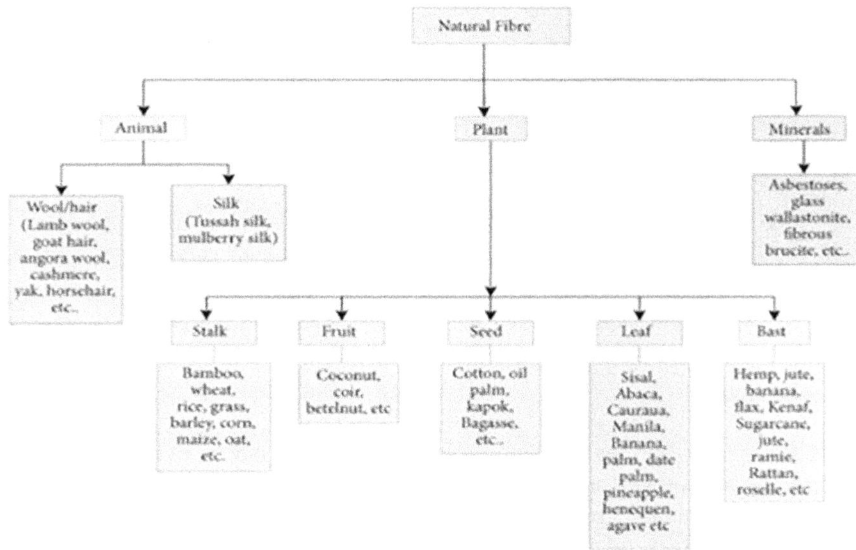

FIGURE 12.11 Types of natural fibers.

Source: Adapted from Gurupranes et al. (2023).

Asbestos, ceramic, and metal fibers are the different categories for mineral fibers. While the latter two mineral fibers are created by combining different natural materials, asbestos is a renewable mineral fiber. Amphiboles, anthophyllite, chrysotile, and serpentine are among the fibers found in asbestos. Aluminum fiber is one kind of metal fiber; ceramic fibers are composed of substances like silicon carbide, boron carbide, and aluminum oxide. The components of cellulose, hemicellulose, and lignin make up plant fibers (de Rosa et al., 2010; Saravana Bavan et al., 2010). Plant fibers are divided into groups based on where they come from, including bast, leaves, seeds, and flowers. While the fibers of monocotyledonous plants run longitudinally across their leaves (Rajeshkumar et al., 2021), bast, also known as stem fibers, are bundles of fibrous material found within the inner bark of plant stems. A few of the instancescotton, hemp, jute, flax, ramie, sisal, banana, hemp, kenaf, ramie, rattan, vine, soybean, and bagasse fiber among plant materials.

12.6 CHARACTERISTICS OF NATURAL FIBERS

The following sections provide a brief summary of the properties—mechanical, chemical, thermal, and electrical.

12.6.1 Physical attributes

The diameter, length, and density of the fiber are its physical characteristics. As Table 12.2 illustrates, this differs depending on the fiber (Todkar et al., 2019).

12.6.2 Molecular formulations

The original fibrils were primarily used in the design of compound composites with spiral orientations. They were made of cellulose suspended in a formless lignin and polyose matrix (de Rosa et al., 2010). Table 12.3 contains a list of the different chemical compositions, including lignin, cellulose, pectin, ash, hemicellulose, wax, and moisture content. Plant tissue location and growth rate affect the percentage of chemical components in fiber (Sreenivasan et al., 2011). It contains

TABLE 12.2
Different fibers

Name of the fiber	Diameter (μm)	Length (mm)	Density(kg/cm3)
Abaca	18.2	4.9	1500
Alfa	5–10	2–5	890
Bagasse	20	1.7	900
Banana	131.76	30	1325
Bamboo	25	2	1500
Coir	17.5	1.25	1250
Cotton	14.5	42	1550
Curaua	170	–	1400
Flax	20	31.45	1450
Hemp	19.9	11.2	1200
Isora	10–20	–	1200
Jute	18.4	2.55	1400
Kapok	25	20	384
Kenaf	19.8	2.35	1300

TABLE 12.3
List of the different chemical compositions

Name of the fiber	Cellulose (%)	Hemi-cellulose (%)	Lignin (%)	Pectin (%)	Waxes (%)
Abaca	62.5	21	12	0.8	3
Alfa	45.4	38.5	14.9	–	2
Bagasse	37	21	22	10	–
Banana	62.4	12.5	7.5	4	–
Bamboo	34.5	20.5	26	–	–
Coir	46	0.3	45	4	–
Cotton	89	4	0.75	6	0.6
Curaua	73.6	5	7.5	4	–
Flax	70.5	16.5	2.5	0.9	–
Hemp	81	20	4	0.9	–
Isora	74	–	23	–	–
Jute	67	16	9	0.2	0.4
Kapok	13.16	–	–	–	–
Kenaf	53.5	21	17	2	–
Pineapple	80.5	17.5	8.3	4	–
Ramie	72	14	0.8	1.95	–
Sisal	60	11.5	8	1.2	–

non-cellulosic substituents (such as hemicellulose, lignin, pectin, and waxes) that weaken the bonding nature of the material, despite having all the components required for binding with a polymer matrix. Pretreatment techniques that included extra controlled factors were employed to get rid of that (Todkar et al., 2019).

In this context, some experimental works based on the extraction of non-cellulosic contents are presented. Multi-layered areca leaf sheath composites treated with 10% NaOH, rinsed with distilled water, and then dried in a micro-oven at 60°C showed better tensile and flexural strength than composites treated with 5% NaOH, according to (Ashok et al., 2020). The 10% NaOH chemical pretreatment affects the crystallinity structure, which in turn modifies the mechanical, physical, and thermal behaviors of the composite, according to research by Jaiswal et al. (2022). Additionally, according to Paiva et al. (2007), the microfibrilalfa fibers were extracted using NaOH, bleached with NaClO, and then dried. This process eliminated any foreign materials and left behind cellulose filaments and some degree of lignin to strengthen the material composite. Furthermore, NaOH concentrations above 10% aid in the disappearance of non-cellulosic contents and cause fiber pull-out, which lowers the composites' mechanical strength. Similarly, Çakir et al. (2014) discovered that treating fibers with 5–10% NaOH has the tendency to remove wax content in higher percentages, strengthening the bond. Nonetheless, based on these investigations, 5–10% NaOH will have a greater impact on the composites' mechanical characteristics.

According to Sever et al. (2012), chemical pre-treatments like fluorocarbon, microemulsion, and alkali can be useful in altering the characteristics of unidirectional-based composite materials. This is especially true when it comes to strengthening their tensile, flexural, and interlaminar shear strengths. By enhancing the interfacial adhesion between the fibers and the matrix, these treatments can produce a composite material that is stronger and more resilient. Moreover, contact angle measurements and X-ray photoelectron spectroscopy can be used to characterize it. Mahbubul Bashar and Khan et al. (2013) investigated the impact of enzymatic degradation and subsequent galacturonic acid analyses on the fiber surface in relation to this study. This kind of surface modification, according to the research, helps to lower the pectin content, which enhances the fibrillation effect. This kind of surface modification, according to the research, helps to lower the pectin content, which enhances the fibrillation effect and lowers porosity and fiber agglomeration (Alomayri et al., 2013; Chokshi et al., 2020).

In order to identify the chemical components of a new class of fibers, Ahmed et al. (2021) studied Elettariacardamomum, also known as cardamom, Epipremnumaureum, also known as golden pothos, maize tassel, Napier grass, and Arundodonax. The researchers discovered that these plants' capacity to aid in the matrix phase's reinforcement was significantly influenced by their high cellulose content (more than 63.12%). These plants' high cellulose content fibers have the potential to be employed in a number of applications where strength and durability are critical parameters, according to the findings. Natural fibers' cellulose content rose when they underwent various chemical treatments. Notably, their surface characteristics changed substantially when compared to fibers that were not treated. Similarly, Martel et al.'s investigation (De et al., 2020) looked into how NaOH treatment affected curauá fibers. The pretreatment improved the fibers' interfacial properties and raised the amount of cellulose in them, the researchers discovered. In comparison to other treatments, the NaOH treatment was found to be more economical and time-efficient, and it also demonstrated better mechanical and thermal properties (Salgado-Ramos et al., 2022; Barba et al., 2021).

According to Sanjay et al. (2018), as illustrated in Figure 12.12, the moisture content of natural fibers influences crystalline alignment, crystallinity level, inflammation, and thermal behavior. It is commonly known that treated fibers with higher cellulose contents have higher values of cellulose-α. Furthermore, compared to the other fibers, the acrylic acid-treated fiber has a lower wax content (0.13 wt %), which enhances the interfacial interaction between the residual and unidirectional fibers. Comparably, findings from Chirayi et al.'s (2014) research show a notable decrease in the amount of ash and wax, which has a strong fire prevention capacity and keeps sensitive chemical groups from reacting, improving thermal stability (Fortunati et al., 2013).

Comparatively speaking, based on studies conducted on date palm in this context, Ghori et al. (2018) reported that composite materials with improved properties were produced by combining date palm fibers with epoxy, polypropylene (PP), and unsaturated polyester polymers. Chemical treatments like NaOH and silane have been used on date palm fibers to improve their surface properties in order to combat their hygroscopic tendencies. Due to their increased adhesion with the polymer matrix, the resultant surface-treated date palm fibers have improved mechanical and thermal properties when used as reinforcement in polymer composites. Similarly, Alotabi et al.'s (2020) study examined the characteristics and makeup of date palm fibrils in combination with polymers.

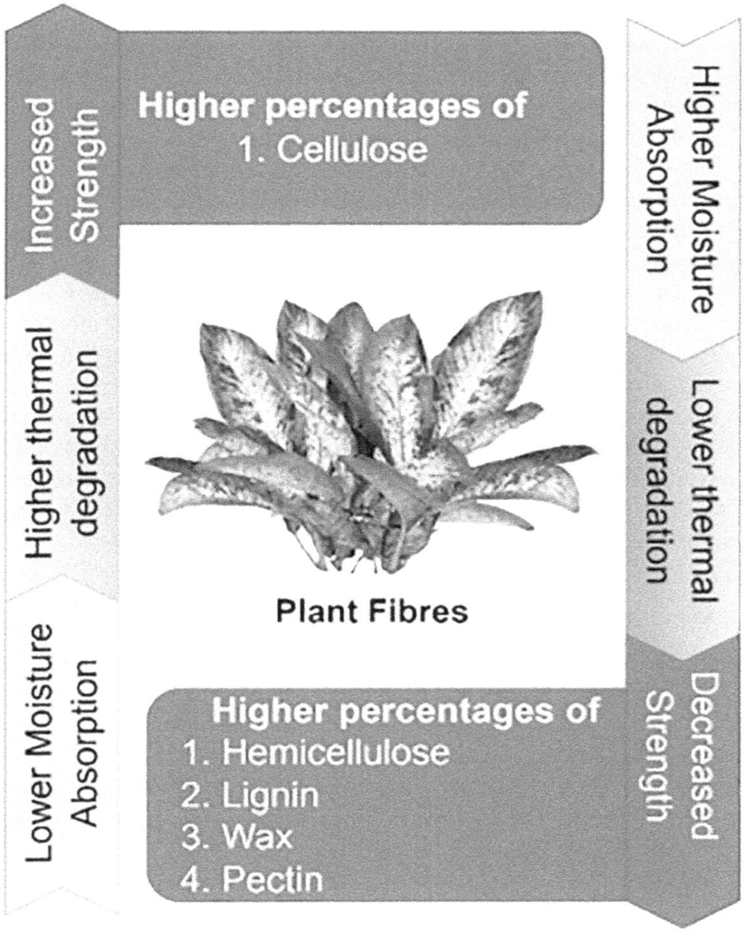

FIGURE 12.12 Chemical components of natural fibers.

Source: Adapted from Gurupranes et al. (2023).

The outcomes demonstrated that the fibrils were mainly composed of cellulose and hemicellulose, with lignin making up only 20% and 60–75% of the weight, respectively. A high percentage of cellulose and hemicellulose led to a 79.4% degree of crystallinity. In addition, compared to the other fiber samples, it displayed superior thermal properties due to its high weight loss (84.15%), low residual weight (15.44%), and high decomposition temperature (364.2°C) (Alotaibi, et al., 2019). The date palm fibrils were also superior in terms of their high weight loss (84.15%), low residual weight (15.44%), and high decomposition temperature (364.2°C). Additionally, date palm biomass's low ash content improved its mechanical and thermal properties when compared to wood pellets, sawdust, and bituminous coal (Hassani et al., 2020). Similar to this, Sreekala et al.'s (2023) study examined the results of pre-treating oil. Oil palm fibers on the final composites' characteristics. The pre-treated fibers had lower moisture and wax concentrations than the untreated fibers, the researchers discovered. Better bonding between the fibers and the matrix material in the composites was the outcome of this decrease in moisture and wax content. The study also discovered that improving the mechanical qualities of the resultant composites was possible by decreasing the percentage of ash in the pre-treated fibers. This implies that oil palm fiber-based composite materials may perform better if ash impurities are removed (Komuraiah et al., 2014).

In a similar vein, some researchers attempted to develop a composite material through the application of a novel variety of plant fiber that experienced surface modifications. Furcraeafoetida is a plant commonly found in the Caribbean and South America. Madival et al. (2022) investigated this plant to see if it could be used as a source of fiber for composite materials. The densities of the raw and chemically treated fibers were measured by the researchers and compared. They discovered that the density of the unprocessed F. foetida was roughly 0.211 g/cm3. But following chemical processing, the fibers' density increased to between 0.228 and 0.362 g/cm3. This density gain is explained by the expansion of the fiber cell walls and the addition of grafted molecules. The mechanical qualities of the fibers were generally improved as a result of these changes to the structure, which suggests that they may find application in composite materials (Z. N. Azwa et al., 2013). Similarly, in order to learn more about the characteristics and possible applications of Arevajavanica fiber, a type of natural fiber that is widely available in Southeast Asia, Ahmed et al. (2019) carried out research on the chemical composition of the fiber. The researchers found that the cellulose content of A. javanica fiber is roughly 72.36 wt %. The fiber's high cellulose content gives it strength and durability. Furthermore, the researchers discovered that wax produces the weak interfacial bonding between the fiber and the matrix and that the fiber contains 10.45 wt % of lignin, which aids in protecting the fiber against biological attack.

12.6.3 Mechanical characteristics

Developing natural fiber composites for structural applications necessitates careful consideration of their mechanical characteristics (Table 12.4), which are crucial for determining the reinforcement of polymer composites. It is desirable to have high cellulose content in the reinforcement to achieve superior mechanical and thermal properties. Improving the mechanical strength of natural fibers can be achieved by modifying their surface, which can reduce their hydrophilic and increase their hydrophobic properties (Todkar et al., 2019).

TABLE 12.4
Mechanical properties of natural fibers

Name of the fiber	Tensile strength (MPa)	Specific strength	Young's modulus (GPA)	Specific Young's Modulus	Failure strain (%)
Abaca	12	–	41	–	3.4
Alfa	350	–	22	–	5.8
Bagasse	290	–	17	–	–
Banana	721.5	534.5	29	22	2
Bamboo	575	383	27	18	–
Coir	140.5	122	6	5.2	27.5
Cotton	500	323	8	5.25	7
Curaua	825	–	9	–	7.5
Flax	700	482.5	60	41	2.3
Hemp	530	360	45	30.5	3
Isora	325	230	37.5	26.5	2.5
Jute	93.3	300	4	12.9	1.2
Kapok	743	–	41	–	–
Kenaf	12	–	41	–	3.4
Pineapple	1020	708.5	71	49.5	0.8
Ramie	925	590	23	15	3.7
Sisal	460	317.5	15.5	–	–

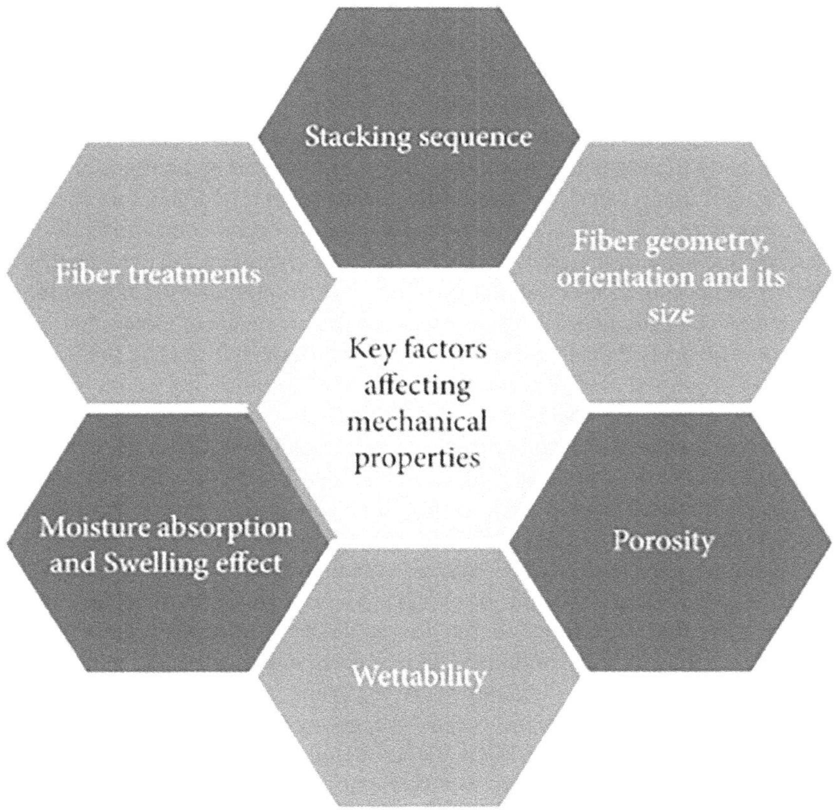

FIGURE 12.13 Key factors affecting mechanical properties of NFRCs.

Source: Adapted from Gurupranes et al. (2023).

Figure 12.13 summarizes some of the key factors affecting the mechanical properties of NFRCs. A novel natural plant fiber from Echinochloafrumentacea was discovered by Rathinavelu and Paramathma et al. (2022). They observed that this fiber had good tensile strength, low density, good crystallinity, and a high cellulose content, which made it suitable for use in a range of temperatures.

It demonstrates that the 60.31% cellulose content created a good fiber-matrix adhesion and surface roughness, resulting in a composite with a higher tensile strength. The tensile strength and tensile modulus of Dioscoreaalata stem fibers treated with NaOH and CH_3COOH, on the other hand, were found to be 151 MPa and 5.7 GPa in the study by Okafor et al. (2022). These values are greater than those of Piliostigmaracemose et al. (2021), Agave americana L. et al. (2014), Juncuseffusus L. et al. (2017), and Kigeliaafricana (2020). This is mostly because of the upkeep temperature of chemical treatment (40 and 60°C) and gauge length (40 and 60 mm). They consequently stated that the fibers treated with NaOH in a dry condition, with a gauge length of 40 mm and a treatment temperature of 60°C, showed improved tensile strength and tensile modulus. Similar to this, Rao et al. (2010) created composites based on banana, bamboo, vakka, and sisal fibers in order to test their tensile strength. They came to the conclusion that, at a fiber volume fraction of 0.37, the tensile strength of vakka fiber composite is comparable to that of bamboo composite and higher than that of sisal and banana composites. The improvement is ascribed to the vakka fiber's superior strength and stronger bonding with the polyester matrix in contrast to sisal and banana. All composites exhibit an increase in tensile modulus with fiber volume fraction along the following bamboo, vakka, banana, and sisal. Because of its lower percentage strain, the tensile modulus of vakka fiber composite is higher than that of sisal and banana composites, and comparable to that of bamboo composite at the same fiber volume fraction. Once more, the goal of Rao et al. was to investigate the tensile properties of fibers extracted from elephant grass using chemical (NaOH) and retting methods. A tensile strength of 237.4 MPa for the retted fiber-based composite and 292.3 MPa for the chemically treated fiber-based composite was obtained by combining up to 31% of the volume of fiber into the composites. The composite consisting of retted fiber and chemically treated fiber differs by approximately 18.1%. The main reason for the retted composite's decreased tensile strength is that the fibers are disastrously extracted from the specimen. Lu et al. (2013) investigated a novel method of combining silane coupling agent and NaOH treatment to improve the mechanical properties of bamboo cellulose fiber/epoxy composites as an extension of mono-chemical treatment. The lignin and amorphous cellulose in the NaOH solution dissolved, causing the fibers to split into smaller sizes. This promoted efficient interfacial adhesion by allowing epoxy resin oligomer to seep into the spaces between the fibers. As a result, the cellulose surface developed chemical bonds Si–O–C and Si–O–Si, which enhanced surface characteristics and raised the composites' tensile strength and elongation break. Similarly, Asim et al. (2013) assessed the mechanical characteristics of hybrid composites made of kenaf phenol formaldehyde and pineapple leaves treated with alkali, silane, and a combination of the two. They noticed that composites with hybridization silane-treated samples showed higher tensile strength, while alkali/silane-treated samples had high interfacial shear strength. Likewise, Dharmalingam et al. (2020) investigated the mechanical properties of luffa/epoxy composites that were functionalized with NaOH at different volume fractions of 2%, 4%, 6%, and 8%. According to their results, the fibers treated with 6 wt % had a significant improvement over untreated fibers in terms of both tensile strength and flexural strength, increasing by 111.5 and 125%, respectively. These findings imply that luffa/epoxy composites' mechanical qualities can be significantly improved by NaOH-amino functionalization, rendering them more appropriate for a range of engineering uses. It is thought that the creation of chemical bonds between the functionalized fibers and the improved mechanical properties strengthens the bond between the two materials as a result of the epoxy resin.

After extracting the fibers, Dawit et al. (2020) used potassium permanganate, stearic acid, benzoyl peroxide, and NaOH to treat them chemically. It was discovered that when the fibers were treated with 20 wt % alkali instead of 10 wt %, their tensile qualities decreased. This result was ascribed to the uneven fiber diameter, with a 25.9% reduction in diameter seen in fibers treated with 20 wt % alkali as opposed to those treated with 10 wt %. The fiber treated with 10 wt % alkali performed better, scoring a tensile strength of 106.81 MPa and a Young's modulus of 6.47 GPa, while the fiber treated with 20 wt % alkali scored a tensile strength of 84.76 MPa and a Young's modulus of 4.10 Pa. However, the Acacia tortilis fiber showed greater tensile performance was better than that of common fibers like ramie fiber (0.3 MPa) and coir fiber (44 MPa), but it was not as strong as the tensile strength of jute fiber (393 MPa). The mechanical characteristics of several natural fibers from different literature sources are shown below.

Similar to tensile strength, Kelly and Tyson's analytical equation was used by Aliotta et al.to determine the interfacial shear strength of short fiber (aspect ratio less than 20) and ultra-short fiber (aspect ratio less than 10)-based NFRCs. They discovered that longer embedding lengths showed better stress transfer with less fluctuation. Because of the distribution of tensions and load transfer mechanisms, short-fiber composites behave mechanically differently from long-fiber composites. Shear stresses at the fiber surfaces—also referred to as edge or end effects—transfer load from the matrix to the fibers. End effects are not significant in long-fiber composites, but they are not to be ignored in short- and very short-fiber composites.

Yan et al.'s study (2016) used alkali-treated coir fibers with varying cross-sectional shapes (circular and noncircular fibers) to create coir/fiber epoxy composites. The researchers discovered that applying a 5% NaOH solution at 20°C for 30 min significantly increased the composite's tensile strength, modulus, flexural strength, fracture energy, and fracture toughness by 17.8%, 6.9%, 16.7%,

7.4%, 550%, and 424%, respectively, in comparison to untreated composites. This is because the fibers' surface became much rougher and cleaner after the alkali treatment. The enhancement of the interfacial adhesion between the epoxy and the fiber is responsible for the reduction in damping ratio and improvement in tensile and flexural properties. This study clearly shows that cross-sectional shapes affect the composite's mechanical properties as well. In a similar vein, Sutradhar et al.'s study (2018) shows that fiber weight ratios also significantly improve mechanical characteristics. Composite materials were made from pp mixed with banana/betelnut fibers in various weight ratios (1:1, 3:1, and 1:3) using a hot-pressing technique. Depending on whether the composite material had been treated, the specimens were split into two groups. The tensile and flexural strength of the composite was enhanced by treating the fibers with 5% NaOH and using a volume proportion of 3:1, according to the results. Conversely, untreated composite materials displayed damage to the fiber structure, including a decrease in the tensile properties due to a rise in deep pores and thinning of the fiber cell walls. These damages might have been brought on by the presence of foreign substrates. The stacking order of composites affects their mechanical properties in addition to chemical treatment and fiber weight ratios. The effect of stacking order on the mechanical properties of jute and hemp hybrid composites was examined in a study by Vinod et al. (2022). With comparable patterns seen in the flexural results, the hemp/jute/hemp hybrid composite demonstrated the highest tensile strength of 65.44 MPa. The study also showed that jute fiber can be used as the core layer and hemp fiber as the skin layer during the hybridization process. This results in a decrease in interlaminar shear strength but an increase in tensile and flexural strength. Hence, a number of variables, such as chemical treatment, fiber weight ratios, and stacking order, affect the mechanical properties of NFRCs. The composites' tensile strength, flexural strength, and interlaminar shear strength are all significantly influenced by these variables. Thus, for the purpose of maximizing the mechanical performance of NFRCs in diverse applications, a comprehensive comprehension of these factors is imperative.

12.7 ROLE OF BIOPOLYMERS

Biopolymers have the ability to enhance the biological activity of other molecules in a product since they are biocompatible and biodegradable. Additionally, they are adaptable to fit a range of possible uses, such as the following.

12.7.1 Sustainability

Chemicals such as additives are frequently added to plastic to improve its qualities, although doing so has an adverse effect on the environment. Reducing the chemical diversity of the plastic is a sustainable method of manufacturing it. Plastic microparticles are typically dispersed throughout the ecosystem by organisms or by forces of nature such as wind, water, birds, or other creatures. They can occasionally obstruct drains and gutters, resulting in issues with water and sewage. Large-scale atmospheric littering is the cause of numerous health problems, including fatalities and injuries to creatures as a result of ingesting microparticles that they wrongly believe to be food. For example, employing low-quality, single-use items or recyclable bags made of natural fibers can help lessen the severity of its detrimental effects. The concept of sustainability satisfies a few fundamentally positive ideas with non-toxic behavior and environmental safety issues. The product's hazardous ingredients can lead to a host of grave issues, including poor workstation surroundings and air quality. A suitable sustainable product needs to satisfy the need for a safe environment for the users. When it comes to bioplastic, farmers cultivate the plants, which manufacturers then polymerize and transform into the finished product. This process is then carried out by the product's transportation to retailers and wholesalers, where it is obtained by consumers. Composting and recycling that don't leave any pollutants behind are end-of-life solutions that preserve the sustainability of nature's equilibrium (Chang et al., 2016).

12.7.2 Plastic waste in India

The country, which is the third-largest producer of polymers worldwide, generates millions of tons of plastic garbage annually as a result of its vast population. Each person produces about 4.38 pounds of plastic garbage. Because of the way plastic doesn't biodegrade, disposing of it has become a big issue. Large-scale plastic recycling is comparatively expensive due to a number of issues, including time-consuming procedures and the need for collection, sorting, transportation, cleaning, and processing. All of the waste is dumped directly into landfills, where it builds up and fills up available space before reacting with water to create dangerous chemicals. Because PET bottles are non-returnable and 80% of Indians sell their own local brands, the country's PET bottle waste has surged significantly.

As per the Swedish Society of Nature Conservation Research, the majority of plastic bottles contain BPA (Bisphenol), which can lead to health problems such as uterine infections and cancer. When water in PE bags is left in them for extended periods of time during the rainy season, diseases like malaria can spread, accounting for almost 50% of pollution in India. When roadside plastic and trash are consumed by street animals, such as cows and bulls, it causes constipation and ultimately death. According to studies, the stomachs of cows and other street animals have been discovered to contain between 30 and 60 kg of plastic garbage. Mumbai, one of the biggest cities in India, discards 3 billion polyethylene bags annually. In 2005, a flood occurred, and the cause was the snaking of plastic bags in the drainage system (Chen et al., 2019).

12.7.3 Method of recycling plastics in India

In India, there are three typical methods for getting rid of plastic waste: littering, incineration, and recycling. The recycling industry is underdeveloped, and the majority of recyclers do not have valid registrations, which allow them to circumvent laws pertaining to worker safety, minimum wage, and taxes. These are illegal and unethical employment circumstances for children. The majority of these recycling industries are manual and operated based on years of experience. When recycling plastic, the first step is to wash the products in soapy water to get rid of all the dirt. After being used repeatedly, the soapy water is directly poured into the drainage system without being treated, which leads to highly contaminated water and more waterborne illnesses. The water must first undergo adequate treatment before being dumped into an open drainage system.

Effects of recycling: Recycling is carried out by unorganized tiny sectors of the economy. Most of the time, illiterate individuals who need money for basic needs such as women, small children, and others work in these facilities. People are sorting and segregating plastics with their bare hands in these regions; therefore, safety precautions are desperately needed. Due to inadequate ventilation, recycled pellets produce a lot of dust during the extrusion process in an enclosed room during recycling, which causes respiratory issues for the workers. One of the hottest countries in the world, India has summer temperatures of up to 50 degrees. Working in such a high temperature with potentially explosive and hazardous chemicals can lead to serious issues, such as lung cancer from constant exposure to carbon black dust, which is inhaled by workers during extraction and deposits itself in their lungs. Government enforcement of appropriate laws and regulations is crucial, as is educating the public about environmental dangers and safety precautions (Jaya Baranwal et al., 2022; Gopal Rao et al., 2014).

12.7.4 3 R's—Reduce, reuse, and recycle

A single plastic bottle will take over 450 years to decompose entirely, according to the findings. It is crucial to recycle plastic for additional beneficial uses. One such usage is to use empty water bottles in indoor flower pots to contain pencils and toothbrushes. Reusing and cutting back on plastic products can help reduce pollution over time. Buyers are required to bring their own reusable fabric bags from home when they go shopping instead of utilizing PE bags. The poly bags are disposable plastic carrying bags that are frequently used again for various additional home uses. It is simple to recycle plastic in factories and businesses, for instance, when a machine produces a lot of goods together with some defective pieces because of pressure, heat, and temperature. Shredders are employed concurrently to recycle those pieces back into granules for future use. To create power, the wasted plastic garbage in municipal waste is gathered in mixed waste and then crushed further.

Procedure: Before the waste is fed into the incinerator boiler, waste cranes in the waste bunker mix it into a uniformly sized mass for at least a week. Through the process of combustion, waste is transformed into energy in the boiler. There have been multiple recoveries of the fly ash from the trash left behind. When "flue gas", which is released during the burning of garbage, combines with lime, it absorbs toxic gases like carbon dioxide and sulfur dioxide. Steam is produced at a temperature of about 320°C by transferring the heat recovered from the flue gases into the district heating water, also known as recycled heat (Emna Chaabouni et al., 2021; Rahul Singh et al., 2014).

12.8 APPLICATIONS WITH HIGH PERFORMANCE

Research focusing mainly on cellulose fiber has investigated the application of lignocellulosic fibers in bioplastics. Raw lignocellulosic fibers have garnered increased interest in bioplastics in recent years (Zhang et al., 2022). The development of high-performance polymeric and composite materials may soon be able to overcome the application challenges of these substantial materials, particularly with regard to their economic viability, in a manner similar to how the use of biomass has advanced. Certain agrobusiness sectors would benefit financially from this development, especially the biofuels sector, which produces a lot of biomass waste (Liu et al., 2016). Polyvinyl alcohol, or PVA, is a biodegradable polymer that has gained popularity as a viable replacement for non-biodegradable petrochemical counterparts in an effort to lessen the environmental impact of the food and pharmaceutical industries. The potential of lignocellulosic cellulose nanofibrils (LCNF) as an inexpensive, multipurpose additive that enhances PVA's qualities for packaging applications is considerable (Zhang et al., 2022). In the current climate, rechargeable energy storage systems are also in high demand. High-performance supercapacitors use activated porous carbon as an excellent electrode material because it is made from biowaste materials based on lignocellulose (Mondal, 2020). This also illustrated the flexible electronics' high mechanical strength, affordability, and sustainability. It was discovered and demonstrated in a study published in Gurupranes et al. (2023) that LCNF are a renewable and durable substrate that can be used to develop appropriate, highly delicate senses.

12.8.1 Natural fibers' innate capabilities for sound absorption

Researchers have created safe, affordable, and easily designed polymeric fibrous materials, both natural and synthetic, to reduce noise in theaters and recording rooms (Wang et al., 2001). Researchers are particularly interested in natural fibers because they are recyclable, biodegradable, and derived from plants or animals. These fibrous materials' primary sources of sound absorption are thermal losses from heat transfer between fibers and viscous effects from friction between air molecules and the pore wall. Using smaller fiber diameters and lower fiber densities can enhance the sound absorption performance.

Cellulose, hemicellulose, and lignin make up the general structure of fibrils made from natural fibers; these components can be further processed to enhance sound absorption. Microfibrils can be produced by converting unprocessed plant fibers into finer fibrils formed, leading to more intricate channels and smaller pores that improve sound energy absorption. This can be accomplished by beating the fibers with hammers or other external forces (Ulrich et al., 2020). NFRCs have historically only been used in structural applications, but as the problem of noise pollution has grown, industry and researchers are now using these materials to reduce noise in the surrounding industrial and residential areas, as Figure 12.14 illustrates.

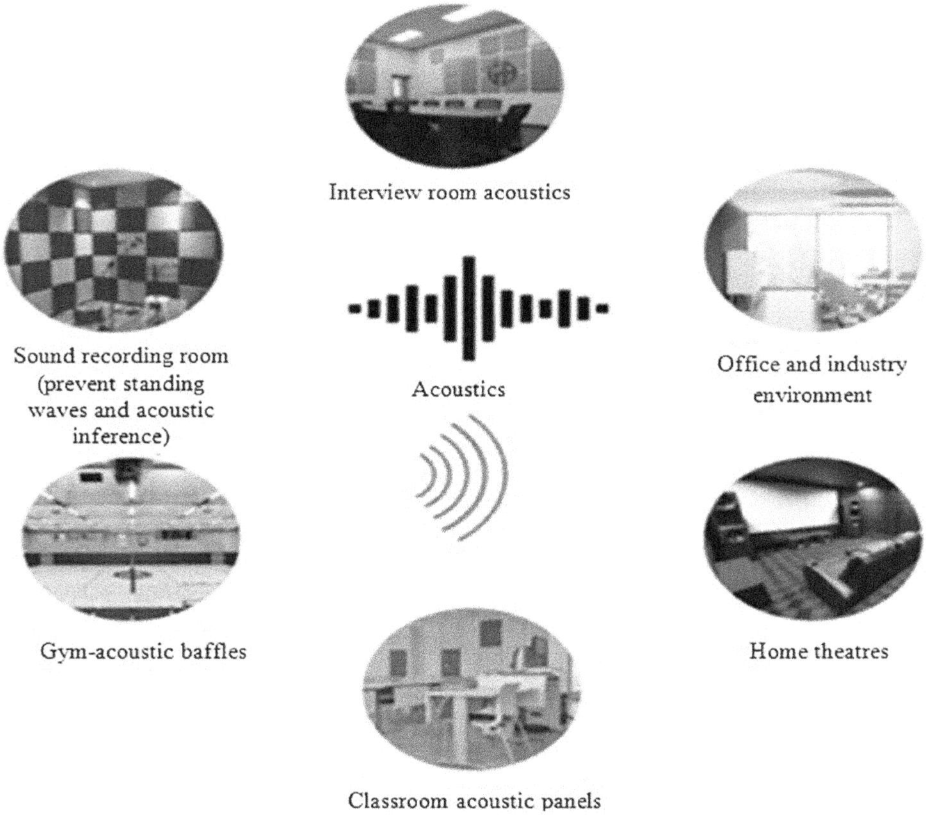

FIGURE 12.14 Application of natural fiber in soundproofing.

Source: Adapted from Gurupranes et al. (2023).

There are currently three types of sound absorption panels in use: single-layer, multi-layer, and sandwich, which have corrugation and honeycomb as the core and low- to medium-density insulators as layers.

Numerous researchers have made various attempts to maximize natural fibers' capacity to absorb sound and to do away with the usage of artificial, non-biodegradable sound-absorbing materials (Asdrubali et al., 2012). In the field of sustainable material development, research on natural fiber-based sound-absorbing materials is emerging.

12.8.2 Organic materials in ballistics

Threats involving firearms have significantly impacted human existence, especially for combatants and active military personnel. A system called the multilayer armor system (MAS) successfully repels a variety of threats. Previously, bulletproof jackets were made of synthetic materials like Kevlar fibers and aluminum. Currently, NFRCs are used in MAS as an additional layer. Pineapple leaf fiber was used in a ballistic analysis by da Luz et al. (2020). The purpose of blending Dyneema plate with Kevlar level IIIA ballistic protective layer vests is to add extra protection. The results of this study show that, in compliance with the international standard for level III security established by the National Institute of Justice (NIJ), this degree of ballistic protection proved effective against 7.62 mm rifle ammunition. Similar to this, Nurazzi et al. (2020) used 7.62 mm bullets to conduct ballistics tests in accordance with NIJ Standard class III and came to the conclusion that composites made with polyester-reinforced woven jute used as a second layer satisfied the ballistic standard requirements. The third layer of aluminum alloy was unable to puncture due to the presence of the jute polyester composite, creating a small indentation in the clay record. As previously mentioned, they also performed the same test using Curaua fiber (Monteiro et al., 2015) in place of woven jute. It was found in this study that the polyester or epoxy matrix composite reinforced with 30 vol.%. Compared to standard aramid fabric plies with an Al2O3 ceramic coat, curaua fiber performed better (it can withstand high-velocity 7.62 mm bullets). The ballistic performance of NFRCs manufactured from cassava fiber was evaluated by Filho et al. (2019). Ballistics testing was conducted using 7.62 mm ammunition, and the composites were created using a 10–50 vol.% mixture. The outcomes showed that piassava fiber composite-based MASs offer sufficient protection. This demonstrates how effectively armor systems can make use of piassava fiber, a sustainable material. Research into a new class of natural fibers is currently very active. The relatively new class of natural fiber known as "Cyperusmalaccensis". De et al. (2020) was studied by Neuba et al. It is a type of sedge fiber that is already used in paper, ropes, and furniture. In a similar vein, the potential of Vernoniaelaeagnifolia and Argyreiaspeciosa waste as waste-to-market products was examined by Shaker et al. (2020).

12.8.3 Performance of Natural Fiber Composite in Crashworthiness

When designing automotive components, crashworthiness is a critical factor because it indicates how well a structure will be able to protect its occupants from death or serious injury in the event of a crash of a certain size.

The energy absorption failure mode, which permits a progressive decline in the load-displacement curve during the energy absorption of structures, determines a vehicle's crashworthiness. Numerous energy-absorbing factors, such as total absorbed energy (EA), specific energy absorption (SEA), peak force (PF), and SEA per unit volume (SEAV), influence crashworthiness characteristics. Figure 12.15 displays various parameters that influence the crashworthiness parameters.

Equation (1) illustrates that the most important parameter to compare the energy absorption of the structures is the SEA, which establishes the energy absorption per unit mass of the absorber.

$$SEA = \frac{E_a}{m}, \tag{1}$$

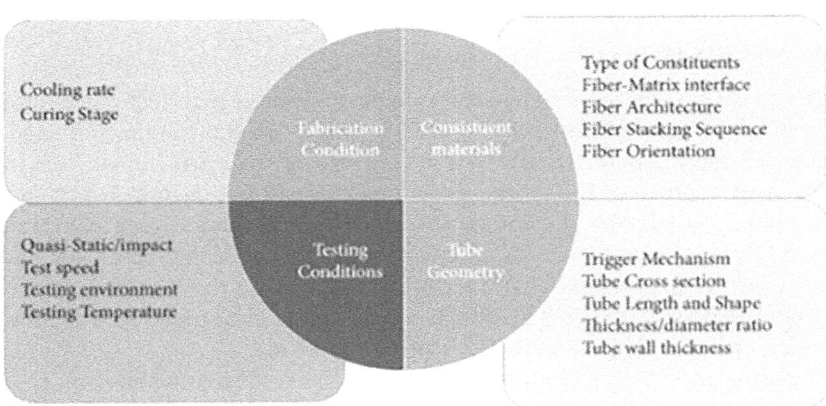

FIGURE 12.15 Factors influencing crashworthiness parameters of NFRCs.

Source: Adapted from Gurupranes et al. (2023).

where, as indicated by Equation (2), m denotes energy absorption during a crash, and E_a is the total energy absorption. Ea can be used to calculate the total energy.

$$E_a = \int_0^d f(x)dx, \tag{2}$$

where the impact force and displacements are denoted by d and f, respectively.

Energy-absorbing capacity controls the rate at which energy disperses during auto collisions. As a result, good crashworthy vehicle collision structures have low PF, high SEA, SEAV, and EA values. It was also discovered that a key factor in improved energy-absorbing capability was the thickness of the tube wall. Generally, quasi-static compression loading is applied in both the axial and lateral directions to conduct crushing tests. In a hydraulic press, natural fiber reinforced concrete tubes are compressed between steel plates at low crosshead speeds, typically ranging from 1 to 20 mm/s. Natural fiber can absorb energy more efficiently than metals, according to a number of studies (Eshkoor et al., 2015). Natural fibers like hemp, jute, silk, and kenaf can fracture instead of deform to absorb energy, in contrast to metal tubing (Ahmad et al., 2023) under axial crushing conditions (Sivagurunathan, 2018).

Several natural fiber failure modes, such as delamination, bending, and local buckling, have been found by Ude et al. (2017) to significantly contribute to energy absorption. Similarly, Wũcławski et al. (2014) investigated the crashworthiness properties of hemp/epoxy composite tubes under quasi-static axial loading through experimentation with various winding directions, such as 10°, 20°, 30°, 60°, and 90°. They discovered that fiber orientation with a 10° orientation showed superior energy absorption with four distinct collapse modes, which are progressive crushing, concertina, diamond shape buckling, and micro buckling. Similar to this, Yan and Chouw L. Yan et al. (2013) assessed the crushing properties under various tube geometries, such as tube thickness, inner diameter, and length-to-diameter ratio, and found that tube geometry significantly impacted superior energy absorption. Using a conical inner core and a circular outer core, Attia et al. (2018) found that this configuration demonstrates superior energy absorption with a low peak load. Eshkoor et al. (2013) presented the trigger mechanism in reference to earlier research in order to examine the axial crushing of silk/epoxy composite tubes. They stated that progressive failures like buckling and delamination have happened along with failure mechanisms like tear onset and tear propagation. To obtain the best impact performance, a suitable material component paired with appropriate tube geometry and triggering mechanism is required (Gao et al. 2022).

12.8.4 Examination of Life Cycle Assessment

Life cycle assessment (LCA) was used to quantify input and output within the functional inventory unit's organizational structure in order to evaluate the environmental sustainability and durability. The environmental impacts were assessed, and the lifecycle analysis and computation were carried out using the Simapro software. The ISO supports a number of LCA methodologies, including ISO 14040, 14041, 14042, and 14043. Determining the ecological effects of harmful elements such as radiation, greenhouse gas emissions, ecotoxicity, climate change, carcinogens, and acidification/eutrophication is part of the process. This is accomplished by using the Intergovernmental Panel on Climate Change guidelines (Shaker et al., 2022) to define functional units, system boundaries, life cycle inventories, and modes of transportation (see Figure 12.16).

When comparing the LCA of synthetic and natural fibers, Navaratnam et al. (2023) discovered that bio-based fiber had lower environmental impacts and lower energy consumption than petroleum-based products. Similar to this, Gupta et al. (2022) introduced green tags that can be applied to specific materials based on a number of criteria, including green manufacturing and the path the material takes to reach the end of its life cycle. Similarly, Ahmad et al.'s analysis Gupta

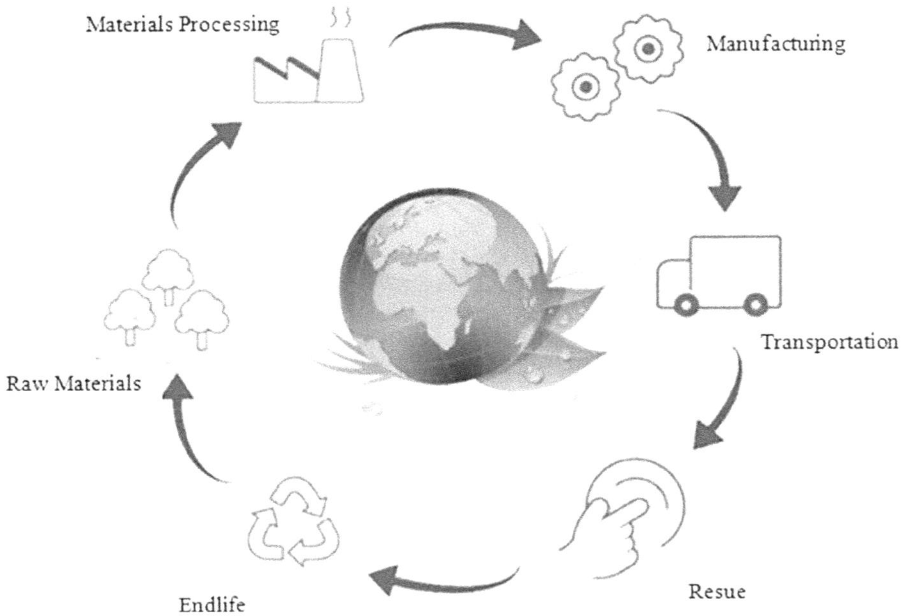

FIGURE 12.16 LCA analysis.

Source: Adapted from Gurupranes et al. (2023).

et al. (2022) of LCA using synthetic and natural fiber revealed that biofiber uses 55% less energy than synthetic materials. Because of this, the environmental footprint of plant-based bio-fiber processing needs to be measured, important environmental factors need to be found, and systems need to be optimized in order to minimize overall effects as well as the expected effects on the environment of supply chain and manufacturing process improvements.

12.9 CONCLUSION

Environmental issues arise from the landfill disposal of biowaste because of the significant amount of CO_2 and NH_3 produced. Given the waste's high sugar, carbohydrate, and cellulose content, the best course of action is to use bacterial fermentation to convert it into an environmentally beneficial and economically viable industrial product. The mutagenesis approach can be used to transform biomass into environmentally beneficial biofuel, biogas, and bio-oil. Due to their high cost, the usage of bioplastics over conventional plastics is limited; however, there are a number of additional ways to economically create bioplastics from biomass feedstock. Because biopolymers are sustainable, their market is expected to grow greatly in the future. Because inorganic resources like petroleum and other mineral sources are running out, green materials are becoming more and more important. Consequently, taking into account the requirements of each type of transportation, replacing the current biocomposite materials with lightweight, recyclable, and renewable materials can satisfy the growing needs for sustainability in the transportation industry. Notwithstanding their many advantages, there are still a number of issues surrounding the usage of biopolymers that need to be resolved. These issues include their sensitivity to water, their expense, and the possibility of biological degradation. All things considered, the use of biopolymers in geotechnical engineering seems to have a bright future because of the large range of biopolymers that are currently accessible, the flexibility with which they may be modified, and the many positive features that they possess. Biopolymers are used to create a range of composites and nanocomposites. Applications for these polymers include biomedical, tissue engineering, automotive, and packaging. Different biopolymers have a wide range of usage in various applications. As a result, biopolymers will be crucial to meeting future demands in human life.

REFERENCES

N.Z. Abd Aziz and R. Mohamed, "Comparison of melt flow and mechanical properties of rice husk and kenaf hybrid composites," *Advanced Materials Research*, vol. 701, pp. 42–46, 2013. https://doi.org/10.4028/www.scientific.net/AMR.701.42

J. Aggarwal, S. Sharma, H. Kamyab, and A. Kumar, "The realm of biopolymers and their usage: An overview," *Journal of Environmental Treatment Techniques*, vol. 8 no. 2, pp. 1005–1016, 2020.

A. Ahmad, A. Moeed, A. Tariq et al., "Effect of hybridization approach on mechanical performance of jute-hemp/epoxy hybrid composite laminates," *Journal of Natural Fibers*, vol. 19, pp. 14449–14460, 2022. https://doi.org/10.1080/15440478.2022.2064398

J. Ahmed, M.A. Balaji, S.S. Saravanakumar, and P. Senthamaraikannan, "A comprehensive physical, chemical and morphological characterization of novel cellulosic fiber extracted from the stem of Elettariacardamomum plant," *Journal of Natural Fibers*, vol. 18, pp. 1460–1471, 2021. https://doi.org/10.1080/15440478.2019.1691121

M.J. Ahmed, M.S. Balaji, S.S. Saravanakumar et al., "Characterization of Arevajavanica fiber – a possible replacement for synthetic acrylic fiber in the disc brake pad," *Journal of Industrial Textiles*, vol. 49, pp. 294–317, 2019. https://doi.org/10.1177/1528083718779446

L. Aliotta and A. Lazzeri, "A proposal to modify the Kelly-Tyson equation to calculate the interfacial shear strength (IFSS) of composites with low aspect ratio fibers," *Composites Science and Technolnology*, vol. 186, p. 107920, 2020. https://doi.org/10.1016/j.compscitech.2019.107920

T. Alomayri, F.U.A. Shaikh, and I.M. Low, "Characterisation of cotton fibre-reinforced geopolymer composites," *Composites Part B: Engineering*, vol. 50, pp. 1–6, 2013. https://doi.org/10.1016/j.compositesb.2013.01.013

M.D. Alotabi, B.A. Alshammari, N. Saba et al., "Microcrystalline cellulose from fruit bunch stalk of date palm: Isolation and characterization," *Journal of Polymers and the Environment*, vol. 28, pp. 1766–1775, 2020. https://doi.org/10.1007/s10924-020-01725-8

M.D. Alotaibi, B.A. Alshammari, N. Saba et al., "Characterization of natural fiber obtained from different parts of date palm tree (Phoenix dactylifera L.)," *International Journal of Biological Macromolecules*, vol. 135, pp. 69–76, 2019. https://doi.org/10.1016/j.ijbiomac.2019.05.102

Ö. Andiç-Çakir, M. Sarikanat, H.B. Tüfekçi et al., "Physical and mechanical properties of randomly oriented coir fiber–cementitious composites," *Composites Part B: Engineering*, vol. 61, pp. 49–54, 2014. https://doi.org/10.1016/j.compositesb.2014.01.029

R. ArunRamnath, S. Murugan, M.R. Sanjay et al., "Characterization of novel natural cellulosic fibers from Abutilon indicum for potential reinforcement in polymer composites," *Polymer Composites*, vol. 44, pp. 340–355, 2023. https://doi.org/10.1002/pc.27100

R.B. Ashok, C.v. Srinivasa, and B. Basavaraju, "Study on morphology and mechanical behavior of areca leaf sheath reinforced epoxy composites," *Advanced Composites and Hybrid Materials*, vol. 3, pp. 365–374, 2020. https://doi.org/10.1007/s42114-020-00169-x

M. Asim, M. Jawaid, K. Abdan, and M.R. Ishak, "Effect of alkali and silane treatments on mechanical and fibre-matrix bond strength of kenaf and pineapple leaf fibres," *Journal of Bionic Engineering*, vol. 13, pp. 426–435, 2016. https://doi.org/10.1016/S1672-6529(16)60315-3

Z.N. Azwa, B.F. Yousif, A.C. Manalo, and W. Karunasena, "A review on the degradability of polymeric composites based on natural fibres," *Materials & Design*, vol. 47, pp. 424–442, 2013. https://doi.org/10.1016/j.matdes.2012.11.025

R.P. Babu, K. O'Connor, and R. Seeram, "Current progress on bio-based polymers and their future trends," *Progress in Biomaterials*, vol. 2, no. 8, pp. 1–16, 2013. https://doi.org/10.1186/2194-0517-2-8

B.G. Babu, D. Princewinston, S.S. Saravanakumar et al., "Investigation on the physicochemical and mechanical properties of novel alkali-treated Phaseolus vulgaris fibers," *Journal of Natural Fibers*, vol. 19, pp. 770–781, 2020. https://doi.org/10.1080/15440478.2020.1761930

R. Balart, D. Garcia-Garcia, V. Fombuena, L. Quiles-Carrillo, and M.P. Arrieta, "Biopolymers from natural resources," *Polymers*, vol. 13, p. 2532, 2021. https://doi.org/10.3390/polym13152532

E. Banachowicz, J. Gapinski, and A. Patkowski. "Solution structure of biopolymers: A new method of constructing a bead model," *Biophysical Journal*, vol. 78, pp. 70–78, 2000. https://doi.org/10.1016/S0006-3495(00)76573-8

J. Baranwal, B. Barse, A. Fais, G.L. Delogu, and A. Kumar, "Biopolymer: A sustainable material for food and medical applications," *Polymers (Basel)*, vol. 14, no. 5, p. 983, 2022 Mar. https://doi.org/10.3390/polym14050983

B.J.D. Barba, J.F. Madrid, D.P. Penaloza Jr. et al., "A review of abaca fiber-reinforced polymer composites: Different modes of preparation and their applications," *Journal of the Chilean Chemical Society*, vol. 65, pp. 4919–4924, 2020.

D.F. Barbin, N.A. Valous, A.P. Dias, J. Camisa, E.Y. Hirooka, and F. Yamashita, "VIS–NIR spectroscopy as a process analytical technology for compositional characterization of film biopolymers and correlation with their mechanical properties," *Materials Science of Engineering: C Materials Biological Application*, vol. 56, pp. 274–279, 2015. https://doi.org/10.1016/j.msec.2015.06.029

M.M. Bashar and M.A. Khan, "An overview on surface modification of cotton fiber for apparel use," *Journal of Polymers and the Environment*, vol. 21, pp. 181–190, 2013. https://doi.org/10.1007/s10924-012-0476-8

M. Beroual, L. Boumaza, O. Mehelli et al., "Physicochemical properties and thermal stability of microcrystalline cellulose isolated from Esparto grass using different delignification approaches," *Journal of Polymers and the Environment*, vol. 29, pp. 130–142, 2021. https://doi.org/10.1007/s10924-020-01858-w

A.B. Bevitori, I.L.A. da Silva, F.P.D. Lopes, and S.N. Monteiro, "Diameter dependence of tensile strength by Weibull analysis: Part II jute fiber," *Matéria*, vol. 15, pp. 117–123, 2010. https://doi.org/10.1590/S1517-70762010000200005

A. Bezazi, A. Belaadi, M. Bourchak et al., "Novel extraction techniques, chemical and mechanical characterisation of Agave americana L. natural fibres," *Composites Part B: Engineering*, vol. 66, pp. 194–203, 2014. https://doi.org/10.1016/j.compositesb.2014.05.014

J.S. Binoj, R.E. Raj, and S. Indran, "Characterization of industrial discarded fruit wastes (TamarindusIndica L.) as potential alternate for man-made vitreous fiber in polymer composites," *Process Safety and Environmental Protection*, vol. 116, pp. 527–534, 2018. https://doi.org/10.1016/j.psep.2018.02.019

R.K Bista, R.F Brucha, and A.M Covingtona. "Infrared spectroscopic study of thermotropic phase behavior of newly developed synthetic biopolymers," *SpectrochimActa Part A*, vol. 81, pp. 583– 589, 2011. https://doi.org/10.1016/j.saa.2011.06.055

B. Blicharska, H. Peemoeller, and M. Witek. "Hydration water dynamics in biopolymers from NMR relaxation in the rotating frame," *Journal of Magnetic Resonance*, vol. 207, no. 2, pp. 287–293. https://doi.org/10.1016/j.jmr.2010.09.012

J.Z. Bozell and G.R. Petersen. "Technology development for the production of biobased products from biorefinery carbohydrates—The US Department of Energy's "Top 10" revisited," *Green Chemistry,* vol. 12, pp. 539–554, 2010. https://doi.org/10.1039/B922014C

L. Calucci, L. Galleschi, M. Geppi, and G. Mollica, "Structure and dynamics of flour by solid state NMR: Effects of hydration and wheat aging," *Biomacromolecules*, vol. 5, pp. 1536–1544, 2004. https://doi.org/10.1021/bm0499177

E. Chaabouni, F. Gassara, and S.K. Brar, "Biopolymers synthesis and application," *Biotransformation of Waste Biomass into High Value Biochemicals*, 415–443, 2014. https://doi.org/10.1007/978-1-4614-8005-1

I. Chang, J. Im, and G.-C. Cho, "Introduction of microbial biopolymers in soil treatment for future environmentally-friendly and sustainable geotechnical engineering," *Sustainability*, vol. 8, pp. 251, 2016. https://doi.org/10.3390/su8030251

C. Chen, L. Wu, M. Perdjon, X. Huang, and Y. Peng, "The drying effect on xanthan gum biopolymer treated sandy soil shear strength," *Construction Building Materials*, vol. 197, pp. 271–279, 2019. https://doi.org/10.1016/j.conbuildmat.2018.11.120

C.J. Chirayil, J. Joy, L. Mathew et al., "Isolation and characterization of cellulose nanofibrils from Helicteresisora plant," *Industrial Crops and Products*, vol. 59, pp. 27–34, 2014. https://doi.org/10.1016/j.indcrop.2014.04.020

S. Chokshi, V. Parmar, P. Gohil, and V. Chaudhary, "Chemical composition and mechanical properties of natural fibers," *Journal of Natural Fibers*, vol. 19, pp. 3942–3953, 2020. https://doi.org/10.1080/15440478.2020.1848738

R. Dalmis Serhan Köktas Köktas, Y.C. Seki Ahmet, R. Kılınç et al., "Characterization of a new natural cellulose based fiber from HierochloeOdarata," *Cellulose*, vol. 27, pp. 127–139, 2020. https://link.springer.com/article/10.1007/s10570-019-02779-1

R. Dash, M. Foston, and A.J. Ragauskas, "Improving the mechanical and thermal properties of gelatin hydrogels cross-linked by cellulose nanowhiskers," *CarbohyPolym*, vol. 91, no. 2 pp. 638–645, 2013. https://doi.org/10.1016/j.carbpol.2012.08.080

P. Davies, C. Morvan, O. Sire, and C. Baley, "Structure and properties of fibres from sea-grass (Zostera marina)," *Journal of Materials Science*, vol. 42, pp. 4850–4857, 2007. https://doi.org/10.1007/s10853-006-0546-1

J.B. Dawit, Y. Regassa, and H.G. Lemu, "Property characterization of Acacia tortilis for natural fiber reinforced polymer composite," *Results in Materials*, 2020, 5, 100054. https://doi.org/10.1016/j.rinma.2019.100054

S.F. De A, N. Chawla, and F.R. De T, "Tensile behavior of high performance natural (sisal) fibers," *Composites Science and Technolnology*, vol. 68, pp. 3438–3443, 2008. https://doi.org/10.1016/j.compscitech.2008.10.001

M.W. De NDR, I.P. Salgado, and F.A. Silva, "The influence of fiber treatment on the morphology, water absorption capacity and mechanical behavior of curauá fibers," *Journal of Natural Fibers*, vol. 19, pp. 642–657, 2020. https://doi.org/10.1080/15440478.2020.1758863

I.M. de Rosa, J.M. Kenny, M. Maniruzzaman et al., "Effect of chemical treatments on the mechanical and thermal behaviour of okra (Abelmoschusesculentus) fibres," *Composites Science and Technolnology*, vol. 71, pp. 246–254, 2011. https://doi.org/10.1016/j.compscitech.2010.11.023

I.M. de Rosa, C. Santulli, and F. Sarasini, "Mechanical and thermal characterization of epoxy composites reinforced with random and quasi-unidirectional untreated Phormiumtenax leaf fibers," *Materials & Design*, vol. 31, pp. 2397–2405, 2010. https://doi.org/10.1016/j.matdes.2009.11.059

S. Dharmalingam, O. Meenakshisundaram, V. Elumalai, and R.S. Boopathy, "An investigation on the interfacial adhesion between amine functionalized luffa fiber and epoxy resin and its effect on thermal and mechanical properties of their composites," *Journal of Natural Fibers*, vol. 18, pp. 2254–2269, 2020. https://doi.org/10.1080/15440478.2020.1726238

D. Divya, I. Suyambulingam, M.R. Sanjay, and S. Siengchin, "Suitability examination of novel cellulosic plant fiber from Furcraeaselloa K. Koch peduncle for a potential polymeric composite reinforcement," *Polymer Composites*, vol. 43, pp. 4223–4243, 2022. https://doi.org/10.1002/pc.26683

M. Elkington, D. Bloom, C. Ward et al., "Hand layup: Understanding the manual process," *Advanced Manufacturing: Polymer and Composites Science*, vol. 1, pp. 138–151, 2015. https://doi.org/10.1080/20550340.2015.1114801

A.M. Fairuz, S.M. Sapuan, E.S. Zainudin, and C.N.A. Jaafar, "Effect of filler loading on mechanical properties of pultrudedkenaffibre reinforced vinyl ester composites," *Journal of Mechanical Engineering and Sciences*, vol. 10, pp. 1931–1942, 2016. https://doi.org/10.1016/j.jmrt.2020.11.103

V. Flaris and G. Singh, "Recent developments in biopolymers," *Journal of Vinyl & Additive Technology*, pp. 1–11, 2009. https://doi.org/10.1002/vnl.20171

C.G. Flores-Hernández, A. Colin-Cruz, C. Velasco-Santos, V.M Castano, J.L. Rivera-Armenta, A. Almendarez-Camarillo, P.E. García-Casillas, and A.L. Martinez-Hernandez. "All green composites from fully renewable biopolymers: Chitosan-starch reinforced with keratin from feathers," *Polymers*, vol. 6, pp. 686–705, 2014. https://doi.org/10.3390/polym6030686

E. Fortunati, D. Puglia, M. Monti et al., "Extraction of cellulose nanocrystals from Phormiumtenaxfibres," *Journal of Polymers and the Environment*, vol. 21, pp. 319–328, 2013. https://doi.org/10.1007/s10924-012-0543-1

R.V. Gadhave, P.A. Mahanwar, and P.T. Gadekar, "Starch-based adhesives for wood/wood composite bonding: Review," *Open Journal of Polymer Chemistry*, vol. 7, pp. 19–32, 2017. https://doi.org/10.4236/ojpchem.2017.72002

W. Ghori, N. Saba, M. Jawaid, and M. Asim, "A review on date palm (phoenix dactylifera) fibers and its polymer composites," *IOP Conference Series: Materials Science and Engineering*, vol. 368, p. 12009, 2018. https://doi.org/10.1088/1757-899X/368/1/012009

M. GopalRao, P. Bharathi, and RM. Akila, "A comprehensive review on biopolymers," *Scientific Reviews & Chemical Communication*, vol. 4, no. 2, pp. 61–68, 2014.

S.V. Gurupranes, I. Rajendran, S. Gokulkumar, M. Aravindh, S. Sathish, and M. Elias Uddin, "Preparation, characteristics, and application of biopolymer materials reinforced with lignocellulosic fibres," *International Journal of Polymer Science*, no. 1, p. 1738967, 2023. https://doi.org/10.1155/2023/1738967

F.-Z. S.A. Hassani, H. Chakchak, M.E. Achaby, R. Bouhfid, and A.E.K. Qaiss, "Date palm fiber extraction and treatment," In *Date Palm Fiber Composites*, M. Midani, N. Saba, and O.Y. Alothman, Eds., Springer. https://doi.org/10.1016/j.ijbiomac.2019.05.102

N. Hernandez, R.C Williams, and E.W Cochran, "The battle for the "green" polymer. Different approaches for biopolymer synthesis: Bioadvantaged vs. bioreplacement," *Organic & Biomolecular Chemistry*, vol. 12, pp. 2834–2849, 2014. https://doi.org/10.1039/C3OB42339E

Y. Ikada, *Integrated Biomaterials Science*, Barbucci, R., Ed. Springer, pp. 1–23, 2002.

R.A. Ilyas and S.M. Sapuan, "Biopolymers and biocomposites: Chemistry and technology," *Current Analytical Chemistry*, vol. 16, no. 5, pp. 500–503, 2020. https://doi.org/10.2174/157341101605200603095311

S. Indran, R. Edwin Raj, and V.S. Sreenivasan, "Characterization of new natural cellulosic fiber from Cissusquadrangularis root," *Carbohydrate Polymers*, vol. 110, pp. 423–429, 2014. https://doi.org/10.1016/j.carbpol.2014.04.051

M. Isik, H. Sardon, and D. Mecerreyes, "Ionic liquids and cellulose: Dissolution, chemical modification and preparation of new cellulosic materials," *International Journal of Molecular Sciences*, vol. 15, pp. 11922–11940, 2014. https://doi.org/10.3390/ijms150711922

D. Jaiswal, G.L. Devnani, G. Rajeshkumar et al., "Review on extraction, characterization, surface treatment and thermal degradation analysis of new cellulosic fibers as sustainable reinforcement in polymer composites," *Current Research in Green and Sustainable Chemistry*, vol. 5, p. 100271, 2022. https://doi.org/10.1016/j.crgsc.2022.100271

F.-L. Jin and S.-J. Park, "Impact-strength improvement of epoxy resins reinforced with a biodegradable polymer," *Materials Science and Engineering: A Review*, vol. 478, no. 1–2, pp. 402–405, 2008. https://doi.org/10.1016/j.msea.2007.05.053

M.K. Kang, W.I. Lee, and H.T. Hahn, "Formation of microvoids during resin-transfer molding process," *Composites Science and Technology*, vol. 60, pp. 2427–2434, 2000. https://doi.org/10.1016/S0266-3538(00)00036-1

M. Kathirselvam, A. Kumaravel, V.P. Arthanarieswaran, and S.S. Saravanakumar, "Characterization of cellulose fibers in Thespesiapopulnea barks: Influence of alkali treatment," *Carbohydrate Polymers*, vol. 217, pp. 178–189, 2019. https://doi.org/10.1016/j.carbpol.2019.04.063

A.Ç. Kılınç, S. Köktaş, Y. Seki et al., "Extraction and investigation of lightweight and porous natural fiber from Conium maculatum as a potential reinforcement for composite materials in transportation," *Composites Part B: Engineering*, vol. 140, pp. 1–8, 2018. https://doi.org/10.1016/j.compositesb.2017.11.059

S. Kitamura, K. Suzuki, and M. Iwatsuki, "Observation of silicon surfaces using ultrahigh vacuum noncontact atomic force microscope," *Japanese Journal of Applied Physics*, vol. 373, pp. 765–3768. https://doi.org/10.1143/JJAP.37.3765

G. Koley, M.G. Spencer, and H.R. Bhangale, "Cantilever effects on the measurement of electrostatic potentials by scanning Kelvin probe microscopy," *Applied Physics Letters*, vol. 79, pp. 545–548, 2001. https://doi.org/10.1063/1.1384004

A. Komuraiah, N.S. Kumar, and B.D. Prasad, "Chemical composition of natural fibers and its influence on their mechanical properties," *Mechanics of Composite Materials*, vol. 50, pp. 359–376, 2014. https://doi.org/10.1007/s11029-014-9422-2

N. Koyama and Y. Doi, "Continuous production of poly(3-hydroxybutymte-co-3-hydroxyvalerate) by Alcaligeneseutrophus," *Biotechnology Letters*, vol. 17, pp. 281–204, 1995. https://doi.org/10.1007/BF01190637

S. Kumar, A. Mukherjee, and J. Dutta, "Chitosan based nanocomposite films and coatings: Emerging antimicrobial food packaging alternatives," *Trends in Food Science & Technology*, vol. 97, pp. 196–209, 2020. https://doi.org/10.1016/j.tifs.2020.01.002

R. Latif, S. Wakeel, N.Z. Khan et al., "Surface treatments of plant fibers and their effects on mechanical properties of fiber-reinforced composites: A review," *Journal of Reinforced Plastics and Composites*, vol. 38, pp. 15–30, 2019. https://doi.org/10.1177/0731684418802022

Y-H Lee, G. Bhattarai, S. Aryal, N-H. Lee, M-H. Lee, T-G Kim, EC. Jhee, H-Y. Kim, and H-K. Yi, "Modified titanium surface with gelatin nano gold composite increases osteoblast cell biocompatibility," *Applied Surface Science*, vol. 256, no. 20, pp. 5882–5887, 2010. https://doi.org/10.1016/j.apsusc.2010.03.069

P. Lehtiniemi, K. Dufva, T. Berg et al., "Natural fiber-based reinforcements in epoxy composites processed by filament winding," *Nature*, vol. 30, pp. 1947–1955, 2011. https://doi.org/10.1177/0731684411431019

Y. Liu, D. Thibodeaux, and G. Gamble, "Characterization of attenuated total reflection infrared spectral intensity variations of immature and mature cotton fibers by two-dimensional correlation analysis," *ApplSpectrosc*, vol. 66, pp. 198–207, 2012. https://doi.org/10.1366/11-06440

C.H. Lovegrove, I. Edwards, I. De Nonic, H. Patel, S.N. El, T. Grassby, C. Zielke, M. Ulmius, L. Nilsson, P.J. Butterworth, P.R Ellis, and P.R. Shewry, "Role of polysaccharides in food, digestion and health," *Digestion and Health, Critical Reviews in Food Science and Nutrition*, pp. 1–65, 2015. https://doi.org/10.1080/10408398.2014.939263

T. Lu, M. Jiang, Z. Jiang et al., "Effect of surface modification of bamboo cellulose fibers on mechanical properties of cellulose/epoxy composites," *Composites Part B: Engineering*, vol. 51, pp. 28–34, 2013. https://doi.org/10.1016/j.compositesb.2013.02.031

M. Maache, A. Bezazi, S. Amroune et al., "Characterization of a novel natural cellulosic fiber from *Juncus effusus* L," *Carbohydrate Polymers*, vol. 171, pp. 163–172, 2017. https://doi.org/10.1016/j.carbpol.2017.04.096

A.S. Madival, D. Doreswamy, S. Maddasani et al., "Processing, characterization of Furcraeafoetida (FF) fiber and investigation of physical/mechanical properties of FF/epoxy composite," *Polymers*, vol. 14, p. 1476, 2022. https://doi.org/10.3390/polym14071476

E. Marsyahyo, Jamasri, R. Hsb, and Soekrisno, "Preliminary investigation on bulletproof panels made from ramie fiber reinforced composites for NIJ level II, IIA, and IV," *Journal of Industrial Textiles*, vol. 39, pp. 13–26, 2009. https://doi.org/10.1177/1528083708098913

L. Mathew, K.U. Joseph, and R. Joseph, "Swelling behaviour of isora/natural rubber composites in oils used in automobiles," *Bulletin of Materials Science*, vol. 29, pp. 91–99, 2006. https://doi.org/10.1007/BF02709362

M.A. Matica, F.L. Aachmann, A. Tøndervik, H. Sletta, and V. Ostafe, "Chitosan as a Wound Dressing Starting Material: Antimicrobial Properties and Mode of Action," *International Journal of Molecular Science*, vol. 20, p. 5889, 2019. https://doi.org/10.3390/ijms20235889

S. Misri, M.R. Ishak, S.M. Sapuan, and Z. Leman, "Filament winding process for kenaffibre reinforced polymer composites," *Manufacturing of Natural Fibre Reinforced Polymer Composites*, pp. 369–383, 2015. https://doi.org/10.1007/978-3-319-07944-8_18

S. Mohan and O.S. Oluwafemi, Nandakumar Kalarikkal, Sabu Thomas, and S.P. Songca, "Biopolymers – Application in nanoscience and nanotechnology," *Recent Advances in Biopolymer*s, pp. 2–30, 2016. https://doi.org/10.5772/62225

S.J. Mohan, P.S.S. Devasahayam, I. Suyambulingam, and S. Siengchin, "Suitability characterization of novel cellulosic plant fiber from Ficusbenjamina L. aerial root for a potential polymeric composite reinforcement," *Polymer Composites*, vol. 43, pp. 9012–9026, 2022. https://doi.org/10.1002/pc.27080

S.N. Monteiro, R.C.M.P. Aquino, and F.P.D. Lopes, "Performance of curaua fibers in pullout tests," *Journal of Materials Science*, vol. 43, pp. 489–493, 2008. https://doi.org/10.1007/s10853-007-1874-5

A.A.M. Moshi, D. Ravindran, S.R.S. Bharathi et al., "Characterization of natural cellulosic fiber extracted from Grewiadamine flowering plant's stem," *International Journal of Biological Macromolecules*, vol. 164, pp. 1246–1255, 2020. https://doi.org/10.1016/j.ijbiomac.2020.07.225

M. Mtibaa, A. Saouab, S. Bouaziz et al., "Numerica modeling of suspension impregnation through a fibrous medium: Application to the CRTM process," *Journal of Reinforced Plastics and Composites*, p. 7316844221142017, 2022. https://doi.org/10.1177/07316844221142017

S.S. Munawar, K. Umemura, and S. Kawai, "Characterization of the morphological, physical, and mechanical properties of seven nonwood plant fiber bundles," *Journal of Wood Science*, vol. 53, pp. 108–113, 2007. https://doi.org/10.1007/s10086-006-0836-x

L.Y. Mwaikambo and M.P. Ansell, "Mechanical properties of alkali treated plant fibres and their potential as reinforcement materials. I. Hemp fibres," *Journal of Materials Science*, vol. 41, pp. 2483–2496, 2006. https://doi.org/10.1007/s10853-006-5098-x

K. Mylsamy and I. Rajendran, "Investigation on physio-chemical and mechanical properties of raw and alkali-treated Agave americana fiber," *Journal of Reinforced Plastics and Composites*, vol. 29, pp. 2925–2935, 2010. https://doi.org/10.1177/0731684410362817

R. Narendar and K. PriyaDasan, "Chemical treatments of coir pith: Morphology, chemical composition, thermal and water retention behavior," *Composites Part B: Engineering*, vol. 56, pp. 770–779, 2014. https://doi.org/10.1016/j.compositesb.2013.09.028

K. Obi Reddy, G. Sivamohan Reddy, C. Uma Maheswari et al., "Structural characterization of coconut tree leaf sheath fiber reinforcement," *Journal of Forestry Research*, vol. 21, pp. 53–58, 2010. https://doi.org/10.1007/s11676-010-0008-0

C.E. Okafor, L.C. Kebodi, C.C. Ihueze et al., "Development of Dioscoreaalata stem fibers as eco-friendly reinforcement for composite materials," *Journal of King Saud University— Engineering Sciences*, 2022. https://doi.org/10.1016/j.jksues.2022.02.003

K. Oksman, "High quality flax fibre composites manufactured by the resin transfer moulding process," *Journal of Reinforced Plastics and Composites*, vol. 20, pp. 621–627, 2016. https://doi.org/10.1177/073168401772678634

M.C. Paiva, I. Ammar, A.R. Campos et al., "Alfa fibres: Mechanical, morphological and interfacial characterization," *Composites Science and Technolnology*, vol. 67, pp. 1132–1138, 2007. https://doi.org/10.1016/j.compscitech.2006.05.019

A. Patti and D. Acierno, "Towards the sustainability of the plastic industry through biopolymers: Properties and potential applications to the textiles world," *Polymers,* vol. 14, p. 692. https://doi.org/10.3390/polym14040692

E.A.O. Paula, R.R. Melo, M.Q. Silva et al., "Characterization of polyester composites reinforced with natural fibers from Luffacylindrica," *Journal of Composite Materials*, vol. 56, pp. 4313–4327, 2022. https://doi.org/10.1177/00219983221130724

X. Peng, M. Fan, J. Hartley, and M. Al-Zubaidy, "Properties of natural fiber composites made by pultrusion process," *Journal of Composite Materials*, vol. 46, pp. 237–246, 2011. https://doi.org/10.1177/0021998311410474

S.J. Pickering, "Recycling technologies for thermoset composite materials—current status," *Composites Part A: Applied Science and Manufacturing*, vol. 37, pp. 1206–1215, 2006. https://doi.org/10.1016/j.compositesa.2005.05.030

V. Placet, "Characterization of the thermo-mechanical behaviour of Hemp fibres intended for the manufacturing of high performance composites," *Composites Part A: Applied Science and Manufacturing*, vol. 40, pp. 1111–1118, 2009. https://doi.org/10.1016/j.compositesa.2009.04.031

D.L. Nichols, M.J. McLaughlin, and M. Benton, "Production intensification and regional specialization: Maguey fibers and textiles in the Aztec city-state of Otumba," Ancient Mesoamerica, vol. 11, pp. 267–291, 2000. PRODUCTION INTENSIFICATION AND REGIONAL SPECIALIZATION: Maguey fibers and textiles in the Aztec city...

M.M. Rababah and F.M. Al-Oqla, "Biopolymer composites and sustainability," *Advanced Processing, Properties, and Applications of Starch and Other Bio-based Polymers*, pp. 1–10, 2020.

A. Rachocki and J. Tritt-Goc. "The molecular origin of nuclear magnetic relaxation in methyl cellulose and hydroxypropylmethyl cellulose," *Journal of Polymer Research*, vol. 13, pp. 201–206, 2006. https://doi.org/10.1007/s10965-005-9026-6

A. Rachocki, J. Kowalczuk, and J Tritt-Goc. "How we can interpret the T1 dispersion of MC, HPMC and HPC polymers above glass temperature?," *Solid State NuclMagnReson,* vol. 30, pp. 192–197, 2006. https://doi.org/10.1016/j.ssnmr.2006.10.001

G. Rajeshkumar, V. Hariharan, S. Indran et al., "Influence of sodium hydroxide (NaOH) treatment on mechanical properties and morphological behaviour of Phoenix sp. fiber/epoxy composites," *Journal of Polymers and the Environment*, vol. 29, pp. 765–774, 2021. https://doi.org/10.1007/s10924-020-01921-6

R. Ramkumar and P. Saravanan, "Characterization of the cellulose fibers extracted from the bark of Piliostigmaracemosa," *Journal of Natural Fibers*, vol. 19, pp. 5101–5115, 2021. https://doi.org/10.1080/15440478.2021.1875356

L. Ranakoti, B. Gangil, P.K. Rajesh et al., "Effect of surface treatment and fiber loading on the physical, mechanical, sliding wear, and morphological characteristics of Tasar silk fiber waste-epoxy composites for multifaceted biomedical and engineering applications: Fabrication and characterizations," *Journal of Materials Research and Technology*, vol. 19, pp. 2863–2876, 2022. https://doi.org/10.1016/j.jmrt.2022.06.024

K.M.M. Rao and K.M. Rao, "Extraction and tensile properties of natural fibers: Vakka, date and bamboo," *Composite Structures*, vol. 77, pp. 288–295, 2007. https://doi.org/10.1016/j.compstruct.2005.07.023

K.M.M. Rao, A.V.R. Prasad, M.N.V.R. Babu et al., "Tensile properties of elephant grass fiber reinforced polyester composites," *Journal of Materials Science*, vol. 42, pp. 3266–3272, 2007. https://doi.org/10.1007/s10853-006-0657-8

K.M.M. Rao, K.M. Rao, and A.R.V. Prasad, "Fabrication and testing of natural fibre composites: Vakka, sisal, bamboo and banana," *Materials & Design*, vol. 31, pp. 508–513, 2010. https://doi.org/10.1016/j.matdes.2009.06.023

R. Rathinavelu and B.S. Paramathma, "Comprehensive characterization of Echinochloafrumentacea leaf fiber as a novel reinforcement for composite applications," *Polymer Composites*, vol. 43, pp. 5031–5046, 2022. https://doi.org/10.1002/pc.26775

D. Rouison, M. Sain, and M Couturier, "Resin transfer molding of hemp fiber composites: Optimization of the process and mechanical properties of the materials," *Composites Science and Technology*, vol. 66, no. 7–8, pp. 895–906, 2006. https://doi.org/10.1016/j.compscitech.2005.07.040

S. Roy and J.-W. Rhim, "Carboxymethyl cellulose-based antioxidant and antimicrobial active packaging film incorporated with curcumin and zinc oxide," *International Journal of Biological Macromolecules*, vol. 148, pp. 666–676, 2020. https://doi.org/10.1016/j.ijbiomac.2020.01.204

A.R. Sahoo, S. Sanket, and S. Pany, "Sanghamitra Pati, Sangram Keshari Samal, Latest development of biopolymers based on polysaccharides," *Processing and Development of Polysaccharide-based Biopolymers for Packaging Applications*, pp. 281–299. https://doi.org/10.1016/B978-0-12-818795-1.00012-5

M. Salgado-Ramos, F.J. Martí-Quijal, A.J. Huertas-Alonso et al., "Almond hull biomass: Preliminary characterization and development of two alternative valorization routes by applying innovative and sustainable technologies," *Industrial Crops and Products*, vol. 179, p. 114697, 2022. https://doi.org/10.1080/15440478.2020.1758863

M.R. Sanjay, P. Madhu, M. Jawaid et al., "Characterization and properties of natural fiber polymer composites: A comprehensive review," *Journal of Cleaner Production*, vol. 172, pp. 566–581, 2018. https://doi.org/10.1016/j.jclepro.2017.10.101

M.R. Sanjay, S. Siengchin, J. Parameswaranpillai et al., "A comprehensive review of techniques for natural fibers as reinforcement in composites: Preparation, processing and characterization," *Carbohydrate Polymers*, vol. 207, pp. 108–121, 2019. https://doi.org/10.1016/j.carbpol.2018.11.083

D. SaravanaBavan and G.C. Mohan Kumar, "Potential use of natural fiber composite materials in India," *Journal of Reinforced Plastics and Composites*, vol. 29, pp. 3600–3613, 2010. https://doi.org/10.1177/0731684410381151

S.S. Saravanakumar, A. Kumaravel, T. Nagarajan, and I.G. Moorthy, "Effect of chemical treatments on physicochemical properties of Prosopisjuliflora fibers," *International Journal of Polymer Analysis and Characterization*, vol. 19, pp. 383–390, 2014. https://doi.org/10.1080/1023666X.2014.903585

K.G. Satyanarayana, K. Sukumaran, P.S. Mukherjee et al., "Natural fibre-polymer composites," *Cement and Concrete Composites*, vol. 12, pp. 117–136, 1990. https://doi.org/10.1016/0958-9465(90)90049-4

P. Senthamaraikannan, S.S. Saravanakumar, M.R. Sanjay et al., "Physico-chemical and thermal properties of untreated and treated Acacia planifrons bark fibers for composite reinforcement," *Materials Letters*, vol. 240, pp. 221–224, 2019. https://doi.org/10.1016/j.matlet.2019.01.024

K. Sever, M. Sarikanat, Y. Seki et al., "Surface treatments of jute fabric: The influence of surface characteristics on jute fabrics and mechanical properties of jute/polyester composites," *Industrial Crops and Products*, vol. 35, pp. 22–30, 2012. https://doi.org/10.1016/j.indcrop.2011.05.020

S.M. Shahril, M.J.M. Ridzuan, M.S.A. Majid et al., "Alkali treatment influence on cellulosic fiber from Furcraeafoetida leaves as potential reinforcement of polymeric composites," *Journal of Materials Research and Technology*, vol. 19, pp. 2567–2583, 2022. https://doi.org/10.1016/j.jmrt.2022.06.002

K. Shaker, M. Umair, S. Shahid, M. Jabbar, R.M.W. Ullah Khan, M. Zeeshan & Y. Nawab, (2022). Cellulosic fillers extracted from Argyreia speciose waste: a potential reinforcement for composites to enhance properties. *Journal of Natural Fibers*, vol. 19(11), pp. 4210–4222, 2022. https://doi.org/10.1080/15440478.2020.1856271

R. Singh, S. Gautam, B. Sharma, P. Jain, and K. DuttChauhan, "Biopolymers and their classifications, biopolymers and their industrial applications from plant," *Animal, and Marine Sources, to Functional Products*, pp. 21–44, 2021. https://doi.org/10.1016/B978-0-12-819240-5.00001-8

R. Siva, T.N. Valarmathi, K. Palanikumar, and A.V. Samrot, "Study on a novel natural cellulosic fiber from Kigeliaafricana fruit: Characterization and analysis," *Carbohydrate Polymers*, vol. 244, p. 116494, 2020. https://doi.org/10.1016/j.carbpol.2020.116494

A.M. Smith, S. Moxon, and G.A. Morris, (2016). *Biopolymers as wound healing materials, wound healing biomaterials,* vol. 2, pp. 261–287. https://doi.org/10.1016/B978-1-78242-456-7.00013-1

K.D. Snell, V. Singh, and S.M. Brumbley. "Production of novel biopolymers in plants: Recent technological advances and future prospects," *CurrOpinBiotechnol*, vol. 32, pp. 68–75, 2015. https://doi.org/10.1016/j.copbio.2014.11.005

A. Soldo, M. Miletić, and M.L. Auad, "Biopolymers as a sustainable solution for the enhancement of soil mechanical properties," *Scientific Reports*, vol. 10, p. 267, 2020. https://doi.org/10.1038/s41598-019-57135-x

R. Somasundaram, R. Rajamoni, I. Suyambulingam et al., "Utilization of discarded Cymbopogonflexuosus root waste as a novel lignocellulosic fiber for lightweight polymer composite application," *Polymer Composites*, vol. 43, pp. 2838–2853, 2022. https://doi.org/10.1002/pc.26580

M.S. Sreekala, M.G. Kumaran, Sabu Thomas, "Oil palm fibers: Morphology, chemical composition, surface modification, and mechanical properties," *Journal of Applied Polymer Science*, 1997.

P.A. Sreekumar, K. Joseph, G. Unnikrishnan, and S. Thomas, "A comparative study on mechanical properties of sisal-leaf fibre-reinforced polyester composites prepared by resin transfer and compression moulding techniques," *Composites Science and Technology*, vol. 67, pp. 453–461, 2007. https://doi.org/10.1016/j.compscitech.2006.08.025

V.S. Sreenivasan, S. Somasundaram, D. Ravindran et al., "Microstructural, physico-chemical and mechanical characterisation of Sansevieriacylindricafibres—an exploratory investigation," *Materials & Design*, vol. 32, pp. 453–461, 2011. https://doi.org/10.1016/j.matdes.2010.06.004

A. Sukan, I. Roy, and T. Keshavarz, "Dual production of biopolymers from bacteria," *Carbohydregan Polymer*, vol. 126, pp. 47–51, 2015. https://doi.org/10.1016/j.carbpol.2015.03.001

A.B.M. Supian, S.M. Sapuan, M.Y.M. Zuhri et al., "Effect of winding orientation on energy absorption and failure modes of filament wound kenaf/glass fibre reinforced epoxy hybrid composite tubes under intermediate-velocity impact (IVI) load," *Journal of Materials Research and Technology*, vol. 10, pp. 1–14, 2021. https://doi.org/10.1016/j.jmrt.2020.11.103

B. Sutradhar, M.B. Mesbah, and M. Hasan, "Effect of fiber ratio and chemical treatment on properties of banana and betel nut fiber reinforced hybrid polypropylene composites," *IOP Conference Series: Materials Science and Engineering*, vol. 438, p. 12006, 2018. https://doi.org/10.1088/1757-899X/438/1/012006

H.R Tang, P.S Belton, A Ng, K.W. Waldron, and P. Ryden, "Solid state H-1 NMR studies of cell wall materials of potatoes," *SpectrochimActa Part A*, vol. 55, pp. 883–894, 1999. https://doi.org/10.1016/S1386-1425(98)00235-2

H.R. Tang, Y.L. Wang, and P.S. Belton, "13C CPMAS studies of plant cell wall materials and model systems using proton relaxation-induced spectral editing techniques," *Solid State NuclMagnReson*, vol. 15, no. 4, pp. 239–248, 2000. https://doi.org/10.1016/S0926-2040(99)00064-8

E.M. Teixeira, A. Campos, J.M. Marconcini, T.J. Bondancia, D. Wood, A. Klamczynski, L.H.C. Mattosoa, and G.M. Glenn, "Starch/fiber/poly (lactic acid) foam and compressed foam composites," *RSC Adviser*, vol. 4, pp. 6616–6623, 2014. https://doi.org/10.1039/C3RA47395C

T. Theophile, editor. "Infrared spectroscopy - Anharmonicity of biomolecules, crosslinking of biopolymers, food quality and medical applications," *InTech*, p. 172, 2015. https://doi.org/10.5772/58483

J.G. Tirrell and D.A Tirrell, "Synthesis of biopolymers: Proteins, polyesters, polysaccharides and polynucleotides," *Current Opinion Solid State and Materials Science*, vol. I, pp. 407–411, 1996. https://doi.org/10.1016/S1359-0286(96)80033-7

S.S. Todkar and S.A. Patil, "Review on mechanical properties evaluation of pineapple leaf fibre (PALF) reinforced polymer composites," *Composites Part B: Engineering*, vol. 174, p. 106927, 2019. https://doi.org/10.1016/j.compositesb.2019.106927

K.J.V. Vardhini, R. Murugan, C. Selvi, and R. Surjit, "Optimisation of alkali treatment of banana fibres on lignin removal," *NIScPR Online Periodicals Repository*, vol. 41, pp. 156–160, 2016.

A. Vedernikov, A. Safonov, F. Tucci et al., "Pultruded materials and structures: A review," *Journal of Composite Materials*, vol. 54, pp. 4081–4117, 2020. https://doi.org/10.1177/0021998320922894

N. Venkateshwaran and A. Elayaperumal, "Banana fiber reinforced polymer composites – a review," *Journal of Reinforced Plastics and Composites*, vol. 29, pp. 2387–2396, 2010. https://doi.org/10.1177/0731684409360578

A. Vinod, J. Tengsuthiwat, Y. Gowda et al., "Jute/hemp bio-epoxy hybrid bio-composites: Influence of stacking sequence on adhesion of fiber-matrix," *International Journal of Adhesion and Adhesives*, vol. 113, p. 103050, 2022. https://doi.org/10.1016/j.ijadhadh.2021.103050

P.C. Williams and K. Norris, editors. *Implementation of near-infrared technology in the agricultural and food industries*, 2nd ed. American Association of Cereal Chemists, St. Paul, 145–169, 2001.

O.C. Wokadala, S.S. Ray, J. Bandyopadhyay, J. Wesley-Smith, and N.M Emmambu, "Morphology, thermal properties and crystallization kinetics of ternary blends of the polylactide and starch biopolymers and nanoclay: The role of nanoclay hydrophobicity," *Polymer*, vol. 71, pp. 82–92, 2015. https://doi.org/10.1016/j.polymer.2015.06.058

L. Yan, N. Chouw, L. Huang, and B. Kasal, "Effect of alkali treatment on microstructure and mechanical properties of coir fibres, coir fibre reinforced-polymer composites and reinforced-cementitious composites," *Construction and Building Materials*, vol. 112, pp. 168–182, 2016. https://doi.org/10.1016/j.conbuildmat.2016.02.182

H.H.I. Yao, M.K.H Hong, and K.J. Drummond, "Haemostasis in neurosurgery: What is the evidence for gelatin-thrombin matrix sealant?" *Journal ClinlNeuro Science,* vol. 20, no. 3, pp. 349–356. https://doi.org/10.1016/j.jocn.2012.09.005

A.A. Yussuf, I. Massoumi, and A. Hassan, "Comparison of polylactic acid/kenaf and polylactic acid/rise husk composites: The influence of the natural fibers on the mechanical, thermal and biodegradability properties," *Journal of Polymers and the Environment*, vol. 18, pp. 422–429, 2010. https://doi.org/10.1007/s10924-010-0185-0

13 Unravelling the multifaceted applications of biofilms for environmental sustainability

Tarun Suryarajan, Naveen Nair, Shivangi Dutta, Swathi Krishnan Venkatesan, Maseed Uddin, Sekaran Ganesan, and Ramani Kandasamy

13.1 INTRODUCTION

Biofilms are multicellular, structured communities of microbial cells formed on an abiotic or biotic surface that are cemented together with an extracellular matrix (Ünal Turhan, 2019). The development of biofilms could be a defence mechanism or a survival strategy to withstand harsh environmental conditions through the biosynthesis of extracellular polymeric substances (EPS) (Shree et al., 2023). Biofilm could either be formed by a single species or by interactions between multiple species, and its composition is reliant on external environmental conditions (Singh, 2020). Most biofilms are associated with detrimental effects such as elevated virulence, antimicrobial resistance, chronic infections in humans, or contamination in the food industry. However, biofilms possess significant potential to be harnessed for several beneficial applications in the fields of bioremediation, bioenergy, and several other fields of biotechnology (Mukhi & Vishwanathan, 2022). Therefore, this chapter delves into the elucidation of the various positive applications of biofilms in fields of environmental sustainability. By understanding and harnessing the beneficial properties of biofilms, we can explore innovative ways to address environmental challenges and promote sustainability in various industries, such as soil remediation, wastewater treatment, microbial fuel cells (MFCs), and the production of bioenergy. Biofilm as a bioremediating agent is a cost-effective and efficient substitute for the detoxification of environmental contaminants.

Owing to their higher resistance to harsh conditions and harmful chemicals, biofilm communities are capable of adsorbing and metabolizing pernicious organic pollutants and toxic heavy metals through the production of extracellular enzymes (Mishra et al., 2022). In addition, biofilms also play a crucial role in wastewater treatment processes such as the ANAMMOX, where nitrifying bacteria and ANAMMOX bacteria symbiotically thrive and reduce nitrogen compounds in the water, making it suitable for discharge into the environment (Philipp et al., 2024). Moreover, biofilms could be employed for both wastewater treatment and energy production through the concept of MFCs. In this innovative approach, the functionality of electro-active biofilms (EAB) is exploited, which are biofilms growing on the surfaces of electrodes (Logan et al., 2006). Moreover, technologies like employing algal biofilm for the production of bioenergy from wastewater are not only eco-friendly but also cost-effective, providing a sustainable solution for both waste treatment and energy generation (Hoh et al., 2016). By utilizing biofilms efficiently in various applications, we can address environmental challenges while also creating valuable resources from waste streams.

Even though biofilm has several benefits, such as being cost-effective and sustainable, it is yet to be widely adopted in mainstream industrial practices due to challenges related to scalability, maintenance, and its time-consuming nature. Therefore, this chapter aims to provide a comprehensive

DOI: 10.1201/9781003500483-13
This chapter has been made available under a (CC-BY-NC-ND) 4.0 license

understanding of the fundamentals of the biofilm development process, along with an elucidation of their signalling system. Additionally, it explores their potential applications in green biotechnology along with the outline of prospective future research.

13.2 FORMATION AND STRUCTURAL ARCHITECTURE OF BIOFILMS

13.2.1 Processes involved in biofilm formation

Biofilm development is a complex sequential process that results in the dissemination of motile nomadic planktonic cells to the sedentary structures of microbial communities. Conventionally, the dynamic growth process can be explained through the five-stage model, which commences with the reversible attachment of planktonic cells, followed by a transition to irreversible attachment, leading to biofilm maturation stages, and finally the dispersion and detachment of cells (Singh, 2020).

The initial attachment of microbial cells is vastly dependent on the formation of a conditioning film (CF) on the surface, which is formed through the adsorption of biomolecules from the surrounding medium (Bhagwat et al., 2021). The elemental composition of these CF varies and is dependent on the organic constituents of the bulk media the surface is exposed to; for instance, CF in the oral cavity constituents of proteinaceous components like albumin, glycoproteins, and lysozymes (Donlan, 2002). CFs primarily function as an anchor that facilitates the initial attachment of cells by altering surface properties like roughness, hydrophobicity/hydrophilicity, charge, and composition (Talluri et al., 2020). After the establishment of CF, the initial attachment of microbes transpires, which further promotes the adhesion of additional planktonic cells, leading to co-aggregation and ultimately resulting in the formation of multiple layers of microbes (Singh, 2020). Studies have reported that the mechanism behind the transport of cells to the substratum could either be passive, like Brownian motion, sedimentation, or convective mass transport. However, initial attachment is attributed to weak forces of interaction like Van der Waals' forces, electrostatic interactions, and hydrophobic interactions, which increase the probability of cell detachment. Therefore, the presence of external appendages like flagella and pili in motile bacteria plays a major role in overcoming the repulsive forces by acting as a linker between the microbe and the surface. This results in the irreversible attachment of microbes, attributed to strong bonds like ionic bonds, hydrogen bonds, etc. (Kumar & Anand, 1998). During this stage, microbes lose their motility and firmly attach to the surface, which results in the formation of cell colonies. Reports suggest that there is a significant enhancement in the biosynthesis of EPS along with the activation of genes encoding for antibiotic resistance during the irreversible stage of attachment. This suggests that the microbes are not cemented to each other and the surface but also develop antibiotic tolerance as an early adaptive response (Sauer et al., 2022). EPS is a critical component in biofilm formation because it strengthens the attachment between cells, thereby forming cell aggregates on the substratum. EPS comprises a wide variety of glycolipids, glycoproteins, and extracellular DNA (e-DNA) (Flemming et al., 2007). It creates a matrix where several microbes and organic and inorganic molecules get embedded and protects the microbial population (Flemming et al., 2023).

After firm attachment to the surface, biofilm maturation takes place, involving complete architecture development. In the initial maturation stage, the microbes start to divide with the help of CF as a bio-augmenting source and form clusters of cells, which are further stabilized by rapid EPS production. Subsequently, after sufficient multiplication of the microbes in the EPS matrix, they form three-dimensional, completely developed microcolonies in the second maturation stage. During this stage, no physical or chemical interactions are involved, and biological processes dominate. Moreover, genetic modification is seen in cells where the growth of surface appendages is limited; however, there is an up-regulation in the production of surface proteins, which impart mechanical stability and protection from environmental fluctuations (Garrett et al., 2008). Quorum sensing plays an important role in this stage, which enables the microbes to regulate their collective

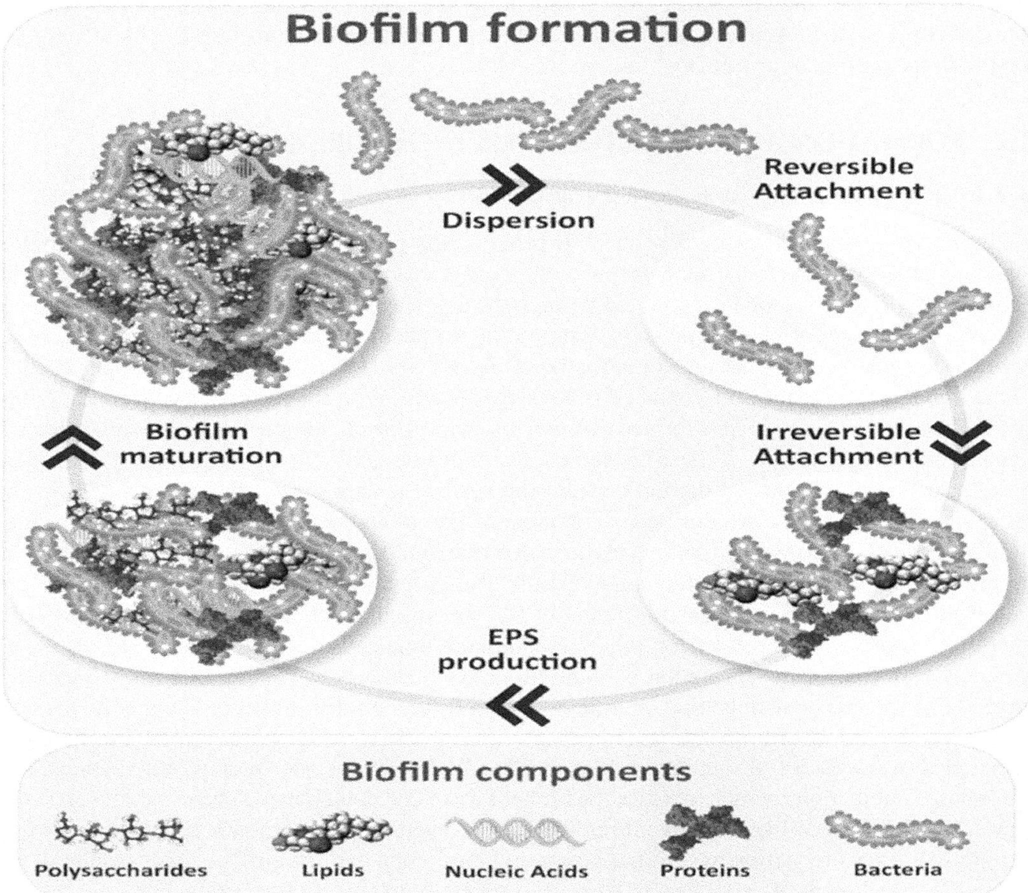

FIGURE 13.1 Stages of biofilm development.

Source: From Balducci et al. (2023), used under creative commons CC-BY license

behaviour. Both Gram-positive and Gram-negative bacteria have different Quorum-inducing molecules, which regulate their gene expression (Otto, 2013).

Dispersion is the final stage in biofilm development where sedentary microbes return to their planktonic free-floating state (Rumbaugh & Sauer, 2020). There are several reasons behind dispersion, such as external environmental stress, limited nutrient supply, and internal bacterial changes that result in the synthesis of degrading enzymes (Zhao et al., 2017). Therefore, after the dispersion of biofilm, these free planktonic cells can colonize a new surface, thereby restarting the cyclic biofilm development process. The schematic representation of stages of the biofilm formations and its components involved is provided in Figure 13.1.

13.2.2 Structure and composition of biofilms

Biofilms consist of two primary components, namely microorganisms and EPS. Among which EPS functions as the matrix in which cells are embedded. EPS are high-molecular-weight polymers synthesized by microbial aggregates, which are composed of polysaccharides, proteins, and nucleic acids (Zhang et al., 2014). However, the chemical constituents of EPS vary depending on the type of microorganisms, age, nutrient availability, and the external environmental conditions. For instance, few studies have reported increased EPS production with slower bacterial growth, while few have demonstrated enhanced production upon interaction with different metal cations and macromolecules (Donlan, 2002).

Polysaccharides are well recognized as the principal components of EPS whose primary function is to maintain the integrity of the matrix. The majority of these compounds are heteropolysaccharides, which can be either charged or neutral. Exopolysaccharides in Gram-negative bacteria are anionic or neutral in nature, comprising elements like uronic acids. In contrast, Gram-positive bacteria have exopolysaccharides that are positive in nature (Vu et al., 2009). The diverse exopolysaccharides serve the dual purpose of safeguarding the biofilm matrix and ensuring sufficient hydration, which protects the biofilm from water fluctuations. Another critical component of EPS is proteins, which are sometimes more abundant than polysaccharides (Fulaz et al., 2019). They can either be structural proteins that facilitate the adhesion of cells or be enzymes that degrade the matrix components, especially in the dispersion stage of biofilm development (Pinto et al., 2020). EPS also comprises extracellular DNA (eDNA), which is universally present in all microbes, irrespective of species and external environment. It has various functions, such as being an integral structural component, facilitating gene transfer, and contributing towards bacterial tolerance (Campoccia et al., 2021).

13.2.3 Factors responsible for biofilm formation

Biofilm production is impacted by a multitude of factors, which can be classified into two primary categories: internal and external factors. Internal factors include cell properties, while external properties include environmental factors and surface properties. Under internal cell surface properties, factors like synthesis of EPS, presence of appendages such as flagella, pili, fimbriae, and cell surface hydrophobicity have impact on biofilm formation. Both the initial attachment of cells through formation of non-specific bonds and also the voluminous growth of biofilm is facilitated by external appendages. Moreover, the biosynthesis of EPS is also critical for the stability and adherence of cells. Therefore, any variation in EPS and external appendages can affect the integrity of biofilm (Zhao et al., 2017). Reports also suggest that cells with higher hydrophobicity attach easily in comparison with hydrophilic cells (Pompilio et al., 2008). Furthermore, studies have reported the critical role of a bacterial secondary messenger called c-di-GMP which controls the regulation from planktonic free-living state to settled structured state (Valentini & Filloux, 2016). Therefore, any alterations in these internal factors can affect the biofilm development process.

Under the external factors category, properties of surface on which biofilm is said to colonize also influences the biofilm formation for instance, increased surface roughness and presence of CF contribute to the advancement of biofilm development. The biofilm formation process is significantly influenced by fluctuations in the surrounding bulk medium, such as variations in temperature, pH, nutrient levels, and ionic strength (Pompilio et al., 2008). Alterations in pH can limit both the initial attachment of bacteria and the efficiency of enzyme activity (Saini et al., 2023). Likewise, changes in temperature can lead to a decrease in the nutritional consumption of microorganisms, thereby causing a decline in the growth of biofilm. This phenomenon is further compounded by the adverse impact on heat-labile compounds within the biofilm (Adetunji & Odetokun, 2012). Furthermore, the presence of adequate oxygen levels is also crucial biofilm development because it is necessary for effective metabolic processes in the microbial cells (Ahn & Burne, 2007). Similarly, if the nutrient concentration is restricted in the media, it will also lead to a hindered development of biofilms. However, in some studies, limited nutrients have resulted in enhancement of biofilms, which could be attributed to the survival strategy of microbes, wherein they consume compounds that they would have otherwise just absorbed. Hence, the production of biofilms can be influenced by several external environmental conditions (Saini et al., 2023).

13.3 INTER-SPECIES INTERACTIONS

13.3.1 Quorum sensing molecules in biofilm formation

Biofilm formation is regulated through a complex mechanism called quorum sensing. This convoluted mechanism involves the secretion and detection of extracellular signalling molecules called autoinducers (Wang et al., 2022). The concentration of these AI molecules is directly dependent on the bacterial population density, with organisms exhibiting different behaviours at different densities. For example, in bacterial species such as *Vibrio cholerae*, biofilm formation occurs at lower cell, whereas in species such as *Pseudomonas aeruginosa*, biofilm formation occurs at a higher cell density (Mukherjee & Bassler, 2019). Every bacterial species employs its own quorum-sensing (QS) system, with the majority of bacterial species possessing several systems. The system consists of a synthase responsible for the production of the autoinducer (AI), along with a matching receptor (Condinho et al., 2023). Gram-negative organisms communicate through acyl-homoserine lactones (AHLs) or molecules that utilize S-adenosylmethionine (SAM) as a substrate. These AIs diffuse through the membrane and receptors that function as transcription factors. This interaction leads to the regulation of gene expression for biofilm formation (Rutherford & Bassler, 2012). Gram-positive organisms, on the other hand, make use of small autoinducer peptides (AIP) which are ribosomally synthesized and post-translationally modified. These AIPs then interact with a histidine-kinase signalling mechanism that regulates the production of biofilm (Prazdnova et al., 2022). Under special conditions, even Gram-negative bacteria have been reported to produce AHL (Biswa & Doble, 2013).

13.3.2 Communication and coordination within biofilms

13.3.2.1 Quorum sensing in Gram-negative bacteria

Gram-negative organisms employ unique signalling molecules known as N-acyl homoserine lactones (AHL), which are distinguished by their acyl chains of varying lengths. The quantity and nature of AHL generated are contingent upon the availability of substrates and the specific AHL synthase. Depending on their length of chain, these molecules can be classified as either long-chain AHLs (C10–C18) or short-chain AHLs (C4–C8) (Flemming et al., 2023). The short-chain AHLs diffuse freely through the cells, while the long-chain AHLs require active transport due to their larger molecular weight. Most Gram-negative organisms employ the homologous LuxR-LuxI system, initially identified, and studied in *Aliivibrio fischeri* where the LuxI protein is responsible for the production of acyl AHLs, while LuxR acts as a receptor to which the AHLs bind and trigger a change in gene expression. AHL is believed to start binding to LuxR only at a critical concentration, which is often achieved depending on factors like environmental conditions and population density. This leads to the subsequent activation of the receptor through conformational changes, followed by the activation of the *lux* box, which induces the transcription of the required factors and the necessary genes (Whitehead et al., 2001). This system is followed by the majority of Gram-negative species. An illustration of this may be seen in the utilization of two synthase genes, *lasI*, and *rhlI*, by *Pseudomonas aeruginosa*, which exhibit homology to the system seen in *Aliivibrio fischeri*. These genes encode for *N*-(3-oxo-dodecanoyl)-l-homoserine lactone (OdDHL) and *N*-butyryl-l-homoserine lactone (BHL), of which the latter is involved in regulating factors that help in the early stages of biofilm formation and virulence, whereas the former system controls other genes that help in biofilm formation (Zhou et al., 2020). Apart from this, two other systems have been identified, *pqs* and *iqs,* which directly affect biofilm formation as illustrated by studies where the null mutation of its genes resulted in decreased biofilm formation and reduced production of key biofilm components such as rhamnolipids, elastase, and pyocyanin (Pompilio et al., 2008). These systems operate in a coordinated way, forming a hierarchical structure that enables sophisticated intercellular communication (Kong et al., 2014). The model of LuxI/LuxR-based QS system is given in Figure 13.2.

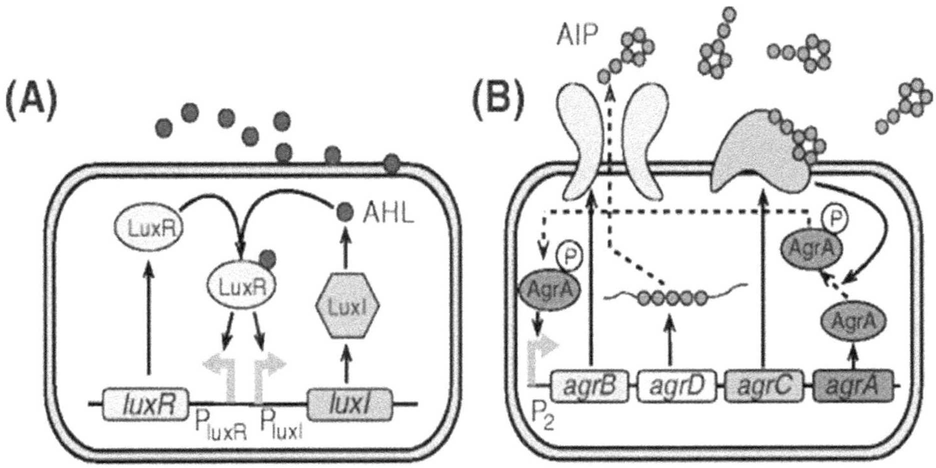

FIGURE 13.2 (a) LuxI/LuxR-based QS system (b) Agr QS system.

Source: From Kong et al. (2014) used under creative commons CC-BY license.

13.3.2.2 Quorum sensing in Gram-positive bacteria

Gram-positive bacteria make use of two major pathways for QS. In the first pathway, QS is achieved through ribosomally synthesized pro-peptides, which are then post translationally modified. These peptides are transported using special ABC transporters, activating the corresponding receptor kinase, leading to its auto-phosphorylation, which leads to the regulation of genes involved in biofilm formation (Bhatt, 2018). One such QS mechanism used by *S. Aureus* employs a two-component AgrA and AgrC system, producing a pro-peptide AgrD, which leads to the phosphorylation of AgrA, and the activation of various promoters that play a major role in the adhering, structuring, and spreading of the biofilm (Philipp et al., 2024). Another QS system Fsr, used by *E. faecalis,* has been demonstrated to regulate GelE, metalloprotease, which helps in the establishment of biofilm formation (Pinkston et al., 2011). The second pathway has been described as a self-signalling pathway, where the post-translationally modified AIPs are synthesized by SecA-dependent systems, activated through modifications, and transported with the help of an oligopeptide transporter system. This involves systems such as *Rap, NprR, PrgX*, and *PlcR* (Bhatt, 2018).

A third QS system, called AI-2, has been recently identified for intra and inter-species communication. This inducer is synthesized by the *luxS* gene, which has been observed in both Gram-positive and Gram-negative species (Zhou et al., 2020). This system is widely used in *Lactobacillus* where it regulates various stages of biofilm growth and stabilization. Multiple organisms, such as *Aggregatibacter actinomycetemcomitans, Sinorhizobium meliloti, Bacillus cereus*, and *Escherichia coli*, have been reported to use a LsrB AI-2 receptor (Pereira et al., 2013). Thus, proving its dominance as a universal signalling molecule. Studies have also reported that manipulating QS systems could allow us to obtain enhanced remediation capabilities. This was achieved through the exogenous addition of C6 and C8 AHL into the bioreactor, which resulted in increased removal of pollutants, remediation, and stability of the operation (Zhou et al., 2020). Another study showed that even the addition of AHL at low concentrations of 10 ng/L showed increased bacterial cell adhesion and biofilm formation, which could translate into better remediation (Prazdnova et al., 2022).

13.3.3 Effect on biofilm architecture and stability

The QS system in organisms can be very complex and regulates multiple factors related to biofilm stability and development, where factors regulated by the LasI/LasR-RhlI/RhlR system include the synthesis of rhamnolipid, lectin, and siderophores (Zhao et al., 2017). Rhamnolipid has been deemed necessary for the formation of open channels and the initial attachment of bacterial cells (Davey et al., 2003), lectins, on the other hand, are directly involved in cell-to-cell interactions, allowing for the crosslinking of galactosides and the formation of microcolonies and mature biofilm. In Gram-negative species, an AIP system, Agr, regulates PSM formation. The overexpression of this compound could also lead to the dispersal of biofilm (Sionov & Steinberg, 2022). Other Gram-positive species, such as *Bacillus cereus,* use a PapR system, where the gene product has been reported to inhibit biofilm formation, thus effectively regulating its growth (Ghosh et al., 2024). Another such QS system, ComCDE, employed by *Streptococcus mutans* was reported to directly affect factors that affect stress response and biofilm formation (Lemos et al., 2019). Therefore, the capacity of these organisms to engage in communication and social interactions with other species has facilitated the development of more organized, adaptable, and enhanced biofilm formation, thereby enabling their utilization for improved remediation.

13.4 MULTIFACETED APPLICATIONS OF BIOFILMS

13.4.1 Biofilms in wastewater treatment

In recent years, urbanization and industrialization have led to the generation of wastewater, which contains loads of organic and inorganic toxins and other recalcitrant compounds. This polluted wastewater is released into the environment from various sources, leading to a significant impact on the ecosystem. Biofilm technologies are incorporated into the treatment of wastewater, where microbial communities have been found to degrade, neutralize, and eliminate various pollutants (Hoh et al., 2016). Industrial effluents are rich in acetonitrile, which is hazardous to living organisms; therefore, a study by Li et al. (2013) demonstrated the functionality of an acetonitrile-degrading bacterium, *Rhodococcus rhodochrous* BX2. In addition, a similar study demonstrated that higher concentrations of acetonitrile (800 mg/L) could be degraded by a recombinant bacterium *B. subtilis* N4-pHT01-nit, within 24 hours in a Moving bed biofilm reactor (Kragh et al., 2016). Biofilm contains more biomass, which facilitates the efficient degradation of toxicants, which can be observed during nitrogen removal in wastewater, which is facilitated by biofilms existing with nitrifiers and denitrifiers in different layers (Saini et al., 2023). Inorganic pollutants such as heavy metals and dyes are present in wastewater and have been reported to be remediated by polysaccharides in the EPS matrix of *Pseudochrobactrum saccharolyticum* LY10 sp., *Arthrobacter* sp., and *P. mendocina* NR802 biofilm (Dey & Paul, 2018). The use of biofilms for wastewater treatment can be attributed to the various advantages it presents, which include smaller reactor sizes, resistance to environmental stress, increased biomass production, and enhanced degradation while producing lower amounts of sludge as well. Currently, two types of biofilm-based treatment methods are employed: (i) dispersed growth systems, where the biomass is grown in a suspended or dispersed form without any surface attachment and (ii) attached growth systems where biofilm is grown on the support medium (Naz, 2016). Biofilm communities actively degrade and metabolize heavy metal and organic contaminants through enzymatic secretions regulated by QS systems. The EPS matrix also allows for the efficient capture of various pollutants, with further stimulating biofilm growth and allowing for enhanced remediation and biosorption (Saini et al., 2023). EPS based barriers have also been reported to help protect cells from the toxicity of heavy metals, while acting as chelating agents against it (Dey & Paul, 2018).

13.4.2 Biofilms in soil remediation

In the current scenario, the rapid industrialization has led to the contamination of soil with various toxic compounds. These hazardous compounds like thalates, halogenated compounds, pesticides, and heavy metals have caused detrimental effects on not only soil health but also the surrounding ecosystem (Henagamage et al., 2022; Huang et al., 2022; Lu et al., 2018). Therefore, biofilm-assisted soil remediation serves as a competent, organized, and viable bio-remediation technology when compared to other treatments (Flemming et al., 2016).

One of the major applications of biofilm-mediated remediation is the removal of hydrocarbons. Biofilms are resistant to the toxic effects of the hydrocarbon, thereby making them a viable option. Biofilms increase the bioavailability and solubility of hydrocarbons like polycyclic aromatic hydrocarbons (PAHs) and thus accelerate their degradation process via the process of biotransformation (Mishra et al., 2022). Similarly, effective degradation of diesel oil in liquid waste was demonstrated by Chandran and Das (2011) through the utilization of a yeast biofilm generated by *Candida tropilcalis*. Mangwani et al. (2014) also exhibited the enhanced biodegradation rate of hazardous hydrocarbons like pyrene and phenanthrene through *Stenotrophomonas acidaminiphila* NCW-702 containing biofilm. Multiple studies have also reported the enhancement of remediation through steady-state biofilm-mediated reactors, which allow for better biofilm growth and improved metabolic rates, which subsequently lead to efficient degradation (R. Singh et al., 2006). In another study, Mangwani et al. (2016) exploited the functionality of two exogenous quorum-sensing molecules, AHLs, which yielded significantly higher degradation of phenanthrene and pyrene by *Pseudomonas aeruginosa*.

Biofilm-mediated degradation of pesticides is also effective and has the potential to restore environmental quality. For instance, bioremediation of organophosphorous pesticides like Profenofos (PF) and Quinalphos (QP) was achieved through *Kosakinia oryzae* VITPSCQ3 biofilm mediation in a circulating Vertical-flow packed-bed biofilm bioreactor (VFPBB) (Dash & Osborne, 2020). Similarly, Lerch et al. (2017) investigated the effect of 2,4-dichlorophenoxyacetic acid (2,4-D) on the bacterial biofilm of *Cupriavidus necator* JMP134 and concluded that the biofilm is utilizing 2,4-D as the sole carbon source, resulting in its biodegradation.

Biofilms also exhibit a promising solution for the remediation of highly toxic heavy metals due to their inherent tolerance towards such substances. Various processes, including immobilization, adsorption, biotransformation, and detoxification, can be employed to remediate these metals (Edwards & Kjellerup, 2013). Reports have showcased the detoxifying capability of fungal-bacteria biofilm made of *Trichoderma harzianum* and *Bacillus subtilis* against cadmium, lead, and zinc-contaminated soil (Henagamage et al., 2022). Similarly, study by Wu et al. (2017) also exhibited the functionality of periphytic biofilm in the purification of soil leachates that contain elevated levels of Cu (II) and Cd (II) in both highly acidic and moderately acidic environments. Therefore, biofilm-mediated removal of heavy metals is remarkably efficient; however, it is dependent on various external parameters that can influence the binding ability of the microbes to the metals (P. Bhatt et al., 2022).

13.4.3 Role of biofilms in microbial fuel cells (MFCs)

MFCs are a sustainable technology that uses biological catalysts, namely, microorganisms such as bacteria, fungus, and algae, to produce electrical energy from naturally existing organic and inorganic substances or waste found in the surrounding environment (Logan et al., 2006). Microbial communities synthesize extracellular substances (proteins, carbohydrates, and lipids) that constitute the biofilm, which are proteinaceous filaments with electrical conductivity termed microbial nanowires, through which electrons are transferred from the cells to the surface (Dumas et al., 2008). In another study by Parameswaran et al. (2013), *Thermincola ferriacetica,* a Gram-positive bacteria form a 38 μm thick layer of biofilm capable of generating a current density of 7–8/Am^{2,} but *Thermincola* potent bacteria, which form a monolayer of biofilm, generate a comparatively lesser current density, thereby suggesting that multi-layer biofilms generate more electricity. Likewise, mixed bacterial cultures in MFCs generate 20% more current density than those of the pure culture MFCs (Ishii et al., 2008). In MFCs, organic substrates such as carbohydrates, proteins, and lipids serve as electron donors to produce energy at the anode. Microorganisms can thrive in MFCs by

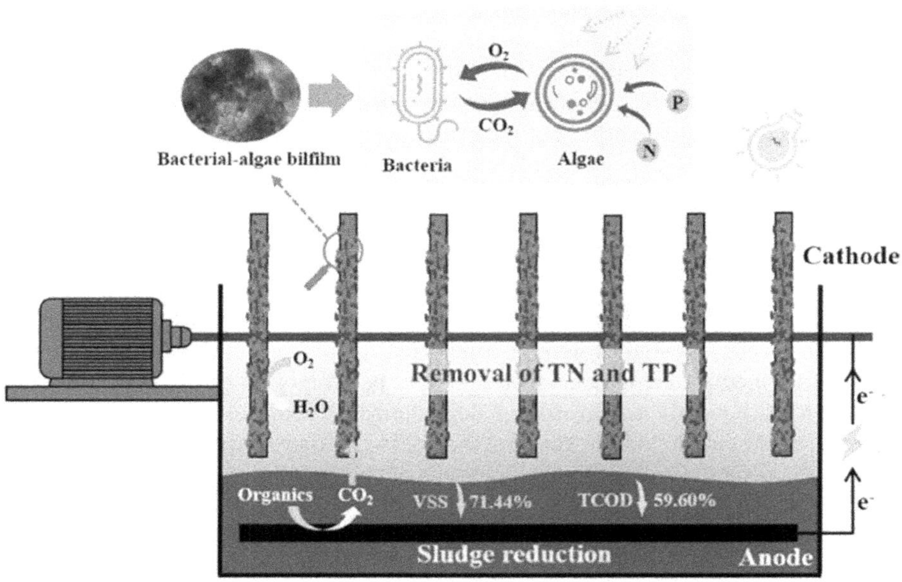

FIGURE 13.3 Microbial fuel cell.

Source: From Chen et al. (2023), used under creative commons CC-BY license.

using various substrates, including nutrients and wastewater sources. The design of MFC is represented in Figure 13.3.

Furthermore, a wide array of microbes exists; however, only those capable of decomposing and oxidizing organic and inorganic substances to generate electrical energy are employed in MFCs. These microbes, which can potentially oxidize substrates, are termed exoelectrogens (Mahmoud et al., 2022). The pathway for degradation or oxidation by the exoelectrogens depends on the type of substrate provided. Subsequently, these complex compounds undergo various processes and are converted to acetyl Co-A, which enters the citric acid cycle. Parallelly, NADH is synthesized from three Nicotinamide Adenine Dinucleotides (NAD^+), and $FADH_2$ is produced via break down of one flavin adenosine dinucleotide (FAD). Post citric acid cycle, CO_2 is released as a by-product, and the Electron Transport Chain (ETC) receives electrons from NADH and $FADH_2$ respectively, converting them into Adenosine Triphosphate (ATP) (Arneth, 2023). The electrons then pass through the proteinaceous filaments and are released as protons at the anode. These are then transported to the cathode through the proton exchange membrane (PEM) and undergo a reaction with oxygen to produce water (Cai et al., 2020).

13.4.3.1 Production of sustainable energy

MFCs can be set up to produce bioelectricity in a sustainable way through the use of wastewater from various households and industries as a substrate for the microorganisms to produce electrons and generate electricity. Furthermore, this approach to utilizing sewage water in MFCs can promote the treatment of chemicals and toxins present in the sewage water, thereby remediating it (Bose et al., 2019). The biofilms used in MFCs are electrochemically active biofilms (EAB), which are found abundantly in various natural sites such as seawater, soil, and different categories of wastewater (Kalathil et al., 2013).

Studies have reported that bacterial species such as *Achromobacter xylosoxidans*, a form of *Betaproteobacteria*, possess the capacity to decompose organic acids and higher levels of chromium present in the wastewater, simultaneously generating bioelectricity (De La Cruz-Noriega et al., 2023). Similarly, generation of bioelectricity was achieved through cellulose and chitin decomposition by *Microbacterium proteolyticum*, a form of *Actinobacteria* (Lewin et al., 2016). Therefore, MFCs provide a sustainable and efficient way to not only treat pollutants but also to generate electricity in a clean and safe.

13.4.4 Biofilms in biofuel generation

Algal biofilms secrete EPS, which possess the potential to generate bioethanol, biodiesel, biogas, and bio-oil (Williams & Laurens, 2010). Agal biomass cultivation is mainly focused on lipid production to generate biofuels (Pulz & Gross, 2004). In one such study, *Chlorella* sp. was cultivated using dairy manure as a growth medium, showing a higher yield of total fatty acids (TFA) content of 9% (w/w), demonstrating its viability as an efficient biodiesel feedstock (Johnson & Wen, 2010). In another study, rotating biological contractors and horizontal biofilm reactors were used to produce biomass for biodiesel generation (Christenson & Sims, 2011). Moreover, biofilm-forming Cyanobacteria are observed to produce 18% (w/w) lipid concentration, and it was also observed that palmitic acid is the main fatty acid of cyanobacterial cultivation, making this a promising biofuel feedstock (Bruno et al., 2012). Many studies have investigated the biogas production potential of algal biofilms of compared to that of conventional feedstocks (Choudhary, 2015).

Bioethanol-producing microbial strains, lignolytic enzymes, and other robust glycosyl hydrolases are incorporated into lignocellulosic waste to yield bioethanol. The effective way to obtain bio-ethanol is by achieving maximum delignification and desaccharification by various microbes (Merklein et al., 2018). For instance, *Sphingomonas paucimobilis* MK1 and *Bacillus circulans* MK2 bacterial strains were used by Chu and Feng (2013) to remove lignin and hemicellulose from used paper under controlled levels of pH and temperature conditions, which yielded 94% improved levels of sugars. Various fungal species are found to possess lignocellulolytic properties, which are used to pretreat lignocellulosic materials, *P. chrysosporium, Pycnoporus cinnabarinus, Ceriporiopsis subvermispora, Pleurotus ostreatus*, and *Cyathus stercoreus* are all white rot fungi that are observed to consume cellulose in the process of degrading lignin. These organisms exhibit greater lignocellulolytic potential at low pH and higher temperature (Taniguchi et al., 2010). Biofilm-based production of biofuel exhibits elevated yield in comparison to suspended systems owing to its high biomass concentration, which corroborates to the condensation of hydrolytic enzymes, which subsequently, increases the reaction rate. Studies have also reported that biofilm containing both fungus and bacteria demonstrates a symbiotic relationship, which leads to simultaneous delignification and saccharification. Moreover, biofilm-assisted technology also provides easier product recovery due to its immobilized state, which also enhances the retention time in fermenter, eventually increasing the yield of biofuel production (Dutta et al., 2022).

13.5 CHALLENGES AND FUTURE PERSPECTIVES

Despite its advantageous nature, biofilm-based applications are often hindered by limited research, especially on factors that regulate biofilm formation. With research throwing light on the working of quorum-sensing systems still in its initial stages, a lot of receptors and their functions still remain unknown. Additionally, biofilm-based applications face challenges such as limited scalability, susceptibility to various toxic compounds, and selective remediation. Biofilm growth is also easily affected by a multitude of factors, such as temperature, oxygen, pH, and the availability of nutrients. More insight into the novel biofilm reactor technologies and lower biofilm formation time are required. Overcoming these challenges will require further research, innovation, and collaboration in order to fully harness the potential of biofilm in various industries, such as healthcare, wastewater treatment, and bioremediation.

13.6 CONCLUSION

The majority of bacterial species utilize the organized structure of biofilms, enabling an array of organisms with intricate variety. It facilitates the dispersion of nutrients and the transfer of genetic material, while playing a crucial role in the organism's survival. A multitude of studies have thoroughly investigated the broad range of applications linked to biofilms. However, there is still a substantial gap in the real-world application of these technologies. The field of biofilm architecture research has undergone a transformation, shifting its focus from primarily exploring strategies preventing biofilm formation to exploring its potential as a viable remediation agent. The manipulation of quorum-sensing systems to enhance biofilm formation and achieve enhanced remediation holds great potential as a viable and cost-effective alternative to current treatment methods. Hence, the adoption of such biofilm-based systems would allow for a safe, efficient, and cost-effective alternative to current methods of treatment.

ACKNOWLEDGMENT

The authors are highly thankful to the Department of Science and Technology, Ministry of Science and Technology, New Delhi, for funding the project under the "Scheme for Young Scientist and Technologists (SYST-SEED)" Project No: SP/YO/2019/1360(G). The authors, Shivangi and Naveen Nair are thankful to Tamil Nadu State Council of Science and Technology (TNSCST), Government of Tamil Nadu (Project code: BS1259) for funding under the "Student Project Scheme".

REFERENCES

Adetunji, V. O., & Odetokun, I. A. (2012). Biofilm formation in human and tropical foodborne isolates of listeria strains. *American Journal of Food Technology*, *7*(9), 517–531. https://doi.org/10.3923/ajft.2012.517.531

Ahn, S.-J., & Burne, R. A. (2007). Effects of oxygen on biofilm formation and the AtlA autolysin of Streptococcus mutans. *Journal of Bacteriology*, *189*(17), 6293–6302. https://doi.org/10.1128/JB.00546-07

Arneth, B. M. (2023). The impact of Krebs Cycle intermediates on the endocrine system and immune system: A comparison. *Endocrines*, *4*(1), 179–193. https://doi.org/10.3390/endocrines4010016

Balducci, E., Papi, F., Capialbi, D. E., & Del Bino, L. (2023). Polysaccharides' structures and functions in biofilm architecture of antimicrobial-resistant (AMR) pathogens. *International Journal of Molecular Science*, *24*(4). https://doi.org/10.3390/ijms24044030

Bhagwat, G., O'Connor, W., Grainge, I., & Palanisami, T. (2021). Understanding the fundamental basis for biofilm formation on plastic surfaces: Role of conditioning films. *Frontiers in Microbiology*, *12*, 687118. https://doi.org/10.3389/fmicb.2021.687118

Bhatt, P., Pandey, S. C., Joshi, S., Chaudhary, P., Pathak, V. M., Huang, Y., Wu, X., Zhou, Z., & Chen, S. (2022). Nanobioremediation: A sustainable approach for the removal of toxic pollutants from the environment. *Journal of Hazardous Materials*, *427*, 128033. https://doi.org/10.1016/j.jhazmat.2021.128033

Bhatt, V. S. (2018). Quorum sensing mechanisms in gram positive bacteria. In *Implication of Quorum Sensing System in Biofilm Formation and Virulence* (pp. 297–311). Springer Singapore. https://doi.org/10.1007/978-981-13-2429-1_20

Biswa, P., & Doble, M. (2013). Production of acylated homoserine lactone by gram-positive bacteria isolated from marine water. *FEMS Microbiology Letters*, *343*(1), 34–41. https://doi.org/10.1111/1574-6968.12123

Bose, D., Gopinath, M., Vijay, P., Sridharan, S., Rawat, R., & Bahuguna, R. (2019). Bioelectricity generation and biofilm analysis from sewage sources using microbial fuel cell. *Fuel*, *255*, 115815. https://doi.org/10.1016/j.fuel.2019.115815

Bruno, L., Di Pippo, F., Antonaroli, S., Gismondi, A., Valentini, C., & Albertano, P. (2012). Characterization of biofilm-forming cyanobacteria for biomass and lipid production. *Journal of Applied Microbiology*, *113*(5), 1052–1064. https://doi.org/10.1111/j.1365-2672.2012.05416.x

Cai, T., Meng, L., Chen, G., Xi, Y., Jiang, N., Song, J., Zheng, S., Liu, Y., Zhen, G., & Huang, M. (2020). Application of advanced anodes in microbial fuel cells for power generation: A review. *Chemosphere*, *248*, 125985. https://doi.org/10.1016/j.chemosphere.2020.125985

Campoccia, D., Montanaro, L., & Arciola, C. R. (2021). Extracellular DNA (eDNA). A major ubiquitous element of the bacterial biofilm architecture. *International Journal of Molecular Science*, *22*(16), 9100. https://doi.org/10.3390/ijms22169100

Chandran, P., & Das, N. (2011). Degradation of diesel oil by immobilized Candida tropicalis and biofilm formed on gravels. *Biodegradation*, *22*(6), 1181–1189. https://doi.org/10.1007/s10532-011-9473-1

Chen, L., Zhang, H., Li, Y., Zhao, C., Liu, L., Li, L., Sun, L., & Li, H. (2023). Sediment microbial fuel cells with algae-assisted cathodes for electricity generation and bio-treatment of sewage sludge. *Fermentation*, *9*(12), 1010. https://doi.org/10.3390/fermentation9121010

Choudhary, P. (2015). Phycoremediation-coupled biomethanation of microalgal biomass. In A. Bhattacharya, S. K. Prajapati, P. Kaushik, & A. Malik, *Handbook of Marine Microalgae* (pp. 483–499). Elsevier. https://doi.org/10.1016/b978-0-12-800776-1.00032-7

Christenson, L., & Sims, R. (2011). Production and harvesting of microalgae for wastewater treatment, biofuels, and bioproducts. *Biotechnology Advances*, *29*(6), 686–702. https://doi.org/10.1016/j.biotechadv.2011.05.015

Chu, K. H., & Feng, X. (2013). Enzymatic conversion of newspaper and office paper to fermentable sugars. *Process Safety and Environmental Protection*, *91*(12), 123–130. https://doi.org/10.1016/j.psep.2011.12.003

Condinho, M., Carvalho, B., Cruz, A., Pinto, S. N., Arraiano, C. M., & Pobre, V. (2023). The role of RNA regulators, quorum sensing and c-di-GMP in bacterial biofilm formation. *Federation of European Biochemical Societies Open Biology*, *13*(6), 975–991. https://doi.org/10.1002/2211-5463.13389

Dash, D. M., & Osborne, W. J. (2020). Rapid biodegradation and biofilm-mediated bioremoval of organophosphorus pesticides using an indigenous Kosakonia oryzae strain -VITPSCQ3 in a Vertical-flow Packed Bed Biofilm Bioreactor. *Ecotoxicology and Environmental Safety*, *192*, 110290. https://doi.org/10.1016/j.ecoenv.2020.110290

Davey, M. E., Caiazza, N. C., & O'Toole, G. A. (2003). Rhamnolipid surfactant production affects biofilm architecture in *Pseudomonas aeruginosa* PAO1. *Journal of Bacteriology*, *185*(3), 1027–1036. https://doi.org/10.1128/jb.185.3.1027-1036.2003

De La Cruz-Noriega, M., Benites, S. M., Rojas-Flores, S., Otiniano, N. M., Sabogal Vargas, A. M., Alfaro, R., Cabanillas-Chirinos, L., Rojas-Villacorta, W., Nazario-Naveda, R., & Delfín-Narciso, D. (2023). Use of wastewater and electrogenic bacteria to generate eco-friendly electricity through microbial fuel cells. *Sustainability*, *15*(13), 10640. https://doi.org/10.3390/su151310640

Dey, S., & Paul, A. K. (2018). Influence of metal ions on biofilm formation by Arthrobacter sp. SUK 1205 and evaluation of their Cr(VI) removal efficacy. *International Biodeterioration & Biodegradation*, *132*, 122–131. https://doi.org/10.1016/j.ibiod.2018.02.015

Donlan, R. M. (2002). Biofilms: Microbial life on surfaces. *Emerging Infectious Diseases*, *8*(9), 881–890. https://doi.org/10.3201/eid0809.020063

Dumas, C., Basseguy, R., & Bergel, A. (2008). Electrochemical activity of Geobacter sulfurreducens biofilms on stainless steel anodes. *Electrochimica Acta*, *53*(16), 5235–5241. https://doi.org/10.1016/j.electacta.2008.02.056

Dutta, B., Nag, M., Lahiri, D., Ghosh, S., Dey, A., Joshi, S., & Ray, R. R. (2022). Biofilms for biofuel production. In *Clean Energy Production Technologies* (pp. 219–237). Springer Nature Singapore. https://doi.org/10.1007/978-981-16-8094-6_13

Edwards, S. J., & Kjellerup, B. V. (2013). Applications of biofilms in bioremediation and biotransformation of persistent organic pollutants, pharmaceuticals/personal care products, and heavy metals. *Applied Microbiology and Biotechnology*, *97*(23), 9909–9921. https://doi.org/10.1007/s00253-013-5216-z

Flemming, H.-C., Neu, T. R., & Wozniak, D. J. (2007). The EPS matrix: The "house of biofilm cells." *Journal Bacteriology*, *189*(22), 7945–7947. https://doi.org/10.1128/JB.00858-07

Flemming, H.-C., van Hullebusch, E. D., Neu, T. R., Nielsen, P. H., Seviour, T., Stoodley, P., Wingender, J., & Wuertz, S. (2023). The biofilm matrix: Multitasking in a shared space. *Nature Reviews Microbiology*, *21*(2), 70–86. https://doi.org/10.1038/s41579-022-00791-0

Fulaz, S., Vitale, S., Quinn, L., & Casey, E. (2019). Nanoparticle-biofilm interactions: The role of the EPS matrix. *Trends Microbiology*, *27*(11), 915–926. https://doi.org/10.1016/j.tim.2019.07.004

Garrett, T. R., Bhakoo, M., & Zhang, Z. (2008). Bacterial adhesion and biofilms on surfaces. *Progress in Natural Science*, *18*(9), 1049–1056. https://doi.org/10.1016/j.pnsc.2008.04.001

Ghosh, B., Dhar, J., Mukhopadhyay, M., & Bhattacharya, D. (2024). Bacillus cereus biofilm: Implications for food and diseases. *The Microbe*, *4*, 100129. https://doi.org/10.1016/j.microb.2024.100129

Henagamage, A. P., Peries, C. M., & Seneviratne, G. (2022). Fungal-bacterial biofilm mediated heavy metal rhizo-remediation. *World Journal of Microbiology and Biotechnology*, *38*(5). https://doi.org/10.1007/s11274-022-03267-8

Hoh, D., Watson, S., & Kan, E. (2016). Algal biofilm reactors for integrated wastewater treatment and biofuel production: A review. *Chemical Engineering Journal*, *287*, 466–473. https://doi.org/10.1016/j.cej.2015.11.062

Huang, D., Zhang, Y., Long, J., Yang, X., Bao, L., Yang, Z., Wu, B., Si, R., Zhao, W., Peng, C., Wang, A., & Yan, D. (2022). Polystyrene microplastic exposure induces insulin resistance in mice via dysbacteriosis and pro-inflammation. *Science of the Total Environment*, *838*, 155937. https://doi.org/10.1016/j.scitotenv.2022.155937

Ishii, S., Watanabe, K., Yabuki, S., Logan, B. E., & Sekiguchi, Y. (2008). Comparison of electrode reduction activities of *Geobacter sulfurreducens* and an enriched consortium in an Air-cathode microbial fuel cell. *Applied and Environmental Microbiology*, *74*(23), 7348–7355. https://doi.org/10.1128/aem.01639-08

Johnson, M. B., & Wen, Z. (2010). Development of an attached microalgal growth system for biofuel production. *Applied Microbiology and Biotechnology*, *85*(3), 525–534. https://doi.org/10.1007/s00253-009-2133-2

Kalathil, S., Khan, M. M., Lee, J., & Cho, M. H. (2013). Production of bioelectricity, bio-hydrogen, high value chemicals and bioinspired nanomaterials by electrochemically active biofilms. *Biotechnology Advances*, *31*(6), 915–924. https://doi.org/10.1016/j.biotechadv.2013.05.001

Kong, W., Celik, V., Liao, C., Hua, Q., & Lu, T. (2014). Programming the group behaviors of bacterial communities with synthetic cellular communication. *Bioresources and Bioprocessing*, *1*(1). https://doi.org/10.1186/s40643-014-0024-6

Kragh, K. N., Hutchison, J. B., Melaugh, G., Rodesney, C., Roberts, A. E. L., Irie, Y., Jensen, P. Ø., Diggle, S. P., Allen, R. J., Gordon, V., & Bjarnsholt, T. (2016). Role of multicellular aggregates in biofilm formation. *mBio*, *7*(2). https://doi.org/10.1128/mbio.00237-16

Kumar, C. G., & Anand, S. K. (1998). Significance of microbial biofilms in food industry: A review. *International Journal of Food Microbiology*, *42*(1–2), 9–27. https://doi.org/10.1016/s0168-1605(98)00060-9

Lemos, J. A., Palmer, S. R., Zeng, L., Wen, Z. T., Kajfasz, J. K., Freires, I. A., Abranches, J., & Brady, L. J. (2019). The biology of streptococcus mutans. *Microbiology Spectrum*, *7*(1). https://doi.org/10.1128/microbiolspec.GPP3-0051-2018

Lerch, T. Z., Chenu, C., Dignac, M. F., Barriuso, E., & Mariotti, A. (2017). Biofilm vs. Planktonic lifestyle: Consequences for pesticide 2,4-D metabolism by cupriavidus necator JMP134. *Frontiers in Microbiology*, *8*. https://doi.org/10.3389/fmicb.2017.00904

Lewin, G. R., Carlos, C., Chevrette, M. G., Horn, H. A., McDonald, B. R., Stankey, R. J., Fox, B. G., & Currie, C. R. (2016). Evolution and ecology of actinobacteria and their bioenergy applications. *Annual Review of Microbiology*, *70*, 235–254. https://doi.org/10.1146/annurev-micro-102215-095748

Li, C., Li, Y., Cheng, X., Feng, L., Xi, C., & Zhang, Y. (2013). Immobilization of Rhodococcus rhodochrous BX2 (an acetonitrile-degrading bacterium) with biofilm-forming bacteria for wastewater treatment. *Bioresource Technology*, *131*, 390–396. https://doi.org/10.1016/j.biortech.2012.12.140

Logan, B. E., Hamelers, B., Rozendal, R., Schröder, U., Keller, J., Freguia, S., Aelterman, P., Verstraete, W., & Rabaey, K. (2006). Microbial fuel cells: Methodology and technology. *Environmental Science Technology*, *40*(17), 5181–5192. https://doi.org/10.1021/es0605016

Lu, L., Wan, Z., Luo, T., Fu, Z., & Jin, Y. (2018). Polystyrene microplastics induce gut microbiota dysbiosis and hepatic lipid metabolism disorder in mice. *Science of the Total Environment*, *631–632*, 449–458. https://doi.org/10.1016/j.scitotenv.2018.03.051

Mahmoud, R. H., Gomaa, O. M., & Hassan, R. Y. A. (2022). Bio-electrochemical frameworks governing microbial fuel cell performance: Technical bottlenecks and proposed solutions. *RSC Advances*, *12*(10), 5749–5764. https://doi.org/10.1039/d1ra08487a

Mangwani, N., Kumari, S., & Das, S. (2016). Effect of synthetic N-acylhomoserine lactones on cell–cell interactions in marine Pseudomonas and biofilm mediated degradation of polycyclic aromatic hydrocarbons. *Chemical Engineering Journal*, *302*, 172–186. https://doi.org/10.1016/j.cej.2016.05.042

Mangwani, N., Shukla, S. K., Kumari, S., Rao, T. S., & Das, S. (2014). Characterization of *Stenotrophomonas acidaminiphila* NCW-702 biofilm for implication in the degradation of polycyclic aromatic hydrocarbons. *Journal of Applied Microbiology*, *117*(4), 1012–1024. https://doi.org/10.1111/jam.12602

Merklein, M., Stiller, B., Vu, K., Madden, S. J., & Eggleton, B. J. (2018). Author Correction: A chip-integrated coherent photonic-phononic memory. *Nature Communications*, *9*(1). https://doi.org/10.1038/s41467-017-02506-z

Mishra, S., Huang, Y., Li, J., Wu, X., Zhou, Z., Lei, Q., Bhatt, P., & Chen, S. (2022). Biofilm-mediated bioremediation is a powerful tool for the removal of environmental pollutants. *Chemosphere*, *294*(133609), 133609. https://doi.org/10.1016/j.chemosphere.2022.133609

Mukherjee, S., & Bassler, B. L. (2019). Bacterial quorum sensing in complex and dynamically changing environments. *Nature Review Microbiology*, *17*(6), 371–382. https://doi.org/10.1038/s41579-019-0186-5

Mukhi, M., & Vishwanathan, A. S. (2022). Beneficial biofilms: A minireview of strategies to enhance biofilm formation for biotechnological applications. *Applied Environment Microbiology*, *88*(3), e0199421. https://doi.org/10.1128/AEM.01994-21

Naz, I. (2016). Role of the biofilms in wastewater treatment. In S. Sehar, *Microbial Biofilms—Importance and Applications*. InTech. https://doi.org/10.5772/63499

Otto, M. (2013). Staphylococcal infections: Mechanisms of biofilm maturation and detachment as critical determinants of pathogenicity. *Annual Review of Medicine*, *64*(1), 175–188. https://doi.org/10.1146/annurev-med-042711-140023

Parameswaran, P., Bry, T., Popat, S. C., Lusk, B. G., Rittmann, B. E., & Torres, C. I. (2013). Kinetic, electrochemical, and microscopic characterization of the thermophilic, anode-respiring bacterium *thermincola ferriacetica*. *Environmental Science & Technology*, *47*(9), 4934–4940. https://doi.org/10.1021/es400321c

Pereira, C. S., Thompson, J. A., & Xavier, K. B. (2013). AI-2-mediated signalling in bacteria. *Federation of European Microbiological Societies Microbiology Reviews*, *37*(2), 156–181. https://doi.org/10.1111/j.1574-6976.2012.00345.x

Philipp, L.-A., Bühler, K., Ulber, R., & Gescher, J. (2024). Beneficial applications of biofilms. *Nature Review Microbiology*, *22*(5), 276–290. https://doi.org/10.1038/s41579-023-00985-0

Pinkston, K. L., Gao, P., Diaz-Garcia, D., Sillanpää, J., Nallapareddy, S. R., Murray, B. E., & Harvey, B. R. (2011). The Fsr quorum-sensing system of Enterococcus faecalis modulates surface display of the collagen-binding MSCRAMM Ace through regulation of gelE. *Journal of Bacteriology*, *193*(17), 4317–4325. https://doi.org/10.1128/JB.05026-11

Pinto, R. M., Soares, F. A., Reis, S., Nunes, C., & Van Dijck, P. (2020). Innovative strategies toward the disassembly of the EPS matrix in bacterial biofilms. *Frontiers in Microbiology*, *11*, 952. https://doi.org/10.3389/fmicb.2020.00952

Pompilio, A., Piccolomini, R., Picciani, C., D'Antonio, D., Savini, V., & Di Bonaventura, G. (2008). Factors associated with adherence to and biofilm formation on polystyrene by Stenotrophomonas maltophilia: The role of cell surface hydrophobicity and motility. *FEMS Microbiology Letters*, *287*(1), 41–47. https://doi.org/10.1111/j.1574-6968.2008.01292.x

Prazdnova, E. V., Gorovtsov, A. V., Vasilchenko, N. G., Kulikov, M. P., Statsenko, V. N., Bogdanova, A. A., Refeld, A. G., Brislavskiy, Y. A., Chistyakov, V. A., & Chikindas, M. L. (2022). Quorum-sensing inhibition by Gram-positive bacteria. *Microorganisms*, *10*(2), 350. https://doi.org/10.3390/microorganisms10020350

Pulz, O., & Gross, W. (2004). Valuable products from biotechnology of microalgae. *Applied Microbiology and Biotechnology*, *65*(6), 635–648. https://doi.org/10.1007/s00253-004-1647-x

Rumbaugh, K. P., & Sauer, K. (2020). Biofilm dispersion. *Nature Review Microbiology*, *18*(10), 571–586. https://doi.org/10.1038/s41579-020-0385-0

Rutherford, S. T., & Bassler, B. L. (2012). Bacterial quorum sensing: Its role in virulence and possibilities for its control. *Cold Spring Harber Perspective in Medicine*, *2*(11), a012427–a012427. https://doi.org/10.1101/cshperspect.a012427

Saini, S., Tewari, S., Dwivedi, J., & Sharma, V. (2023). Biofilm-mediated wastewater treatment: A comprehensive review. *Materials Advances*, *4*(6), 1415–1443. https://doi.org/10.1039/d2ma00945e

Sauer, K., Stoodley, P., Goeres, D. M., Hall-Stoodley, L., Burmølle, M., Stewart, P. S., & Bjarnsholt, T. (2022). The biofilm life cycle: Expanding the conceptual model of biofilm formation. *Nature Reviews Microbiology*, *20*(10), 608–620. https://doi.org/10.1038/s41579-022-00767-0

Shree, P., Singh, C. K., Sodhi, K. K., Surya, J. N., & Singh, D. K. (2023). Biofilms: Understanding the structure and contribution towards bacterial resistance in antibiotics. *Medicine Microecology*, *16*(100084), 100084. https://doi.org/10.1016/j.medmic.2023.100084

Singh, M. P. (2020). Microbial biofilms: Development, structure, and their social assemblage for beneficial applications. In P. Singh, H.- B. Li, Q.- Q. Song, & R. K. Singh, *New and Future Developments in Microbial Biotechnology and Bioengineering: Microbial Biofilms* (pp. 125–138). Elsevier. https://doi.org/10.1016/b978-0-444-64279-0.00010-4

Singh, R., Paul, D., & Jain, R. K. (2006). Biofilms: Implications in bioremediation. *Trends in Microbiology*, *14*(9), 389–397. https://doi.org/10.1016/j.tim.2006.07.001

Sionov, R. V., & Steinberg, D. (2022). Targeting the holy triangle of quorum sensing, biofilm formation, and antibiotic resistance in pathogenic bacteria. *Microorganisms*, *10*(6), 1239. https://doi.org/10.3390/microorganisms10061239

Talluri, S. N. L., Winter, R. M., & Salem, D. R. (2020). Conditioning film formation and its influence on the initial adhesion and biofilm formation by a cyanobacterium on photobioreactor materials. *Biofouling*, *36*(2), 183–199. https://doi.org/10.1080/08927014.2020.1748186

Taniguchi, M., Takahashi, D., Watanabe, D., Sakai, K., Hoshino, K., Kouya, T., & Tanaka, T. (2010). Effect of steam explosion pretreatment on treatment with Pleurotus ostreatus for the enzymatic hydrolysis of rice straw. *Journal of Bioscience and Bioengineering*, *110*(4), 449–452. https://doi.org/10.1016/j.jbiosc.2010.04.014

Ünal Turhan, E. (2019). Beneficial biofilm applications in food and agricultural industry. In Z. Erginkaya, M. Korukluoğlu, & G. Konuray, *Health and Safety Aspects of Food Processing Technologies* (pp. 445–469). Springer International Publishing. https://doi.org/10.1007/978-3-030-24903-8_15

Valentini, M., & Filloux, A. (2016). Biofilms and cyclic di-GMP (c-di-GMP) Signaling: Lessons from Pseudomonas aeruginosa and Other Bacteria. *Journal of Biologyical Chemistry*, *291*(24), 12547–12555. https://doi.org/10.1074/jbc.R115.711507

Vu, B., Chen, M., Crawford, R. J., & Ivanova, E. P. (2009). Bacterial extracellular polysaccharides involved in biofilm formation. *Molecules*, *14*(7), 2535–2554. https://doi.org/10.3390/molecules14072535

Wang, Y., Bian, Z., & Wang, Y. (2022). Biofilm formation and inhibition mediated by bacterial quorum sensing. *Applied Microbiology Biotechnology*, *106*(19–20), 6365–6381. https://doi.org/10.1007/s00253-022-12150-3

Whitehead, N. A., Barnard, A. M. L., Slater, H., Simpson, N. J. L., & Salmond, G. P. C. (2001). Quorum-sensing in gram-negative bacteria. *FEMS Microbiology Review*, *25*(4), 365–404. https://doi.org/10.1111/j.1574-6976.2001.tb00583.x

Williams, P. J. L. B., & Laurens, L. M. L. (2010). Microalgae as biodiesel & biomass feedstocks: Review & analysis of the biochemistry, energetics & economics. *Energy & Environmental Science*, *3*(5), 554. https://doi.org/10.1039/b924978h

Wu, Y., Yang, J., Tang, J., Kerr, P., & Wong, P. K. (2017). The remediation of extremely acidic and moderate pH soil leachates containing Cu (II) and Cd (II) by native periphytic biofilm. *Journal of Cleaner Production*, *162*, 846–855. https://doi.org/10.1016/j.jclepro.2017.06.086

Zhang, P., Fang, F., Chen, Y.-P., Shen, Y., Zhang, W., Yang, J.-X., Li, C., Guo, J.-S., Liu, S.-Y., Huang, Y., Li, S., Gao, X., & Yan, P. (2014). Composition of EPS fractions from suspended sludge and biofilm and their roles in microbial cell aggregation. *Chemosphere*, *117*, 59–65. https://doi.org/10.1016/j.chemosphere.2014.05.070

Zhao, X., Zhao, F., Wang, J., & Zhong, N. (2017). Biofilm formation and control strategies of foodborne pathogens: Food safety perspectives. *RSC Advance*, *7*(58), 36670–36683. https://doi.org/10.1039/c7ra02497e

Zhou, L., Zhang, Y., Ge, Y., Zhu, X., & Pan, J. (2020). Regulatory mechanisms and promising applications of quorum sensing-inhibiting agents in control of bacterial biofilm formation. *Frontiers in Microbiology*, *11*, 589640. https://doi.org/10.3389/fmicb.2020.589640

14 Nanocomposites for clean water

Radha K.V. and Selvi V. S.

14.1 INTRODUCTION

A nanocomposite is a solid material composed of multiple phases, where at least one of the phases has one, two, or three dimensions in the nanometer range. The nanoscale phase process achieves the goal of synergy between different constituents. Nanomaterials included in nanocomposites are nanoparticles (NPs), nanofibers, and nanoclays. The properties of the material change when the size of the material constituents is below a certain size, which is known as the critical size (Nikolaeva et al., 2023). When the material dimensions are reduced to the nanometer level, interactions occur at the phase boundaries, which are very important for improving the material properties. The ratio between the surface area and the volume of the reinforced material used in the production of nanocomposites is directly involved in understanding the structure-property relationship. The nanocomposite material (at least one nanometer-scale (10–9 m) component) composed of nonmetallic, metallic, and polymeric materials by a special process has the added advantage of retaining primary properties to overcome defects and express some new properties (Wongvasana et al., 2023).

Such a material represents a multiphase hybrid of matrix material and reinforcing material. The reinforcing material is a dispersed phase, usually fibrous materials such as glass fibers, organic fibers, etc., and nanocomposites represent a new alternative to overcome the current limitations of micro composites and monoliths and are becoming materials of the future. The main advantages of nanocomposites over other composites are high surface-to-volume ratio, which allows small filler size and spacing between fillers; better mechanical properties; high ductility without loss of strength, scratch resistance; and improved optical properties (light transmission depends on particle size). Nanocomposites are classified into various groups (Omanović-Mikličanin et al., 2020). Some of the types of nanocomposites along with their processing methods, advantages, disadvantages, and applications are tabulated in Table 14.1.

Nanocomposites are suitable materials to meet the emerging demands for next step in our progress. Today, different processing methods (CMNC, MMNC, and PMNC) are available, but limitations and drawbacks request search for new opportunities techniques and engineering. They offer improved performance over monolithic and microcomposite counterparts, and they are suitable candidates to overcome the limitations of many currently existing materials and devices (Ferreira et al., 2018). Today, applications of nanocomposites do exist, but the full potential is still not discovered. Properties such as very high mechanical endurance even at low loading of reinforcements, gas barrier, and flame-related properties create potential applications and market for these materials (Singh and Agarwal, 2016).

Due to the high corrosion susceptibility of metals used in oil and gas pipelines and the failure rate of conventional materials, the importance of nanocomposites cannot be overstated. Nanocomposites are materials with a nanoscale structure that improve the macroscopic properties of products. Mechanically, nanocomposites differ from conventional composites in the exceptionally high surface-to-volume ratio of the reinforcing phase and/or their exceptionally high aspect ratio. The reinforcing material may consist of particles (e.g., minerals), sheets (e.g., expanded clay stacks), or fibers (e.g., carbon nanotubes [CNTs] or electrospun fibers).

DOI: 10.1201/9781003500483-14
This chapter has been made available under a (CC-BY-NC-ND) 4.0 license

TABLE 14.1
Types of nanocomposites and its applications

	Ceramic matrix nanocomposites	Polymer matrix nanocomposites	Metal matrix nanocomposites
Processing methods	Powder process, polymer precursor process, and sol-gel process	In situ intercalative polymerization, melt intercalation, and template synthesis	Spray pyrolysis, liquid infiltration, Sol-gel, rapid solidification, RSP with ultrasonics
Examples	Si_3N_4/SiC, Al_2O_3/SiC, $B4_C/TiB_2$, $Al_2O_3/NdAlO_3$	Nylon-montmorillonite nanocomposite and thermoplastics, thermoplastic nanocomposites, and double-layer hydroxide-based nanocomposites	W/Cu, Fe/MgO, Pb/Cu, W/Cu/Nb/Cu, Pb/Fe Nb/Fe,Fe/SiO_2, Ag/Au, Au/Fe/Au, Al/X/Zr (X = Si, Cu, Ni), Al/Pb
Advantages	Higher resistance/hardness, improved toughness/durability, decreased elasticity and ductility and reduces rejection risk	Tethering effect through which linking is enabled, promote dispersion of the silicate layers in a one-step process, without presence of the onium ion.	Effective and versatile, processing temperature low, good chemical homogeneity, rigorous stoichiometry control, high purity products.
Disadvantages	Rate of formation and phase dispersion is low, agglomeration occurs and requirement of high temperatures	Promote dispersion of the silicate layers in a one-step process, without presence of the onium ion.	Drawback with metal-metal nanocomposites; due to agglomeration and non-homogeneous formation
Applications	SiO_2/Fe-High performance catalysts and data storage technology. $BaTiO_3$/SiC, PZT/Ag -Electronic industry, ferroelectric property. SiO_2/Ni-chemical sensors. $Al_2O_3/NdAlO_3$ and $Al_2O_3/LnAlO_3$-Solid state laser media, phosphors, and optical amplifiers. $PbTiO_3/PbZrO_3$-microelectronic and micro-electromechanical systems.	Gas barriers for packaging and sports goods. Energy storage systems. Optical glass and membranes. Electronics and automobile sectors. Coatings.	Fe/MgO-Catalysts, magnetic devices. Ni/PZT-Wear resistant and thermally graded coatings. Ni/TiN, Ni/ZrN, Cu/ZrN-Industrial high -speed machinery, optics and magnetic storage materials. $Fe/Fe_{23}C_6/Fe_3B$-Structural materials. Cu/Al_2O_3-Electronic packaging. Nb/Cu-structural materials for high temperature application.

The area of the interface between the matrix and the reinforcing phase(s) is typically an order of magnitude larger than that of conventional composites. The properties of the matrix material are significantly affected near the reinforcement. In their study, Ajayan et al. (2003) found that for polymer nanocomposites, properties related to local chemistry, degree of cure, polymer chain mobility, polymer chain conformation, degree of polymer chain ordering, or crystallinity can vary significantly and continuously from the interface with the reinforcement into the bulk of the matrix (Miao et al., 2019). This large reinforcement surface area means that a relatively small amount of nanoscale reinforcement can have a remarkable effect on the macroscopic properties of the composite. For example, the addition of CNTs improves electrical and thermal conductivity. Other types of NPs can result in improved optical properties, dielectric properties, heat resistance, or mechanical properties such as stiffness, strength, and resistance to wear and damage (Mittal et al., 2018).

Generally, the nano reinforcement is dispersed into the matrix during processing. The weight percentage (called mass fraction) of the introduced NPs can remain very low (on the order of 0.5 to 5%) due to the low percolation threshold of the filler, especially for the most used non-spherical fillers with high aspect ratio (e.g., nanometer-thin platelets such as clay or nanometer-diameter cylinders such as CNTs) (Harito et al., 2019).

Nanocomposites can significantly improve the properties of materials by leading to the formation of nanoscale aluminide secondary phases in aluminum alloys, thereby increasing their strength and corrosion resistance. He further explained that magnetic multilayered materials are one of the most important aspects of nanocomposites, as they have led to significant advances in storage media (Okpala, 2014).

14.2 NEED FOR WASTEWATER TREATMENT

In developing countries, industrial wastewater management is one of the greatest dilemmas of our time. In these countries, industrial effluents are discharged directly into the natural drainage system, into the sewerage system, into an internal septic tank, or into a nearby field. Some of these industrial effluents are inadequately treated or not treated at all before they enter the sewer system. In recent years, urbanization and industrial activities in developing countries have led to environmental degradation, and the quality of industrial wastewater is responsible for the degradation of receiving waters (Dutta et al., 2021). This is because inadequately treated or untreated industrial wastewater can lead to eutrophication of receiving waters and create favorable conditions for toxin-producing pathogens in the water. Although it appears to be abundant on the Earth's surface, water is a rare and precious commodity, and only a vanishingly small fraction of the Earth's water reserves (about 0.03%) represents the water resource available for human activities (Kanu et at., 2011). The growth of the world's population and industry has led to an ever-increasing demand for water out of proportion to the available supply, which remains constant. Therefore, it is necessary to minimize water consumption and return water to the environment with minimal contamination, as the capacity of self-purification is limited. This is why wastewater treatment is so important (Kehrein et al., 2020).

In wastewater treatment, there are four classifications of treatment. Pretreatment includes the removal of large particles as well as solids in wastewater. The second classification is primary treatment, in which organic and inorganic solids are removed by a physical process, and the resulting wastewater is called primary effluent. The third treatment is called secondary treatment. Here, suspended, residual organic matter, and compounds are broken down. Secondary treatment includes biological (bacterial) degradation of unwanted products. The fourth is tertiary treatment, which is usually a chemical process and very often includes residual disinfection (Gómez et al., 2007). The worldwide interest for quality water, whether for reasons for drinking, sterilization, water system, and modern use, has been on a nonstop ascent, and there has been overpowering worry in ongoing years about water treatment and reuse requiring the strictest principles. The drug business is assailed with high-esteem, low volume multiproduct plants on one hand, which are for the most part group activities wherein the emanating is blended and treated. There are some devoted clumps, semi batch, also, and nonstop interaction plants delivering mass medications. These plants make use of a variety of reactants, such as solvents, solids, (homogeneous) catalysts, water, and special machinery (Strade et al., 2020). In these kinds of units, the significant expense of the medication relies upon the sort of contamination instead of on the virtue of the medication. In this way, partition processes assume an extremely fundamental part in this industry. The presence, result, and poisonousness of chemical deposits in the oceanic climate present challenges. Hence, recuperation of high-esteem programming interface and drugs from weaken streams, rather than treatment, should be considered while managing this issue. Antibiotics, analgesics, antihistamines, and other antituberculosis (TB) medications are among the most frequently prescribed generic medications (Chakraborty et al., 2022). As a result, most of the spread and effects of these moieties' presence in the environment are unknown and unclear. These compounds have been recognized in a wide

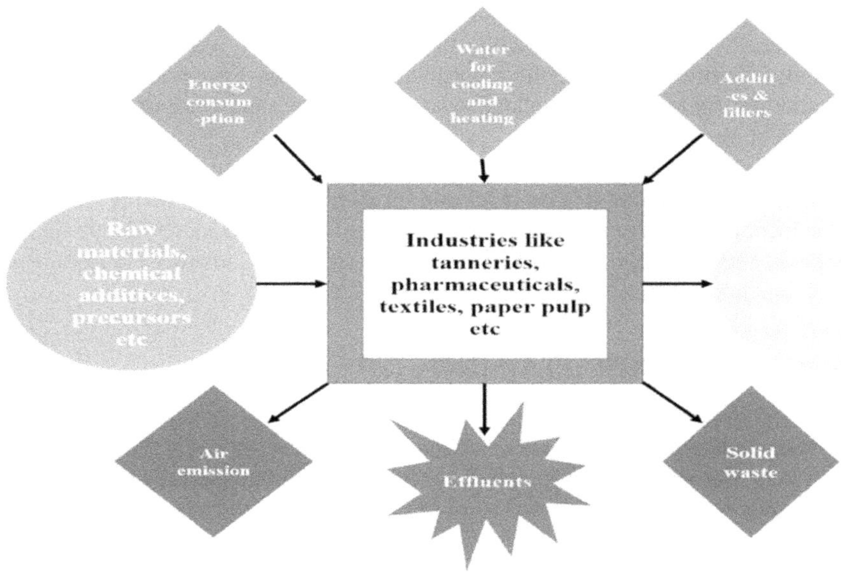

FIGURE 14.1 Schematic diagram showing the generation of effluents in industries.

assortment of ecological tests including sewage, surface waters, groundwater, and consumable water; their focuses by and large reach from a couple of parts per trillion to parts per billion levels (Vasilachi et al., 2021). Nanomaterials are ordinarily characterized as materials less than 100 nm in somewhere around one aspect. At this scale, materials frequently have novel size-subordinate properties unique in relation to their enormous partners, a significant number of which have been investigated for applications in water and wastewater treatment. A portion of these applications use the easily versatile size-subordinate properties of nanomaterials, which connect with the high unambiguous surface region, like quick disintegration, high reactivity, and solid sorption. Others exploit their irregular properties, for example, super paramagnetism, restricted surface plasmon reverberation, and quantum control impact (Singha and Mishrab, 2020).

14.3 SYNTHESIS STRATEGIES FOR NANOCOMPOSITES

Nanocomposites address a significant class of nanomaterials, and there have been a few entrancing turns of events around here in the previous ten years. One of the significant difficulties in the combination of nanocomposites is the way to plan and set up the ideal design with different capabilities, for example, reactant, attractive, electronic, and optical properties, as well as surface usefulness combined with biocompatibility, low poisonousness, and high strength. As a significant group of nanocomposites, attractive nanocomposites with attractively responsive centers and useful shells certainly stand out due to their extraordinary usefulness and distinctness.

Attractive NPs have expected applications in attractive fluids, catalysis, biotechnology/biomedicine, attractive reverberation imaging (X-ray), information capacity, and ecological remediation. Notwithstanding, a few inescapable issues are related with attractive NPs, for example, their characteristic flimsiness over extensive stretches because of their inclination to total to lessen their surface energy, as well as the simplicity with which they are oxidized in air. The conglomeration of attractive NPs can significantly decline their interfacial region, in this manner bringing about the deficiency of attraction and dispersibility (Anik et al., 2021). It is consequently pivotal to foster new techniques to balance out the stripped attractive NPs against debasement artificially during or after the engineered processes. Research has shown that coatings of polymer, silica, or different materials over the attractive NPs can forestall total and functionalize the attractive NPs to broaden their applications in catalysis what's more, biomedicine. Magnetic NPs have been coated and stabilized with a variety of materials, including surfactant, dextran, polyethylene glycol (PEG), dimercaptosuccinic acid, poloxamers, polyoxoamines, metal oxide, silica, and carbon (Yeap et al., 2017).

Among the materials read up for covering, silica and carbon are especially alluring as they display high biocompatibility and strength, low harmfulness, and straightforward usefulness. The disclosure of the supramolecular self-get-together of mesoporous materials has started escalated interest in different research regions. With appealing properties, like enormous surface regions, uniform pore sizes, and tunable intermittent designs, mesoporous silicas and carbons are promising competitors as nanoreactors and huge particle conveyance vehicles (Castillo et al., 2019).

Magnetic mesoporous materials have received a lot of attention for their ability to combine a mesoporous structure with magnetic properties to achieve magnetic response, a large surface area, high pore volume, and ease of functionalization. Profoundly permeable attractive materials could be used in the capacity and conveyance of little atoms, for example, fluorescent colors; furthermore, drugs, as well as huge atoms like nucleotides and proteins. The attractive nanocomposites with mesoporous designs can be eliminated after use by applying an attractive field, and designated conveyance can likewise be accomplished by utilizing an outer attractive field (Brigante et al., 2016). To work on the usefulness of attractive nanocomposites, different strategies have been created to tailor the morphology of the nanocomposites and present utilitarian gatherings on a superficial level. Consequently, attractive mesoporous nanocomposites are exceptionally encouraging for application as medication/quality/RNA conveyance transporters, multimodal imaging specialists, water treatment adsorbents, and as impetuses for different responses.

Then again, ongoing investigations have shown that the synergistic coupling among nanomaterials and graphene can prompt upgraded execution or even another property that isn't found in the singular parts. In perspective on these, a much exertion has been given to the plan, furthermore, controlled manufacture of graphene-based nanocomposites (Kewat et al., 2024). By and large, two distinct techniques have been laid out. The first includes the immediate development of nanocrystals on the surface of graphene nanosheets with the forerunner salts adsorbed on their basal planes (in situ development), while the other includes the earlier blend of nanocrystals with wanted aspects and morphologies, and afterward appending them to the outer layer of graphene sheets (the self-gathering approach). Nonetheless, the fine control of the size what's more, circulation of the practical nanomaterials on graphene sheets is yet a significant test to the improvement of graphene-based nanocomposites for inescapable applications, furthermore, little examination has been centered around the correlation of these two unique manufactured procedures (Wu et al., 2012). High-quality phosphors, up-conversion materials, time-resolved fluorescence labels, and other applications rely heavily on rare earth oxides because of their outstanding optical and catalytic properties. As one of the most responsive intriguing earth metal oxides, CeO_2 has gotten a lot of consideration due to its expansive scopes of uses in catalysis, metal cleaning specialists, UV hindering, oxygen sensors, what's more, oxygen particle guides in strong oxide energy components (Xu et al., 2014).

Also, a few investigations have demonstrated the way that CeO_2 could be photoactivated by close UV-vis illumination and break down organics in the watery stage under apparent light or sunlight-based illumination, which makes CeO_2 a promising material for photocatalytic applications. It was proposed that an aqueous technique for the blend of a graphene/CeO_2 nanocomposite and explored its electrochemical properties as a potential anode material for lithium particle batteries (Mishra and Ahmaruzzaman, 2021). Li and collaborators fostered an in-situ strategy for the blend of a graphene/CeO_2 NP nanocomposite, which shows a high unambiguous capacitance and power thickness in supercapacitors. However, little research has been done on RGO/CeO_2 nanocomposites. Two approaches have employed for RGO-upheld CeO_2 NP composites, viz., in situ development and the self-gathering approach. The impacts of these two methodologies and the surfactant poly (vinylpyrrolidone) (PVP) on the dissemination, furthermore, size control of CeO_2 NPs on RGO nanosheets were efficiently explored. Besides, photocatalytic corruption of methylene blue (MB) was utilized as a model response to assess the synergistic movement of the RGO/CeO_2 nanocomposites (Ojha et al., 2017). Nanocomposites can be synthesized through various methods, and some of them are tabulated in Table 14.2. Researchers use various methods for synthesis, and methodology varies accordingly (Liu et al., 2011).

TABLE 14.2
Methods for the synthesis of nanocomposites

S.no	Method of synthesis	Description
1	Coprecipitation	Coprecipitation is an exceptionally successful strategy for the planning of nanocomposites. It very well may be ready in fluid arrangements by the coprecipitation of metal salts under basic circumstances at encompassing temperature, or at raised temperatures with the security of a dormant gas. The fundamental benefit of the coprecipitation cycle is that iron oxide NPs can be helpfully incorporated on a huge scale. Be that as it may, control of the molecule size circulation is restricted on the grounds that the development of nanocrystals is administered by motor elements. Using a coprecipitation reaction, monodisperse iron oxide magnetic NPs can be produced through a short nucleation burst followed by controlled, slow growth.
2	Thermal decomposition	Nanocomposites can be made through the warm decay of organometallic precursors in high-limit natural solvents containing unsaturated fats or amines as balancing out surfactants. This technique gives size-controllable and monodisperse attractive nanocrystals with a customary and great crystallite morphology. Nonetheless, a high response temperature is expected to instigate nucleation and resulting nanoparticle development. Warm disintegration of organometallic antecedents, in which the metal is zero-valent, can at first lead to the arrangement of metal NPs. However, high-quality monodisperse metal oxides can be produced through oxidation. Then again, the disintegration of precursors with cationic metal places can lead straight forwardly to attractive metal oxide NPs.
3	Microemulsion- or nanoemulsion-based synthetic methods	A microemulsion is defined as a thermodynamically stable isotropic scattering of two immiscible fluids, in which the microdomain of one or the other or the two fluids has been stabilized by an interfacial film of surface-dynamic atoms. Attractive particles can be ready by scattering attractive components in a natural stage containing an organosoluble initiator, blending the scattering in with a watery arrangement made of water and emulsifier, homogenizing the blend to give micrometer beads in the natural stage, and finally polymerizing the homogenized blend after the expansion of monomer, if essential. The dispersion of the droplets (and consequently of the polymer particles) is a component of the extent of emulsifier present in the fluid arrangement, and the proportion of the natural to the fluid stage. The size distribution of the polymer particles acquired by this cycle is wide.

(*Continued*)

TABLE 14.2 (*Continued*)
Methods for the synthesis of nanocomposites

S.no	Method of synthesis	Description
4	Hydrothermal and solvothermal synthetic methods	Aqueous amalgamation of nanocomposites has been generally discussed in literatures. Aqueous responses are handled under high tension (> 2000 psi) and high temperature (> 200°C) in reactors or autoclaves. Through a fluid (ethanol-linoleic corrosive) strong (metal linoleate) arrangement (water-ethanol) response, there is a wide range of nanocrystals by utilizing the aqueous strategy. By embracing bimetal forerunners in certain mole proportions, composite oxide nanocrystals, for example, attractive metal/ceramic nanocomposites can be ready through coprecipitation responses following a fluid strong arrangement stage move and separation strategy. This strategy is based on a general phase-transfer and separation mechanism that takes place at the interfaces of the liquid, solid, and solution phases during the synthesis. The uniform iron nanoparticles that result from the solvothermal decomposition of the iron complex are controlled oxidized to form the highly crystalline and monodisperse nanocrystallites.
5	Assembly of small nanocrystals into large magnetic nanoclusters by surfactants	The assembly of tiny magnetic nanocrystals can produce magnetic nanoclusters. Tween 20 (Polysorbate 20) was utilized as an optional surfactant to gather the hydrophobic attractive NPs into sphere-like "attractive totals" with higher attractive extents.

14.4 PREPARATION OF NANOCOMPOSITE-BASED ADSORBENT

Material selection, synthesis of nanoscale components, fabrication of the composite, and characterization of the resulting adsorbent are typical steps in the preparation of adsorbents based on nanocomposites (Chang et al., 2013). The majorly classified adsorbents based on nanocomposites are given in Table 14.3.

The incorporation of NPs into polymeric or inorganic membranes provides a route to multifunctional and synergistic effects, boosting membrane performance and efficiency in a variety of applications (Esfahani et al., 2019).

Metal oxide NPs that are hydrophilic include Al_2O_3, TiO_2, and Zeolite. The incorporation of hydrophilic metal oxide NPs increases the hydrophilicity of the membrane surface. This lowers fouling while improving flow and overall membrane performance. NPs can be utilized to modify the membrane's pore size and distribution, allowing for molecular size-based selective filtering or separation. Water purification, desalination, and wastewater treatment are just a few of the applications concerned with effluent treatment with hydrophilic nanocomposites. Another type of nanocomposites includes antimicrobial nanocomposites (e.g., Nano-Ag, with CNTs). Antimicrobial NPs like nano-silver (Ag) and CNTs are effective in inhibiting the growth of bacteria and microorganisms on the membrane surface (Radha et al., 2025). By incorporating these NPs into the membrane, biofouling can be minimized, leading to longer membrane lifespan and better performance. These are often used in medical filtration, food and beverage processing, and other applications where maintaining a sterile environment is crucial (Ma et al., 2024). Catalytic nanomaterials include Bi-Metallic NPs, TiO_2. When exposed to light or certain reactants, (photo) catalytic nanomaterials can break down organic pollutants. They are employed in water treatment to improve the breakdown of organic pollutants. Photocatalytic compounds such as TiO_2 allow membranes to self-clean by

TABLE 14.3
Different types of adsorbents

Type of adsorbent	Selection of material	Synthesis	Preparation of composite	Application	References
Graphene oxide- metal oxide nanocomposite	Graphene oxide (a nanoscale component), metal oxide nanoparticles (for example, iron oxide, titanium dioxide), and a suitable matrix (e.g., polymers).	Hummers' method is used to make graphene oxide. Metal oxide nanoparticles can be created via sol-gel or precipitation techniques.	Using solution blending or in situ polymerization, combine graphene oxide and metal oxide nanoparticles with a polymer matrix.	In contaminated water, the composite will be used for heavy metal ion adsorption. The graphene oxide has a wide surface area, and nanoparticles of metal oxides improve heavy metal specific adsorption.	Khan et al. (2015)
Carbon nanotubes (CNT)-based polymer nanocomposite	Carbon nanotubes (CNTs) with multiple walls, a polymer matrix (e.g., polyethylene, polypropylene), and an appropriate crosslinking agent.	Improve CNT adsorption and dispersion in the polymer matrix by functionalizing them.	Melt blending or solution mixing can be used to incorporate them into the polymer.	Adsorption of organic contaminants (e.g., dyes, phenols) from water is tested using the composite. Because of their huge surface area and unique structure, carbon nanotubes improve adsorption.	Yin et al. (2020)
Metal-organic framework-based polymer nanocomposites	ZIF-8 and MIL-101 polyvinyl alcohol and a crosslinking agent.	MOF nanoparticles (such as ZIF-8 and MIL-101) are combined with a polymer matrix (such as polyvinyl alcohol) and a crosslinking agent.	Using in situ polymerization or solution blending, create MOF nanoparticles and scatter them into the polymer matrix.	Due to the high porosity and specific surface area given by the MOF nanoparticles, evaluate the composite for gas adsorption (e.g., CO_2, CH_4).	Jafarian et al. (2023)

degrading organic debris and fouling agents. Their applications include water treatment, wastewater treatment, and air purification (Pasinszki et al., 2020). These NPs can be integrated into membranes in a variety of ways, including blending them with the membrane material during production, surface modification, or post-treatment techniques. This method enables the modification of membrane properties to specific filtration, separation, or purification requirements. Overall, the introduction of NPs into membranes has improved membrane performance, selectivity, and durability, making

TABLE 14.4
Types of adsorbents

S.no	Type of adsorbent
1	Xerogels and aerogels
2	Hydrogels
3	Ferrogels
4	Iron oxide and ferrites
5	Nano zero valent iron
6	Adsorbents based on carbon matrix
7	Adsorbents based on silica
8	Adsorbents based on zeolites
9	Adsorbents based on polymers
10	Adsorbents based on biomolecules

these modified membranes useful tools in a variety of industries ranging from healthcare to environmental cleanup (Zhao et al., 2017). Table 14.4 describes the various types of adsorbents, and their synthesis steps and examples are discussed below.

Select appropriate precursors for xerogel and aerogel. Typical forerunners consolidate silica, alumina, or other metal oxides. Blend the picked forerunner in with a reasonable dissolvable and an impetus (normally a corrosive or base) to make a sol-gel arrangement. Stir and heat the sol-gel mixture to start it gelling and forming a gel. To eliminate the dissolvable, dry the gel under controlled conditions (frequently at elevated temperatures), resulting in a permeable xerogel. Repeat the sol-gel process as for the xerogel anyway using different drying conditions (Dincer Yilmaz, 2021). The profoundly permeable design of the gel can be saved by drying it utilizing a supercritical drying strategy, like supercritical carbon dioxide, to create an aerogel. Mix the xerogel and aerogel in legitimate degrees to approach a composite material. To guarantee that the parts are conveyed consistently, completely homogenize the combination. If important, play out a cross-interfacing or change push toward work on the hidden decency and strength of the nanocomposite (Ali et al., 2022).

Making hydrogel-based nanocomposites includes consolidating NPs or nanomaterials into a hydrogel network to upgrade its properties for different applications. Pick a hydrogel type considering the ideal properties and application. Polyacrylamide, polyvinyl alcohol, PEG, alginate, and chitosan are all common hydrogels. Choose nanomaterials or NPs that are suitable for the intended use. Normal decisions incorporate NPs of metals (e.g., silver, gold), metal oxides (e.g., titanium dioxide, silica), carbon-based NPs (e.g., graphene, CNTs), or mud NPs (e.g., montmorillonite) (Wahid et al., 2020). Disperse the picked NPs in a reasonable dissolvable or distributing specialist to make a stable NP suspension. Blend the hydrogel forerunner arrangement in with the NP scattering. Mix or sonicate the blend to guarantee even scattering of NPs inside the hydrogel forerunner arrangement. Start the cross-connecting process for the hydrogel antecedent to shape a hydrogel structure while consolidating NPs. Start gelation or polymerization of the hydrogel forerunner utilizing reasonable techniques, like warm, substance, or photochemical commencement (Jiao et al., 2015).

Integrate or get iron oxide NPs utilizing a reasonable strategy like co-precipitation or warm decay. Change the outer layer of the iron oxide NPs with a covering to upgrade solidness and forestall collection. Scatter the iron oxide NPs in a reasonable dissolvable (e.g., water) to get a stable NP scattering. Mix the NP dispersion with the hydrogel precursor solution to ensure an even distribution. Add the cross-connecting specialist and initiator to the blend. Start polymerization by applying the proper improvement (e.g., warm, substance, or photochemical inception) to frame the ferrogel nanocomposite.

Iron oxide and ferrite-based nanocomposites include consolidating iron oxide NPs (e.g., magnetite, maghemite) and ferrite NPs into a lattice material (Khaleelullah et al., 2017). Ferrites are mixtures of iron and different metals (e.g., zinc, nickel) with a particular gem structure, frequently displaying attractive properties. Incorporate or acquire iron oxide and ferrite NPs utilizing suitable strategies like co-precipitation, warm decay, or sol-gel techniques. Change the outer layer of the NPs to further develop soundness, forestall conglomeration, or upgrade similarity with the framework material (Radha and Balajee, 2022). Scatter the iron oxide and ferrite NPs independently in appropriate solvents or distributing specialists to acquire stable NP scatterings. Combine the dispersed iron oxide and ferrite NPs in the desired quantities with the matrix material. Homogenize the blend to guarantee a uniform dispersion of NPs inside the lattice. For polymer-based networks, add cross-connecting specialists and initiators to start polymerization and structure the nanocomposite. For earthenware-based lattices, follow suitable sintering or handling strategies to shape the nanocomposite (Suresh et al., 2021).

Nano zero-valent iron (nZVI)-based nanocomposites are generally utilized in ecological remediation, water treatment, and different applications because of their amazing reactivity and proficiency in treating toxins. Get ready nZVI utilizing suitable strategies like compound decrease of iron salts (e.g., $FeCl_3$ or $FeSO_4$) with a lessening specialist, for example, sodium borohydride. The response ought to be done under controlled conditions to get NPs of the ideal size and properties. Adjust the outer layer of the nZVI to further develop solidness and forestall agglomeration, frequently through the expansion of settling specialists or coatings. Blend the nZVI NPs with the picked framework material, guaranteeing a homogenous scattering of NPs inside the network. Add balancing out specialists or useful gatherings to upgrade the dependability and reactivity of the nZVI inside the nanocomposite. Sonicate the blend to guarantee uniform scattering and circulation of nZVI inside the framework material. Start the arrangement of the nanocomposite structure by proper techniques relying upon the grid material. Chemical reduction, for instance, is required to produce a stable composite structure in the case of nanocomposites based on graphene oxide (Ansari et al., 2021).

Adsorbents with a carbon matrix are widely used in environmental remediation, air pollution control, gas separation, and water purification. Carbon-based adsorbents commonly have high surface regions and porosities, making them viable for adsorbing many contaminations. Normal antecedents incorporate initiated carbon, CNTs, graphene oxide, carbon dark, or biomass-determined materials. Heat the chose forerunner material in a dormant climate (e.g., nitrogen) at high temperatures (normally 600–900°C) to carbonize the material and eliminate non-carbon parts. Actuate the carbonized material utilizing physical or substance initiation methods to build its porosity and surface region. Steam activation, chemical activation with activating agents like KOH or H_3PO_4, and physical activation with CO_2 or air are all common methods of activation (Marzeddu et al., 2022). Integrate different materials, for example, metal NPs, metal oxides, or polymers, into the carbon lattice to upgrade its adsorption properties. Blend the forerunner materials or impregnate the carbon framework with the ideal substances. Functionalize the carbon surface with explicit useful gatherings (e.g., - COOH, - NH_2) to upgrade its adsorption abilities for explicit contaminations. To get rid of any residues or impurities, wash the carbon-based material that has been prepared with a suitable solvent. Dry the material completely to eliminate dampness and any leftover dissolvable (Sajid et al., 2022). Due to their high surface area, porosity, and chemical stability, silica-based adsorbents are widely used in a variety of applications, such as catalyst supports, environmental remediation, and gas and liquid phase separations. Pick a reasonable silica forerunner in view of the expected application. Normal antecedents incorporate tetraethyl orthosilicate (TEOS), sodium silicate, and silica gel. Set up a sol-gel arrangement by blending the silica forerunner in with a reasonable dissolvable (e.g., ethanol, water) and an impetus (e.g., ammonium hydroxide) to start the gelation cycle. Permit the sol-gel blend to go through gelation, shaping a gel structure (Ahmad et al., 2017). Control the maturing time and temperature to accomplish the ideal pore construction and properties. Dry the gel under controlled conditions (e.g., surrounding air, broiler drying) to eliminate the dissolvable and make a permeable xerogel. Change the drying conditions to control the pore structure and size. Play out a calcination step at raised temperatures (commonly 400–800°C) to eliminate any leftover natural materials and work on the adsorbent's surface region and pore structure. Enhance the adsorption properties of certain pollutants by functionalizing the silica surface through the introduction of functional groups (such as -NH_2, -COOH) through post-synthesis treatments (Zeb et al., 2016).

Adsorbents considering biomolecules are frequently gotten from regular sources, like proteins, catalysts, polysaccharides, and other naturally determined compounds. These biomolecules offer explicit associations and high selectivity, making them great for adsorption applications. Based on the intended application, select the appropriate biomolecules. Normal biomolecules incorporate proteins (e.g., egg whites), chemicals (e.g., lipase), polysaccharides (e.g., chitosan), and nucleic acids. Detach or extricate the ideal biomolecule from the normal source utilizing reasonable procedures like extraction, refinement, or maturation. Alter or functionalize the disconnected biomolecule to upgrade its adsorption properties (Gong et al., 2019). This might include compound adjustments, cross-connecting, or adding explicit practical gatherings to tailor its cooperation with target atoms. To make an adsorbent, immobilize the modified biomolecule on a suitable support material. Normal help materials incorporate NPs, enacted carbon, silica, or other permeable materials. Cross-connect the biomolecule or embody it inside a framework to balance out the adsorbent and forestall draining or denaturation (Kulal et al., 2021).

14.5 ORGANIC WASTE MATERIALS FOR THE PREPARATION OF ADSORBENT

Natural waste materials are normal or plant-based substances that come from living creatures and can be separated by natural cycles. These materials are biodegradable and essentially comprise carbon-based mixtures like starches, proteins, fats, and nucleic acids. They are a huge part of city strong waste and are produced from different sources, including families, businesses, farming, and food handling. Agricultural byproducts and residues are produced by farming activities. This incorporates crop deposits (stalks, leaves), straw, husks, stems, and other unused plant parts. Natural waste begins from the readiness, cooking, and utilization of food. It incorporates extras, ruined food, strips, centers, and terminated items. Natural waste from finishing and planting exercises. This incorporates grass clippings, tree decorations, leaves, branches, and other plant squander. Natural waste from animals and poultry cultivating. Natural materials utilized in bundling that are biodegradable, for example, plant-based plastics and compostable bundling (Joshi and Gururani, 2022). A combination of natural and inorganic waste is produced from families, organizations, and establishments. It incorporates food squander, yard squander, paper, plastics, metals, glass, and the sky is the limit from there (Maqbool et al., 2022).

Food and agricultural wastes are high-volume, low-value materials that are highly susceptible to microbial spoilage, which restricts their use. Legal restrictions and the costs of collection, drying, storage, and transportation can also prevent further exploitation. Along these lines, for the most part, at present these materials are either utilized as creature feed (not satisfactory all the time because of hardships in appropriately adjusting the nourishing necessities), ignition feedstock or then again arranged to landfill causing major ecological issues (e.g., discharge of huge amounts of unpredictable natural mixtures on account of ignition and tainting of groundwater on account of landfill). These materials normally contain elevated degrees of cellulose, hemicellulose, lignin, and proteins and as such can comprise inexhaustible normal assets for a plenty of cheap eco-accommodating and reasonable materials. Instances of such modest materials are minimal expense adsorbents (Nadeem et al., 2021).

Adsorption has been considered one of the most mind-blowing procedures for the expulsion of natural and inorganic toxins of wastewaters and of unfortunate substance parts in the agri-food industry. In view of their astounding adsorption capacity, enacted carbons are the most generally utilized sorbents and have been utilized in the agri-food industry for a variety of utilizations like the decolorization of sugar and vegetable oils, the evacuation of copper particles and unwanted organics in the refined cocktails industry and others (Madima et al., 2020). However, even though activated carbon is by far the most popular sorbent, its widespread use is constrained by its inherent high cost (primarily due to the costs of the precursor material and the energy-intensive production processes). As a result, low-cost adsorbents have recently been intensively sought. To work on the seriousness of any adsorbent in a business market, three key measures should be satisfied: (a) a low cost of production; (b) a high yield of the product; and (c) a high removal efficiency or adsorption capacity.

Zinc oxide (ZnO) NPs are one of the most normally fabricated nanomaterials and a constituent of numerous items, for example, sunscreen, antimicrobials, and so forth. ZnO NPs can likewise be utilized for adsorption of pollutants in view of their high liveliness, huge surface region and being harmless to the ecosystem. In any case, it is expensive if ZnO NPs are exclusively utilized yet regardless this issue can be settled by consolidating ZnO NPs with biochar. The capability of utilizing biochar in poison expulsion has been reported in a few examinations (Liou et al., 2021). Biochar can be acquired from endless sources, for example, bamboo, natural product strips, and rice husk; biochar produced from rice husk has been accounted for to display different capabilities, furthermore, be a minimal expense material. Numerous studies used rice husk biochar to remove a variety of pollutants from water and wastewater. The elimination of reactive red dye (RR195) with rice husk biochar was also performed previously. Rice husk biochar was additionally applied to adsorb methylene blue and methyl orange. To further develop execution, later concentrates on zeroed in on altering rice husk biochar prior to applying it for eliminating colors. Congo red and other dyes were adsorbed using alkaline-modified rice husk biochar and rice husk-derived magnetic biochar (Wang et al., 2016).

Normally happening silica particularly that viewed as in rural waste can give an elective source to costly business silica forerunners in the combination of mesoporous silica. Rice husk is the most used farming waste to be changed over completely to more important silica inferred results. Rice (*Oryza sativa*), which covers 1% of the world's surface, is an essential wellspring of nourishment for billions of individuals. Internationally, around 600 million tons of rice are created every year. Rice husk, which is the covering of rice grains, is made from half cellulose, 25–30% lignin, and 15–20% silica. During milling, the primary waste product, 0.28 kg of rice husk are produced for every kilogram of rice produced. At the point when the rice husk is scorched at a temperature over 500°C, the natural parts decay and rice husk debris is gotten. The SiO_2 present in rice husk debris has a virtue of 94–96% with minor pollutants like K_2O, Na_2O, and Fe_2O_3. If the rice husk is subjected to pretreatments like leaching in acids like HCl, HNO_3, H_3PO_4, and H_2SO_4, which assist in the removal of the impurities, the purity of the SiO_2 that is obtained through the incineration of rice husk can be further improved to 98–99% (Liou et al., 2021).

14.6 REACTORS FOR TREATING WASTEWATER USING BIO-NANOCOMPOSITES

Utilizing nanocomposite adsorbents in reactors for emanating treatment is a creative methodology pointed toward improving the productivity and viability of wastewater treatment processes. Nanocomposite adsorbents consolidate the advantages of nanomaterials and conventional adsorbents, offering higher surface region, further developed adsorption limit, selectivity, and, in general, execution. Treatment of effluents is a crucial issue for reducing environmental pollution. Nanocomposite adsorbents, joining nanomaterials and regular adsorbents, grandstand improved adsorption properties and make ready for practical wastewater treatment (Sharifi et al., 2021).

The studies conducted indicate that two types of reactors are typically considered for the photocatalytic process: fluidized-bed and fixed-bed reactors. A fixed-bed reactor can be utilized as a proper cycle in water purging and wastewater treatment. This technique enjoys various benefits and some impediments. The effective surface of nanocomposites is diminished when the particles of composites are immobilized on a suitable substrate. In addition, because the reaction only takes place at the liquid-solid interface, mass transfer from the liquid bulk to the catalyst surface has little effect on the reaction rate (Natarajan et al., 2023). This is because the fluidized-bed reactor is more efficient than this one. In any case, it ought to be noticed that, in this technique, in light of the fact that the adsorbent is immobilized on the substrate, no impetus can go into the fluid mass during the cycle. Subsequently, by taking out the filtration step, costs connected with the detachment of impetus from arrangement are saved, while this stage is expected for fluidized-bed reactors. Then again, adsorbent outflow is forestalled, and the administrators are less presented to nanocomposite particles. Additionally, the adsorbent could be utilized for a longer time (Agboola et al., 2021).

Different investigations likewise recommend the utilization of pressed-bed reactors, while nanocomposite adsorbent is packed on various types of reactors. The utilization of adsorbent in photocatalytic reactors has additionally been recommended for the treatment of modern wastewater. The techniques utilized for packing the adsorbent incorporate twist covering, shower covering, sol gel plunge covering, electrophoretic affidavit, and faltering have been presented for substrate covering. Be that as it may, the utilization of these techniques is normally time what's more, energy-consuming, and every technique requires unique and expensive hardware.

Various sorts of bioreactor frameworks have been tried for effluent treatment and precipitation of biogenic molecules including persistently blended tank reactor, stuffed bed reactor (PBR), up-stream anaerobic slime cover reactor, and layer biofilm bioreactor. Nonetheless, recuperation couldn't be accomplished utilizing these reactors because natural molecules encourage halfway onto the biomass. Thusly, a strong fluid partition step is frequently required in the downstream of such bioreactor frameworks, yet without heightening the expense of activity. In this specific situation, a promising bioreactor setup for effluent treatment decrease and recuperation in a solitary unit is the backwards fluidized bed reactor containing low-thickness floatable bio support material, which is fluidized descending. In this reactor framework, biofilm creates over the bio support material, and it stays at the highest point of the reactor, though that encourages shaped get isolated from the biomass because of fluidization and settle at the base, accordingly empowering a simple recuperation of the bio precipitates (Oliveira et al., 2014). In any case, fixed bed reactor has not been accounted for up to this point for selenite evacuation and recuperation as NPs. Various kinds of bio support materials were recently announced for their utilization in fixed bed reactors framework, for example, polystyrene globules, wipe solid shapes, squander lignocellulosic materials, and so on.

In contrast, these materials, which are commonly used in moving bed biofilm reactors, have a large surface area and high biomass maintenance capacities (Sharififard et al., 2018). Depending on the requirements and particular application, reactors that use bio-nanocomposites for wastewater treatment might have different designs and modes of operation. Some of such reactors include.

- Fixed bed reactors
- Fluidized bed reactors
- Membrane bioreactors
- Suspended growth reactors
- Trickling filters
- Sequential batch reactors

14.6.1 Fixed Bed Reactors

In fixed-bed reactors, a solid substance is placed inside a vessel to serve as the bio-nanocomposite's support matrix. Inert materials like sand or specially made carriers can be used as the solid material to increase surface area and assist the growth of microorganisms. This support matrix immobilizes the bio-nanocomposite, which is made up of nanomaterials like NPs or nanofibers and biological elements like bacteria, biofilms, or enzymes. The fixed-bed reactor receives wastewater either constantly or sporadically (Heidarzadeh-Samani et al., 2021). It passes through the reactor's densely packed bed, giving the bio-nanocomposite material close contact. Because of their high surface area and unique surface chemistry, the nanomaterials incorporated in the bio-nanocomposite enable the adsorption of pollutants from the wastewater onto their surfaces. Enzymes and microbes are examples of biological components that catalyze biochemical reactions that break down or change pollutants into less hazardous chemicals. Depending on the oxygen content of the reactor, these biological activities may involve either anaerobic or aerobic breakdown.

The retention time, a term used to describe the length of time that wastewater must stay in touch with the bio-nanocomposite in order for successful pollutant removal, is guaranteed by the design of fixed-bed reactors. Reactor dimensions, flow rate, and the properties of the bio-nanocomposite all have an impact on the retention period. The nature and concentration of contaminants in the wastewater, the reactor's operating parameters (such as flow rate, temperature, and pH), and the characteristics of the bio-nanocomposite (such as adsorption capacity and enzyme activity) all affect how well fixed-bed reactors treat wastewater. The fixed-bed reactor's performance is maximized by monitoring and controlling parameters including pH, temperature, and flow rate. To evaluate treatment effectiveness and spot any operational problems, pollutant levels in the influent and effluent streams should be regularly monitored. Bio-nanocomposites in fixed-bed reactors may lose their activity or get saturated with pollutants over time because of fouling or deterioration. The bio-nanocomposite may be revitalized through periodic regeneration procedures such as chemical cleaning, biological rejuvenation, or backwashing (Chkirida et al., 2019). The wastewater that has been processed and is referred to as effluent is released from the reactor. Regulations governing suspended particles, chemical oxygen demand (COD), biochemical oxygen demand (BOD), and specific pollutants must be satisfied by the effluent's quality.

14.6.2 Fluidized Bed Reactors

Fluidized bed reactors are dynamic devices where aeration or an upward flow of wastewater suspends and fluidizes bio-nanocomposite particles. This is an explanation of the operation of bio-nanocomposites-based fluidized bed reactors for the treatment of wastewater. Fluidized bed reactors are made up of a distribution system for adding wastewater or aeration and a vessel filled with bio-nanocomposite particles. To spread the wastewater or air flow uniformly, the reactor's bottom may have a porous plate or distributor. The bio-nanocomposite is made up of nanomaterials (such as NPs or nanofibers) mixed with biological components (like bacteria, biofilms, or enzymes). These elements are rendered immobile inside a matrix of support, creating particles that are appropriate for fluidization (Liu et al., 2011).

The reactor's bottom is filled with wastewater, which causes a liquid to flow upward. The bio-nanocomposite particles are suspended and fluidized inside the reactor vessel when the liquid velocity rises over the minimum fluidization velocity. The bio-nanocomposite's incorporated nanomaterials offer a large surface area for the adsorption of pollutants found in the wastewater. Biochemical reactions that break down or change pollutants into less dangerous chemicals are catalyzed by biological components. Improved mass transfer rates and efficient contact between pollutants and the bio-nanocomposite are guaranteed by the fluidized environment (Mougnol et al., 2023).

The bio-nanocomposite particles' fluidized form makes mass transfer and mixing easier, which makes it possible for pollutants to be transported effectively to the active areas for adsorption or biological degradation within the particles. In fluidized bed reactors, the residence time distribution can be tuned by varying the bed height and flow rate. This makes it possible to optimize the retention period and guarantee that the wastewater and the bio-nanocomposite have enough time to come into contact for efficient treatment. To maximize treatment performance, operational parameters including pH, temperature, and flow rate are tracked and managed. Frequent influent and effluent quality monitoring aids in determining treatment effectiveness and enables necessary operating condition adjustments (Romero-Cedillo et al., 2020).

14.6.3 Membrane Bioreactors

Membrane filtration units are attached to a biological reactor vessel in a membrane bioreactor, which treats wastewater. Bio-nanocomposites are either immobilized on the membrane surface or integrated into the bioreactor itself. When biomaterials like NPs or nanofibers are coupled with biological elements like bacteria, biofilms, or enzymes, the result is a bio-nanocomposite that is employed in MBRs. In order to create particles appropriate for usage in the bioreactor or membrane surface coating, these elements are immobilized within a support matrix. Wastewater is fed into the bioreactor, which is a biological reactor that uses bio-nanocomposites to support biological processes. Depending on the availability of oxygen, the microorganisms in the bio-nanocomposites either use aerobic or anaerobic mechanisms to destroy organic pollutants (Sheen Mers et al., 2022).

Membrane filtering devices sort treated water (permeate) from suspended particulates and biomass while wastewater is treated in the bioreactor. Bio-nanocomposites immobilized on the membrane surface can improve the rejection of pollutants and decrease fouling to improve filtration performance. Through adsorption onto their surfaces and biological breakdown aided by embedded enzymes or microorganisms, bio-nanocomposites help to remove contaminants. The bio-nanocomposites' nanomaterials offer a large surface area for adsorption, and the biological elements catalyze the biochemical reactions. During operation, pollutants and biomass can foul membranes, decreasing the effectiveness of filtration. By extending the lifespan of membranes and mitigating fouling, bio-nanocomposites with enzymatic activity or antifouling qualities may lower the need for frequent membrane replacement or cleaning.

To maximize treatment performance, operational factors like flow rate, aeration, and mixed liquor suspended solids (MLSS) concentration are tracked and managed. Input and effluent quality monitoring aids in determining treatment effectiveness and enables necessary operating condition adjustments. In order to sustain the activity and performance of bio-nanocomposites within the MBR, periodic maintenance and regeneration procedures could be necessary. This could involve replenishing depleted components, cleaning the membrane, or rejuvenating the bio-nanocomposite.

14.6.4 Suspended growth reactors

Typically, suspended growth reactors are made up of a tank or basin that is used to continuously or sporadically mix bio-nanocomposite particles with wastewater. Either mechanical agitation or aeration is used to maintain these particles suspended in the water column. Utilizing nanomaterials like NPs or nanofibers along with biological components like bacteria, biofilms, or enzymes, bio-nanocomposites are employed in suspended growth reactors. For the purpose of creating particles appropriate for suspension in wastewater, these constituents are immobilized inside a support matrix. Wastewater is added to the reactor and mixes with the suspended particles of the bio-nanocomposite. The suspended biomass undergoes biological processes that are aided by the bio-nanocomposites, which cause the pollutants in the wastewater to break down or change (Besharati Vineh et al., 2024).

Because the bio-nanocomposites' nanomaterials have a large surface area, pollutants can more easily adsorb onto them and be removed from the wastewater. Biochemical processes involving biological components catalyze the degradation or transformation of pollutants into less hazardous compounds. Nanomaterials may be able to boost microbial growth or enzyme activity in these reactions, which take place in the suspended biomass. In order to promote mixing and mass transfer of pollutants to the active areas within the biomass, mechanical agitation or aeration is used to guarantee that bio-nanocomposite particles are uniformly suspended throughout the reactor. By modifying reactor capacity or flow rates, wastewater residence time—also referred to as the hydraulic retention time (HRT)—can be managed within the reactor. In order to accomplish effective treatment, this permits an adequate amount of contact time between the wastewater and the bio-nanocomposites. Treatment performance is maximized by monitoring and regulating operational parameters like temperature, pH, dissolved oxygen concentration, and biomass concentration. It is easier to evaluate treatment effectiveness and make necessary operating condition adjustments when influent and effluent quality are regularly monitored (Garg et al., 2023).

14.6.5 Trickling filters

Wastewater is sprayed or trickled through a bed of support media (such as pebbles, plastic media, or biofilm carriers) in a trickling filter (Spychała et al., 2023). To improve treatment efficiency, bio-nanocomposites are added to the filter media's surface or to biofilm carriers. Biomolecules (enzymes, bacteria, or biofilms) are mixed with nanomaterials (NPs or nanofibers) to create bio-nanocomposites, which are utilized in trickling filters. To create particles appropriate for attachment to the filter media or carriers, these constituents are immobilized within a support matrix (Russo et al., 2021).

The bio-nanocomposites' nanomaterials offer a large surface area for pollutants to adsorb onto the carriers or filter media, making it easier to remove them from wastewater. Biochemical reactions that break down or change pollutants into less dangerous chemicals are catalyzed by biological components. Nanomaterials may be able to increase microbial growth or enzyme activity in these reactions, which take place inside the biofilm that is adhered to the filter media or carriers. A thin layer of water is formed by the distribution of wastewater across the filter media's surface, and this water runs through the bed and downhill. Contaminants in the wastewater are broken down or transformed by biological activities taking place inside the biofilm that is adhered to the filter media or carriers and supported by the bio-nanocomposites (Sharma et al., 2021).

The flow rate or the depth of the filter bed can be modified to alter the HRT, which is the amount of time wastewater takes to pass through the trickling filter. In order to accomplish effective treatment, this permits an adequate amount of contact time between the wastewater and the bio-nanocomposites. The wastewater flows slowly through the bed, and the filter media or carriers have a wide surface area, which allows for enough contact time between the wastewater and the bio-nanocomposites attached to the media or carriers for successful treatment (Tripathy et al., 2024).

14.6.6 Sequential batch reactors

A single treatment tank that runs in batch mode makes up a sequential batch reactor. A series of treatment stages, including filling, reaction, settling, decanting, and idle phases, are cycled through the reactor. To aid in the removal of contaminants, bio-nanocomposites are added to the reactor during the reaction phase. Wastewater is added to the reactor until it reaches a set level during the filling phase. To guarantee the consistent distribution of wastewater and bio-nanocomposites inside the reactor, mixing or aeration devices may be installed. The bio-nanocomposites suspended in the wastewater aid in the destruction or transformation of pollutants in the wastewater during the reaction phase. The suspended biomass contains biological activities that are catalyzed by embedded enzymes or microorganisms, with the assistance of nanomaterials that promote microbial growth or enzyme activity (Deng et al., 2020). Following the reaction phase, gravity or the lack of mixing causes the suspended solids to sink to the reactor's bottom. Supernatant, or treated water, can be separated from suspended solids and biomass during the settling process. The treated water is carefully taken from the reactor's top and released for additional treatment or disposal during the decanting phase. Pumps, weirs, or other hydraulic devices can be used to regulate the decanting process and guarantee that only cleared water is removed. After decanting, the reactor goes into an idle phase, where it stays that way until the next cycle begins. Any leftover biomass settles down even further during the idle phase, and the reactor may be maintained or prepared for the subsequent cycle.

14.7 CONCLUSION

Wastewater treatment with nanocomposites has emerged as a very effective and promising solution to the rising water pollution challenge. Nanocomposites, which blend NPs with a matrix material, have distinct benefits for wastewater treatment. Because of the incorporation of NPs, nanocomposites have a large surface area and an abundance of active sites. This considerably improves adsorption capacity and catalytic activity, resulting in more effective removal of contaminants from wastewater as compared to traditional treatment approaches. Nanocomposites have proven to be extremely successful at removing a wide range of pollutants from wastewater, including heavy metals, organic compounds, colors, medications, and pathogens. Because of the unique features of NPs, many nanocomposites have increased oxidation or catalytic activities.

By tailoring the surface qualities and composition of NPs in nanocomposites, certain contaminants may be removed selectively. This selectivity guarantees tailored treatment, which reduces overall environmental effect while optimizing resource utilization in the treatment process. NPs' tiny size and high surface-to-volume ratio result in fast adsorption kinetics and response rates. This shortens treatment timeframes and increases treatment capacity by speeding up the wastewater treatment process. The use of nanocomposites frequently allows for the creation of compact and efficient wastewater treatment systems. Nanocomposites' high adsorption capacity and catalytic activity minimize the amount of adsorbent/material required, resulting in smaller reactor sizes and lower resource usage. Nanocomposites may be engineered for reusability, which contributes to wastewater treatment sustainability. Efficient regeneration systems can support several treatment cycles, lowering operational costs and waste creation. For complete wastewater treatment, nanocomposites can be incorporated into hybrid systems that include adsorption, catalysis, filtration, and other approaches. These hybrid systems use the advantages of multiple technologies to improve pollutant removal and overall treatment efficiency. Nanocomposites have the ability to purify water at the point of use, particularly in rural or decentralized regions where centralized treatment is not practical. Portable and economical nanocomposite-based treatment systems can enable decentralized access to clean water. Because of the inclusion of NPs, nanocomposites frequently have a larger surface area and more accessible active sites. When compared to typical adsorbents, this results in higher adsorption capacity, allowing for the adsorption of a greater amount of target contaminants. Surface characteristics of nanocomposites may be adjusted by varying NP content, size, and surface functionalization. This tailoring allows for selectivity and efficiency in adsorbing certain contaminants, making nanocomposites useful for a variety of adsorption applications. NPs in nanocomposites have quick adsorption kinetics due to their nanoscale size and high surface area-to-volume ratio. Adsorption methods utilizing nanocomposites frequently achieve equilibrium faster than bulk materials, enhancing total adsorption efficiency.

Nanocomposites are materials that can integrate numerous functions into a single substance. They can, for example, have catalytic, magnetic, or photocatalytic activities in addition to adsorption capabilities. This synergy enables simultaneous pollutant removal and treatment, resulting in an all-encompassing approach to environmental cleanup. Nanocomposites may be made to be generable and reusable, making the adsorption process more cost-effective and sustainable. The adsorbent may be regenerated and utilized for several adsorption cycles without substantial loss of efficiency by optimizing the composite structure and surface changes. Adsorption using nanocomposites contributes to environmental sustainability by removing pollutants in an efficient, low-energy, and less intrusive manner. The utilization of nanocomposites can result in less waste, less energy consumption, and less chemical usage during the adsorption process. Adsorption employing nanocomposites provides substantial benefits and opens up new avenues for efficient and environmentally friendly adsorption procedures. Nanocomposites, which are materials made up of NPs plus a matrix material, have unique features that improve adsorption capacities.

Ongoing research is looking at novel NP-matrix combinations, surface changes, and optimization approaches to improve the adsorption effectiveness of nanocomposites. Prospects for the future include the development of nanocomposites with enhanced characteristics and multi-functionality to solve increasing environmental concerns. In future, it is aimed at enhancing nanocomposite-based wastewater treatment, including the exploration of novel NPs, the optimization of composite structures, the development of scalable manufacturing techniques, and the study of long-term environmental effects. Future innovation is predicted to result in ever more efficient and environmentally friendly wastewater treatment methods.

ACKNOWLEDGMENT

This chapter was made possible through the support of Anna University, Chennai for carrying out the work in Bio Products Laboratory, Department of Chemical Engineering. The authors also acknowledge all of the contributors whose work is referenced in this chapter.

REFERENCES

Agboola, O., Fayomi, O. S. I., Ayodeji, A., Ayeni, A. O., Alagbe, E. E., Sanni, S. E., & Oni, B. A. (2021). A review on polymer nanocomposites and their effective applications in membranes and adsorbents for water treatment and gas separation. *Membranes*, *11*(2), 139. https://doi.org/10.3390/membranes11020139

Ahmad, I., Siddiqui, W. A., & Ahmad, T. (2017). Synthesis, characterization of silica nanoparticles and adsorption removal of Cu2+ ions in aqueous solution. *International Journal of Emerging Technology and Advanced Engineering*, *7*(8), 439–445.

Ajayan, P. M. (2003). Bulk metal and ceramics nanocomposites. *Nanocomposite Science and Technology*, 1–75. https://doi.org/10.1002/3527602127

Ali, I., Neskoromnaya, E. A., Melezhik, A. V., Babkin, A. V., Kulnitskiy, B. A., Burakov, A. E., ... & Alsubaie, A. (2022). Magnetically active nanocomposite aerogels: Preparation, characterization and application for water treatment. *Journal of Porous Materials*, *29*(2), 545–557. https://doi.org/10.1007/s10934-021-01175-0

Anik, M. I., Hossain, M. K., Hossain, I., Mahfuz, A. M. U. B., Rahman, M. T., & Ahmed, I. (2021). Recent progress of magnetic nanoparticles in biomedical applications: A review. *Nano Select*, *2*(6), 1146–1186. https://doi.org/10.1002/nano.202000162

Ansari, A., Siddiqui, V. U., Akram, M. K., Siddiqi, W. A., Khan, A., Al-Romaizan, A. N., ... & Puttegowda, M. (2021). Synthesis of atmospherically stable zero-valent iron nanoparticles (nZVI) for the efficient catalytic treatment of high-strength domestic wastewater. *Catalysts*, *12*(1), 26. https://doi.org/10.3390/catal12010026

Besharati Vineh, M., Poostchi, A. A., Kordestani, D., Qushehbolagh, M. K., & Saboury, A. A. (2024). Mechanically stirred enzymatic membrane reactor containing HRP immobilized on Tau-SiO2@ Fe3O4-GO nanocomposite for removal of tetracycline in synthetically concocted wastewater. *Biodegradation*, 1–16. https://doi.org/10.1007/s10532-023-10066-x

Brigante, M., Pecini, E., & Avena, M. (2016). Magnetic mesoporous silica for water remediation: Synthesis, characterization and application as adsorbent of molecules and ions of environmental concern. *Microporous and Mesoporous Materials*, *230*, 1–10. https://doi.org/10.1016/j.micromeso.2016.04.032

Castillo, R. R., & Vallet-Regí, M. (2019). Functional mesoporous silica nanocomposites: Biomedical applications and biosafety. *International Journal of Molecular Sciences*, *20*(4), 929. https://doi.org/10.3390/ijms20040929

Chang, H., & Wu, H. (2013). Graphene-based nanocomposites: Preparation, functionalization, and energy and environmental applications. *Energy & Environmental Science*, *6*(12), 3483–3507. https://doi.org/10.1039/C3EE42518E

Chkirida, S., Zari, N., Qaiss, A. E. K., & Bouhfid, R. (2019). Nanocomposite materials based on TiO 2/clay for wastewater treatment. *Advanced Research in Nanosciences for Water Technology*, 363–380. https://doi.org/10.1007/978-3-030-02381-2_16

Deng, R., Huang, D., Wan, J., Xue, W., Wen, X., Liu, X., & Zhang, Q. (2020). Recent advances of biochar materials for typical potentially toxic elements management in aquatic environments: A review. *Journal of Cleaner Production*, *255*, 119523. https://doi.org/10.1016/j.jclepro.2019.119523

Deng, D., Lamssali, M., Aryal, N., Ofori-Boadu, A., Jha, M. K., & Samuel, R. E. (2020). Textiles wastewater treatment technology: A review. *Water Environment Research*, *92*(10), 1805–1810. https://doi.org/10.1002/wer.1437

De Oliveira, D. V. M., Rabelo, M. D., & Nariyoshi, Y. N. (2014). Evaluation of a MBBR (moving bed biofilm reactor) pilot plant for treatment of pulp and paper mill wastewater. *International Journal Environment Moniter Analysis*, *2*, 220–225. https://doi.org/10.11648/j.ijema.20140204.15

Dincer Yilmaz, N. E. (2021). Characterization of nano-composite thermites containing metal and sol-gel synthesized iron oxide xerogels. *In AIAA Propulsion and Energy 2021 Forum* (p. 3337) https://doi.org/10.2514/6.2021-3337

Dutta, D., Arya, S., & Kumar, S. (2021). Industrial wastewater treatment: Current trends, bottlenecks, and best practices. *Chemosphere*, *285*, 131245. https://doi.org/10.1016/j.chemosphere.2021.131245

Esfahani, M. R., Aktij, S. A., Dabaghian, Z., Firouzjaei, M. D., Rahimpour, A., Eke, J., & Koutahzadeh, N. (2019). Nanocomposite membranes for water separation and purification: Fabrication, modification, and applications. *Separation and Purification Technology, 213*, 465–499. https://doi.org/10.1016/j.seppur.2018.12.050

Fan, Y., Yang, R., Lei, Z., Liu, N., Lv, J., Zhai, S., & Wang, L. (2016). Removal of Cr (VI) from aqueous solution by rice husk derived magnetic sorbents. *Korean Journal of Chemical Engineering, 33*, 1416–1424. https://doi.org/10.1007/s11814-015-0248-y

Ferreira, F. V., Dufresne, A., Pinheiro, I. F., Souza, D. H. S., Gouveia, R. F., Mei, L. H. I., & Lona, L. M. F. (2018). How do cellulose nanocrystals affect the overall properties of biodegradable polymer nanocomposites: A comprehensive review. *European Polymer Journal, 108*, 274–285. https://doi.org/10.1016/j.eurpolymj.2018.08.045

Garg, A., Chauhan, A., Agnihotri, C., Singh, B. P., Mondem, V., Basu, S., & Agnihotri, S. (2023). Sunlight active cellulose/g-C3N4/TiO2 nano-photocatalyst for degradation of industrial dye and pharmaceutical drug in real wastewater. https://doi.org/10.21203/rs.3.rs-2442588/v1

Gómez, M., Plaza, F., Garralón, G., Pérez, J., & Gómez, M. A. (2007). A comparative study of tertiary wastewater treatment by physico-chemical-UV process and macrofiltration–ultrafiltration technologies. *Desalination, 202*(1–3), 369–376. https://doi.org/10.1016/j.desal.2005.12.076

Gong, C., Sun, S., Zhang, Y., Sun, L., Su, Z., Wu, A., & Wei, G. (2019). Hierarchical nanomaterials via biomolecular self-assembly and bioinspiration for energy and environmental applications. *Nanoscale, 11*(10), 4147–4182. https://doi.org/10.1039/C9NR00218A

Goswami, L., Kumar, R. V., Borah, S. N., Manikandan, N. A., Pakshirajan, K., & Pugazhenthi, G. (2018). Membrane bioreactor and integrated membrane bioreactor systems for micropollutant removal from wastewater: A review. *Journal of Water Process Engineering, 26*, 314–328. https://doi.org/10.1016/j.jwpe.2018.10.024

Harito, C., Bavykin, D. V., Yuliarto, B., Dipojono, H. K., & Walsh, F. C. (2019). Polymer nanocomposites having a high filler content: Synthesis, structures, properties, and applications. *Nanoscale, 11*(11), 4653–4682. https://doi.org/10.1039/C9NR00117D

Hassan, F. F., & Karam, F. F. (2021). Preparation and characterization of MWCNTs-Chitosan Composite. In *IOP Conference Series: Earth and Environmental Science* (Vol. 790, No. 1, p. 012008). IOP Publishing. https://doi.org/10.1088/1755-1315/790/1/012008

Heidarzadeh-Samani, M., Behzad, T., & Mehrabani-Zeinabad, A. (2021). Development of a continuous fixed–bed column to eliminate cadmium (II) ions by starch-g-poly (acrylic acid)/cellulose nanofiber bionanocomposite hydrogel. *Environmental Science and Pollution Research, 28*(41), 57902–57917. https://doi.org/10.1007/s11356-021-14567-1

Jafarian, H., Firouzjaei, M. D., Aktij, S. A., Aghaei, A., Khomami, M. P., Elliott, M., & Rahimpour, A. (2023). Synthesis of heterogeneous metal organic Framework-Graphene oxide nanocomposite membranes for water treatment. *Chemical Engineering Journal, 455*, 140851. https://doi.org/10.1016/j.cej.2022.140851

Jiao, T., Guo, H., Zhang, Q., Peng, Q., Tang, Y., Yan, X., & Li, B. (2015). Reduced graphene oxide-based silver nanoparticle-containing composite hydrogel as highly efficient dye catalysts for wastewater treatment. *Scientific Reports, 5*(1), 11873. https://doi.org/10.1038/srep11873

Joshi, N. C., & Gururani, P. (2022). Advances of graphene oxide based nanocomposite materials in the treatment of wastewater containing heavy metal ions and dyes. *Current Research in Green and Sustainable Chemistry, 5*, 100306. https://doi.org/10.1016/j.crgsc.2022.100306

Kanu, I., & Achi, O. K. (2011). Industrial effluents and their impact on water quality of receiving rivers in Nigeria. *Journal of Applied Technology in Environmental Sanitation, 1*(1), 75–86.

Kehrein, P., Van Loosdrecht, M., Osseweijer, P., Garfí, M., Dewulf, J., & Posada, J. (2020). A critical review of resource recovery from municipal wastewater treatment plants–market supply potentials, technologies and bottlenecks. *Environmental Science: Water Research & Technology, 6*(4), 877–910. https://doi.org/10.1039/C9EW00905A

Kewat, H. L., Sharma, R. K., Sidiqi, U., & Ghosh, P. (2024). Graphene and graphene-based nanocomposites: From synthesis to applications. In *Handbook of Materials Science, Volume 1: Optical Materials* (pp. 517–543). Springer Nature Singapore.

Khaleelullah, M. M. S. I., Dheivasigamani, T., Natarajana, P.,Masuda, Y., Inamib, W., Kawataa, Y., & Hayakawa, Y., (2017). Size controlled synthesis of silver sulfide nanostructuresby multi-solvent thermal decomposition method. *Journal of Crystal Growth, 468*, 119–124. ISSN 0022-0248, https://doi.org/10.1016/j.jcrysgro.2016.10.081.

Khan, M., Tahir, M. N., Adil, S. F., Khan, H. U., Siddiqui, M. R. H., Al-warthan, A. A., & Tremel, W. (2015). Graphene based metal and metal oxide nanocomposites: Synthesis, properties and their applications. *Journal of Materials Chemistry A, 3*(37), 18753–18808. https://doi.org/10.1039/C5TA02240A

Kulal N, Vetrivel R, Chinnakonda S. Gopinath, Rahul K. R, Vinod N. R, Manjunath Shetty, Shrikanth R, Dinesh R,& Ganapati V. S.(2021). Green route for carbonylation of amines by CO2 using Sn-Ni-O bifunctional catalyst and theoretical study for finding best suited active sites.*Chemical Engineering Journal*, *419*, 129439, ISSN 1385-8947, https://doi.org/10.1016/j.cej.2021.129439.

Liu, J., Qiao, S. Z., Hu, Q. H., & Lu, G. Q. (2011). Magnetic nanocomposites with mesoporous structures: Synthesis and applications. *small*, *7*(4), 425–443. https://doi.org/10.1002/smll.201001402

Liou, T. H., Tseng, Y. K., Liu, S. M., Lin, Y. T., Wang, S. Y., & Liu, R. T. (2021). Green synthesis of mesoporous graphene oxide/silica nanocomposites from rich husk ash: Characterization and adsorption performance. *Environmental Technology & Innovation*, *22*, 101424. https://doi.org/10.1016/j.eti.2021.101424

Ma, X., Tian, Y., Yang, R., Wang, H., Allahou, L. W., Chang, J., Williams, G., Knowles, J. C., & Poma, A. (2024). Nanotechnology in healthcare, and its safety and environmental risks. *Journal of Nanobiotechnology*, *22*(1), 715. https://doi.org/10.1186/s12951-024-02901-x. PMID: 39548502; PMCID: PMC11566612.

Madima, N., Mishra, S. B., Inamuddin, I., & Mishra, A. K. (2020). Carbon-based nanomaterials for remediation of organic and inorganic pollutants from wastewater. A review. *Environmental Chemistry Letters*, *18*, 1169–1191. https://doi.org/10.1007/s10311-020-01001-0

Maqbool, Q., Barucca, G., Sabbatini, S., Parlapiano, M., Ruello, M. L., & Tittarelli, F. (2022). Transformation of industrial and organic waste into titanium doped activated carbon–cellulose nanocomposite for rapid removal of organic pollutants. *Journal of Hazardous Materials*, *423*, 126958. https://doi.org/10.1016/j.jhazmat.2021.126958

Marzeddu, S., Décima, M. A., Camilli, L., Bracciale, M. P., Genova, V., Paglia, L., … & Boni, M. R. (2022). Physical-chemical characterization of different carbon-based sorbents for environmental applications. *Materials*, *15*(20), 7162. https://doi.org/10.3390/ma15207162

Miao, C., & Hamad, W. Y. (2019). Critical insights into the reinforcement potential of cellulose nanocrystals in polymer nanocomposites. *Current Opinion in Solid State and Materials Science*, *23*(4), 100761. https://doi.org/10.1016/j.cossms.2019.06.005

Mishra, S. R., & Ahmaruzzaman, M. (2021). Cerium oxide and its nanocomposites: Structure, synthesis, and wastewater treatment applications. *Materials Today Communications*, *28*, 102562. https://doi.org/10.1016/j.mtcomm.2021.102562

Mittal, G., Rhee, K. Y., Mišković-Stanković, V., & Hui, D. (2018). Reinforcements in multi-scale polymer composites: Processing, properties, and applications. *Composites Part B: Engineering*, *138*, 122–139. https://doi.org/10.1016/j.compositesb.2017.11.028

Mougnol, J. B. B., Maswanganyi, S., Gusain, R., Kumar, N., Fosso-Kankeu, E., Ray, S. S. & Waanders, F. (2023). Recent advances in photoreactors for water treatment. In *Photoreactors in Advanced Oxidation Processes* (eds E. Fosso-Kankeu, S. Pandey and S.S. Ray). https://doi.org/10.1002/9781394167289.ch7

Natarajan, B., Kannan, P., Rather, J. A., & Sheikh, R. A. (2023). Recent developments in metal nanoparticles functionalized nanocomposite adsorbents for heavy metals removal from wastewaters. *Journal of the Taiwan Institute of Chemical Engineers*, *147*, 104942. https://doi.org/10.1016/j.jtice.2023.104942

Nikolaeva, A. L., Bugrov, A. N., Sokolova, M. P., Kuntsman, I. V., Vlasova, E. N., Ivan'kova, E. M., & Gofman, I. V. (2023). Synergistic effect of metal oxide and carbon nanoparticles on the thermal and mechanical properties of polyimide composite films. *Polymers*, *15*(10), 2298. https://doi.org/10.3390/polym15102298

Ojha, G. P, Pant, B., Park, S. J., Park, M. & Kim, H. Y. (2017). Synthesis and characterization of reduced graphene oxide decorated with CeO_2-doped MnO_2 nanorods for supercapacitor applications. *Journal of Colloid and Interface Science, 494*, 338–344. https://doi.org/10.1016/j.jcis.2017.01.100. Epub 2017 Jan 28. PMID: 28167422.

Okpala, C. C. (2014). The benefits and applications of nanocomposites. *International Journal of Advanced Engineering and Technology*, *12*, 18.

Omanović-Mikličanin, E., Badnjević, A., Kazlagić, A., & Hajlovac, M. (2020). Nanocomposites: A brief review. *Health and Technology*, *10*(1), 51–59.https://doi.org/10.1007/s12553-019-00380-x

Pasinszki, T., & Krebsz, M. (2020). Synthesis and application of zero-valent iron nanoparticles in water treatment, environmental remediation, catalysis, and their biological effects. *Nanomaterials*, *10*(5), 917. https://doi.org/10.3390/nano10050917

Radha, K. V., & Balajee, L. (2022). Strategic approach on flow characteristics of magnetic nano adsorbent on treatment of dye wastewater. *Environmental Quality Management*, *32*(1), 13–25. https://doi.org/10.1002/tqem.21800

Radha, K. V., Selvi, V. S., & Aarcha, J. (2025). Silver nanofiber membranes for indoor air pollution treatment. *Sustainable Chemistry for Climate Action*, 100056. https://doi.org/10.1016/j.scca.2025.100056

Romero-Cedillo, L., Poggi-Varaldo, H. M., Santoyo-Salazar, J., Escamilla-Alvarado, C., Matsumoto-Kuwabara, Y., Ponce-Noyola, M. T & García-Rocha, M. (2020). Biological synthesis of iron nanoparticles using hydrolysates from a waste-based biorefinery. *Environmental Science and Pollution Research*, *27*, 28649–28669. https://doi.org/10.1007/s11356-020-08729-w

Russo, T., Fucile, P., Giacometti, R., & Sannino, F. (2021). Sustainable removal of contaminants by biopolymers: A novel approach for wastewater treatment: Current state and future perspectives. *Processes*, *9*(4), 719. https://doi.org/10.3390/pr9040719

Sajid, M., Asif, M., Baig, N., Kabeer, M., Ihsanullah, I., & Mohammad, A. W. (2022). Carbon nanotubes-based adsorbents: Properties, functionalization, interaction mechanisms, and applications in water purification. *Journal of Water Process Engineering*, *47*, 102815. https://doi.org/10.1016/j.jwpe.2022.102815

Sharifi, M. J., Nouralishahi, A., Hallajisani, A., & Askari, M. (2021). Magnetic chitosan nanocomposites as adsorbents in industrial wastewater treatment: A brief review. *Group*, *60*, 61.

Sharififard, H., Rezvanpanah, E., & Rad, S. H. (2018). A novel natural chitosan/activated carbon/iron bio-nanocomposite: Sonochemical synthesis, characterization, and application for cadmium removal in batch and continuous adsorption process. *Bioresource Technology*, *270*, 562–569. https://doi.org/10.1016/j.biortech.2018.09.094

Sheen Mers, S. V., Manju, V., Kamaraj, S. K., & Pérez, M. G. L. (2022). Sustainable bio-polymer-based nanocomposites for wasterwater treatment. In *Functional Polymer Nanocomposites for Wastewater Treatment* (pp. 115–144). Springer International Publishing. https://doi.org/10.1007/978-3-030-94995-2_4

Singh, N. B., & Agarwal, S. (2016). Nanocomposites: An overview. *Emerging Materials Research*, *5*(1), 5–43. https://doi.org/10.1680/jemmr.15.00025

Singha, I., & Mishrab, P. K. (2020). Nano-membrane filtration a novel application of nanotechnology for waste water treatment. *Materials Today: Proceedings*, *29*, 327–332 https://doi.org/10.1016/j.matpr.2020.07.284

Spychała, M., Kruszelnicka, I., Ginter-Kramarczyk, D., & Michałkiewicz, M. (2023). Waste materials and composites as a trickling filter filling. *Desalination and Water Treatment*, *303*, 132–141. https://doi.org/10.5004/dwt.2023.29720

Strade, E., Kalnina, D., & Kulczycka, J. (2020). Water efficiency and safe re-use of different grades of water-Topical issues for the pharmaceutical industry. *Water Resources and Industry*, *24*, 100132. https://doi.org/10.1016/j.wri.2020.100132

Suresh, R., Rajendran, S., Hoang, T. K., Vo, D. V. N., Siddiqui, M. N., & Cornejo-Ponce, L. (2021). Recent progress in green and biopolymer based photocatalysts for the abatement of aquatic pollutants. *Environmental Research*, *199*, 111324. https://doi.org/10.1016/j.envres.2021.111324

Tripathy, J., Mishra, A., Pandey, M., Thakur, R. R., Chand, S., Rout, P. R., & Shahid, M. K. (2024). Advances in nanoparticles and nanocomposites for water and wastewater treatment: A review. *Water*, *16*(11), 1481. https://doi.org/10.3390/w16111481

Vasilachi, I. C., Asiminicesei, D. M., Fertu, D. I., & Gavrilescu, M. (2021). Occurrence and fate of emerging pollutants in water environment and options for their removal. *Water*, *13*(2), 181. https://doi.org/10.3390/w13020181

Wahid, F., Bai, H., Wang, F. P., Xie, Y. Y., Zhang, Y. W., Chu, L. Q., …& Zhong, C. (2020). Facile synthesis of bacterial cellulose and polyethyleneimine based hybrid hydrogels for antibacterial applications. *Cellulose*, *27*, 369–383. https://doi.org/10.1007/s10570-019-02806-1

Wu, D., Zhang, F., Liang, H., & Feng, X. (2012). Nanocomposites and macroscopic materials: Assembly of chemically modified graphene sheets. *Chemical Society Reviews*, *41*(18), 6160–6177. https://doi.org/10.1039/C2CS35179J

Wongvasana, B., Thongnuanchan, B., Masa, A., Saito, H., Sakai, T., & Lopattananon, N. (2023). Reinforcement behavior of chemically unmodified cellulose nanofiber in natural rubber nanocomposites. *Polymers*, *15*(5), 1274. https://doi.org/10.3390/polym15051274

Xu, C., & Qu, X. (2014). Cerium oxide nanoparticle: A remarkably versatile rare earth nanomaterial for biological applications. *NPG Asia Materials*, *6*(3), e90–e90. https://doi.org/10.1038/am.2013.88

Yeap, S. P., Lim, J., Ooi, B. S., & Ahmad, A. L. (2017). Agglomeration, colloidal stability, and magnetic separation of magnetic nanoparticles: Collective influences on environmental engineering applications. *Journal of Nanoparticle Research*, *19*, 1–15. https://doi.org/10.1007/s11051-017-4065-6

Yin, Z., Cui, C., Chen, H., Duoni, Yu, X., & Qian, W. (2020). The application of carbon nanotube/graphene-based nanomaterials in wastewater treatment. *Small*, *16*(15), 1902301. https://doi.org/10.1002/smll.201902301

Zeb, F., Sarwer, W., Nadeem, K., Kamran, M., Mumtaz, M., Krenn, H., & Letofsky-Papst, I.(2016). Surface spin-glass in cobalt ferrite nanoparticles dispersed in silica matrix. *Journal of Magnetism and Magnetic Materials*, *407*, 241–246,ISSN 0304-8853. https://doi.org/10.1016/j.jmmm.2016.01.084.

Zhao, Y. Y., Kong, F. X., Wang, Z., et al. (2017). Role of membrane and compound properties in affecting the rejection of pharmaceuticals by different RO/NF membranes. *Frontiers of Environmental Science & Engineering*, *11*, 20. https://doi.org/10.1007/s11783-017-0975-x

Zhu, J., Luo, B., Qian, Y., Sotto, A., Gao, C., & Shen, J. (2019). Three-dimensional stable cation-exchange membrane with enhanced mechanical, electrochemical, and antibacterial performance by in situ synthesis of silver nanoparticles. *ACS omega*, *4*(15), 16619–16628. https://doi.org/10.1021/acsomega.9b02537

15 An overview of cathode development for microbial fuel cell

Neeraj V. S., Muthukumar K., and Samsudeen Naina Mohamed

15.1 INTRODUCTION

The global community endeavours to achieve the sustainable development goal (SDG) by 2030. Clean water and sanitation (SDG 6) and affordable and clean energy (SDG 7) for all are two primary goals that are of great concern (Pradhan et al., 2017). Microbial fuel cells (MFCs) are a key to achieving these sustainable goals. MFCs can be used for wastewater treatment, mean time it can generate electricity. The increasing demand for energy along with the overexploitation of all non-renewable resources, led to the search for new energy, which started and ended up in MFC, which is safe and environmentally friendly; moreover, it's a renewable resource. In general, MFCs exploit electroactive microorganisms to convert biomass energy to electric energy by decomposition and generate electrons at the anode. These electrons are accepted by electron acceptors and reduced at the cathode (Das, 2017). This cycle makes a complete redox reaction, which releases energy in the form of electric energy. Many advanced bioelectrochemical systems are developed that can produce other byproducts like methanol, ethanol, hydrogen peroxide, and hydrogen. The primary components of an MFC are an anode, cathode, and proton exchange membrane (PEM). PEM separates the anodic compartment and cathodic compartment. The electroactive microorganisms in the anodic chamber convert the organic pollutants in the wastewater into protons, electrons, and carbon dioxide. The electrons are moved to the cathodic through external circuits, and the protons generated move to the anodic chamber via PEM and reduction occurs (Vidhyeswari et al., 2016). The schematic diagram of a simple dual-chamber MFC is shown in Figure 15.1. The reaction involved is as follows.

$$\text{Anode: } CH_3COOH + 2H_2O \rightarrow 2CO_2 + 8H^+ + 8e^- \quad (1)$$

$$\text{Cathode: } 2O_2 + 8H^+ + 8e^- \rightarrow 4H_2O \quad (2)$$

$$\text{Overall reaction: } CH_3COOH + 2O_2 \rightarrow 2H_2O + 2CO_2 \quad (3)$$

The key factors that impact the performance of the MFC are as follows:

- Microorganisms, metabolism, and electron transfer mechanisms
  The microorganism residing in the anodic chamber plays a vital role in electron transfer and oxidation of pollutants. The metabolic activities of microorganisms generate electrons.

DOI: 10.1201/9781003500483-15
This chapter has been made available under a (CC-BY-NC-ND) 4.0 license

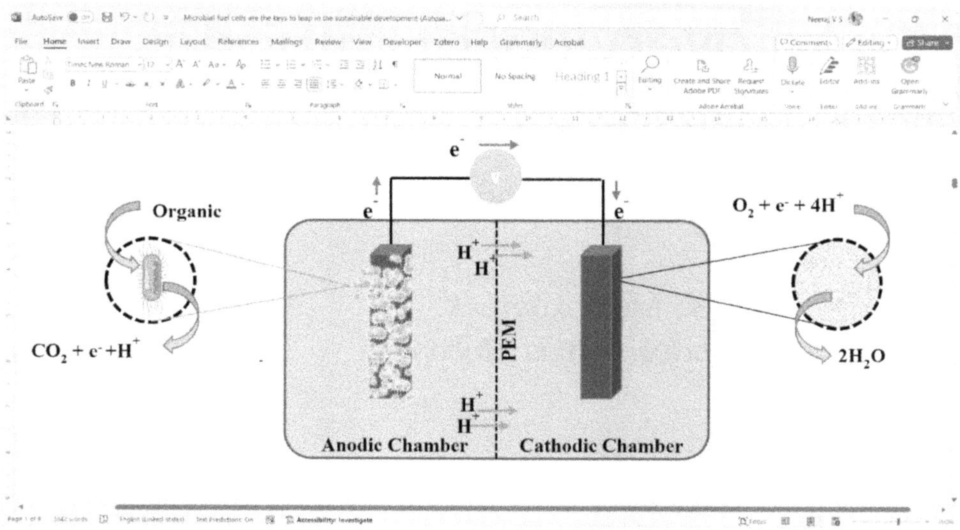

FIGURE 15.1 Schematic diagram of dual-chamber MFC.

Efficient electron transfer from microorganisms is essential for maximizing the power generation of MFC. The understanding of the metabolic activities of the microorganisms helps in the optimization of MFC performance and enhances the electron transfer efficiency.

- **Membranes**
  The membrane facilitates a critical role in MFC by imparting selective ionic transport and acts as a barrier for oxygen transport from cathode to anode. Thus, the selection of a proper membrane material allows an efficient electron transfer and prevents the crossover of anolyte and catholyte.
- **Substrate and operating conditions**
  Substrate is another important crucial factor. Wastewater is generally served as the source of the rich medium in MFC. The organic-rich substrates facilitate microbial growth by oxidizing the organic matter and generating electrons. Maintaining the pH, temperature, ionic strength, and salinity at optimum can improve microbial activity, thereby facilitating electron transfer and power generation. The electron mediators in the substrate can also facilitate the electron transfer process.
- **Electrode materials and design**
  The selection of suitable electrode materials and the design with proper configuration and spacing significantly impact the MFC performance. It aids electron transfer efficiency and power generation. Also, it includes the distribution of microorganisms in the anodic chamber, which can further improve the power generation and wastewater treatment capability of MFCs.

With careful consideration and optimization of these key factors, many researchers improved the overall efficiency of MFCs. Despite this progress, the relatively low power density and higher capital cost are the primary setbacks for the MFC advancement and scale-up. Major studies are to maximize power generation and columbic efficiency by choosing a highly sustainable, low-cost and scalable material as anode and cathode. The selection of the electrode material is critical to the performance of MFCs. High-performance anodes were the main focus of these studies. Only limited literature is available related to the cathode. This chapter comprehensively analyses the recent advancement in cathodic materials by critically analysing the overall efficacy, design, and potential applications of cathodic materials, which assist in the high-level application of MFC technology.

15.2 CATHODE

Oxygen reduction reaction (ORR) is the primary reaction occurring at the cathode. The reaction progresses through two different pathways, namely, four-electron pathways and two-electron pathways. In four-electron pathways, O_2 is directly converted into H_2O molecules using four electrons (Eq. 4). In two-electron pathways, O_2 is converted to H_2O molecules by using two electrons generating intermediate hydrogen peroxides (Eqs. 5 and 6).

$$O_2 + 4H^+ + 4e^- \uparrow 2H_2O \tag{4}$$

$$O_2 + 2H + + \ 2e- \rightarrow H_2O_2 \tag{5}$$

$$H_2O_2 + 2H + +2e^- \rightarrow 2H_2O \tag{6}$$

The high cathodic overpotential resulting from the activation loss, ohmic loss, and limiting mass transport resulted in the overall performance loss of MFCs by hindering the ORR pathways. In order to improve the MFC performance, the cathode should possess specific properties in addition to the general properties needed for the electrodes, such as electrical conductivity, non-corrosiveness, high specific surface area, easy scale-up, and low cost. Electrocatalytic property and enhancement of the triple-phase ORR are needed for cathode materials. In the past two decades, many studies have been carried out to overcome these limitations to maximize power generation and columbic efficiency by choosing a highly sustainable, low-cost, and scalable material as anode and cathode. These losses can also be reduced by the addition of effective ORR electrocatalysts and electron acceptors, which help in the reduction of activation energy for the reduction reaction as well as reduce the electron transfer resistance. Oxygen is mainly preferred as an electron acceptor due to its ability to reduce to water. However, the poor reaction kinetics of ORR results in the use of Platinum (Pt) and Platinum group metals(PGM). Since these electrodes are expensive and the scale-up of these systems is challenging, the search for alternative cathodic materials ends up with other metallic, carbonaceous, and hybrid electrode materials.

15.3 CLASSIFICATION OF CATHODE MATERIAL

Most of the anodic material can also be used as cathode material, but the catalytic property, which helps in decreasing activation energy for the reduction reaction, is the primary requirement. Also, in the study made by Rozendal et al, on the cost estimation of laboratory-scale preparation of MFC, the cost estimation of the cathode is higher when compared with other components of MFC (Rozendal et al., 2008). It limits the scale-up of the technology as well as the finding of high-level applications. So, selection of the cathodic material highly depends on the overall performance of MFC and its application. A wide range of materials has been reported in the past two decades that can be used as cathodes. Also, these reported materials have merits as well as demerits. In general, cathodes can be classified broadly into three categories: air cathode, aqueous air cathode, and bio cathodes; catalytic materials used in these cathodes are classified as metallic, carbon-based cathodes, and bio-cathodes.

15.3.1 Metallic cathodic material

Metallic materials are the pioneering materials used as cathodes in the MFC. In the beginning, platinum (Pt) and Pt-based materials were mainly used since it has high electrocatalytic properties for ORR; the long-term stability of these electrodes ensures consistent MFC operation and longevity in a prolonged operating system. ORR can occur at relatively low potential, ensuring energy conversion efficiency, non-corrosive nature ensures structural integrity. It minimizes the degradation under extreme environmental conditions, and compatibility with standard electrochemical techniques helps in facilitating accurate electrochemical characteristics.

In the early 1980s, numerous works on bioelectrochemical systems are studied. In the majority of the works, the cathode used was Pt and PGMs (Bennetto et al., 1983; Davis et al., 1983; Delaney et al., 1984; Patchett et al., 1988; Tanisho et al., n.d.). However, these systems primarily focused on anodic material, microorganisms, and substrates. The power densities in these systems are very low. Davis et al. (1983) reported a power density of 20 mW/m^2 (Davis et al., 1983). Later on, improvement in the cathode takes place by replacing pure Pt and PGMs with these coatings on other suitable substrates. The Pt performance is high in the acidic medium when compared with neutral and alkaline medium; this is due to the strong binding action of anions onto the Pt surface.

However, the high cost, material scarcity, application in scale-up, and the depolarization of electrodes make way for new electrode materials. The other metallic materials include metal oxides (Prakash et al., 2020), iron (Nwaokocha et al., 2020), and stainless steel (Pushkar and Mungray, 2020). The performance of these electrodes also depends upon the nature of the feed wastewater. pH, temperature, and metal ion concentration. Typically, the reported metal electrodes can be used in a wide range of pH and temperature. However, a direct comparative study of the metal electrode material has yet to be reported for the cathode. The corrosive resistance and durability, along with the scale-up of the electrode system is a significant setback. Recently, Chen et al. (2024) developed a novel CoS_2/TiO_2 attaching Fe-based metal-organic frameworks grown on NiFe-layered double hydroxide as cathode and reported a power density of 75 mW/m^2 (Chen et al., 2024).

15.3.2 Carbon-Based Electrodes

Carbon and carbonaceous materials are good alternatives for metal-based electrode materials due to their low cost, high electric conductivity, and availability. However, the ORR activities of these materials in raw form are comparatively low. So, in recent studies, many modified carbonaceous materials have been reported, which give better properties and results when compared with metal electrodes. The study made by Deng et al. (2010) shows the comparison of carbon paper with modified carbon paper. It shows more than 10 times the effectiveness of modified carbon as electrode materials. During modification, the material consists of 3 parts. Diffusion layer, catalyst/binder layer, and conductive supporting material. The commonly used binders are PTFE, Nafion, etc. They bind the catalytic material over the base material. In carbon-based electrodes, the conductive supporting layer is carbon, and the catalysts are coated over the carbon material using binders. As stated earlier these carbon materials can be, carbon paper (Yu et al., 2018), carbon cloths (Dehghani et al., 2016; Khan et al., 2020; Wang et al., 2016; Xiao et al., 2012), carbon fibre brush (Deng et al., 2010; Wang et al., 2017), carbon fibre paper (Zhou et al., 2019), carbon felt (Mousset et al., 2016), activated carbon, graphite paper (Mousset et al., 2016; Yao et al., 2021; Zhang et al., 2018), graphite felt (Liang et al., 2020; Liu et al., 2017), etc. The durability and stability of conventionally used binding materials are very less since the electrodes are always dipped in the liquid medium. Over time, the binding material will peel off from the base material. In recent studies, many advanced methods have been introduced to modify the electrodes without using this binder. The nanotechnology advancement also improvises the modification of raw carbon electrodes like electrospinning (Eom et al., 2020) and vapor deposition (Amaral-Labat et al., 2013).

Pt catalyst coated in carbon material is the commonly used electrode. Pt coated over carbon cloth is the most commonly used electrode, which is also commercially available. However, the amount of Pt loading in carbon cloth is much higher. Other carbon material such as carbon fibre, activated carbon, and CNT coated with Pt decreases the plating loading to a great extent. Even though the system gives higher results, the cost of platinum, the durability of binding the platinum over the electrode, and slow ORR kinetics are significant demerits.

Other metallic materials like Co (Xue et al., 2020), Fe (Xue et al., 2020), MnO_2 (Divya Priya et al., 2020; Hirose et al., 2023; Zhang and Liu, 2021), TiO_2 (Zhang and Liu, 2021), polypyrrole MoO_2 (Geetanjali et al., 2019; Karthick and Haribabu, 2020) coated with carbon-based material and vice versa (Jiang et al., 2020; Zhang et al., 2021). They are also studied, which shows a high-power density generation or a comparable power output and oxygen reaction activity, which is comparable with a conventional carbon-coated Pt catalyst. The heteroatom (Shi et al., 2012; Xue et al., 2020; Zhuang et al., 2020). Doped carbon materials are even more efficient and generate higher power output than regular Pt electrodes. The reason for the tremendous change in these heteroatom electrodes is currently under study. The nitrogen-doped heteroatom electrodes are showing much more interest now since they provide higher output along with high stability and durability. These materials can replace the Pt electrode completely.

The performance of the modified carbon material with conventional carbon material is studied by Mashkour and Rahimnejad (2015). Keeping the anode material as graphite electrode and varying the cathode electrode, graphite, carbon paper, carbon cloth and carbon paper coated with carbon nanotube and Pt (CNT/Pt), the resultant power densities are 0.937, 2.26, 3.35, and 16.26, respectively. The high-power density is due to the mixed action of CNT and Pt together. As CNT increases, the surface area and Pt increase the electric conductivity and ORR. The modification of conventional cathode material can improve the performance. Co_2P embedded in nitrogen-doped carbon nano-framework to modify the activated carbon on Stainless steel mesh is used, and the maximum power density is 2001 ± 48 mW/m^2 (Lin et al., 2021).

One of the comparative studies of carbon cloth cathode material with modified carbon cloth material by Huang et al. (2021). Carbon nanotube-modified carbon cloth and graphene-modified carbon cloth are studied with uncoated carbon cloth; the graphene-modified carbon cloth shows a high power density of 199 mW/m^2. Since the graphene material has better electrocatalytic activity, specific surface area, and excellent electron transport characteristics. Also, this graphene-modified carbon cloth shows the lowest internal resistance of 0.66 ohms. Table 15.1. shows some of the carbon-based cathode materials with their power densities. The results show that carbon-based material typically has a lower power density, but due to the activation and addition of the catalyst enhances the power density.

TABLE 15.1
List of some of the carbon-based cathode materials with their power densities

S. no	Cathode material	Anode material	P_{max} (mW/m^2)	References
1	Carbon foam	Carbon fibre	190	Pushkar and Mungray (2020)
2	Carbon cloth	Polyaniline/SnO_2 in carbon cloth	523	Khan et al. (2020)
3	Carbon paper	Carbon paper	708	Yu et al. (2018)
4	Carbon paper	Carbon felt	67	Deng et al. (2010)
5	Activated carbon fibre felt	Carbon felt	784	Deng et al. (2010)
6	Carbon fibre paper	Graphene modified CFP	1158	Zhou et al. (2019)
7	Activated carbon/SS.	Carbon felt	2000	Jiang et al. (2020)
8	Porous iron nitrogen-doped carbon nanospheres	Carbon felt	1913	Zhang et al. (2021)
9	Pd/PAN carbon nanofibre	PAN/CNF	367.9	Eom et al. (2020)
10	Graphite felt	Graphite felt with CNT.		Liang et al. (2020)
11	Nickel foam/GO	Nickel foam/GO	36.4	Zhang et al. (2018)

15.3.3 Biocathodes

Biocathodes are another advancement in cathode material development. As we know, ORR in cathode catalysts is required. The conventionally used cathodes are expensive. Therefore, the microbes present in the electrode will act as biocatalysts. Mostly, carbon-based biocathodes are available. In recent studies, metal-based biocathodes have also been reported. Carbon paper (Zhang et al., 2012), carbon cloth (Khater et al., 2023), carbon felt (Shi et al., 2023; Yang et al., 2020; Zhuang et al., 2023), carbon brush (K. Shi et al., 2023), graphite granules (Freguia et al., 2008; Zhang et al., 2011), graphite felt (Zhang et al., 2012), and graphite fibre brush (Zhang et al., 2011) and granular activated carbon (Gurung et al., 2023; Thapa et al., 2024) are mainly used. Most of these studies are focused on heavy metal removal. The power output is much better than the conventional electrodes. It also reported the graphite fibre having high output since it's having a relatively higher specific area, low ohmic resistance, and unclogging. The nanoparticle-doped carbon-based electrodes are also reported, which show a significant improvement in the power density (Marzorati et al., 2019). Metal-based biocathodes are also reported (Apollon et al., 2024). The comparative study of stainless steel with modified graphite material shows a lower output in stainless steel biocathode. It is due to the lower specific surface area and also due to the lower interaction between microbes. Used Cladophora sp. as a photosynthetic biocathode in a membrane-free biochemical system and generated a power density of 619.1 mW/m^2 (Taşkan and Taşkan, 2022). It is one of the best reported power densities using biocathodes.

Catholytes, it's another development in enhancing the cathodic property. The cathodic ohmic loss can be minimized by increasing the ionic strength/conductivity of the electrolyte. Oxygen has higher redox potential, but the poor interaction between the electrodes causes the rate of reduction to decrease. This cathodic reaction is enhanced by adding an electron acceptor called catholyte. The extreme ionic strength of the catholyte can inactivate the metal-based catalyst and bio-catalyst (Rismani-Yazdi et al., 2008). The ionic strength of the catholyte should be maintained such that the output power should be higher.

Ferricyanide, permanganate, hydrogen peroxide, iron, copper, chromium, and carbon dioxide are the most reported catholytes. Potassium ferricyanide is a suitable electron acceptor since the redox potential is lower than oxygen. It can produce output compared to oxygen (Forrestal et al., 2014). They are toxic to the aquatic environment, which is a drawback. Potassium permanganate (Deng et al., 2010; Wang et al., 2019; You et al., 2006). It is another widely used electron acceptor. Its performance depends on the pH of the medium. Controlling the pH for the effectual power output is a demerit. The substantial oxidizing property of hydrogen peroxide is used as a catholyte (Silveira et al., 2020). The usage of hydrogen peroxide shows that when compared with air, the power output is 3-fold higher when using hydrogen peroxide. Since the concentration of available oxygen is higher in hydrogen peroxide, the performance will increase.

15.4 FUTURE SCOPE AND CONCLUSION

The past 2 decades have made many developments in improving the performance of MFCs. All these modifications and developments are made in the MFC's materials to improve the functional properties and performance of MFCs. These improvising properties only focus on power generation. The high cost and stability of electrodes are still a big challenge in the scale-up of MFCs on an industrial scale. The scale-up of the carbon-based electrode causes a high ohmic loss; this high ohmic loss can be overcome by modification using metal coating or metal supports. In virtue of minimizing the capital cost of the MFCs, the cost of electrodes must be minimized. As the estimated total cost of a laboratory scale, MFC's overall cost depends on the cathode electrode. This can be reduced by using the most available and low-cost cathode parts. The use of noble metals like Pt can be replaced by stainless steel or other metal oxides. As the studies show, these give a comparable result with Pt-based electrodes. Nanotechnology improves the material properties to increase the specific surface area and electric conductivity. The application of catholyte helps in decreasing the ohmic loss in MFC. The application of catholyte on a large scale is challenging. The test for durability and stability of high-performance, low-cost electrodes needs to be studied better, which is another major setback in the future scope of MFCs. Most of the laboratory MFCs are studied in a short span of a maximum of one year. As industrial and large-scale application comes into the picture, the durability and stability of electrodes are significant factor, which increases the maintenance cost of the MFCs. So, it is evident that electrode manufacturing and design are significant challenges in the MFC. It requires more studies on the commercial application of modified, energy-efficient, and cost-effective electrodes in MFC technology for better sustainable development.

REFERENCES

Amaral-Labat, G., Zollfrank, C., Ortona, A., Pusterla, S., Pizzi, A., Fierro, V., and Celzard, A., 2013. Structure and oxidation resistance of micro-cellular Si-SiC foams derived from natural resins. *Ceramics International* 39, 1841–1851. https://doi.org/10.1016/j.ceramint.2012.08.032

Apollon, W., Kamaraj, S.-K., Rodríguez-Fuentes, H., Gómez-Leyva, J.F., Vidales-Contreras, J.A., Mardueño-Aguilar, M.V., and Luna-Maldonado, A.I., 2024. Bio-electricity production in a single-chamber microbial fuel cell using urine as a substrate. *Biofuels* 15, 665–675. https://doi.org/10.1080/17597269.2023.2277991

Bennetto, H.P., Stirling, J.L., Tanaka, K., and Vega, C.A., 1983. Anodic reactions in microbial fuel cells. *Biotech & Bioengineering* 25, 559–568. https://doi.org/10.1002/bit.260250219

Chen, J., Li, X., Li, Yingxuan, Li, Yao, Du, Y., Li, S., Wang, R., Yang, Y., and Liu, Y., 2024. Enhanced bio-electrochemical performance of CoS2/TiO2 attaching Fe-based metal organic frameworks grown on NiFe-layered double hydroxide as cathode catalyst in microbial fuel cell. *International Journal of Hydrogen Energy* 72, 124–132. https://doi.org/10.1016/j.ijhydene.2024.05.389

Das, D., 2017. Microbial fuel cell: A bioelectrochemical system that converts waste to watts, microbial fuel cell: A bioelectrochemical system that converts waste to watts. https://doi.org/10.1007/978-3-319-66793-5

Davis, G., Hill, H.A.O., Aston, W.J., John Higgins, I., and Turner, A.P.F., 1983. Bioelectrochemical fuel cell and sensor based on a quinoprotein, alcohol dehydrogenase. *Enzyme and Microbial Technology* 5, 383–388. https://doi.org/10.1016/0141-0229(83)90013-3

Dehghani, S., Rezaee, A., Moghiseh, Z., and Mohebrad, B., 2016. Performance of bioelectrochemical process using steel wool and carbon cloth electrodes to remove phenol in the aquatic environment. *Koomesh* 18, 380–387.

Delaney, G.M., Bennetto, H.P., Mason, J.R., Roller, S.D., Stirling, J.L., and Thurston, C.F., 1984. Electron-transfer coupling in microbial fuel cells. 2. performance of fuel cells containing selected microorganism—mediator—substrate combinations. *Journal of Chemistry Technology Biotechnol* 34, 13–27. https://doi.org/10.1002/jctb.280340104

Deng, Q., Li, X., Zuo, J., Ling, A., and Logan, B.E., 2010. Power generation using an activated carbon fiber felt cathode in an upflow microbial fuel cell. *Journal of Power Sources* 195, 1130–1135. https://doi.org/10.1016/j.jpowsour.2009.08.092

Divya Priya, A., Deva, S., Shalini, P., and Pydi Setty, Y., 2020. Antimony-tin based intermetallics supported on reduced graphene oxide as anode and MnO2@rGO as cathode electrode for the study of microbial fuel cell performance. *Renewable Energy* 150, 156–166. https://doi.org/10.1016/j.renene.2019.12.109

Eom, H., Joo, H.J., Kim, S.C., and Kim, S.S., 2020. Properties of carbon-based nanofiber with Pd and its application to microbial fuel cells electrode. *Environmental Technology and Innovation* 19, 100800. https://doi.org/10.1016/j.eti.2020.100800

Forrestal, C., Huang, Z., and Ren, Z.J., 2014. Percarbonate as a naturally buffering catholyte for microbial fuel cells. *Bioresource Technology* 172, 429–432. https://doi.org/10.1016/j.biortech.2014.09.014

Freguia, S., Rabaey, K., Yuan, Z., and Keller, J., 2008. Sequential anode-cathode configuration improves cathodic oxygen reduction and effluent quality of microbial fuel cells. *Water Research* 42, 1387–1396. https://doi.org/10.1016/j.watres.2007.10.007

Geetanjali, Rani, R., and Kumar, S., 2019. High-capacity polyaniline-coated molybdenum oxide composite as an effective catalyst for enhancing the electrochemical performance of the microbial fuel cell. *International Journal of Hydrogen Energy* 44, 16933–16943. https://doi.org/10.1016/j.ijhydene.2019.04.201

Gurung, A., Thapa, B.S., Ko, S.-Y., Ashun, E., Toor, U.A., and Oh, S.-E., 2023. Denitrification in Microbial fuel cells using Granular activated carbon as an effective biocathode. *Energies* 16, 709. https://doi.org/10.3390/en16020709

Hirose, S., Takasugi, K., Nakamoto, T., and Taguchi, K., 2023. Cobalt-intercalated birnessite-type manganese oxide catalysts for low-cost cathodes in microbial fuel cells. *Resourceedings* 3, 17–22. https://doi.org/10.21625/resourceedings.v3i3.1025

Huang, S.J., Ubando, A.T., Wang, C.Y., Su, Y.X., Culaba, A.B., Lin, Y.A., and Wang, C.T., 2021. Modification of carbon based cathode electrode in a batch-type microbial fuel cells. *Biomass and Bioenergy* 145, 105972. https://doi.org/10.1016/j.biombioe.2021.105972

Jiang, M., Xu, T., and Chen, S., 2020. A mechanical rechargeable small-size microbial fuel cell with long-term and stable power output. *Applied Energy* 260, 114336. https://doi.org/10.1016/j.apenergy.2019.114336

Karthick, S., and Haribabu, K., 2020. Bioelectricity generation in a microbial fuel cell using polypyrrole-molybdenum oxide composite as an effective cathode catalyst. *Fuel* 275, 117994. https://doi.org/10.1016/j.fuel.2020.117994

Khan, N., Anwer, A.H., Ahmad, A., Sabir, S., and Khan, M.Z., 2020. Investigating microbial fuel cell aided bio-remediation of mixed phenolic contaminants under oxic and anoxic environments. *Biochemical Engineering Journal* 155, 107485. https://doi.org/10.1016/j.bej.2019.107485

Khater, D.Z., Amin, R.S., Fetohi, A.E., Mahmoud, M., and El-Khatib, K.M., 2023. Insights on hexavalent chromium(VI) remediation strategies in abiotic and biotic dual chamber microbial fuel cells: electrochemical, physical, and metagenomics characterizations. *Science Reprint* 13, 20184. https://doi.org/10.1038/s41598-023-47450-9

Liang, Y., Zhai, H., Liu, B., Ji, M., and Li, J., 2020. Carbon nanomaterial-modified graphite felt as an anode enhanced the power production and polycyclic aromatic hydrocarbon removal in sediment microbial fuel cells. *Science of the Total Environment* 713, 136483. https://doi.org/10.1016/j.scitotenv.2019.136483

Lin, Z., Su, W., Zhang, S., Zhang, M., Li, K., and Liu, J., 2021. Co2P embedded in nitrogen-doped carbon nanoframework derived from Co-based metal-organic framework as efficient oxygen reduction reaction electrocatalyst for enhanced performance of activated carbon air-cathode microbial fuel cell. *Journal of Electroanalytical Chemistry* 895, 115355. https://doi.org/10.1016/j.jelechem.2021.115355

Liu, D., Zheng, T., Buisman, C., and Ter Heijne, A., 2017. Heat-treated stainless steel felt as a new cathode material in a methane-producing bioelectrochemical system. *ACS Sustainable Chemistry and Engineering* 5, 11346–11353. https://doi.org/10.1021/acssuschemeng.7b02367

Marzorati, S., Cristiani, P., Longhi, M., Trasatti, S.P., and Traversa, E., 2019. Nanoceria acting as oxygen reservoir for biocathodes in microbial fuel cells. *Electrochimica Acta* 325, 134954. https://doi.org/10.1016/j.electacta.2019.134954

Mashkour, M., and Rahimnejad, M., 2015. Effect of various carbon-based cathode electrodes on the performance of microbial fuel cell. *Biofuel Research Journal* 2, 296–300. https://doi.org/10.18331/BRJ2015.2.4.3

Mousset, E., Wang, Z., Hammaker, J., and Lefebvre, O., 2016. Physico-chemical properties of pristine graphene and its performance as electrode material for electro-Fenton treatment of wastewater. *Electrochimica Acta* 214, 217–230. https://doi.org/10.1016/j.electacta.2016.08.002

Nwaokocha, C.N., Giwa, S.O., Layeni, A.T., Kuye, S.I., Samuel, O.D., Ogunbona, C.K., Adebayo, J.K., Sosanya, A., and Babalola, A., 2020. Microbial fuel cell: Bio-energy production from Nigerian corn starch wastewater using iron electrodes. *Materials Today: Proceedings.* https://doi.org/10.1016/j.matpr.2020.09.345

Patchett, Roy A., Kelly, Alison F., Kroll, and Rohan, G., 1988. Use of a microbial fuel cell for the rapid enumeration of bacteria. *Applied Microbiology and Biotechnology* 28. https://doi.org/10.1007/BF00250492

Pradhan, P., Costa, L., Rybski, D., Lucht, W., Kropp, J.P., 2017. A systematic study of Sustainable Development Goal (SDG) interactions. *Earth's Future* 5, 1169–1179. https://doi.org/10.1002/2017EF000632

Prakash, O., Mungray, A., Chongdar, S., Kailasa, S.K., and Mungray, A.K., 2020. Performance of polypyrrole coated metal oxide composite electrodes for benthic microbial fuel cell (BMFC). *Journal of Environmental Chemical Engineering* 8, 102757. https://doi.org/10.1016/j.jece.2018.11.002

Pushkar, P., and Mungray, A.K., 2020. Exploring the use of 3 dimensional low-cost sugar-urea carbon foam electrode in the benthic microbial fuel cell. *Renewable Energy* 147, 2032–2042. https://doi.org/10.1016/j.renene.2019.09.142

Rismani-Yazdi, H., Carver, S.M., Christy, A.D., and Tuovinen, O.H., 2008. Cathodic limitations in microbial fuel cells: An overview. *Journal of Power Sources* 180, 683–694. https://doi.org/10.1016/j.jpowsour.2008.02.074

Rozendal, R.A., Hamelers, H.V.M., Rabaey, K., Keller, J., and Buisman, C.J.N., 2008. Towards practical implementation of bioelectrochemical wastewater treatment. *Trends in Biotechnology* 26, 450–459. https://doi.org/10.1016/j.tibtech.2008.04.008

Shi, K., Cheng, W., Cheng, D., Xue, J., Qiao, Y., Gao, Y., Jiang, Q., and Wang, J., 2023. Stability improvement and the mechanism of a microbial electrolysis cell biocathode for treating wastewater containing sulfate by quorum sensing. *Chemical Engineering Journal* 455, 140597. https://doi.org/10.1016/j.cej.2022.140597

Shi, X., Duan, Z., Jing Wang, Zhou, W., Jiang, M., Li, T., Ma, H., and Zhu, X., 2023. Simultaneous removal of multiple heavy metals using single chamber microbial electrolysis cells with biocathode in the micro-aerobic environment. *Chemosphere* 318, 137982. https://doi.org/10.1016/j.chemosphere.2023.137982

Shi, X., Feng, Y., Wang, X., Lee, H., Liu, J., Qu, Y., He, W., Kumar, S.M.S., and Ren, N., 2012. Application of nitrogen-doped carbon powders as low-cost and durable cathodic catalyst to air-cathode microbial fuel cells. *Bioresource Technology* 108, 89–93. https://doi.org/10.1016/j.biortech.2011.12.078

Silveira, G., de Aquino Neto, S., and Schneedorf, J.M., 2020. Development, characterization and application of a low-cost single chamber microbial fuel cell based on hydraulic couplers. *Energy* 208, 118395. https://doi.org/10.1016/j.energy.2020.118395

Tanisho, S., Kamiya, N., and Wakao, N., n.d. Microbial fuel cell using Enterobacter aerogenes.

Taşkan, B., and Taşkan, E., 2022. Sustainable bioelectricity generation using *Cladophora* sp. as a biocathode in membrane-less microbial fuel cell. *Bioresource Technology* 347, 126704. https://doi.org/10.1016/j.biortech.2022.126704

Thapa, B.S., Pandit, S., Gurung, A., Ashun, E., Ko, S.-Y., and Oh, S.-E., 2024. Granular activated carbon assisted biocathode for effective electrotrophic denitrification in microbial fuel cells. *Chemosphere* 352, 141341. https://doi.org/10.1016/j.chemosphere.2024.141341

Vidhyeswari, A. Surendhar, Jerold, M., and Sivasubramanian, V., 2016. Microbial fuel cell technology: a sustainable energy producer from wide variety of waste sources. In V. Sivasubramanian (Ed.), *Environmental Sustainability using Green Technologies*. Boca Raton: CRC Press. (ISBN 9781498753050). https://www.taylorfrancis.com/chapters/edit/10.1201/9781315364339-22/microbial-fuel-cell-technology-sustainable-energy-producer-wide-variety-waste-sources?context=ubx&refId=a6071d22-f7c9-4dbd-952e-d11c2d24ac1d (accessed 4.29.24).

Wang, J., Song, X., Wang, Y., Zhao, Z., Wang, B., and Yan, D., 2017. Effects of electrode material and substrate concentration on the bioenergy output and wastewater treatment in air-cathode microbial fuel cell integrating with constructed wetland. *Ecological Engineering* 99, 191–198. https://doi.org/10.1016/j.ecoleng.2016.11.015

Wang, Q., Huang, L., Pan, Y., Zhou, P., Quan, X., Logan, B.E., and Chen, H., 2016. Cooperative cathode electrode and in situ deposited copper for subsequent enhanced Cd(II) removal and hydrogen evolution in bioelectrochemical systems. *Bioresource Technology* 200, 565–571. https://doi.org/10.1016/j.biortech.2015.10.084

Wang, S., Tian, S., Zhang, P., Ye, J., Tao, X., Li, F., Zhou, Z., and Nabi, M., 2019. Enhancement of biological oxygen demand detection with a microbial fuel cell using potassium permanganate as cathodic electron acceptor. *Journal of Environmental Management* 252, 109682. https://doi.org/10.1016/j.jenvman.2019.109682

Xiao, L., Damien, J., Luo, J., Jang, H.D., Huang, J., and He, Z., 2012. Crumpled graphene particles for microbial fuel cell electrodes. *Journal of Power Sources* 208, 187–192. https://doi.org/10.1016/j.jpowsour.2012.02.036

Xue, W., Zhou, Q., and Li, F., 2020. The feasibility of typical metal–organic framework derived Fe, Co, N co-doped carbon as a robust electrocatalyst for oxygen reduction reaction in microbial fuel cell. *Electrochimica Acta* 355, 136775. https://doi.org/10.1016/j.electacta.2020.136775

Yang, H.Y., Wang, Y.X., He, C.S., Qin, Y., Li, W.Q., Li, W.H., and Mu, Y., 2020. Redox mediator-modified biocathode enables highly efficient microbial electro-synthesis of methane from carbon dioxide. *Applied Energy* 274, 115292. https://doi.org/10.1016/j.apenergy.2020.115292

Yao, J., Huang, Y., Hou, Y., Yang, B., Lei, L., Tang, X., Scheckel, K.G., Li, Z., Wu, D., and Dionysiou, D.D., 2021. Graphene-modified graphite paper cathode for the efficient bioelectrochemical removal of chromium. *Chemical Engineering Journal* 405, 126545. https://doi.org/10.1016/j.cej.2020.126545

You, S., Zhao, Q., Zhang, J., Jiang, J., and Zhao, S., 2006. A microbial fuel cell using permanganate as the cathodic electron acceptor. *Journal of Power Sources* 162, 1409–1415. https://doi.org/10.1016/j.jpowsour.2006.07.063

Yu, F., Wang, C., and Ma, J., 2018. Capacitance-enhanced 3D graphene anode for microbial fuel cell with long-time electricity generation stability. *Electrochimica Acta* 259, 1059–1067. https://doi.org/10.1016/j.electacta.2017.11.038

Zhang, G.D., Zhao, Q.L., Jiao, Y., Zhang, J.N., Jiang, J.Q., Ren, N., and Kim, B.H., 2011. Improved performance of microbial fuel cell using combination biocathode of graphite fiber brush and graphite granules. *Journal of Power Sources* 196, 6036–6041. https://doi.org/10.1016/j.jpowsour.2011.03.096

Zhang, Q., and Liu, L., 2021. Cathodes of membrane and packed manganese dioxide/titanium dioxide/graphitic carbon nitride/granular activated carbon promoted treatment of coking wastewater in microbial fuel cell. *Bioresource Technology* 321, 124442. https://doi.org/10.1016/j.biortech.2020.124442

Zhang, X., Lin, Z., Liang, B., Zhong, M., Zhang, M., and Li, K., 2021. Highly efficient improvement of power generation and waste removal in microbial fuel cell by associating activated carbon with a novel porous iron-nitrogen-doped carbon nanosphere. *Journal of Power Sources* 498, 229883. https://doi.org/10.1016/j.jpowsour.2021.229883

Zhang, Y., He, Q., Xia, L., Li, Y., and Song, S., 2018. Algae cathode microbial fuel cells for cadmium removal with simultaneous electricity production using nickel foam/graphene electrode. *Biochemical Engineering Journal* 138, 179–187. https://doi.org/10.1016/j.bej.2018.07.021

Zhang, Y., Sun, J., Hu, Y., Li, S., and Xu, Q., 2012. Bio-cathode materials evaluation in microbial fuel cells: A comparison of graphite felt, carbon paper and stainless steel mesh materials. *International Journal of Hydrogen Energy* 37, 16935–16942. https://doi.org/10.1016/j.ijhydene.2012.08.064

Zhou, S., Lin, M., Zhuang, Z., Liu, P., and Chen, Z., 2019. Biosynthetic graphene enhanced extracellular electron transfer for high performance anode in microbial fuel cell. *Chemosphere* 232, 396–402. https://doi.org/10.1016/j.chemosphere.2019.05.191

Zhuang, S., Shao, C., Ye, J., Li, B., and Wang, X., 2020. Enhancing oxygen reduction reaction in air-cathode microbial fuel cells treating wastewater with cobalt and nitrogen co-doped ordered mesoporous carbon as cathode catalysts. *Environmental Research* 191, 110195. https://doi.org/10.1016/j.envres.2020.110195

Zhuang, X., Tang, S., Dong, W., Xin, F., Jia, H., and Wu, X., 2023. Improved performance of Cr(vi)-reducing microbial fuel cells by nano-FeS hybridized biocathodes. *RSC Advances* 13, 6768–6778. https://doi.org/10.1039/D3RA00683B

Index

abiotic 224
acetogenesis 185
Achromobacter xylosoxidans 281
acidogenesis 221
activated carbon adsorption 26
activated sludge 227
adsorption isotherm 103
adsorption process 131
advanced oxidation processes (AOPs) 27
aerobic biodegradation 215
aerobic process 220
agar gum 240
Air-L-Shaped Bioreactor 59
algae 179
anaerobic biodegradation 215
anaerobic digestion 227
anaerobic dynamic membrane bioreactor 189
Anaerobic Fixed Bed 189
anaerobic fluidized bed reactor 189
anaerobic process 220
autoinducer peptides 276

bacteria 7
bioactive compounds 64
bioadsorption 32
bioaugmentation 219
bioaugmentation and biostimulation 231
biocatalysts 62
biocathode 76
biochar 92
biodegradation 215, 218, 219
biodegradation deterioration 216
bioeconomy 127
bioelectrodes 72
bioethanol 173
biofilm based treatment 278
biofilm development 273
biofilm maturation 273
biofilms 272
biofuels 161
biogas 183
biohydrogen 180
biomineralization 32
biophotolysis 180
biopolymers 238
biorefinery 127
bioremediation 208
biosorption 60
biostimulation 219
biotic 224
BOD (biochemical oxygen demand) reduction 220
butanol fermentation 178

carbon (C) 228
carbonaceous materials 312
carrageenan 116
casein 240
catholytes 314
cellulose 106, 241
chemisorption 102
chitin 55, 243
chitosan 110, 243
chromophore 8
collagen 244
composting 215
continuous fermentation 178
coprecipitation 292
cyanobacteria 36

dark fermentation 181
denitrification 220
direct biophotolysis 180
direct electron transfer 77
direct oxidation 204
direct Transesterification 168

electrocatalytic oxidation 204
electro-Fenton (EF) process 30
electropermeabilization 79
electroporation 79
emerging contaminants 10
emerging pollutants (EPs) 25, 231
exopolysaccharides 275

facultative process 220
fenton process 27, 205
fermentation 221
ferrites 295
fluidized bed reactors 300
FT-IR 246
fungal extracellular enzymes 62
fungi 34, 55

gelatin 114, 240
genetic engineering 231
Grey H_2 179

half-saturation constant (Kr) 221
hetero-polysaccharides 239
highly reactive species 207
homo-polysaccharides 239
hydraulic Retention time 223
hydrolysis 221

indirect oxidation 204
indirect photolysis 180
industrial effluents 278
integrated microbial electrolysis cell 190
interstitial adsorption 103

laminar composite 249
lignin 118

lignocellulosic wastes 188
lipids 163
liquidstate fermentation (SmF) 55

macroalgae 160
matrix phase 249
maximum specific growth rate (αmax) 220
membrane bioreactor 59
mesophilic 188
methanogenesis 221
microalgae 161
microbial electrolysis 183
microbial fuel cells 279
microemulsion 292
microplastics 202
mineralization 221
molasses 178
Mucor circinelloides 166
mycoprotein 63
mycoremediation 13

N-acyl homoserine lactones 276
nanocomposite 287
natural attenuation 219
natural biopolymers 105
natural fiber reinforced composites (NFRCs) 249
nitrification 220
nitrogen (N) 228
NMR spectroscopy 247
non-polarizable electrodes 74
nutrient availability 221

organic matter 55
oxidation 221
oxygen reduction reaction 311

particulate matter 249
pectin 240
phosphorus (P) 228
photo fermentation 181
photocatalysis 205
photocatalytic oxidation 205
photo-Fenton process 28
photolysis 206
physisorption 102
polarizable electrodes 74
pollutant diversity 231
polylactide 243
polymeric biomaterials 244
primary MPs 201
primary treatment 227
psychrophilic 188
Pt catalyst 312
pyrolysis 97

quartenary recycling 204
quorum sensing 276

reaction rate kinetics 220
recycling methods 203
reductive dechlorination 205
reinforcement phase 249
response surface methodology 60
retention time 223

Scanning Kelvin Probe Microscopy (SKPM) 248
seaweeds 160
secondary MPs 201
secondary recycling 203
secondary treatment 227
single cell oils 166
sodium alginate 111
spores 55
starch 113, 241
stimulator electrodes 73
surface adsorption 103
surfactants 167
suspended growth reactors 301

tertiary microorganisms 7
tertiary recycling 203
tertiary treatment 227
thermal decomposition 292
thermophilic 188
thermoplastics 201
thermosets 201
trickling filters 227
Turquoise hydrogen 179
two-phase methane fermentation process 190

ultrasonic waves 185
ultrasonication 185
upflow anaerobic sludge blanket reactor 188
UV-C 207
UV radiation 207

VIS–NIR spectroscopy 246

wastewater 1

Xray diffraction techniques 247

Yoon-Nelson model 221

For Product Safety Concerns and Information please contact our EU
representative GPSR@taylorandfrancis.com
Taylor & Francis Verlag GmbH, Kaufingerstraße 24, 80331 München, Germany

www.ingramcontent.com/pod-product-compliance
Ingram Content Group UK Ltd.
Pitfield, Milton Keynes, MK11 3LW, UK
UKHW052051230926
475702UK00025B/1097
* 9 7 8 1 0 3 2 7 9 6 8 4 0 *